CANINE
INTERNAL
MEDICINE
SECRETS

CANINE INTERNAL MEDICINE SECRETS

Stanley I. Rubin, DVM, MS, Diplomate ACVIM
Director
Veterinary Teaching Hospital
Western College of Veterinary Medicine
University of Saskatchewan
Saskatoon, Saskatchewan, Canada

Anthony P. Carr, Dr. med. vet., Diplomate ACVIM
Associate Professor
Department of Small Animal Clinical Sciences
Western College of Veterinary Medicine
University of Saskatchewan
Saskatoon, Saskatchewan, Canada

With more than 60 illustrations

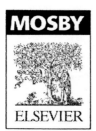

11830 Westline Industrial Drive
St. Louis, Missouri 63146

CANINE INTERNAL MEDICINE SECRETS

ISBN-13: 978-1-56053-629-1
ISBN-10: 1-56053-629-2

Notice

Knowledge and best practice in this field are constantly changing. As new research and experience broaden our knowledge, changes in practice, treatment and drug therapy may become necessary or appropriate. Readers are advised to check the most current information provided (i) on procedures featured or (ii) by the manufacturer of each product to be administered, to verify the recommended dose or formula, the method and duration of administration, and contraindications. It is the responsibility of the practitioner, relying on their own experience and knowledge of the patient, to make diagnoses, to determine dosages and the best treatment for each individual patient, and to take all appropriate safety precautions. To the fullest extent of the law, neither the Publisher nor the Authors assume any liability for any injury and/or damage to persons or property arising out or related to any use of the material contained in this book.

The Publisher

Library of Congress Cataloging-in-Publication Data
Canine internal medicine secrets/[edited by] Stanley I Rubin, Anthony P. Carr
   p. cm.
   Includes index.
ISBN-13: 978-1-56053-629-1 (sc)   ISBN-10: 1-56053-629-2 (sc)
1. Dogs—Diseases—Miscellanea. I. Rubin, Stanley I. (Stanley Ian), 1954- II. Carr, Anthony, P., 1960-
SF991.C236 2006
636.7'0896—dc22

          2006047245

ISBN-13: 978-1-56053-629-1
ISBN-10: 1-56053-629-2

Publishing Director: Linda L. Duncan
Publisher: Penny Rudolph
Managing Editor: Teri Merchant
Publishing Services Manager: Patricia Tannian
Project Manager: Claire Kramer
Designer: Jyotika Shroff

Printed in the United States of America

Last digit is the print number: 9 8 7 6 5 4 3

Working together to grow
libraries in developing countries

www.elsevier.com | www.bookaid.org | www.sabre.org

ELSEVIER   BOOK AID International   Sabre Foundation

Contributors

Jonathan A. Abbott, DVM, Diplomate ACVIM (Cardiology)
Associate Professor
Department of Small Animal Clinical Sciences
Virginia Maryland Regional College of Veterinary Medicine
Virginia Tech, Blacksburg, Virginia

Charles W. Brockus, DVM, PhD
Assistant Professor
Department of Veterinary Pathology
College of Veterinary Medicine
Iowa State University, Ames, Iowa

Clay A. Calvert, DVM, Diplomate ACVIM
Professor
Department of Small Animal Medicine
College of Veterinary Medicine
University of Georgia, Athens, Georgia

Anthony P. Carr, Dr. med. vet., Diplomate ACVIM
Associate Professor
Department of Small Animal Clinical Sciences
Western College of Veterinary Medicine
University of Saskatchewan
Saskatoon, Saskatchewan, Canada

John Crandell, DVM
Internist
Akron Veterinary Referral and Emergency Center
Akron, Ohio

Mala Erickson, DVM, MVSc
Monterey Peninsula Veterinary Emergency & Specialty Center
Monterey, California

Leslie E. Fox, DVM, MS
Associate Professor
Department of Veterinary Clinical Sciences
College of Veterinary Medicine
Iowa State University, Ames, Iowa

David Clark Grant, DVM, MS, Diplomate ACVIM (Internal Medicine)

Assistant Professor
Department of Small Animal Clinical Sciences
Virginia Maryland Regional College of Veterinary Medicine
Virginia Tech, Blacksburg, Virginia

Karen Dyer Inzana, DVM, PhD, Diplomate ACVIM (Neurology)

Professor, Section Chief
Department of Small Animal Clinical Sciences
Virginia Maryland Regional College of Veterinary Medicine
Virginia Tech, Blacksburg, Virginia

Catherine Kasai, DVM

Internal Medicine Resident
Department of Veterinary Clinical Sciences
College of Veterinary Medicine
Iowa State University, Ames, Iowa

Robert R. King, DVM, PhD

Senior Clinician
Department of Veterinary Clinical Sciences
College of Veterinary Medicine
Iowa State University, Ames, Iowa

Dawn D. Kingsbury, DVM

Internal Medicine Resident
Department of Veterinary Clinical Sciences
College of Veterinary Medicine
Iowa State University, Ames, Iowa

Jo Ann Morrison, DVM

Clinician
Department of Veterinary Clinical Sciences
College of Veterinary Medicine
Iowa State University, Ames, Iowa

Astrid Nielssen, DVM, Diplomate ACVIM

Canada West Veterinary Specialists and Critical Care Hospital
Vancouver, British Columbia, Canada

David L. Panciera, DVM, MS, Diplomate ACVIM (Internal Medicine)

Professor
Department of Small Animal Clinical Sciences
Virginia-Maryland Regional College of Veterinary Medicine
Virginia Tech, Blacksburg, Virginia

Erin M. Portillo, DVM
Internal Medicine Resident
Department of Veterinary Clinical Sciences
College of Veterinary Medicine
Iowa State University, Ames, Iowa

Klaas Post, DVM, MVetSc
Professor and Head
Department of Small Animal Clinical Sciences
Veterinary Teaching Hospital
Western College of Veterinary Medicine
Saskatoon, Saskatchewan, Canada

Michelle A. Pressel, DVM, Diplomate ACVIM
Mid Coast Veterinary Internal Medicine
Arroyo Grande, California

Laura Gaye Ridge, DVM, MS, Diplomate ACVIM
Internist, Upstate Veterinary Specialists
Greenville, South Carolina

**John H. Rossmeisl, Jr., DVM, MS, Diplomate ACVIM
(Internal Medicine and Neurology)**
Assistant Professor
Department of Small Animal Clinical Sciences
Virginia-Maryland Regional College of Veterinary Medicine
Virginia Tech, Blacksburg, Virginia

Stanley I. Rubin, DVM, MS, Diplomate ACVIM
Director, Veterinary Teaching Hospital
Western College of Veterinary Medicine
University of Saskatchewan
Saskatoon, Saskatchewan, Canada

Elizabeth Streeter, DVM
Clinician
Department of Veterinary Clinical Sciences
College of Veterinary Medicine
Iowa State University, Ames, Iowa

**Gregory C. Troy, DVM, MS, Diplomate ACVIM
(Internal Medicine)**
Professor
Department of Small Animal Clinical Sciences
Virginia-Maryland Regional College of Veterinary Medicine
Virginia Tech, Blacksburg, Virginia

Michelle Wall, DVM, Diplomate ACVIM
Upstate Veterinary Specialists
Small Animal Oncology Service
Greenville, South Carolina

**Wendy A. Ware, DVM, MS, Diplomate ACVIM
  (Cardiology)**
Professor
Departments of Veterinary Clinical Sciences and Biomedical
  Sciences
College of Veterinary Medicine
Iowa State University, Ames, Iowa
Staff Cardiologist
Veterinary Teaching Hospital
Iowa State University, Ames, Iowa

Preface

Why write another reference text on internal medicine? Simply, we wanted to provide the reader with a quick reference to find the essentials of canine internal medicine. These are the same topics and facts that are discussed during rounds and that appear on examinations, including board examinations.

This book, which we hope is a useful learning tool for students, will also be a vital reference for the practicing clinician. The book contains a great deal of clinical information that can be applied on a daily basis. It is not meant to replace the detail provided in reference textbooks. Our authors have worked to distill the essence of what the clinician is looking for into something that is user friendly.

We believe that the question-and-answer approach used in the *Secrets Series* is a logical and efficient way to tackle clinical problems. This complements a problem-based approach to medicine.

Small animal internal medicine has been blessed with an abundance of high-quality textbooks. These, along with current journals, monographs, and proceedings, serve to provide the clinician with a large amount of information. Where does one start? *Canine Internal Medicine Secrets* is different in that it relies on experienced authors to begin with a question that may be asked on an examination or in clinical rounds and is followed with a response that is based on the author's experience and factual knowledge. The book is not meant to be comprehensive; there are many standard textbooks that can serve this role. The goal of this book is to provide readers with an efficient means to find key information that will give them direction in the management of their cases. Just as in veterinary school, we encourage readers to continue reading other texts to further gain a better understanding of their canine internal medicine problem.

We are proud to have authors who are not only well credentialed but also highly experienced in their chosen fields. Their sections are interesting, up to date, and concise. We would like to acknowledge our colleagues' efforts in completing this text; their contributions are greatly appreciated.

We are also indebted to Teri Merchant, Managing Editor, at Elsevier. Without her, this project would not have happened.

We thank our wives, Diane and Suzette, and our children, Olivia, Kyle, Luke, Sophie, Clara, and Joe. We could not have done this without their support.

Stanley I. Rubin, DVM, MS, DACVIM
Anthony Carr, Dr. med. vet., DACVIM

Contents

I. NEUROLOGY AND NEUROMUSCULAR DISEASE
Karen Dyer Inzana
1. Neurologic Examination and Lesion Localization, *Karen Dyer Inzana,* 1
2. Seizures, *Karen Dyer Inzana,* 8
   Felbamate (Febatol), 13
   Gabapentin (Neurontin), 13
   Zonisamide, 13
   Levetiracetam (Keppra), 13
3. Peripheral Nerve Disease, *Karen Dyer Inzana,* 14
4. Inflammatory Intracranial Diseases: The Meningoencephalitides, *John H. Rossmeisl, Jr.,* 18
   Bacterial Meningoencephalitis, 19
   The Rickettsioses, 20
   Intracranial Mycotic Infections, 21
   Idiopathic (Noninfectious) Meningoencephalitides, 23
   Protozoal Meningoencephalitides, 25
   Viral Diseases, 27
5. Diseases of the Spinal Cord, *John H. Rossmeisl, Jr.,* 30
   Congenital and Hereditary Anomalies and Disorders, 32
   Degenerative Diseases, 36
   Inflammatory and Infectious Diseases, 47
   Vascular Disorders, 54

II. CARDIOLOGY
Jonathon A. Abbott
6. Acquired Valvular Disease, *Jonathon A. Abbott,* 59
7. Pericardial Disease, *Wendy A. Ware,* 71
8. Management of Heart Failure, *Jonathon A. Abbott,* 81
   Controversy, 91
9. Congenital Heart Disease, *Jonathon A. Abbott,* 93
10. Canine Myocardial Disease, *Jonathon A. Abbott,* 107
    Controversy, 116
11. Infective Endocarditis, *Clay A. Calvert and Michelle Wall,* 118
12. Canine Heartworm Disease, *Clay A. Calvert and Laura Gaye Ridge,* 125

III. PULMONARY DISEASE
Robert R. King
13. Canine Rhinitis, *Charles W. Brockus,* 143
    Bacterial Rhinitis, *Charles W. Brockus,* 145

Mycotic Rhinitis, *John Crandell,* 146

Allergic Rhinitis, *Charles W. Brockus,* 151

Lymphoplasmacytic Rhinitis, *Charles W. Brockus,* 152

14. Conformational Disorders, *Dawn D. Kingsbury,* 154
15. Tumors of the Nasal and Paranasal Sinuses, *Leslie E. Fox,* 159
16. Upper Airway Disorders, *Jo Ann Morrison,* 167

     Brachycephalic Airway Syndrome, *Elizabeth Streeter,* 168

     Laryngeal Paralysis, *Elizabeth Streeter,* 171

17. Laryngeal Tumors, *Leslie E. Fox,* 173
18. Tracheal Tumors, *Leslie E. Fox,* 175
19. Large Airway Disorders, *Jo Ann Morrison,* 177
20. Small Airway Disorders, *Jo Ann Morrison,* 184
21. Parenchymal Disorders and Diseases, *Elizabeth Streeter,* 192

     Viral Diseases, *Erin M. Portillo,* 194

     Bacterial Diseases, *Robert R. King and Michelle A. Pressel,* 196

     Parasitic and Protozoal Diseases, *Catherine Kasai,* 204

22. Pulmonary Thromboembolism, *Erin M. Portillo,* 208
23. Pleural Space Diseases, *Robert R. King and Michelle A. Pressel,* 211
24. Lower Respiratory Tract Tumors, *Leslie E. Fox,* 219

IV. ENDOCRINE DISEASE

David L. Panciera

25. Diabetes Mellitus, 229

     Diabetic Ketoacidosis, 234

26. Hypoadrenocorticism, 237
27. Hyperadrenocorticism, 241
28. Hypothyroidism, 246
29. Hyperthyroidism, 249
30. Hypercalcemia, 250
31. Hypocalcemia, 253
32. Hypoglycemia, 255
33. Central Diabetes Insipidus, 258

V. GASTROINTESTINAL PROBLEMS

Anthony P. Carr

34. The Approach to Vomiting and Regurgitation, 261
35. The Approach to Diarrhea, 263

     Acute Diarrhea, 265

     Viral Diarrhea, 266

     Bacterial Diarrhea, 267

     Fungal Disease, 268

     Parasites, 269

     Adverse Reactions to Food, 270

     Inflammatory Bowel Disease, 270

Protein-Losing Enteropathy, 271
Neoplasia, 272
36. The Approach to Ascites, 273
37. Esophageal Disease, 275
38. Diseases of the Stomach, 279
Gastric Dilation Volvulus, 279
Stomach Tumors, 282
Helicobacter, 282
Gastric Motility Disorders, 284
39. Diseases of the Rectum and Anus, 285
40. Pancreas and Pancreatitis, 288
41. Exocrine Pancreatic Insufficiency, 292
42. Liver, 293
Approach to the Dog with Icterus, 293
Liver Disease Basics, 295
Chronic Inflammatory Liver Disease, 296
Copper Storage Hepatopathies, 298
Toxic Liver Disease, 299
Hepatic Encephalopathy, 299
Portosystemic Shunts, 300
Diseases of the Gallbladder, 303

VI. URINARY SYSTEM
Stanley I. Rubin
43. Acute Renal Failure, *Stanley I . Rubin and Mala Erickson,* 305
44. Chronic Renal Failure, *Mala Erickson and Stanley I. Rubin,* 312
45. Glomerular Disease, *Mala Erickson and Stanley I. Rubin,* 319
46. Urolithiasis, *Mala Erickson and Stanley I. Rubin,* 324
47. Urinary Incontinence, *Stanley I. Rubin and Mala Erickson,* 331
48. Urinary Tract Neoplasia, *Stanley I. Rubin and Mala Erickson,* 334
49. Urinary Tract Infection, *Mala Erickson and Stanley I. Rubin,* 336

VII. REPRODUCTIVE PROBLEMS
Klaas Post
50. Cystic Endometrial Hyperplasia/Pyometra Complex, *Klaas Post,* 341
51. Infertility in the Female Dog, *Klaas Post,* 343
52. Brucellosis, *Klass Post,* 345
53. Prostatic Disease, *Stanley I. Rubin and Mala Erickson,* 348
Benign Prostatic Hyperplasia, 350
Bacterial Prostatitis, 351
Acute Prostatitis, 352
Chronic Prostatitis, 352
Prostatic Cysts, 352
Prostatic Neoplasia, 353

VIII. POLYSYSTEMIC PROBLEMS
Astrid Nielssen

54. Polysystemic Problems: Fever, 355
55. Lymphadenopathy, 358
56. Joint Disease, 359
57. Edema, 362
58. Paraneoplastic Syndromes, 364

IX. HEMOLYMPHATIC DISORDERS
Astrid Nielssen

59. Canine Lymphoma, 367
60. Hemangiosarcoma, 370
61. Approach to the Bleeding Dog, 372
62. Anemia, 373
63. Polycythemia, 375
64. Neutropenia, 377
65. Thrombocytopenia, 378
66. Immune-Mediated Hemolytic Anemia, 381
67. Coagulopathies, 384
   Acquired, 384
   Inherited, 386

X. INFECTIOUS DISEASES
Gregory C. Troy

68. Antifungal Therapy, *Gregory C. Troy and David Clark Grant,* 389
69. Canine Infectious Disease, *David Clark Grant and Gregory C. Troy,* 394
   Viral Diseases, 399
   Rickettsial Diseases, 404
   Bacterial Diseases, 409
   Fungal Diseases, 414

Index, 423

Section I
Neurology and Neuromuscular Diseases
Section Editor: Karen Dyer Inzana

1. Neurologic Examination and Lesion Localization
Karen Dyer Inzana

1. Where do I start when performing a neurologic examination?

Always start by looking at the animal across the room. Look for abnormal body postures (i.e., head tilt or turn), abnormal movements (circling, head tremors), or behaviors that you would not expect from an animal in the hospital environment (dementia, excessive solumnence or extreme agitation). If any of these things are observed, then the problem must involve the brain lesion (above the foramen magnum).

2. How will changes in gait help localize lesions?

After observing the animal across the room, next watch the animal walk, preferably on a nonslippery surface. Look again for abnormal head postures or movements, but then concentrate on gait. Is there one side that appears weaker than the other? Is there a similar amount of coordination in the front and rear limbs? If the front limbs are abnormal, are they more or less abnormal than the rear limbs? Because the brachial intumescence in most dogs is located between C6 to T2 spinal cord segments, normal to near normal gait in the front limbs with poor coordination in the rear limbs suggests a lesion caudal to the second thoracic spinal cord segment (T2). If the front limbs are as weak or weaker than the pelvic limbs, then the problem likely resides within the cervical intumescence. If the front limbs are abnormal, but appear stronger than the pelvic limbs, this usually indicates a lesion rostral to C6. If one side (thoracic and pelvic limbs) appears weaker than the other (hemiparesis), the same rules apply as previously described, but one side of the spinal cord or brain is more severely affected than the other.

3. How can you be sure that an abnormal gait is caused by neurologic disease rather than an orthopedic condition?

Sometimes it can be difficult to differentiate between neurologic and orthopedic diseases. The best way to do this is with a series of tests referred to as postural reactions. Postural reactions are a series of maneuvers that place the animal's feet in an abnormal position to bear weight. The animal must first recognize that the foot is in an abnormal position (sensory systems) and then have the strength to replace the foot in a more normal position (motor systems). Animals with orthopedic disease can accomplish most postural reactions. Occasionally animals with orthopedic disease will resist the postural reactions that require a lot of movement on the weight-bearing limb (e.g., hemiwalking, hopping, wheelbarrowing). However, it is extremely rare that all postural reactions are abnormal in an animal with only orthopedic disease. The following are the more common postural reactions.

- **Conscious proprioception:** Gently support the animal's weight and turn one foot onto its dorsal surface. I place a hand under the pelvis when evaluating the pelvic limbs, and under the chest when examining the thoracic limbs. All four limbs should be examined. A normal response is to immediately flip the paw over onto the normal weight-bearing surface. Abnormal responses include leaving the foot in the abnormal position, repositioning it slowly or repositioning it incompletely (i.e., leaving one or more toes turned over).

- **Wheelbarrowing:** Support the animal's pelvic limb with all of the weight on the thoracic limbs. Push the animal forward so it must take several steps with the thoracic limbs to maintain balance. This is often accomplished first with the head and neck in a normal position, then repeated with the head and neck elevated. Abnormal responses include delayed positioning of one or both thoracic limbs or exaggerated placement. Exaggerated placement may suggest an abnormality in the cerebellum or caudal brain stem.
- **Extensor postural thrust:** Lift the animal off the floor and gently lower it onto the pelvic limbs. A normal animal will often extend the limbs in anticipation of contact and then take several steps backwards to position the limbs correctly. An alternative technique for dogs that are too big to be picked up is to lift the front legs and push them backwards. I have rarely found this alternative helpful.
- **Hemistanding and hemiwalking:** Lift both front and rear limbs on one side so that one side supports all of the animal's weight. Most normal animals can then accomplish lateral hopping movements with the supporting limbs.
- **Hopping:** This reaction is similar to hemiwalking, but all of the animal's weight is concentrated on one limb. Again, normal animals can make lateral hopping movements in the one supporting limb.
- **Visual and tactile placing:** For small animals that are easily supported, bring the animal close to a tabletop while the examiner supports most of its weight. A normal response is for the animal to see the table and reach for it with the closest limb. A similar tactile response can be elicited by covering the animal's eyes and advancing the animal so one limb brushes the side of the table. Again, a normal animal will attempt to place the limb in a position to bear weight.

4.   When do you test spinal reflexes?

After completing the postural reactions, I have a good idea if the gait abnormality is orthopedic or neurologic in origin. If it is neurologic, I use the same information regarding localization of gait abnormalities that I described previously. Spinal reflexes help determine if the problem involves the intumescence (either cervical or pelvic) or is "upstream" of the intumescence. As previously mentioned, the cervical intumescence resides within spinal cord segments C6-T2, whereas the pelvic intumescence resides within spinal cord segments L4-S3. The intumescences contain the cell bodies for the lower motor neurons that innervate the thoracic or pelvic limbs, respectively. Injury to the lower motor neurons will cause spinal reflexes to be decreased or absent. Because the predominate clinical feature is caused by injury to the lower motor neuron, paresis or paralysis with decreased or absent spinal reflexes is frequently referred to as lower motor neuron clinical signs. Alternatively, if the lower motor neuron is intact but the problem resides in one or more neurons upstream or closer to the motor center in the brain, then spinal reflexes will still be intact and may be exaggerated even though the animal has lost some or all voluntary motor ability in that limb. Paresis or paralysis with normal to increased spinal reflexes if often referred to as upper motor neuron clinical signs that reflect that the injury is upstream from the lower motor neurons.

5.   Do spinal reflexes help distinguish between neurologic and nonneurologic diseases?

Rarely. Postural reactions do a better job of answering the question, Is the problem neurologic or nonneurologic in origin? Spinal reflexes are strongly influenced by the temperament and anxiety level of the animal. If the animal is anxious, then the muscles are tense, and spinal reflexes often will appear exaggerated in an otherwise normal animal. If reflexes are abnormal, I will repeat postural reactions. It would be most unusual for neuronal injury severe enough to cause abnormal spinal reflexes to not also affect postural reactions.

6. Is it correct that spinal reflexes primarily distinguish between upper motor neuron and lower motor neuron injury?
Yes, this is the primary value of spinal reflexes in a neurologic examination.

7. How do you perform spinal reflexes and what should they look like?
Thoracic limb reflexes include the following:

- *Flexor reflex, withdrawal reflex, pedal reflex:* Pinching the toe (or other noxious stimuli) causes prompt flexion or withdrawal of the limb. The afferent branch varies with the area pinched; the efferent nerves are those that mediate flexion of the limb (axillary, musculocutaneous, median, and ulnar).
- *Biceps reflex:* This reflex is initiated by percussion of the biceps tendon (near its insertion on the craniomedial aspect of the forearm) and both afferent and efferent axons are carried in the musculocutaneous nerve (spinal cord segments C6-C8). The appropriate response is flexion of the elbow. However, this is often hard to see when holding the limb, so often you only see a visible contraction of the biceps muscle.
- *Triceps reflex:* This reflex is initiated by percussion of the triceps tendon near the olecranon. Both afferent and efferent axons are carried in the radial nerve (spinal cord segments C7-T2) and the appropriate response is extension of the elbow. This is the most difficult reflex to see in the front leg.
- *Extensor carpi radialis response:* Percussion directly over the belly of the extensor carpi radialis elicits extension of the carpus. Whereas they are both direct effects on the skeletal muscle and stimulation of stretch receptors (and associated myotatic reflex), a normal response requires an intact radial nerve. The appropriate response is extension of the carpus.

8. Pelvic limb reflexes include the following:

- *Flexor reflex:* This reflex is initiated by noxious stimulation of the limb. Afferents are carried in either the femoral nerve (if the medial surface of the limb is stimulated) or sciatic nerve. The efferent axons are carried in the sciatic nerve (L6-S1). The appropriate response is flexion of the limb.
- *Patellar reflex:* Percussion of the patellar tendon elicits a brisk extension of the stifle. The peripheral nerve controlling this reflex is the femoral nerve (spinal cord segments L4-L6).
- *Perineal reflex:* Noxious stimulation of the perineum results in constriction of the anal sphincter and flexion of the tail (spinal cord segments S2-S3).
- *Gastrocnemius reflex:* Percussion of the Achilles tendon causes contraction of the gastrocnemius muscle and extension of the hock. It requires an intact tibial branch of the sciatic nerve (spinal cord segments L6-L7, S1).
- *Cranial tibial response:* Percussion directly over the cranial tibial muscle causes flexion of the hock. Again this response is mediated by a combination of direct muscle contraction and a myotatic stretch reflex. A normal response requires an intact peroneal branch of the sciatic nerve (spinal cord segments L6-L7, S1).

9. What would a lesion between L4 and S3 spinal cord segments look like?
The animal would have gait abnormalities in the pelvic limbs. Postural reactions should be decreased in the pelvic limbs and normal in the thoracic limbs. Spinal reflexes should be decreased to absent in the pelvic limbs. In addition, the limb would feel flaccid and muscle atrophy would occur quickly.

10. What would a lesion between T2 and L4 spinal cord segments look like?
The animal would have gait abnormalities in the pelvic limbs. Postural reactions should be decreased in the pelvic limbs and normal in the thoracic limbs. Spinal reflexes should be increased in the pelvic limbs and, occasionally, you may see abnormal reflexes. The limb should not feel flaccid; muscle atrophy occurs slowly from disuse.

11. What do you mean by abnormal reflexes?

There are several reflexes that are typically masked and only become apparent when the upper motor neuron has been injured. These include a crossed extensor reflex and Babinski's reflex.

The crossed extensor reflex is seen with the animal in lateral recumbency and appears as an involuntary extension of the opposite limb during the flexor reflex. This is a normal reflex when the animal is standing, but inhibited by descending spinal pathways in a recumbent animal. The presence of this reflex is reliable evidence that these descending pathways have been injured.

Babinski's reflex is elicited by stroking the caudolateral surface of the hock, beginning at the hock and continuing to the digits. An abnormal response is extension of the digits. This reflex is also an indicator of injury to inhibitory descending spinal pathways.

12. Does the presence of abnormal reflexes indicate a worse prognosis?

Abnormal reflexes become more prominent over time. Therefore their presence is an indication that the problem has existed for weeks to months. Obviously, a more chronic lesion would have a worse prognosis. However, the ability to consciously recognize painful stimulation to areas caudal to the lesion is the most reliable prognostic indicator. Animals without conscious pain sensation caudal to the lesion have a much worse prognosis than those that can still feel their limbs.

13. Can you localize a lesion between the T2 and L4 spinal cord segments more precisely with a clinical examination?

It is difficult to be extremely accurate with localization in areas other than the intumescences. However, the panniculus reflex may be helpful. The panniculus reflex is caused by contraction of the cutaneous trunci muscle in response to a sensory stimulus of the skin. Dorsal cutaneous afferent nerves are stimulated. The impulse is transmitted up the spinal cord in ascending superficial pain pathways that synapse on the lateral thoracic nerve (located between the C8 and T2 spinal segments). The response is blocked in segments caudal to the injury. For example, an animal with injury at T13-L1 would have a normal response cranial to the level, but the response would be absent caudal to this point. This can be helpful in narrowing the localization within the spinal cord. However, this is not the most reliable response and may still be present in animals with severe spinal injury and absent in some with mild injury.

A focal area of pain (hyperpathia) can be a more sensitive lesion localizer. For example, an animal with a type I disk herniation at T13-L1 may or may not have a panniculus response that corresponds to this lesion. However, deep palpation in this area will often appear to cause pain. Focal hyperpathia is only useful for animals with lesions that cause meningeal or periosteal irritation. The spinal cord does not have pain receptors and so lesions that are confined to neural parenchyma alone are not painful.

14. How would a lesion between the C6 and T2 spinal cord segments appear clinically?

The animal would have upper motor neuron signs to the pelvic limbs that would be indistinguishable from the previous case. However, the thoracic limbs would also be affected and would show lower motor neuron clinical signs because this is in the area of the cervical intumescence. Occasionally, injury between C8 and T2 will also damage the sympathetic innervation to the head because the first efferent neuron in the sympathetic chain is located in this area. Clinical signs would include miosis, ptosis, and enophthalmus of the ipsilateral eye.

15. How would a lesion between the C1 and C6 spinal cord segments appear clinically?

These animals would be weak in all four limbs and spinal reflexes should be normal to increased. As previously mentioned, the animals generally appear worse in the pelvic limbs than in the thoracic limbs. It is rare to see an animal completely paralyzed with a cervical spinal lesion because severe injury will cause paralysis of the respiratory muscles and death.

16. Where would you localize the lesion in an animal with paralysis of all four limbs and decreased spinal reflexes?

This would be the typical presentation of an animal with generalized peripheral nerve or neuromuscular junction injury.

17. If an animal has a head tilt, where does this place the lesion?

An abnormal head posture is seen with injury rostral to the foramen magnum. Generally, the head tilt is toward the side of the lesion. With careful observation, you will see that animals with injury to the caudal portions of the brain have a typical head tilt that changes as you move rostrally to a head turn. This is a subtle point and not always reliable, but it can be helpful at times.

18. If all lesions in the brain cause a head deviation, then how can you localize lesions within the brain?

Postural reactions are extremely helpful here. With focal lesions in the central nervous system caudal to the midbrain, postural reactions will be abnormal on the same side as the lesion. With focal lesions rostral to the midbrain, postural reactions will be abnormal on the side opposite the lesion. It is easy to remember that this changes in the middle of the brain. Within the midbrain itself, lesions in the caudal midbrain produce ipsilateral postural reaction deficits, whereas lesions in the rostral midbrain, especially those rostral to the red nucleus, produce postural reaction deficits on the side opposite the lesion. Because the head tilt is usually to the side of the lesion, an animal with a right head tilt and postural reaction deficits on the right side has a lesion in the midbrain or caudal. If an animal has a right head tilt and postural reaction deficits on the left side, then the lesion is midbrain or rostral.

19. Can you localize lesions more precisely within the brain?

Cranial nerves can help localize lesions to very specific regions of the brain. Cranial nerves V through XII are located in the metencephalon (pons) and myelencephalon (medulla); cranial nerves III and IV are located in the mesencephalon (midbrain). Cranial nerve II is intimately associated with the ventral diencephalon (thalamus, hypothalamus).

20. What do cranial nerves do?

Cranial nerve I is the olfactory nerve and mediates the sense of smell. It is difficult to clinically evaluate this nerve.

Cranial nerve II is the optic nerve. You can often determine visual function from earlier parts of the examination. By covering each eye of the animal and making a menacing gesture toward each eye, you can evaluate vision in each eye. Unfortunately, other lesions such as facial nerve paralysis or cerebellar disease may also alter the menace reaction. Pupillary light reactions are also helpful in establishing optic nerve function. With injury to cranial nerve II, there will be no direct pupillary light response on the abnormal side, and no consensual response in the other eye.

Cranial nerve III carries parasympathetic innervation to the pupil. Injury to cranial nerve III will cause the pupil on the same side to be dilated and not constrict with bright light. With a pure cranial nerve III injury, the dog is still visual so menace reaction is still normal.

Cranial nerves III, IV, and VI (occulomotor, trochlear, and abducens nerves) innervate the extraocular eye muscles. Injury to any one of these three will result in the eye being permanently deviated to one side.

Cranial nerve V is the trigeminal nerve. It provides motor innervation to the muscles of mastication and sensation to the entire face. Injury to this nerve often results in atrophy of the ipsilateral temporalis muscle and analgesia to the ipsilateral side of the face.

Cranial nerve VII is the facial nerve. It controls the muscle of facial expression. Injury to this nerve causes inability to blink or retract the lip. The nose may be deviated toward the normal side with early facial nerve injury and the nostril on the affected side will not flare with inhalation. The facial nerve also carries the sensory fibers for taste, but this is rarely tested in practice.

Cranial nerve VIII is the vestibulocochlear nerve. It has two branches. The cochlear nerve relays sensory impulses associated with sound. Bilateral injury results in deafness, but unilateral injury can be difficult to detect without special electrophysiologic testing. The vestibular portion of cranial nerve VIII mediates the sense of balance and orientation of the head and body with respect to gravity. Deficits in this branch result in marked head tilt, and staggering or falling to the side of the lesion. The vestibular nerve also plays an important role in coordinating eye movement; therefore vestibular nerve injury often results in nystagmus and intermittent strabismus.

Cranial nerves IX, X, and XI (glossopharyngeal, vagus, and accessory nerves) provide motor innervation to the pharynx, larynx, and palate. Injury to these nerves causes inability to swallow, a poor gag reflex, and inspiratory stridor because of laryngeal paralysis. The accessory nerve also provides motor innervation to the trapezius muscle and parts of the sternocephalicus and brachiocephalicus muscles. Denervation atrophy in these muscles can be seen with careful examination.

Cranial nerve XII (hypoglossal nerve) provides motor innervation to the muscles of the tongue. Injury results in paralysis of the ipsilateral side of the tongue.

21. How do you evaluate cranial nerves?

Cranial nerve evaluation is simple. I look at the animal's pupils for asymmetry and evaluate pupillary light reflexes (cranial nerve II, parasympathetic and sympathetic innervation), then elicit a menace reaction from each eye (cranial nerves II and VII).

I move the animal's head from side to side to be sure it can move the eyes in all positions (cranial nerves III, IV, and VI), then touch its face by the eye, nose, and lip to be sure it has normal sensation (cranial nerve V) and movement of the face (cranial nerve VII).

I open the animal's mouth to evaluate jaw tone (cranial nerve V) and stimulate the pharynx with my hand to evaluate gag reaction (cranial nerve IX, X, and XII) and look at its tongue to be sure it has normal motor (cranial nerve XII).

For cranial nerve VIII, I look for abnormal body postures during the earlier parts of my examination and carefully examine the eyes to be sure that there is normal conjugate eye movement. This is best done while you position the animal for evaluation of spinal reflexes.

22. How would a lesion in the pons and medulla appear?

The animal would have a head tilt toward the side of the lesion with ipsilateral postural reaction deficits. You should also observe deficits in cranial nerves V through XII on the same side of the lesion.

23. How would a lesion in the midbrain appear?

The animal would have a head tilt to the side of the lesion, postural reaction deficits may be ipsilateral or contralateral, but deficits in cranial nerves III and IV should be on the same side of the lesion. In my experience, focal midbrain injury is rare.

24. How would a lesion in the thalamus appear?

The animal would have a head tilt toward the side of the lesion, postural reaction deficits on the side opposite the head tilt, and often it will have seizures. Complete loss of cranial nerve II function will be present only if the lesion is in the ventral portions of the hypothalamus near the optic chiasm. If the injury is in other areas of the thalamus, the pupils may appear asymmetrical, but the deficits will not appear complete.

25. How would a lesion in the cerebrum appear?
Lesions in the cerebrum are often indistinguishable from lesions in the thalamus. If the injury affects the occipital lobes of the cerebrum, then the animal may not have a menace on the opposite side, but pupillary light reactions will be normal. Because these areas often appear clinically the same, the cerebrum and thalamus-hypothalamus are often collectively referred to as the forebrain.

26. Do seizures occur only with injury to the thalamus-hypothalamus or cerebrum?
Yes, seizure activity is a sign of forebrain disease.

27. We left out the cerebellum. What do lesions in the cerebellum look like?
The cerebellum is a complex structure that coordinates movement throughout the body. Portions of the cerebellum are involved with the vestibular apparatus, and selective lesions in this region will appear similar to cranial nerve VIII deficits. Lesions in other areas will cause movements to appear incoordinated. The animal's limbs may appear hypermetric or hypometric during movement. Often the animal's head will tremor when it is concentrating on some activity such as eating or drinking.

28. Does injury to the cerebellum cause postural reaction deficits?
A lesion that only affects the cerebellum (e.g., cerebellar hypoplasia) will not cause postural reactions to be absent, but they may be performed poorly or with exaggerated movements. However, it is more common for the cerebellum to be injured along with the underlying pons and medulla in which case postural reactions will be diminished or absent.

29. Can you have vestibular disease without postural reaction deficits?
Yes, if you injure any cranial nerve outside the calvaria, you will see loss of function of that nerve, but the motor and sensory tracts in the brain stem will still be intact. Peripheral injury to cranial nerve VIII commonly occurs with ear infections, some toxins, and idiopathic causes. In this case, the animal will have a head tilt (to the side of injury) and a tendency to fall or roll to that side. Sometimes they are so disorientated that postural reactions are difficult to evaluate. However, if you are careful and persistent, you will find that postural reactions are still intact. Another interesting feature of peripheral vestibular disease is that the nystagmus is always in the same direction. It generally is horizontal with the fast phase away from the head tilt, although it can be rotatory as well. What I mean by "always in the same direction" is you may not see abnormal eye movements in all body positions, but when you do see it, the movement is always the same. With injury to brain stem or cerebellar structures, the nystagmus often changes direction when the animal is rolled in other body positions. We should note that both the facial nerve and sympathetic innervation to the face pass through the inner ear and are also often injured with inner ear infections. Cranial nerve VII is close to cranial nerve VIII in the brain stem and these are often injured by a single lesion, but it is rare to see Horner's syndrome with a lesion in the central nervous system.

30. I feel comfortable with localizing lesions outside the brain, but I never seem to be able to localize problems within the brain. Is this unusual?
Honestly, most of the intracranial diseases encountered in small animal practice are multifocal or diffuse in nature. Things such as metabolic encephalopathies, toxic encephalopathies, or infectious or inflammatory diseases typically affect more than one area of the brain and so they are not readily localizable. Diseases that tend to be focal include tumors and infarcts; these can be difficult to localize if they are large enough that they put pressure on large parts of the brain. It is important to be able to localize lesions, though; otherwise you would not know that the problem is multifocal or diffuse.

2. Seizures

Karen Dyer Inzana

1. What is a seizure?

A seizure is a clinical sign of cerebral dysfunction. It results from a usually transient, hypersynchronous electrical activity of neurons. The outward manifestation of this electrical event varies with the number and location of neurons involved. Partial seizures are a manifestation of dysrhythmia occurring in only a limited number of neurons, whereas generalized seizures arise from simultaneous activation of neurons in both cerebral hemispheres.

2. What causes a seizure?

Anything that lowers the brain's ability to prevent hypersynchronous electrical activity will cause a seizure. Many refer to this ability as the seizure threshold. Every animal is capable of having a seizure, but there is a mechanism that prevents this from happening in a normal animal. Exactly what constitutes this mechanism is not entirely clear, but most likely represents a balance between excitatory and inhibitory influences (both ionic and neurotransmitter levels).

Below is a list of differentials for seizures and the age that they are most likely to occur (Table 2-1). Note that a young dog (younger than 6 months of age) is more likely to have seizures as a result of a congenital disorder (hydrocephalus, lissencephaly, portosystemic shunt), intoxication, or infectious disease, whereas an older dog (older than 6 years of age) is more likely to have neoplastic disease. Epilepsy is more likely to occur in middle-age animals.

Table 2-1 *Common Causes of Seizures in Dogs by Age of First Seizure*

CAUSE	< 1 YEAR	1-5 YEARS	> 5 YEARS
Degenerative			
Storage disease	X	X	X (uncommon)
Anomalous			
Hydrocephalus	X		
Lissencephaly	X		
Primary epilepsy		X	
Metabolic			
Portosystemic shunts	X		
Acquired liver disease			X
Hypoglycemia	X		X
Hyperlipoproteinemia		X	X
Electrolyte imbalance	X	X	X
Neoplastic (brain tumors)			X
Infectious	X	X	X
Inflammatory without infectious cause*		X	
Trauma (secondary epilepsy)	X	X	X
Toxic	X	X	X

*Granulomatous meningoencephalitis in dogs, nonsuppurative meningoencephalitis in cats.

3.   What is epilepsy?

By definition, recurrent seizures from an unknown cause are considered epilepsy. Although this is the most accepted definition, it includes most of the diseases listed previously. It is often more convenient to consider epilepsy as recurrent seizures from a nonprogressive intracranial disease process. This limits the definition to conditions that cause abnormal electrical activity within the brain, but do not themselves cause progressive disease and can only be treated with anticonvulsants. Most neurologists then divide epilepsy into two forms: primary and secondary.

4.   What is primary epilepsy?

Primary epilepsy (also known as congenital epilepsy, inherited epilepsy, or functional epilepsy) is a congenital disorder that results in an abnormally lowered seizure threshold. In some experimental models, abnormal ion channels on neuronal membranes that keep them closer to threshold cause this. The exact cause of the condition in dogs is not known. However, there are three characteristics of seizures that occur in primary epilepsy: the first seizure generally occurs between 6 months and 5 years of age (most between 10 and 20 months of age); seizures are generally isolated at first, but become more frequent and longer in duration over time; and the seizures are generalized from the onset. This last criterion is probably the weakest, because families of dogs have been identified that have what appears to be partial seizures.

5.   What is secondary epilepsy?

Secondary epilepsy (also known as acquired or structural epilepsy) results from an acquired lesion in the brain. This lesion may be from previous trauma or infection that has resolved, but left a glial scar that develops an abnormal electrical generator. Because these are acquired, they can begin at any age and may appear focal in onset. As with primary epilepsy, these seizures often become more frequent and more intense over time.

6.   If epilepsy is a nonprogressive disease, then why do the seizures intensify over time?

Recurrent seizures lower the seizure threshold and make it easier for the brain to develop more hypersynchronous electrical activity. This phenomenon is referred to as kindling or development of mirror foci. Therefore, seizures typically become more frequent and intense over time. Clinically, the interictal period between seizures becomes shorter and eventually isolated seizures become cluster seizures and eventually status epilepticus.

7.   What are cluster seizures and how do they differ from status epilepticus?

With cluster seizures, multiple seizures occur in a short period, generally 24 hours, but the animal regains consciousness between seizures. In status epilepticus, the seizure discharge continues for longer periods without intervening periods of consciousness. No one has clearly defined how long a seizure must go on before it is considered status epilepticus. Borrowing from the human literature, it is a continuous seizure that lasts longer than 20 minutes.

8.   Are either cluster seizures or status epilepticus dangerous to the animal?

Yes, both are serious conditions that warrant immediate treatment. Experimentally, it takes longer than 20 minutes of continuous seizure activity to result in visible lesions in the brain. However, chemical and metabolic changes occur before structural lesions; these can result in prolonged dementia and lessen the chances of controlling the seizure.

9.   How are seizures treated?

The most important first step is to rule out progressive diseases. The diagnostic steps will vary with the signalment and clinical signs. Most animals require a complete blood cell count (CBC), biochemical profile, urinalysis, and liver function test such as bile acids. It is a good idea to obtain baseline values for these tests even in animals with epilepsy because many of the anticonvulsants can affect liver function. Neuroimaging (computed tomography or magnetic resonance imaging) is often recommended for both young and older animals and cerebrospinal fluid analysis with titers for infectious diseases is helpful in animals suspected of having encephalitis. I do not routinely request either computed tomography/magnetic resonance images or cerebrospinal fluid evaluation in animals with a signalment or history that suggest epilepsy.

After you have established the diagnosis of epilepsy, then the goal is to raise the seizure threshold to the point where seizures only occur at infrequent intervals, if at all. Estrus lowers the seizure threshold in intact females and neutering will often result in a lower seizure incidence. However, most require anticonvulsant therapy.

10. How do you decide if seizure frequency is occurring too often and anticonvulsant therapy should be initiated?

There is no clear definition of acceptable or unacceptable seizure frequency. There are some clients that consider any seizure unacceptable, whereas others can manage an animal that is having isolated seizures at infrequent intervals. I always recommend keeping a diary and considering anticonvulsant therapy if the interictal period shortens or the seizures become more intense. After this, it becomes a judgment call. Personally, I begin anticonvulsant therapy in large-breed dogs earlier than smaller breeds because of previous difficulty in gaining seizure control in some of these dogs. I generally recommend anticonvulsant therapy in any animal that has cluster seizures, or if the seizures are occurring more frequently than every 3 months. However, there are no firm rules and the decision is based largely on the client's ability to tolerate the seizures. I do advise clients that anticonvulsants will raise the seizure threshold and reduce the frequency of seizures, but they will not eliminate seizures completely in all animals.

11. Which anticonvulsants are best?

Ideally, serum concentrations of anticonvulsants should not fluctuate between dosing. Pharmacologically, to maintain steady serum concentrations, a drug should be given at least twice within its half-life. There are only two anticonvulsants with a dosing frequency that makes routine care practical. These are phenobarbital and potassium bromide.

Phenobarbital has been used the longest, so most clinicians have experience with this drug. It is highly effective at raising the seizure threshold and thereby controlling seizures, and is inexpensive. Unfortunately, about 5% of dogs on high doses for long periods develop hepatocellular injury. Because phenobarbital is metabolized in the liver via glucuronide conjugation, it alters the metabolism of many other drugs that the animal is likely to receive during its lifetime. The half-life of phenobarbital in most dogs is approximately 48 hours. Therefore it can be administered twice daily. Because it requires five half-lives to reach steady-state concentration, phenobarbital reaches steady-state serum concentrations within 2 weeks of administration.

Potassium bromide is a salt. It is excreted unchanged by the kidneys and has no known deleterious effects on any organ system. It also does not interfere with other drug metabolism. The half-life of potassium bromide is between 20 and 28 days and so in theory only requires administration once per week. Unfortunately, it is a gastric irritant and so it is typically dosed once or twice daily to lower the amount that is given in any one dose. Because of its long half-life, it does not reach steady-state serum concentrations for 4-5 months with routine dosing. Therefore many clinicians give an initial loading dose to achieve therapeutic serum concentrations within the first week before beginning maintenance therapy. It too is highly effective and inexpensive. There are two drawbacks to potassium bromide. First, because of its long half-life, dosage adjustments are not reflected in serum concentrations very quickly and second, it is not as effective as phenobarbital in some animals.

12. What about primidone; is it an effective anticonvulsant?

Yes, primidone is an effective anticonvulsant. However, primidone is rapidly metabolized to phenylethylmalonic acid and phenobarbital. Although all three have anticonvulsant activity, the short elimination half-lives of both primidone and phenylethylmalonic acid probably render them ineffective in seizure management. Therefore phenobarbital is thought to account for at least 85% of the anticonvulsant effects of primidone. Dosing is higher than phenobarbital (15-35 mg/kg), but adjustments in dose are based on serum concentrations of phenobarbital.

13. What is the dose of phenobarbital?

The best dose of any anticonvulsant is the lowest dose that will reduce seizure frequency to an acceptable level. I typically begin with 2.2 mg/kg of phenobarbital twice daily. If seizures continue, I will measure the serum concentration and adjust it so that it is within the therapeutic concentration of 20-40 µg/dl. The formula (new dose = current dose × (target concentration/ measured concentration) is helpful at achieving this desired serum concentration.

14. What if the owner complains of sedation after starting phenobarbital?

It is not uncommon for dogs to appear sedated when beginning phenobarbital therapy. Unless the dog is unusually sedate, I recommend waiting for 2 weeks before adjusting the dosage.

15. How often do you recommend rechecking the animal?

Occasionally, idiosyncratic reactions occur such as pancytopenia. These typically occur within 2 weeks of beginning therapy. Therefore, a recheck about 2 weeks after starting therapy is indicated. I will check a CBC and draw a baseline phenobarbital level. If there are no further problems, I recommend reevaluating the dog every 6 months for the first year and then yearly thereafter. Obviously, if seizures continue, then more frequent evaluation of serum concentrations is warranted.

16. How long after the last dose of phenobarbital do you recommend waiting before checking serum concentrations?

Because phenobarbital maintains steady serum concentrations throughout the day, the time of serum collection is of little concern. It is true that there will be some slight fluctuation in concentrations throughout the day, but generally not enough to make a difference in treatment recommendations. Therefore, collecting the serum when it is convenient for both doctor and client is satisfactory.

17. How do you evaluate hepatic function in dogs on phenobarbital?

CBC, biochemical profile, and serum phenobarbital concentration is measured during each recheck. Hepatic enzyme levels are typically difficult to evaluate because these enzymes are induced by phenobarbital. Unless alkaline phosphatase or alanine amino transferase levels are very high, or have risen dramatically from the last evaluation, little significance is placed on these values. Certainly a low albumin or elevated bilirubin would be of concern. Bile acids are a reliable indicator of liver function and should be evaluated in any animal with suspect liver indices. However, on a more practical level, phenobarbital concentration itself is a useful measure of liver function. If the dosage had remained the same, then serum concentrations should remain relatively constant. The concentration will often be lower after the first 6 months of therapy as the liver becomes more efficient at metabolizing the drug. It should remain constant thereafter.

18. If a dog continues to have seizures while receiving phenobarbital, when is something else tried, and what is the next step?

I continue to increase the dose of phenobarbital until the serum concentration is around 30 µg/dl. You can continue to increase the dose until closer to 40 µg/dl, but generally increasing the dose beyond this point only increases hepatotoxicity but gaining little more seizure control. Therefore when the serum concentration approaches 30 to 35 µg/dl, I add potassium bromide as a secondary anticonvulsant.

If the seizure frequency is every 3 months or longer, I will simply begin maintenance therapy with potassium bromide at 20 to 40 mg/kg daily. If the seizure interval is shorter, I will load the dog with bromide by administering 500 mg/kg over 3 to 5 days. This is generally accomplished by administering 100 mg/kg in 5 doses every 12 to 24 hours. As previously mentioned, potassium bromide is hypertonic and irritates the gastric mucosa if too much volume is administered at once. Most dogs tolerate smaller doses at more frequent intervals. Maintenance therapy is continued after the loading dose is completed.

Unfortunately, the sedative effects of phenobarbital and potassium bromide are additive. If serum concentration of phenobarbital is higher than 20 µg/dl, then I will often lower the phenobarbital dose when adding potassium bromide.

If seizures continue, I increase the dose of potassium bromide gradually until the owner complains of excessive sedation. This state of stupor induced by excessive levels of bromide is referred to as bromism and once exhibited, it does not wear off without reducing the dosage of one or both anticonvulsants as phenobarbital did initially.

19. If the dog is doing well on the combination of phenobarbital and potassium bromide, then how often do you perform rechecks?

I reevaluate the animal initially at 6-month intervals and yearly thereafter. During recheck appointments I perform a CBC, biochemical profile, and measure serum phenobarbital and potassium bromide. Published serum concentrations for potassium bromide are 15 to 300 mg/dl. Unfortunately, these values have been extracted from the human literature and at this time have little therapeutic value for animals. Perhaps this will change as more information is gained. Because toxic effects from bromide use in dogs other than bromism previously mentioned are not recognized, then high serum concentrations are of academic interest only. You can no longer increase the dose of bromide when the dog appears excessively sedated.

20. Is it true that some dogs will have pancreatitis or skin eruptions while receiving potassium bromide?

There are several reports of dogs that had pancreatitis or cutaneous lesions while receiving potassium bromide. However, these occur so infrequently that they do not preclude the use of this drug. If an animal has either pancreatitis or cutaneous lesions while receiving potassium bromide, the drug should be discontinued.

21. Is sodium bromide safer?

Bromide has the anticonvulsant properties of any bromide salt. There may be times when an animal has difficulty maintaining physiologic concentrations of potassium while receiving potassium bromide. In this case, switching to sodium bromide is warranted. Dosing of potassium and sodium bromide differs. The molecular weight of sodium is lower than potassium, which results in more bromide per gram of sodium bromide than potassium bromide. The conversion generally is 1 mg potassium bromide = 0.8 mg sodium bromide.

22. If you choose to begin potassium bromide as the sole anticonvulsant before trying phenobarbital, how would management differ?

If I choose to begin anticonvulsant therapy with potassium bromide rather than phenobarbital, I would begin with either maintenance or loading therapy described previously and continue with maintenance therapy. If the dog continued to have seizures despite achieving a serum bromide concentration of 300 mg/dl, I would then add phenobarbital.

23. What do you try if both phenobarbital and potassium bromide do not result in satisfactory seizure control?

The prognosis for effective seizure control is significantly worse in animals that are refractory to both phenobarbital and potassium bromide. There are several additional anticonvulsants listed in the following section that are being tried. However, that there is no universal recommendation at this point indicates that none of these therapies has proved beneficial in a large number of dogs.

FELBAMATE (FEBATOL)

The half-life of felbamate is relatively short in dogs (approximately 6 hours). It therefore is not effective at maintaining serum concentrations and is recommended as adjunct therapy for bromide. Felbamate is metabolized by the liver and hepatotoxicity is exacerbated by concurrent phenobarbital therapy. Therefore the goal is to replace phenobarbital with felbamate in refractory epileptics while still maintaining bromide therapy. The dosage of felbamate is 15 to 60 mg/kg every 8 hours.

GABAPENTIN (NEURONTIN)

Gabapentin has a half-life of only 3 to 4 hours in the dog. As with felbamate, it is not suitable alone for seizure control. However, gabapentin is excreted unchanged in the urine and has few toxic side effects. It can be added to existing phenobarbital/bromide therapy at a dosage of 10 to 20 mg/kg every 8 hours.

ZONISAMIDE

This is another anticonvulsant with a half-life of only 6 to 9 hours. It has hepatic metabolism, but appears well tolerated with anorexia and sedation being the primary complications. Recommended dosage is 8 to 12 mg/kg every 8 hours.

LEVETIRACETAM (KEPPRA)

Levetiracetam is a new anticonvulsant that has primary renal excretion. The half-life is only 3 to 4 hours in the dog, but it may be added onto phenobarbital and bromide combination therapy at a dose of 20 mg/kg every 8 hours.

24. How do you manage status epilepticus?

If the animal presents in status without a previous history of seizures, then metabolic conditions such as hypoglycemia or hypocalcemia should be considered. Hypoglycemia can be treated with 50% glucose at a dose of 2 mg/kg intravenously; hypocalcemia can be treated with 10% calcium gluconate at a dose of 4 mg/kg intravenously slowly to effect.

Most animals require anticonvulsants. The ideal anticonvulsant to use in status epilepticus is one that has excellent anticonvulsant properties, rapidly crosses the blood-brain barrier and exerts its effect, and has minimal cardiovascular or respiratory depressant effects. The drug that best fulfills these criteria is diazepam. A dose of 0.5 mg/kg should be administered intravenously. If seizures continue after 5 minutes, this dose should be repeated two more times.

25. What should you do if the animal continues to be in status epilepticus after you have administered diazepam?

If seizures continue despite three doses of diazepam, then another rapidly acting anticonvulsant should be used. The two best choices in this situation is pentobarbital or propofol. Pentobarbital should be administered at a dose of 3 to 15 mg/kg intravenously slowly to effect. Because pentobarbital is a potent respiratory depressant, the clinician should be prepared to assist ventilation. Propofol is much more expensive than pentobarbital and must be administered in a constant rate infusion of 4 to 8 mg/kg/hr. Propofol may cause apnea and hypovolemia. However, the level of anesthesia can be more carefully controlled and recovery is much smoother with propofol than pentobarbital. Anesthesia should be maintained for 4 hours with propofol. If seizures resume after this interval, then propofol should be continued for an additional 12 hours before trying to discontinue use.

26. How do you manage an animal that responds initially to diazepam, but seizures resume after about 20 minutes?

Diazepam has a half-life of approximately 20 minutes, so it is not uncommon for seizures to resume after 20 minutes. There are several choices at this point.

Administer phenobarbital along with another dose of diazepam.

Phenobarbital takes approximately 20 minutes to cross the blood-brain barrier and exert its effect. Therefore it is not a good choice during the initial treatment, but it works well in animals that can be controlled with diazepam for 20 minutes. Therefore, administer another dose of diazepam with phenobarbital. If the dog has never previously received phenobarbital, then the initial dose is 15 mg/kg intravenously. However, if the dog is a refractory epileptic that should have a measurable serum concentration of phenobarbital, then a more conservative dose is indicated. If possible, serum should be collected for phenobarbital concentrations before additional drug is administered. If the serum can be analyzed quickly, then 1 mg/kg of phenobarbital can be administered for each 1 μg/ml you wish to increase the serum concentration. However, if serum concentrations are not readily available, then 2 mg/kg can usually be safely administered three times.

Administer a continuous benzodiazepine infusion.

If seizures resume a short period after diazepam and phenobarbital administration, a continuous infusion of diazepam may be helpful. Diazepam can be added hourly to an inline burette at a rate of 0.1-0.5 mg/kg/hr. There are several disadvantages to this technique. Diazepam will adhere to the plastic tubing used in the administration set, so the actual dose administered is unknown. Furthermore, diazepam does not readily go into solution, and a fine precipitate is usually present in the diluted preparation. Despite these limitations, diazepam infusion may effectively control status epilepticus in some animals. Midazolam (Versed) a newer benzodiazepine, has the advantage of being water soluble and is an effective anticonvulsant. Unfortunately, it is five times more expensive than diazepam. Note that rapid withdrawal of benzodiazepines can induce seizures, so infusion should be reduced by 50% every 6 hours for a minimum of 12 hours before discontinuing.

27. If a dog has frequent bouts of status epilepticus at home, what can the owner do until he or she can obtain veterinary assistance?
Benzodiazepines can be administered both rectally and intranasally at a dose of 1 mg/kg of diazepam. It takes approximately 15 minutes to reach peak plasma concentrations with this route and can be given up to three times in a 24-hour period.

3. Peripheral Nerve Disease
Karen Dyer Inzana

1. What clinical signs do you associate with peripheral nerve disease?
Injury to a single or group of peripheral nerves (i.e., brachial plexus) causes weakness or paralysis of the muscles innervated by those nerves, loss of spinal reflexes, and rapid muscle atrophy. If the injury occurred before muscle atrophy is noticeable, the muscles will feel flaccid when palpated.

Animals with generalized peripheral nerve disease appear weak and poorly muscled, and have diminished or absent spinal reflexes. With the exception of the optic nerve, cranial nerves are peripheral nerves and are susceptible to the same diseases as spinal nerves. Therefore laryngeal paralysis, weak gag responses, facial paralysis, atrophy of the muscles of mastication, and abnormal pupillary light reflexes may be seen as well.

2. How can you distinguish peripheral nerve diseases from generalized muscle disease?
The clinical signs of generalized peripheral nerve disease and muscle disease overlap considerably. It often requires laboratory testing to distinguish between these. With most, but not all muscle diseases, there will be increased serum concentrations of creatine kinase. Electrophysiologically, both neuropathies and myopathies cause abnormal electromyographic spontaneous activity. However, nerve conduction velocities are normal in myopathies. If electrophysiologic tests are not available, muscle biopsy histology will distinguish the two. With peripheral nerve injury, there will be angular atrophy of both type I and type II myofibers. With primary muscle disease, pathology specific to the type of myopathy will be seen.

3. What are the most common causes of monoparesis in dogs?
It is best to break these down into acute or chronic in onset. With acute monoparesis, trauma is the most common cause. This can be due to specific nerve injury or to avulsion of the brachial plexus during extreme abduction of the limb. Avulsion of the pelvic plexus is much less common.
In cases of chronic, progressive monoparesis, neoplastic infiltration by nerve sheath tumors or entrapment of the peripheral nerves by surrounding neoplastic growths is common.

4. If an isolated peripheral nerve is injured, can it be repaired by suturing the severed ends?
Yes and no. Certainly peripheral axons are capable of regeneration. However, they do so slowly, at the rate of about 1 to 2 mm per day. Therefore functional regeneration is more likely with distal injuries. Injuries in which the nerve is not completely severed (e.g., crush injury or stretch injury) have a much better prognosis than complete transections mainly because the conduits through which regenerating axons can regrow are still intact. If the nerve has been completely transected, it is very difficult for regenerating axons to find appropriate channels to enable functional regrowth.

5. Are all cases of brachial plexus avulsion hopeless?
For a limb to be functional, the radial nerve must be intact. Unfortunately, this nerve is usually injured with cranial plexus avulsions (injuring nerve roots C6-C8) or caudal plexus avulsions (injuring nerve roots C8-T2) and complete avulsions. In all cases of closed peripheral nerve trauma, there are some fibers that are stretched, but not transected. It is therefore important to wait for a minimum of 4 to 6 weeks to see how much functional return will occur. If the animal is unable to fix the elbow in extension, then salvage procedures for the limb are of little use. Limb amputation should be considered if self-mutilation or trauma occurs in areas without sensation.

6. With chronic monoparesis cases, how can you distinguish nerve tumors from orthopedic injuries?
In the early stages, nerve sheath tumors can easily be confused with orthopedic problems. Presence of a Horner's syndrome or loss of panniculus response on the side of the lameness generally indicates nerve damage. Denervation muscle atrophy can be distinguished from disuse muscle atrophy electromyographically.

7. How can you confirm the diagnosis of nerve sheath tumor, and what treatment options are available?
Computed tomography has been helpful in identifying tumors of peripheral nerves. Occasionally, enlarged nerve roots can be identified with ultrasonography. However, a definitive diagnosis requires surgical exploration and biopsy of the nerves involved. Wide surgical excision

has resulted in complete cures in isolated cases. However, tumors usually recur because not all neoplastic cells can be removed. Radiation therapy has been proposed to decrease the incidence of recurrence. However, the efficacy of this therapy is not known.

8. What are the most common causes of acute generalized peripheral nerve disease in dogs?

There are three common neuropathies with an acute onset of clinical signs: tick paralysis, botulism, and coonhound paralysis. Rarely, an acute toxicity or acute fulminant myasthenia gravis could be confused with these three syndromes.

9. What is tick paralysis?

Tick paralysis is caused by a neurotoxin released from the salivary gland of a female *Dermacentor* tick. This toxin prevents the release of acetylcholine at the nerve terminal. Diagnosis is based on finding a tick on the animal and response to removal. Most cases of tick paralysis are much improved within 24 hours and are normal within 48 hours.

10. What is Coonhound paralysis?

Coonhound paralysis is the term originally used to describe acute polyradiculoneuritis. The first cases were described in Coonhounds that had received a raccoon bite, but it has been reported subsequently in other breeds. This appears to be caused by an immune-mediated destruction of myelin and axons in ventral nerve roots. Although raccoon saliva is recognized as an antigenic stimulant for this immune reaction, other cases without exposure to raccoons have been described. Several electrophysiologic techniques have been described to confirm that the primary injury has occurred in ventral nerve roots. However, it can be difficult to confirm this diagnosis antemortem. Spontaneous remission may begin as early as 1 week after the onset of clinical signs, but other animals remain paralyzed for several months. It is difficult to know if all cases would eventually improve, because long-term supportive care is not tenable for many cases. Therapy for this disease is supportive care. Despite the probable immune-mediated pathogenesis of this disease, immunosuppressive therapy usually increases the incidence of secondary infections and muscle atrophy.

11. What is botulism?

Botulism is an acute generalized polyneuropathy that results from ingestion of the endotoxin produced by *Clostridium botulinum*. This toxin is produced under anaerobic conditions, generally in carrion. After it is ingested, it binds to nerve terminals and prevents the release of acetylcholine. Unlike the toxin that causes tick paralysis, botulinum endotoxin binds irreversibly to the nerve terminal. Improvement occurs by sprouting of distal axons and regeneration of nerve terminals. This generally takes at least 4 weeks. Diagnosis of botulism can be confirmed by identifying botulinum toxin in ingesta. Treatment is largely supportive. An antitoxin is available that will inactivate unbound toxin, but will not influence already bound toxin. The antitoxin must also be specific for the type of botulism toxin. There are eight antigenically distinct types of botulism neurotoxins. However, most cases in dogs are caused by type C. Recommended antitoxin dosage is 10,000 to 15,000 U administered intravenously or intramuscularly twice at 4-hour intervals. Anaphylaxis is possible, so an intradermal test injection is advisable.

12. What are the most likely causes of generalized peripheral nerve disease with a more insidious onset and progressive course?

Systemic diseases that present as chronic progressive neuropathies include diabetes mellitus (usually only clinical in cats), hypoglycemia/insulinoma, hypothyroidism, and paraneoplastic syndrome typically associated with carcinomas. Therefore any adult animal that presents with chronic progressive neuropathy should be screened for these conditions. Unfortunately, the cause of a large percentage of neuropathies is never identified and is classified as idiopathic.

13. Is there anything that can be used to treat idiopathic neuropathies?
In recent clinical trials, researchers have used the Prosaptide TX14(A), a neurotropic peptide, to aid in the regeneration of peripheral nerves. Preliminary results suggest that this drug may help some dogs with peripheral nerve disease. This drug is available through Myelos Corporation at 4940 Carroll Canyon Road, Suite M, San Diego, CA 92121 and at *www.myelos.com.*

14. Are there breed-related, inherited neuropathies in dogs?
Yes, several different breeds of dogs have been identified with peripheral nerve disease. A complete discussion of these is available in the chapter "Peripheral Nerve Disease" in the *Textbook of Veterinary Internal Medicine*, 5th edition (S. Ettinger, E. Feldman, editors, Philadelphia, 1999, WB Saunders, pp 662-684). Breeds that have neuropathies before 6 months of age include Cairn Terriers, German Shepherds, Pointers, Rottweilers, Brittany Spaniels, Swedish Lapland Dogs, Boxers, Golden Retrievers, Tibetan Mastiffs, and Dachshunds. Breeds that have neuropathies after 6 months of age include Rottweilers, Brittany Spaniels, Alaskan Malamutes, Siberian Huskies, and Dalmatians.

15. Is myasthenia gravis a peripheral nerve disease?
Technically, myasthenia gravis is a muscle disease. It is caused by a reduction in acetylcholine receptors on the postsynaptic muscle membrane. Inefficient neuromuscular transmission results in generalized weakness that worsens with exercise and improves with rest. There are two forms of the disease: congenital and acquired. Acquired myasthenia is much more common.

16. Do all cases of myasthenia gravis look the same?
Three major categories have been identified in dogs: focal, chronic generalized, and acute fulminant generalized. The focal form occurs in approximately 36% of recognized cases and consists of variable degrees of facial, pharyngeal, laryngeal, and esophageal dysfunction. Subclinical evidence of appendicular muscle involvement has been demonstrated in some focal myasthenics. The two generalized forms are distinguished primarily by the rate with which clinical signs develop. It is important to note that between 89% and 90% of dogs with generalized myasthenia also have megaesophagus.

17. How do I diagnose myasthenia gravis?
Supportive evidence for the diagnosis of myasthenia can be made by the demonstration of increased muscle strength after administration of the short-acting acetylcholinesterase agent edrophonium chloride (Tensilon, 0.1-0.2 mg/kg intravenously). Electrophysiologic testing may be helpful if there is a decrementing response to repetitive muscle stimulation. However, the primary criterion for diagnosis of all forms of acquired myasthenia is identifying elevated concentrations of serum antibodies to acetylcholine receptors.

18. How do I treat myasthenia gravis?
Pyridostigmine bromide (Mestinon) when given at 1 to 3 mg/kg every 8 to 12 hours improves skeletal muscle strength, but has minimal effect on esophageal motility. Therapy should begin at the low end of the scale and gradually increase to desired effect. Alternatively, injectable neostigmine (Prostigmin) has been recommended at a dosage of 0.04 mg/kg every 6 hours intramuscularly to bypass the problem of oral administration of medication in regurgitating animals. Immunosuppressive therapy should also be considered to reduce antibody titers. Rapid administration of immunosuppressive doses of prednisone (1 mg/kg twice daily) often exacerbates weakness so a more conservative approach is recommended. I often begin with an antiinflammatory dose of prednisolone (0.25 mg/kg twice daily) and gradually increase the dosage to reach immunosuppressive doses over 3 to 4 weeks.

19. What is the prognosis for myasthenia gravis?

Approximately 50% of animals die within the first 2 weeks of aspiration pneumonia. Feeding in an upright position and holding the animals in an elevated position for 5 to 10 minutes after feeding can reduce the risk of aspiration pneumonia. In my experience, percutaneous gastrotomy tube feeding does not reduce the incidence of aspiration. After antibody titers are reduced, esophageal motility improves, which greatly improves the prognosis.

---

4. Inflammatory Intracranial Diseases: The Meningoencephalitides

John H. Rossmeisl, Jr.

---

1.   What is meningoencephalitis?

Meningoencephalitis is the generic term used to describe any inflammatory central nervous system (CNS) disorder involving the meninges (meningitis) and brain parenchyma (encephalitis). Because of the intimate anatomic relationship between the meninges and brain parenchyma, inflammatory intracranial diseases often involve both tissues, prompting the use of the inclusive term *meningoencephalitis*. Many of the inflammatory intracranial diseases can also originate in or extend to involve the spinal cord parenchyma and meninges, in which case the disease process would be referred to as meningoencephalomyelitis.

2.   Are there specific clinical signs that should increase my clinical suspicion that meningoencephalitis is present?

The meningoencephalitides are typically acute in onset and, in the absence of specific therapy, progressive in nature. Ultimately, the clinical manifestations of inflammatory intracranial disease are dependent on the neuroanatomic location of the lesions. Classically, the animal with meningoencephalitis will present with evidence of multifocal or diffuse intracranial disease on the neurologic examination. However, one study reported that approximately 66% of dogs with inflammatory CNS disease presented with clinical signs referable to a focal neuroanatomic area. The results of the neurologic examination are rarely specific for the etiology of the meningoencephalitis.

The antemortem identification of the cause of the meningoencephalitis can be difficult, and has remained elusive in approximately one third of dogs in one study.

3.   Do most animals with meningoencephalitis have systemic signs of illness?

Many animals with meningoencephalitis have no extraneural signs of disease. Dogs with viral, bacterial, and granulomatous meningoencephalitis (GME) have been reported to commonly have a fever and funduscopic abnormalities at presentation. Animals with CNS disease from fungal infections can also have extraneural signs of disease, notably in the respiratory, lymphatic, integumentary, and ocular systems. A complete ophthalmic examination is indicated in any animal with suspected meningoencephalitis.

4.   What ancillary diagnostics aids are helpful in determining the cause of meningoencephalitis?

Results of the complete blood cell counts, biochemical profiles, and urinalyses rarely provide specific information, but are useful in screening for the presence of concurrent systemic disease.

Cerebrospinal fluid (CSF) examination, often performed in conjunction with advanced intracranial imaging, serologic assays, and cultures, is the most commonly used method to establish an antemortem diagnosis of meningoencephalitis. In many cases, definitive diagnosis of meningoencephalitis requires histopathologic examination of brain tissue. Recent studies have shown that both computed tomography (CT)-guided and open surgical brain biopsy techniques are safe and valuable diagnostic tools.

5.   Are there any abnormalities present in CSF that are specific for the cause of meningoencephalitis?

Animals with meningoencephalitis often will have a CSF pleocytosis, an increase in the number of leukocytes. The type and number of CSF leukocytes present may provide additional information regarding the specific cause, such as bacterial, viral, or fungal disease, but in most cases, the identification of pleocytosis is a nonspecific finding. Occasionally, analysis of CSF can provide a definitive diagnosis, as is the case with cytologic identification of cryptococcal organisms.

6.   Besides routine analysis, should I save CSF for any other ancillary tests?

If CSF collection is performed, a small volume should be saved for the performance of immunologic, serologic, or microbiologic tests. Selection of these adjunctive tests should be based on the animal's neurologic condition and results of the initial gross, biochemical, and cytologic examination of CSF.

BACTERIAL MENINGOENCEPHALITIS

7.   What bacterial species are commonly associated with bacterial meningoencephalitis?

Streptococcus, Escherichia coli, Klebsiella, Nocardia, Actinomyces, and *Staphylococcus* are frequently identified aerobes in clinical cases. Various anaerobic species have also been incriminated.

8.   How do animals typically acquire bacterial meningoencephalitis?

Small animals with bacterial meningoencephalitis usually acquire the causative organism from their own endogenous flora. CNS bacterial infection can occur through several general mechanisms: direct traumatic inoculation, hematogenous spread from a systemic septic focus, opportunistic colonization of mucosal surfaces, progression of an infected local anatomic structure (e.g., orbit, inner ear, sinus), or by congenital or acquired communication of the CSF with body surfaces.

9.   Are systemic signs of infectious disease seen in cases of bacterial meningoencephalitis?

Yes. Systemic signs of illness, such as fever, vomiting, diarrhea, pulmonary crackles, and dyspnea can be variably present. The animal should be examined for signs of local infections in anatomic structures in proximity to the head. However, the absence of systemic signs of illness does not exclude a diagnosis of bacterial meningoencephalitis.

10.   What are common neurologic manifestations of CNS bacterial infections?

Seizures, cranial nerve deficits, behavioral change, altered mentation, and cervical rigidity are common. Signs of focal intracranial disease may be present in cases of abscessation.

11.   What are the most common laboratory abnormalities?

Results of a complete blood count can reveal an inflammatory leukogram, thrombocytopenia, or leukopenia. Serum biochemical abnormalities are present in 70% of dogs with bacterial meningoencephalitis, but are variable and nonspecific.

12. How is a diagnosis of bacterial meningoencephalitis made?

The diagnosis is most often made based on results of CSF analysis, which often reveals a moderate to severe neutrophilic pleocytosis. The further identification of degenerate neutrophils and the finding of intracellular bacterial organisms in CSF confirm the diagnosis. Gram stain preparations of CSF samples may facilitate visualization of bacteria and guide empirical therapy. Culture of CSF with these characteristics is always indicated, but is frequently negative. In one study, a positive antemortem CSF culture was obtained in only 13% of dogs with bacterial meningoencephalitis. CT and magnetic resonance (MR) imaging scans of the brain may also reveal changes consistent with inflammatory disease.

13. How should bacterial meningoencephalitis be treated?

When possible, treatment should be based on culture and sensitivity results. Considering the high frequency of negative CSF cultures despite known infections, treatment is often empiric. Ideally, broad-spectrum, bactericidal antibiotics with the ability to penetrate the blood-brain barrier should be chosen.

Metronidazole, fluoroquinolones, and potentiated sulfonamides are good empirical first choices. Successful treatment of brain abscessation requires both surgical drainage and chronic antimicrobial therapy.

14. What is the prognosis for animals with bacterial meningoencephalitis?

The prognosis associated with bacterial meningoencephalitis is variable. Many animals that survive experience residual neurologic dysfunction or clinical relapses.

THE RICKETTSIOSES

Rocky Mountain Spotted Fever

15. What is the causative agent of Rocky Mountain spotted fever (RMSF)?

RMSF is caused by the obligate intracellular parasite, *Rickettsia rickettsii*. RMSF is a tick-transmitted disease. *Dermacentor* tick species are primarily responsible for maintenance of sylvatic disease cycle and transmission to animals and humans in the United States.

16. What neurologic signs are seen in animals with RMSF?

Clinical evidence of neurologic disease occurs in approximately one third of dogs with RMSF. Seizures, alterations in consciousness, vestibular disease, and signs referable to spinal cord dysfunction (e.g., spinal hyperpathia, ataxia, paresis) are commonly noted. Systemic evidence of illness may or may not be present, and is reviewed in Chapter 69.

17. How does RMSF cause neurologic disease?

RMSF is endotheliotropic, with a predilection for small arteries and veins of all body systems. The resulting necrotizing vasculitis is responsible for the clinical and biochemical manifestations.

18. How is RMSF diagnosed?

Because RMSF is an acute clinical disease, initial diagnosis is often made based on tick exposure, physical examination, compatible clinical and laboratory abnormalities, and response to treatment. Serologic diagnosis is dependent on a single elevated serum titer, or demonstration of seroconversion between acute and convalescent serum samples. Polymerase chain reaction genetic testing has also been reportedly used as a diagnostic tool.

19. How is RMSF treated?

Tetracycline, doxycycline, chloramphenicol, and enrofloxacin are all effective antimicrobials for the treatment of RMSF. Antibiotic therapy should be continued for 2 to 3 weeks in animals with neurologic signs. In cases with severe multisystemic involvement, intensive supportive care and monitoring is also necessary.

20. What is the prognosis for animals with RMSF?

Animals with RMSF that have mild clinical signs or that are treated early in the course of the disease can often make a complete recovery. Most cases will demonstrate clinical improvement within 48 hours of initiation of treatment. In some cases of RMSF, continual neurologic deterioration is seen despite appropriate therapy. Rapidly progressive necrotizing meningoencephalitis, intracranial hemorrhage, or thrombosis of CNS vasculature may be responsible for these refractory neurologic signs. Some animals that survive may have residual neurologic deficits or experience a prolonged neurologic recovery.

Ehrlichiosis

21. What causes ehrlichiosis?

Several species of ehrlichial organisms can infect small animals. Most commonly, *Ehrlichia canis* has been incriminated in canine cases. Ehrilichial infections can occur throughout the year in endemic temperate areas, and clinical disease can be acute, subacute, or chronic in nature.

22. What percentage of dogs with ehrlichiosis will have neurologic signs?

Approximately 33% of dogs with ehrlichiosis will have neurologic signs, which are similar to those described for RMSF. Neurologic disease is primarily caused by inflammation and bleeding of meningeal vessels. Meningitis can be found on postmortem examination of many animals with ehrlichiosis, even in the absence of clinical signs.

23. What are the diagnostic tests available for ehrlichiosis?

Serologic testing, immunoblotting procedures, and genetic (polymerase chain reaction) testing are all used for diagnosis and to distinguish between the ehrlichial species capable of causing clinical disease. CSF analysis of animals with ehrlichiosis typically reveals mononuclear pleocytosis. Occasionally, ehrlichial morulae have been identified in CSF leukocytes. Serology can also be performed on CSF to confirm the diagnosis.

24. How is ehrlichiosis treated?

Tetracycline, doxycycline, oxytetracycline, imidocarb diproprionate, minocycline, and chloramphenicol can be used to treat ehrlichiosis. In some cases, concurrent usage of corticosteroids is necessary to control signs of polysystemic inflammation, and in particular meningitis, which likely has an immune-mediated component.

25. What is the prognosis for animals with neurologic disease attributable to ehrlichiosis?

The overall prognosis is good to fair with early recognition and appropriate treatment. Animals that have systemic evidence of overt bleeding diatheses may develop refractory neurologic signs.

INTRACRANIAL MYCOTIC INFECTIONS

Cryptococcosis

26. What organism causes cryptococcosis?

The dimorphic fungus, *Cryptococcus neoformans* var neoformans most often causes clinical disease. Several antigenic variants of cryptococcal species have also been reported to cause disease with lesser frequency.

27. How do animals acquire cryptococcosis?

In the warm climates of the southern and southeastern United States, cryptococcosis is ubiquitous in the environment, especially in areas where pigeon excrement is found. The presumed method of infection is via inhalation and hemolymphatic dissemination, or possibly through direct extension of the organism through the cribiform plate.

28. What are the common clinical signs associated with cryptococcosis?

Dogs with cryptococcosis are often young adult, are large breeds, and have presenting complaints referable to the eye or CNS disease. In dogs, neurologic signs are often multifocal and commonly involve the brain stem (vestibular dysfunction, facial paralysis, ataxia), forebrain (seizures, circling), cervical spinal cord (tetraparesis, spinal hyperpathia, ataxia), or optic nerves (optic neuritis).

29. How is the diagnosis best established?

Demonstration of the cryptococcal organism in cytologic or histologic tissue samples is the preferred method of diagnosis. Samples obtained from cutaneous lesions, respiratory exudates, enlarged lymph nodes, CSF, and ocular paracentesis will often contain organisms. Diagnostic imaging studies often provide additional information that supports the diagnosis and can aid the clinician in the selection of tissues to aspirate or biopsy. Miliary interstitial infiltrates are often seen on thoracic radiographs. CT or MR imaging of the brain can reveal focal or multiple mass lesions, meningeal enhancement, or evidence of diffuse disease.

Serologic testing can be beneficial in cases in which the organism cannot be demonstrated. The latex agglutination cryptococcal capsular antigen test can be performed on serum or CSF, and is sensitive and specific. False-negative serologic results can sometimes be seen in animals with sequestered CNS infections.

30. How is cryptococcosis treated?

Ketoconazole, itraconazole, amphotericin B, and flucytosine have all been used with variable results for the treatment of cryptococcosis. Considering the prevalence of CNS involvement in dogs, fluconazole, a triazole antifungal agent with the ability to penetrate the blood-brain barrier, may be the preferred therapeutic agent. Chronic medical treatment is often necessary for several months. Treatment should be continued for 1 to 2 months beyond the resolution of all clinical signs, or preferably until the serum titer is negative.

31. Are there any prognostic indicators for animals with cryptococcosis?

A decrease in the magnitude of serially measured titers by tenfold over a 60-day period was a favorable prognostic indicator in one study. It is unknown if the organisms can be ever truly eliminated from immunoprivileged sites such as the CNS.

Cerebral Phaeohyphomycosis

32. What is the etiologic agent of cerebral phaeohyphomycosis?

The phaeohyphomycoses are infections caused by a group of opportunistic, saprophytic, pathogenic molds that share the common ability to form pigmented hyphal elements in living tissue. The encephalitic form of phaeohyphomycosis is most often associated with *Xylohypha* (previously *Cladosporium*) species.

33. How are animals infected with phaeohyphomycosis?

The portal of entry into the CNS is not known, but has been postulated to occur through inhalation of spores with secondary hematologic dissemination. Animals with disseminated disease may also develop CNS foci of infection.

34. What neurologic signs are seen with phaeohyphomycosis?

Most described cases have had clinical evidence of multifocal neurologic disease. Cerebral (seizures, central blindness), brain stem (central vestibular disease, cranial nerve deficits), and spinal cord signs (tetraparesis) have been reported.

35. How is phaeohyphomycosis diagnosed?

Cerebral phaeohyphomycosis is most commonly diagnosed at necropsy, by demonstration of hyphal tissue invasion and culture. Brain imaging with CT or MR may reveal mass lesions with imaging features consistent with an inflammatory granuloma. A clinical diagnosis was established using CT-guided brain biopsy in one dog with phaeohyphomycosis. CSF analysis is variable—mononuclear and suppurative inflammation can be seen.

36. What treatment options are available?

CNS phaeohyphomycosis is a severe and almost invariably fatal infectious disease in both people and animals. Surgical resection of lesions in combination with systemic antifungal treatment is recommended. At this time, there are no antifungal agents with proven efficacy against the phaeohyphomycoses. Fluconazole therapy, in conjunction with subtotal debulking of a cerebral granuloma, was used in one dog with phaeohyphomycosis that was eventually euthanized because of progressive neurologic disease.

IDIOPATHIC (NONINFECTIOUS) MENINGOENCEPHALITIDES

Granulomatous Meningoencephalitis

37. What is granulomatous meningoencephalitis (GME)?

GME is a descriptive term for a clinically distinct, idiopathic inflammatory CNS disease of dogs. GME is named after the neuropathologic features that are considered the hallmark of the disease: perivascular accumulations of macrophages, lymphocytes, and plasma cells.

38. What are possible causes of GME?

Because GME is still considered an idiopathic inflammatory disease, its cause is unknown. Viral encephalitic infections have been postulated to be the cause of GME, but efforts have not proven an association between GME and infectious agents. Some researchers believe that GME is not a distinct clinical syndrome, but a variant of CNS neoplastic reticulosis. Recent evidence suggests that GME may be an immune-mediated hypersensitivity reaction.

39. Are there any readily identifiable predisposing factors?

GME can affect any sex, breed, or age of dog. The classic signalment of a dog with GME is a young to middle-age, small-breed dog. Some studies have reported higher prevalence in female dogs, and breed predilections for Poodles and Terriers.

40. What are the clinical manifestations of GME?

Three distinct clinical forms of GME are recognized:
1. Ocular: acute onset of blindness; clinical and fundoscopic evidence of optic neuritis.
2. Focal: space-occupying, coalescing granulomatous lesions most often noted in the cerebral or brain stem white matter; clinical signs are indicative of the neuroanatomic location of the lesion. The focal form of the disease may have a more chronic onset and progression.
3. Diffuse: clinical signs suggest a multifocal neurologic disease; clinical disease is typically acute in onset and rapidly progressive.

GME can cause virtually any neurologic sign. Seizures, vestibular deficits, ataxia, paresis, cervical pain, and behavioral change are some of the most common presenting complaints.

41. What is the preferred method of diagnosing GME?

GME is primarily diagnosed in the routine clinical setting by excluding other possible causes of meningoencephalomyelitis. CSF analysis is beneficial in cases of GME and typically is characterized by a moderate to marked mononuclear pleocytosis and elevated CSF protein. However, animals with GME can have primarily a neutrophilic pleocytosis and a wide variety of CSF cytologic abnormalities. Some animals have normal CSF. Imaging of the brain can be useful for the identification of single (Fig. 4-1) or multiple mass lesions, but these findings are not specific for GME. Advanced imaging of the brain is crucial if brain biopsy is being considered. Ultimately, a definitive diagnosis requires microscopic examination of affected nervous tissue.

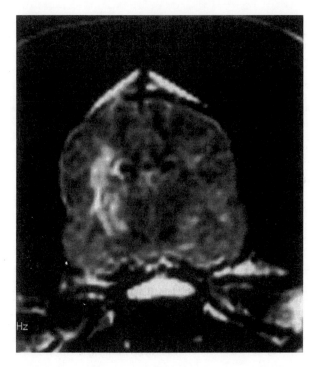

Figure 4-1. T1-weighted, postgadolinium, axial magnetic resonance image of the brain at the level of the thalamus demonstrating an enhancing lesion involving the right cerebrum, lateral ventricle, and thalamus of a 5-year-old, female Poodle with generalized seizures. Necropsy examination revealed the lesion to be consistent with granulomatous meningoencephalitis.

42. What treatments are available for animals with GME?

Immunosuppressive doses of corticosteroids may offer temporary palliation. Radiation therapy has also been shown to be effective treatment for GME. Chemotherapeutic protocols combining a cytotoxic drug (e.g., procarbazine, cytosine arabinoside, lomustine, or carmustine) with prednisone have been shown in preliminary reports to be well tolerated and superior to steroid treatment alone.

43. Are there any prognostic indicators in dogs with GME?

The prognosis for complete and permanent recovery is poor for animals with GME. One study examining prognostic indicators reported that dogs with focal clinical signs live significantly longer (median survival, 114 days) when compared with those with multifocal neurologic deficits (median, 8 days). In addition, dogs with focal telencephalic signs were reported to live longer (median, survival greater than 395 days) than those animals with evidence of focal disease in other neuroanatomic locations (median, 59 days). This same study also reported a statistically significant survival benefit when radiation was used as a treatment in dogs with focal forebrain disease.

Pug Encephalitis

44. What is the cause of Pug encephalitis?

Pug encephalitis is a necrotizing, nonsuppurative meningoencephalitis whose pathogenesis is unknown. As evident from the name of the disease, Pug dogs are commonly affected, but Yorkshire Terriers and Maltese dogs can be affected by a similar disease.

45. How is Pug encephalitis different from GME?

Clinically, Pug encephalitis can appear identical to GME with forebrain involvement. However, the two diseases can be distinguished based on their pathologic features. Pug encephalitis is unique in that it is a nonsuppurative, necrotizing encephalitis with a predilection for the forebrain. Pug encephalitis can result in large foci of malacia and necrosis in the absence of inflammation, which would be unusual for GME.

46. What are the clinical features of Pug encephalitis?

The disease can affect dogs of all ages, but typically occurs in the young. Two distinct clinical courses are recognized: an acute fulminant disease with severe neurologic dysfunction occurring within 2 to 3 weeks of the onset of clinical signs, and a chronic, insidiously progressive disease with a temporal course of several months. Clinical signs seen with the acute disease include seizures, behavioral change, blindness, and ataxia. The chronic form of the disease initially manifests as recurrent seizures, with interictal neurologic deficits such as blindness, circling, and behavioral change gradually developing as the disease progresses.

47. What are the diagnostic features of Pug encephalitis?

Diagnosis is usually made based on the signalment, clinical features, and CSF analysis. Pug encephalitis is associated with a moderate to severe lymphocytic CSF pleocytosis. CT or MR imaging of the brain can identify focal areas of necrosis, edema, and inflammation. Definitive diagnosis requires histopathologic examination of brain tissue.

48. How is Pug encephalitis treated?

Immunosuppressive chemotherapeutics, as described for GME, in conjunction with anticonvulsants, can result in temporary improvement in some cases of pug encephalitis. The prognosis for longevity is poor, especially in dogs with acute, fulminant disease.

PROTOZOAL MENINGOENCEPHALITIDES

Toxoplasmosis and Neosporosis

49. What are the causative agents of these two diseases?

Toxoplasmosis is caused by the obligate intracellular coccidian parasite *Toxoplasma gondii*. *Neospora caninum* is the causative agent of neosporosis. These two diseases are discussed together because they are morphologically similar and have similar clinical features.

50. What are the definitive hosts for these two diseases?

Domestic cats are a definitive host for *Toxoplasma gondii*, as are some other wild-type felids. Dogs serve as a definitive and intermediate host for *N. caninum*. The complete life cycle of neosporosis is still unknown.

51. How do animals acquire protozoal meningoencephalitis?

Toxoplasmosis can be transmitted via three major mechanisms: congenital transplacental transmission, ingestion of infected tissues from an intermediate host, or consumption of food or water sources contaminated with cat feces containing sporulated oocysts.

Infection with neosporosis can occur through ingestion of infective oocysts shed in dog feces, by transplacental propagation, and ingestion of tissue stages found in organs of intermediate hosts.

52. What clinical signs are associated with protozoal meningoencephalomyelitis?

Generalized toxoplasmosis is usually seen in puppies younger than 1 year of age. Pyrexia, respiratory, gastrointestinal, and neurologic signs are common. Adult dogs with toxoplasmosis most often have neuromuscular disease, with specific signs being reflective of the location of the lesions. Toxoplasmosis can affect any area of the nervous system.

In dogs, neosporosis is also capable of causing polysystemic disease, but neuromuscular signs are usually predominant. Infected young dogs characteristically develop an ascending paralytic disease, with the pelvic limbs more severely affected. Affected puppies will often have marked pelvic limb muscle atrophy and contracture. Neosporosis usually causes multifocal intracranial or spinal cord disease in older dogs, and occasionally polymyositis.

53. Are there any known factors that predispose an animal to the development of clinical disease?

It is unknown why some exposed animals develop disease and others do not. Important factors likely include the age, species, general health, and immune status of the host, as well as pathogenicity of the strain, infective dose, and stage of the protozoan. Reactivation of latent, subclinical toxoplasmosis infections acquired early in life may occur secondary to stress, vaccination, immunosuppressive therapy, or concurrent infections. These factors may also play a role in dogs with neosporosis, but concurrent illness and immunodeficiencies have not been consistently identified in previously described cases.

54. What are the best methods of diagnosis?

Detection of toxoplasmosis tachyzoites in tissues or body fluids is possible during acute clinical illness. When present, body cavitary effusions have a high diagnostic yield. Toxoplasmosis tachyzoites are rarely found in CSF. *N. caninum* stages may also be detected in CSF or other cytologic tissue samples. Muscle biopsy specimens are also helpful for detecting organisms in dogs with neosporosis (Fig. 4-2).

Serologic testing is valuable in the diagnosis of both toxoplasmosis and neosporosis. Serum antibodies of *N. caninum* and *T. gondii* generally do not cross-react under most laboratory conditions. Demonstration of serum antibodies to neosporosis helps confirm disease in animals with consistent clinical signs. Serology may be performed on CSF, but titers are generally lower than those in serum.

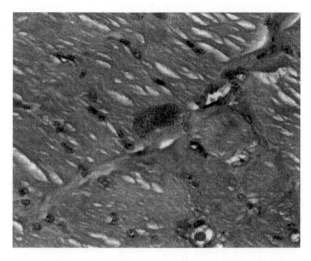

Figure 4-2. Muscle biopsy specimen obtained from triceps of a 3-year-old Labrador with clinical evidence of polymyositis. A focus of *Neospora* organisms can be seen the center of the field. Hematoxylin and eosin stain ×200.

The definitive serologic antemortem diagnosis of clinical toxoplasmosis is difficult, because tissue cysts persist for life in infected animals. A clinical diagnosis is often established based on fulfillment of the following criteria:
1. Clinical presentation consistent with the disease
2. Exclusion of other causes based on appropriate diagnostics
3. Serologic evidence of active infection
   -High serum immunoglobulin M (IgM) titer
   -Fourfold or greater increase in serially measured serum IgG
4. Positive clinical response to antiprotozoal therapy

Ancillary serologic testing of CSF can be helpful in documenting CNS disease.

55. What is an antibody coefficient, and what is its role in diagnosis?

Calculation of an antibody coefficient (AC) value theoretically allows for differentiation of intrathecally produced antibody from antibodies diffusing across a damaged blood-brain barrier.

$$AC = \frac{T.\ gondii\ \text{CSF IgG}}{T.\ gondii\ \text{serum IgG}} \times \frac{\text{Other agent-specific serum IgG}}{\text{Other agent-specific CSF IgG}}$$

AC values greater than 1 are suggestive of intrathecal antibody production.

56. How are the protozoal meningoencephalitides treated?

Toxoplasmosis and neosporosis are treated identically. Clindamycin, trimethoprim-sulfonamide, and combinations of pyrimethamine and a sulfonamide have all been used successfully. In young puppies with clinical neosporosis, it is prudent to treat the entire litter, even if only a single animal is affected. Most animals will show dramatic clinical improvement within the first week of treatment. The prognosis is poor for animals with rapid, ascending paralytic disease and extensive muscular contractures.

57. What preventive measures are available for protozoal diseases?

The best methods of preventing toxoplasmosis in small animals are designed to reduce the incidence of feline infections and subsequent shedding of oocysts. Outdoor cats should be isolated from food-producing animals. Primarily indoor dwelling cats should be fed a commercial cat food and prevented from hunting. If meat products are a part of the daily ration, they should be thoroughly cooked.

Toxoplasmosis is a zoonotic disease with the potential to cause severe disease in both human adults and feti. The most severe, and possibly life-threatening, human disease occurs from fetal infections acquired in the first half of gestation and in immunosuppressed adults. The risk of human exposure can be minimized through the practice of routine sanitary habits, prompt and proper disposal of cat excrement, regular disinfection of litter pans, and the cooking of meat before consumption.

Until the complete life cycle of neosporosis is elucidated, the ideal means of prevention are unknown. Bitches that have produced infected puppies should be withdrawn from breeding programs, because current medical treatments will not prevent transplacental infections. Because *N. caninum* is also a major cause of bovine abortions, dogs that coexist with cattle should be prevented from defecating in grazing or feeding areas and from consuming bovine placentas or aborted feti.

VIRAL DISEASES

Canine Distemper Viral Encephalitis

58. What causes canine distemper viral (CDV) encephalitis?

CDV encephalitis is caused by a single-stranded RNA Morbillilovirus in the *Paramyxoviridae* family.

59. How is CDV transmitted?
Susceptible animals usually acquire CDV after exposure to aerosolized respiratory secretions from infected animals. Rare cases of vaccine induced CDV have been reported after administration of modified live vaccinal strains.

60. What is the pathophysiology of CNS infection with CDV?
The type and severity of CDV encephalitis is dependent on many host and viral factors, especially the immunocompetence of the host animal and the pathogenicity of the infecting viral strain. Young, unvaccinated, or immunocompromised dogs that mount a poor or absent antiviral immune response will often develop severe, acute encephalitis and polysystemic disease. Neurologic dysfunction in acute CDV encephalitis is principally the result of direct viral destruction of neurons, resulting in primarily a polioencephalomalacia of the cerebrum and thalamus. Mature dogs that have a delayed or partial antiviral immune response develop chronic CDV encephalitis, which classically causes a leukoencephalomyelomalacia, with a predilection for the white matter of the brain stem and spinal cord. Both inflammatory and noninflammatory types of subacute encephalitis have also been reported.

61. What are the clinical neurologic manifestations of CDV?
Neurologic signs are dependent on the area of the CNS affected, and may coincide with the development of systemic disease or appear days to months after recovery from clinical or subclinical systemic infection. Dogs with acute encephalitis commonly have generalized or "chewing gum" type seizures, ataxia, or paresis. Chronic CDV encephalitis is often associated with vestibular signs and gait deficits. Myoclonus, the spontaneous, rhythmic, repetitive twitching of a single or group of muscles, is seen in less than half of animals with CDV encephalitis.

62. Is the presence of myoclonus pathognomonic for CDV encephalomyelitis?
No. Although CDV infection is the most commonly recognized cause of myoclonus, other inflammatory CNS diseases can also cause myoclonus.

63. How is CDV encephalomyelitis diagnosed?
Acute CDV encephalitis is often presumptively diagnosed in young dogs with consistent historical and clinical examination findings. In dogs with signs compatible with chronic CDV encephalomyelitis, definitive antemortem diagnosis can be difficult.

Cerebrospinal fluid abnormalities seen with CDV encephalitis typically include an increase in protein concentration and a mild to moderate lymphocytic pleocytosis. Dogs with the noninflammatory forms of CDV encephalitis may have normal CSF. Identification of anti-CDV specific antibody in CSF is useful for documenting CNS infection, but interpretation is often complicated in dogs that have been previously vaccinated against distemper by contamination of CSF with peripheral blood during collection. Calculation of an AC, as described for toxoplasmosis, is helpful in documenting intrathecally produced anti-CDV antibody.

A diagnosis of CDV can also be made after demonstration of CDV antigen in tissues from affected dogs with immunofluorescent techniques. Cytologic specimens obtained from respiratory epithelium, conjunctiva, or lymphoid tissue as well as biopsies from the spleen, lymph nodes, tonsils, lung, gastrointestinal tract, and brain can be used for immunofluorescent testing. A negative result from an immunofluorescent test does not rule out infection, but a positive test result is diagnostic. It has been previously reported that antigen could be identified in the conjunctiva in over 50% of dogs with CDV encephalomyelitis.

The quantification of CDV antibodies in serum alone is of extremely limited diagnostic use and only serves to inform the clinician that the dog has been recently or previously exposed to or vaccinated against CDV. Serum antibodies are best used in conjunction with CSF analysis during calculation of an AC.

Occasionally, cerebrocortical atrophy and white matter lesions can be detected on diagnostic imaging studies performed in dogs with CDV, but these findings are nonspecific.

CDV genetic material can be amplified from a variety of tissues from infected dogs with polymerase chain reaction assays and is an additional adjunctive diagnostic method. Polymerase chain reaction testing has been useful for the retrospective diagnostic conformation of CDV in cases in which immunologic results have been conflicting. In addition, genetic testing offers the potential advantage of differentiation between infective viral strains, which could provide significant insight into the epidemiology and pathogenesis of CDV.

64. What treatments are available for CDV encephalomyelitis?

Treatment is nonspecific and primarily supportive. Neurologic signs are primarily treated symptomatically, with anticonvulsant administration often being required. Dogs with significant chorioretinitis or optic neuritis may benefit from corticosteroid therapy. Myoclonus is a persistent and irreversible condition, but is often well tolerated. Several drugs, including procainamide, have been used anecdotally to treat myoclonus, but have largely been unsuccessful.

65. What is "old dog encephalitis," and is it caused by CDV?

Old dog encephalitis is a rare and poorly understood clinical and neuropathologic syndrome caused by CDV. Clinical manifestations are seen in middle aged to geriatric dogs and include insidiously progressive dementia, visual deficits, circling, and ataxia.

BIBLIOGRAPHY

Anor S, Sturges BK, Lafranco L et al: Systemic phaeohyphomycosis (Cladophialophora bantiana) in a dog—clinical diagnosis with stereotactic computed tomographic-guided brain biopsy, *J Vet Int Med* 15:257-261, 2001.

Berthelin CF, Legendre AM, Bailey CS et al: Cryptococcosis of the nervous system in dogs, part 2: diagnosis, treatment, monitoring, and prognosis, *Prog Vet Neurol* 5:136-146, 1994.

Bleck TP: Central nervous system involvement in rickettsial diseases, *Neurol Clin* 17:801-812, 1999.

Cordy DR, Holliday TA: A necrotizing meningoencephalitis of Pug dogs, *Vet Pathol* 26:191-194, 1989.

Foley JE, Lapointe JM, Koblik P et al: Diagnostic features of clinical neurologic feline infectious peritonitis, *J Vet Int Med* 12:415-423, 1998.

Foley JE, Leutenegger C: A review of coronavirus infection in the central nervous system of cats and mice, *J Vet Int Med* 15:438-444, 2001.

Gerds-Grogan S, Dayrell-Hart B: Feline cryptococcosis: a retrospective evaluation, *J Am Anim Hops Assoc* 33:118-122, 1997.

Jacobs GJ, Medleau L, Calvert C et al: Cryptococcal infection in cats: factors influencing treatment outcome, and results of sequential serum antigen titers in 35 cats, *J Vet Int Med* 11:1-4, 1997.

Lindsay DS, Blagburn BL, Dubey JP: Feline toxoplasmosis and the importance of the Toxoplasma gondii oocyst, *Comp Cont Educ Pract Vet* 19:448-461, 1997.

Lindsay DS, Dubey JP, McAllister M: Neopsora caninum and the potential for parasite transmission, *Comp Cont Educ Pract Vet* 21:317-321, 1999.

Mariani CL, Platt SR, Scase TJ et al: Cerebral phaeohyphomycosis caused by Cladosporium spp. in two domestic shorthair cats, *J Am Anim Hosp Assoc* 38:225-230, 2002.

Munana KR: Encephalitis and meningitis, *Vet Clin North Am Small Anim Pract* 26:857-874, 1996.

Munana KR, Luttgen PJ: Prognostic factors for dogs with granulomatous meningoencephalomyelitis: 42 cases (1982-1996), *J Am Vet Med Assoc* 212:1902-1906, 1998.

Platt SR, Radelli ST: Bacterial meningoencephalomyelitis in dogs: a retrospective study of 23 cases (1990-1999), *J Vet Int Med* 16:159-163, 2002.

Ruehlmann D, Podell M, Oglesbee M et al: Canine neosporosis: a case report and literature review, *J Am Anim Hosp Assoc* 31:174-183, 1995.

Thomas WB: Inflammatory diseases of the central nervous system in dogs, *Clin Tech Sm Anim Pract* 13:167-178, 1998.

Thomas WB, Sorjonen DC, Steiss JE: A retrospective evaluation of 38 cases of canine distemper encephalomyelitis, *J Am Anim Hosp Assoc* 29:129-133, 1993.

Tipold A: Diagnosis of inflammatory and infectious diseases of the central nervous system in dogs: a retrospective study, *J Vet Int Med* 9:304-314, 1995.

Tipold A, Vandevelde M, Jaggy A: Neurologic manifestations of canine distemper virus infection, *J Sm Anim Pract* 33:466-470, 1992.

5. Diseases of the Spinal Cord

John H. Rossmeisl, Jr.

LOCALIZATION OF AND FREQUENTLY ASKED QUESTIONS ABOUT SPINAL CORD DISEASES

1. **List the four major neuroanatomic segments of the spinal cord that are used for localization of spinal cord diseases.**
    1. C1-C5—cervical
    2. C6-T2—cervical intumescence
    3. T3-L3—thoracolumbar
    4. L4-S3—cauda equina

2. **Are there specific signs that are common to all animals with spinal cord disease?**
    Yes. Animals with spinal cord disease, regardless of specific neuroanatomic location, can have variable degrees of altered muscle tone (spasticity or flaccidity), abnormalities in sensory function (ataxia, depressed or absent conscious pain perception), loss of voluntary movement (paresis/plegia), and abnormal spinal reflexes (depressed-hyporeflexia, absent-areflexia, or exaggerated-hyperreflexia).

3. **What clinical signs are seen with diseases affecting each neuroanatomic segment of the spinal cord?**
    See Tables 5-1 through 5-4.

4. **What is the Schiff-Sherrington sign?**
    Animals with the Schiff-Sherrington signs have opisthotonus (extension of the head and neck), spastic thoracic limbs, and paraplegia. Schiff-Sherrington posture can result from any spinal cord lesion caudal to T2.

5. **Is the Schiff-Sherrington sign associated with a poor prognosis?**
    Although the Schiff-Sherrington sign is indicative of severe spinal cord injury, it does not have any prognostic value.

Table 5-1	*Clinical Signs of C1-C5 Spinal Cord Disease*
Gait	Ataxia of all limbs; tetraparesis
Postural reactions	Depressed/absent in all limbs
Muscle tone	Normal to spastic
Muscle atrophy	Absent
Spinal reflexes	Normal to upper motor neuron in all limbs
Other signs	Cervical pain/rigidity (common)
	Phrenic nerve paralysis/respiratory compromise (C5-C7)
	Horner's syndrome (rare)
	Root signature

Table 5-2   Clinical Signs of C6-T2 Spinal Cord Disease

Gait	Ataxia of all limbs; tetraparesis
Postural reactions	Depressed/absent in all limbs
Muscle tone	Normal to decreased in thoracic limbs
	Normal to spastic in pelvic limbs
Muscle atrophy	± Neurogenic atrophy of forelimbs
Spinal reflexes	Normal or lower motor neuron in thoracic limbs
	Normal or upper motor neuron in pelvic limbs
Other signs	Cervical pain/rigidity (common)
	Phrenic nerve paralysis/respiratory compromise (C5-C7)
	Horner's syndrome (T1-T3)
	Loss of cutaneous trunci reflex (C8-T1)
	Root signature

Table 5-3   Clinical Signs of T3-L3 Spinal Cord Disease

Gait	Pelvic limb ataxia; paraparesis/paraplegia
Postural reactions	Normal in thoracic limbs
	Depressed or absent in pelvic limbs
Muscle tone	Normal to spastic in thoracic limbs (Schiff-Sherrington sign)
	Normal to spastic in pelvic limbs
Muscle atrophy	Absent
Spinal reflexes	Normal in thoracic limbs
	Normal or upper motor neuron in pelvic limbs
Other signs	Focal spinal hyperpathia (common)
	Loss of cutaneous trunci caudal to level of focal lesion
	Schiff-Sherrington sign
	Upper motor neuron bladder (common)
	Depressed or absent pelvic limb pain sensation

Table 5-4   Clinical Signs of L4-S3/Cauda Equina Disease

Gait	Pelvic limb ataxia; paraparesis/paraplegia
Postural reactions	Normal in thoracic limbs
	Depressed or absent in pelvic limbs
Muscle tone	Normal to spastic in thoracic limbs (Schiff-Sherrington sign)
	Normal to depressed in pelvic limbs, tail, anus, bladder
Muscle atrophy	± Pelvic limbs
Spinal reflexes	Normal in thoracic limbs
	Normal or lower motor neuron in pelvic limbs, anus
Other signs	Focal spinal hyperpathia (common)
	Schiff-Sherrington sign (occasional)
	Fecal/urinary incontinence (common)
	Depressed or absent pelvic limb pain sensation

6. **What neuroanatomic structures in the spinal column are responsible for generation of pain?**
    Pain can be associated with disease of the paraspinal musculature, intervertebral discs, vertebral bone, meninges, spinal nerve roots, and articular facet joints.

7. **Provide two potential risks associated with myelography.**
    1. Postmyelographic seizures—more common in large breeds, dogs with Wobbler disease, and dogs undergoing cervical myelography.
    2. Deterioration in neurologic status after myelography—this is usually a transient phenomenon.

8. **Why is the loss of deep pain sensation a negative prognostic indicator in animals with spinal cord disease?**
    Pain perception is transmitted by small myelinated and unmyelinated nerve fibers that are diffuse, multisynaptic, and positioned deep within the spinal cord parenchyma. These small fibers are more resistant to compressive injury than larger, more superficially located myelinated ascending nerve fibers. Thus in an animal with a transverse myelopathy, loss of deep pain implies that the damage involves a significant portion of the spinal cord diameter in that area.

9. **Provide three general principles of conservative management of spinal cord diseases.**
    1. Enforced cage rest. This is the most important component of conservative treatment. Most diseases will require the animal to be confined for 3 to 6 weeks to allow for complete recovery, depending on the specific cause.
    2. Provision of analgesia. Because many spinal cord diseases are associated with clinical signs of pain, administration of analgesics is often necessary. Nonsteroidal antiinflammatory drugs and opioids are popular and effective analgesics.
    3. Provision of supportive and hygienic care. Animals will often require manual bladder expression, padded bedding, frequent turning to prevent decubitus; daily bathing; and nutritional support.

CONGENITAL AND HEREDITARY ANOMALIES AND DISORDERS

Atlantoaxial Instability

10. **What is atlantoaxial instability (AAI)?**
    AAI is a generic term used to describe any congenital or acquired disease process that allows for excessive flexion of the atlantoaxial joint. This abnormal mobility of the joint results in clinical signs consistent with a compressive cervical myelopathy due to displacement of the axis dorsally into the vertebral canal.

11. **What types of specific lesions are associated with AAI?**
    AAI can result from the following:
    1. Malformations of the odontoid process (dens) including agenesis and hypoplasia.
    2. Nonunion of the odontoid process with C2.
    3. Absence or traumatic disruption of the supporting ligaments of C1, most commonly the transverse ligament.
    4. Traumatic fracture of the odontoid process.
    5. Combinations of traumatic injuries and congenital anomalies.

12. **Is there a typical signalment of a dog with AAI?**
    Anatomic malformations resulting in AAI are commonly seen in toy dogs or small dog breeds during the first 2 years of life. Animals with anomalous C1-C2 articulations can also be asymptomatic until experiencing what appears to be a minor traumatic incident. Traumatic lesions can affect any age, breed, or sex of dog or cat.

13. What are the clinical signs associated with AAI?

Clinical signs are referable to a focal C1-C5 myelopathy with severity ranging from mild cervical pain or sensory ataxia to tetraplegia with or without respiratory compromise. Evidence of dysfunction of some cranial nerves with nuclei residing in the medulla, in particular the vestibular nuclei, is present in some animals.

14. What radiographic criteria are used to diagnose AAI?

Radiographic indicators of AAI that can be obtained from a lateral view of the cervical spine include a widened space between the dorsal arch of C1 and the C2 spinous process and dorsocranial displacement of the body of C2 into the vertebral canal. Ventrodorsal and oblique views may reveal the anomalies or fractures of the odontoid process. The clinician should exercise extreme caution when manipulating, sedating, or anesthetizing animals with suspected AAI to prevent additional spinal cord compression. Additional radiographic techniques, such as the flexed lateral and open mouth views, have been described as being valuable diagnostic tools, but are not routinely recommended because of their potential to cause further neurologic dysfunction. Computed tomographic and magnetic resonance imaging is also beneficial in the diagnosis of AAI.

15. What treatments are available for AAI?

Animals with clinical signs of acute AAI should receive corticosteroid therapy (see the section on acute spinal cord trauma). Animals with clinical evidence of mild neurologic dysfunction (pain and ataxia) may be candidates for conservative management, which includes external coaptation (neck brace) and strict confinement for 4 to 6 weeks. Proper application of a neck brace is reportedly successful in some dogs. In animals with moderate to severe neurologic signs, or recurrence after conservative therapy, surgical stabilization is recommended. Several different surgical techniques using both dorsal and ventral approaches have been described.

16. What is the prognosis for animals with AAI?

The prognosis for animals with AAI is variable. Some positive prognostic indicators in dogs with AAI treated surgically include: age of onset of clinical signs at younger than 2 years, mild to moderate preoperative neurologic deficits, and duration of clinical signs for less than 10 months.

Dermoid Sinus

17. What is a dermoid sinus?

A dermoid sinus is an invagination of the skin covering the dorsum of the spinal column into the underlying tissues. It is a congenital defect that results from a faulty separation of the skin from the neural tube during development.

18. Are there other terms used to describe dermoid sinuses?

Dermoid sinuses have also been referred to as pilonidal sinuses and dermoid cysts.

19. How are dermoid sinuses classified?

There are five different types of dermoid sinuses. Classification is dependent on the depth to which the sinus penetrates into the underlying tissue.

1. Type I—sinus extends to the level of the supraspinous ligament
2. Type II—sinus is more superficial and cystic than Type I and is attached to supraspinous ligament by a fibrous cord
3. Type III—contains a superficial cystic (sac-like) portion as in Type II with no attachment to the supraspinous ligament
4. Type IV—sinus extends to the dura mater and may communicate with the subarachnoid space
5. Type V—this is a true cyst with a closed complete epithelial lining

20. What breeds have been reported to have dermoid sinuses?
Rhodesian Ridgebacks are most commonly affected, but Cocker Spaniels, Boxers, Terriers, and other breeds have been reported. In one survey of Rhodesian Ridgeback owners, 67 of 1263 (5.3%) dogs were affected with a dermoid sinus.

21. What clinical signs can be seen in dogs with a dermoid sinus?
Signs are variable and can range from asymptomatic to severe neurologic dysfunction if the sinus communicates with the subarachnoid space. Some dogs will have clinical signs resulting from infection of the sinus and surrounding skin.

22. How are dermoid sinuses diagnosed?
Dermoid sinuses are frequently detected during routine examinations. Dermoid sinuses occur most commonly in the cervical or craniothoracic regions, but can occur in the sacrococcygeal area and head. Multiple dermoid sinuses can occur in a single individual. In Rhodesian Ridgebacks, dermoid sinuses typically do not occur within the confines of the "ridge" of hair. Sinuses can be difficult to detect unless the haircoat is shaved, or sometimes may be palpated as a cord of tissue along the midline. Sacrococcygeal sinuses are more likely to present with dural communications. Diagnosis is further supported by plain radiography or contrast enhanced fistulography.

23. What treatment options are available for dermoid sinuses?
Treatment is often not necessary unless the sinus is infected or communicates with the dura. Surgical excision of the sinus is the treatment of choice, with some surgeons recommending a course of antibiotic treatment to resolve concurrent infection prior to excision. Cephalosporins are good empirical first choice antibiotics.

24. Can dermoid sinuses be prevented?
The mode of inheritance is still unknown. However, because dermoid sinuses are considered a serious defect by many Rhodesian Ridgeback breeders and special interest organizations, breeding of affected dogs is not recommended.

Globoid Cell Leukodystrophy

25. What is globoid cell leukodystrophy?
Globoid cell leukodystrophy is a lysosomal storage disease resulting from a deficiency of β-D-galactocerebrosidase, and is inherited as an autosomal recessive disorder in dogs.

26. Which breeds can be affected with globoid cell leukodystrophy?
Globoid cell leukodystrophy has been reported most often in the Cairn and West Highland White Terriers, but also in the Beagle and Poodle.

27. What are the neuropathologic features of globoid cell leukodystrophy?
Pathologic findings typically include bilaterally symmetric demyelination of white matter and the perivascular accumulation of large foamy macrophages (globoid cells). White matter lesions can be of variable severity in different locations throughout the neuraxis, but typically involve the corona radiata, corpus callosum, optic tracts, peripheral subpial spinal cord parenchyma, and peripheral nerves.

28. What clinical syndromes are associated with globoid cell leukodystrophy?
Clinical signs are usually seen within the first few months of life, but can occasionally manifest after several years. Neurologic dysfunction, after it is clinically apparent, is progressive in nature. In dogs, the disease has two distinct clinical appearances. The first syndrome is dominated by a progressive upper motor neuron paraparesis. The second manifestation is primarily typified by

evidence of cerebellar disease and is the most common clinical presentation in cats. Behavioral change, blindness, and hyporeflexia with muscular atrophy may also be seen in some animals. The clinical course of the disease is variable, ranging from one to several months, but is more rapidly debilitating in cats.

29. What diagnostic methods are available for globoid cell leukodystrophy?

A specific DNA-based genetic test is available for globoid cell leukodystrophy. A clinical diagnosis can also be supported by finding globoid cells in cerebrospinal fluid (CSF), demonstrating characteristic lesions in a brain or peripheral nerve biopsy specimens, or by identifying demyelinating lesions using magnetic resonance (MR) imaging techniques. Before genetic testing, a presumptive diagnosis was often made on the basis of the appropriate signalment, history, and exclusion of other causes.

30. Are there any treatments available for globoid cell leukodystrophy?

At this time, treatment for this disease is not available.

Myelodysplasia

31. What is myelodysplasia?

Myelodysplasia is the nonspecific term used to refer to a multitude of spinal cord malformations that are hypothesized to be the result of failure of development or incomplete closure of the neural tube.

32. Are there particular types of defects that occur with myelodysplasia?

Individual reported defects consist of segmental spinal hypoplasia and anomalies of the central canal, including duplication, hydromyelia, syringohydromyelia, absence of a ventral median fissure, and abnormal morphologic distribution of neural elements. Several defects can occur simultaneously.

33. What are the clinical signs of myelodysplasia?

Myelodysplasia is an inherited disease in the Weimaraner and has been sporadically reported in several other breeds of dogs and cats.

Clinical signs usually suggest a thoracolumbar myelopathic process of variable severity that is first apparent at ambulation. Affected dogs may have a characteristic, symmetric "bunny-hopping" gait.

34. What tests are helpful to diagnose myelodysplasia?

The diagnosis is made based on the signalment, history, and neurologic examination findings. Advanced diagnostic imaging modalities such as MR and computed tomography (CT) may provide further insight into the particular structural anomalies that may be present.

35. What is the prognosis for animals with myelodysplasia?

Currently, there is no treatment, and the prognosis is variable and dependent on the severity of the neurologic dysfunction present. The disease is not progressive in all cases, and affected animals, especially Weimaraners, may be suitable pets.

Syringohydromyelia

36. What is syringohydromyelia?

Syringohydromyelia is a collective term used to describe the abnormal intraspinal accumulation of fluid. Syringomyelia specifically denotes a fluid focus (i.e., syrinx) within the spinal cord parenchyma, whereas hydromyelia refers to dilatation of the central canal. Because of the difficulties associated with clinical differentiation between syringomyelia and hydromyelia, the terms are often combined and referred to as a singular entity.

37. Is the pathophysiology behind the development of syringohydromyelia known?

Syringohydromyelia is a relatively recently recognized clinical entity in veterinary medicine, and our understanding of this condition is limited. There are several potential pathophysiologic mechanisms that may contribute to the development of syringohydromyelia. Very simplistically, these can be divided into disorders that affect normal CSF flow dynamics, resulting in altered CSF pressures, or diseases resulting in a congenital or acquired loss of normal neural parenchyma with resultant replacement with abnormal fluid accumulations.

38. Are there any conditions associated with the development of syringohydromyelia?

Traumatic spinal cord injury or myelitis may result in the formation of syrinxes. Hydrocephalus and Chiari-type malformations have also been recognized in dogs with syringohydromyelia.

39. What is a Chiari-type malformation?

Chiari-type malformations are congenital or acquired abnormalities of the foramen magnum area that result in variable degrees of extension of the caudal cerebellum into the foramen magnum and caudal displacement of the medulla oblongata and fourth ventricle into the cervical spinal canal. It is the obstruction of CSF flow that results from these malformations that is thought to cause syringohydromyelia.

40. Is syringohydromyelia associated with any specific clinical manifestations?

No; the clinical signs are related to the location of the lesion; however, although syringohydromyelia is an intraspinal disease, discomfort can be apparent. In a report of seven dogs with syringohydromyelia, cervical pain, otic pain, and thoracic limb pain were common findings. Possible sources of the pain include inflammation or hemorrhage associated with the syringohydromyelia. Dogs with syringohydromyelia may also have scoliosis or signs consistent with central cord syndrome—paresis that is more pronounced in the thoracic limbs because of selective damage to the thoracic limb pathways that are more medially located within the spinal cord. Syringohydromyelia can also be subclinical and detected as an incidental finding.

41. What methods are available to confirm a diagnosis of syringohydromyelia?

Because syringohydromyelia is an intraspinal disease, diagnosis requires visual inspection of the spinal cord parenchyma, which is ideally done with MR imaging. Occasionally, during myelography, an abnormally dilated central canal may be injected with contrast material and allow identification of syringohydromyelia. Myelography can be normal in cases in which cystic abnormalities do not communicate with the central canal and are focal, or altered CSF flow dynamics do not allow for filling of the defect.

42. Are there medical treatment options for animals with syringohydromyelia?

Clinical signs have been reported to improve after the administration of antiinflammatory doses of corticosteroids or with the use of nonsteroidal antiinflammatory drugs.

43. What surgical options are available to treat syringohydromyelia?

The surgical management of syringohydromyelia is controversial, and will likely remain so until the pathophysiology of the condition is more thoroughly understood. Decompressive procedures involving the foramen magnum and vertebrae, cystic lesion drainage and marsupialization, and CSF fluid diversion through a variety of shunting procedures have all been attempted.

DEGENERATIVE DISEASES

Intervertebral Disc Disease

44. What is the intervertebral disc?

The intervertebral disc is an anatomic structure located between each pair of vertebrae of the spinal column, with the exception of C1-C2, whose physiologic role is to provide resistance against deforming loads placed on the spinal column while simultaneously allowing for some flexibility. Each intervertebral disc consists of an outer annulus fibrosus, an inner portion called the nucleus pulposus, and two cartilaginous endplates.

45. List the defining features of Hansen Type I and Hansen Type II disc disease.
1. Hansen Type I disc herniations are most common in chondrodystrophoid dogs (e.g., Dachshunds, Poodles, Beagles, Cocker Spaniels) and are characterized by extrusion of portions of the nucleus pulposus through the dorsal annulus, which results in clinical signs of acute spinal cord compression.
2. Hansen Type II disc disease results in dorsal protrusion of the annulus into the spinal canal, is associated with fibrous metaplasia of the disc, and occurs in nonchondrodystrophic breeds of dogs.

46. What is Type III disc disease?
Type III disc disease is a clinical term used to describe an explosive herniation of a small amount of disc material that spreads a large distance within the epidural space. This type of disc disease is often associated with significant amount of epidural and subarachnoid hemorrhage, and often does not result in a large amount of spinal cord deformation. Type III disc disease is unrelated to the specific forms of intervertebral disc disease (IVDD) described by Hansen.

47. Provide five differential diagnoses for IVDD.
1. Meningomyelitis
2. Trauma
3. Discospondylitis
4. Neoplasms of the spinal cord or vertebral column
5. Ischemic myelopathy

48. List five survey radiographic signs of IVDD.
1. Narrowing of the intervertebral disc space
2. Wedging of the intervertebral disc space
3. Collapse or narrowing of the articular facets
4. Opacification of the intervertebral foramen
5. Deformation or size reduction of the intervertebral foramen (Fig. 5-1)

49. What are the myelographic features of IVDD?
Myelography is the most commonly used imaging technique used to diagnose IVDD. The classic myelographic features of IVDD noted on a lateral radiographic projection are elevation of

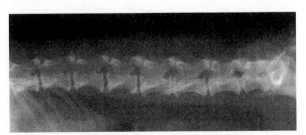

Figure 5-1.   Lateral lumbar radiograph obtained from a mixed breed dog with paraplegia demonstrating some of the survey radiographic features of IVDD. At the L1-L2 location, the following abnormalities can be seen: wedging and narrowing of the disc space, opacification of the intervertebral foramen, and collapse of the articular facet joint.

the ventral contrast column by an extradural mass lesion and thinning or absence of the dorsal contrast column in the same region. In some cases, the spinal cord will be severely swollen, resulting in a loss of the contrast columns over several disc spaces, which can complicate identification of the precise site of the lesion. Ventrodorsal and oblique views are used to confirm the location of the disc disease and attempt to lateralize the lesion to facilitate surgical planning.

50. Are there other imaging modalities used to diagnose IVDD?
Yes; CT and MR (Fig. 5-2) imaging are also useful for diagnosing IVDD. CT is often used after myelography (Fig. 5-3) in an effort to provide a more precise localization of the lesion when myelographic results are questionable.

51. How common is cervical disc disease, and which sites are usually affected?
The incidence of cervical IVDD is variable but has been reported to be as high as 25% of all disc lesions. C2-C3 is reportedly the most commonly affected disc, with the incidence decreasing at each successive disc caudal to C2-C3.

52. Provide three indications for medical treatment of cervical IVDD.
1. First episode consisting of cervical pain only
2. Cervical pain and mild, ambulatory paresis present
3. Financial limitations of owner

53. What is the recurrence rate of cervical IVDD in conservatively managed dogs?
Up to one third of dogs managed conservatively may have a recurrence of clinical signs.

54. What are indications for surgical management of cervical IVDD?
1. Cervical pain persists despite appropriate medical management
2. Moderate to severe neurologic deficits present

55. Name the two most commonly used decompressive surgical procedures used to manage cervical IVDD.
Ventral slot decompression is the most commonly used surgical technique. Some surgeons also use a dorsal laminectomy technique.

56. Provide three potential complications associated with cervical decompressive surgery.
1. Operative hemorrhage associated with disruption of the vertebral venous plexus or other vascular structures
2. Cardiac arrhythmias due to manipulation of the vagosympathetic trunk
3. Respiratory arrest

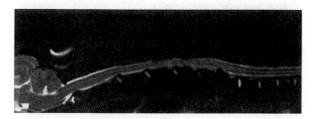

Figure 5-2.   Sagittal T2-weighted MR image from a Fox Terrier with tetraparesis. Note signal void in the C6-C7 disc space and corresponding ventral extradural compression of the spinal cord associated with a Type I disc herniation, and the normally high signal intensity that can be seen in the nucleus pulposus of normal discs (C2-C3, C3-C4, C4-C5).

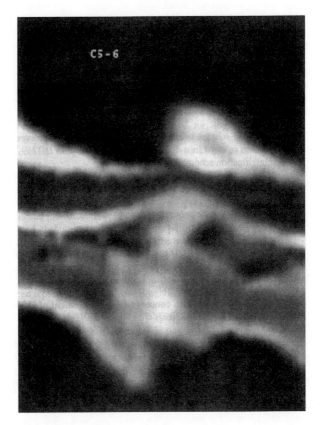

Figure 5-3. Sagittal/myelogram appearance of C5-C6 IVDD. There is a hyperdense ventral extradural lesion resulting in significant compression of the spinal cord.

57. What is the prognosis associated with surgical treatment of cervical IVDD?
The prognosis for functional recovery is excellent in dogs with cervical pain or mild to moderate neurologic dysfunction after successful surgical decompression.

58. How common is thoracolumbar IVDD?
IVDD is the most common clinical cause of neurologic dysfunction referable to the thoracolumbar region and accounts for up to 85% of all disc lesions.

59. Provide the most common neuroanatomic sites of Type I thoracolumbar disc herniation.
T12-T13 is the most common site of disc herniation, followed closely by T13-L1 and L1-L2. Lesions at these sites account for nearly 65% of all Type I disc lesions.

60. Can large-breed dogs have Type I thoracolumbar IVDD?
Yes, and the L1-L2 space is most frequently affected in nonchondrodystrophic, large-breed dogs with Type I IVDD.

61. Why is IVDD rare in the T2-T10 area?
The intercapital ligament, which extends across the vertebral canal over the T2-T10 disc spaces to connect the rib heads, prevents dorsal extrusion of disc material in this area.

62. What is the significance of the radiographic identification of in situ disc mineralization?
Although mineralized disc material in situ suggests that degenerative disc disease is present, it does not imply that the particular disc is the cause of the clinical signs.

63. Is there a useful grading scheme available to clinically classify the severity of neurologic dysfunction present in a dog with thoracolumbar IVDD?
A frequently used classification scheme is as follows:
1. Grade 1—spinal hyperpathia (pain) only
2. Grade 2—ataxia and ambulatory paraparesis
3. Grade 3—ataxia and nonambulatory paraparesis
4. Grade 4—paraplegia with intact sensorium (deep pain present)
5. Grade 5—paraplegia with absent deep pain perception

64. What dogs with thoracolumbar IVDD are candidates for conservative management?
Conservative management is indicated in dogs with Grade 1 or 2 clinical disease or in dogs whose owners decline surgery.

65. What is the prognosis associated with conservative management of IVDD?
The prognosis is variable but, in general, dogs with Grade 1 or 2 deficits have a good (>80%) prognosis for functional recovery. The prognosis is guarded for animals with paraplegia (40%-50% recovery rate). Recurrence rates as high as 40% have been reported for animals treated conservatively.

66. What role do steroids have in the acute emergency treatment of thoracolumbar IVDD?
The use of corticosteroids for the treatment of IVDD remains controversial in veterinary medicine. Methylprednisolone is the only corticosteroid with proven efficacy in the treatment of acute spinal cord injury in humans, and is beneficial in animals that are able to receive treatment within 8 hours of spinal cord injury (see the section on acute spinal cord trauma). A similar benefit has not been proven in dogs.

67. When is surgery recommended?
Surgery is recommended for all animals with no voluntary motor function (Grades 3-5). There are some surgeons who do not routinely recommend surgery for animals with Grade 5 deficits that have been present for longer than 48 hours because of the questionable benefit of surgical intervention.

68. Name three surgical techniques described for the treatment of thoracolumbar IVDD.
1. Hemilaminectomy (most common)
2. Dorsal laminectomy
3. Pediculectomy (minihemilaminectomy)

69. What is fenestration and when is it indicated?
Fenestration is the surgical removal, laser ablation, or chemical dissolution of the nucleus pulposus of the intervertebral disc. Historically, fenestration has been used prophylactically and therapeutically in dogs with IVDD. Some surgeons and neurologists perform fenestration concomitantly during decompressive surgery with the intent of reducing future recurrence of

IVDD at other sites. Fenestration, when used as a sole technique, does not address the spinal cord compression that results from disc herniation. Fenestration is a subject of continual debate among veterinarians. It is not universally used by all neurosurgeons because the risks and benefits of this procedure have not yet been evaluated in a controlled study.

70. What is the prognosis for dogs with thoracolumbar IVDD treated surgically?

In dogs with intact pain perception, the prognosis for recovery is generally considered to be good to excellent (80%-90%), although overall reported success rates range from 60% to 95%. A longer recovery period is usually required for dogs with more severe neurologic disability. Most dogs that have voluntary motor function will regain ambulatory ability within 2 weeks after successful surgery, compared with the 4 to 8 weeks that is often required for paraplegic dogs.

71. What is the prognosis for dogs with absent deep pain perception?

Although the absence of deep pain implies severe spinal cord injury and has traditionally been a negative prognostic indicator, this remains a controversial subject for animals with IVDD. It is generally accepted that animals with no pain perception have a poor to grave prognosis, depending on the duration of the sensory loss. Recovery rates as high as 76% have been reported in dogs with absent pain sensation that are operated on within 12 to 36 hours, and the prognosis is usually more favorable for those dogs whose duration of sensory loss has been less than 12 hours. Dogs with negative pain perception that regain sensory function within 2 weeks of surgery have been reported to have a good prognosis for eventual recovery.

Cervical Spondylomyelopathy (Wobbler Syndrome)

72. Are there additional terms used to describe this syndrome?

Yes, in addition to Wobbler syndrome, cervical spondylomyelopathy has been referred to as cervical vertebral stenosis, cervical spondylolisthesis, cervical vertebral instability, and caudal cervical malformation-malarticulation.

73. When the term "Wobbler" is used what is being implied?

Wobbler syndrome is a generic reference often used to describe large-breed dogs with any degree of tetraparesis and proprioceptive ataxia resulting from cervical spinal cord disease, regardless of the specific underlying cause.

74. Are there pathologically distinct manifestations of Wobbler syndrome?

Yes. Traditionally, five different pathologic manifestations have been described based on the location and anatomic basis of the compressive lesion within the cervical spine. These include the following:

1. Chronic, degenerative disc disease
2. Congenital bony malformations of the vertebrae
3. Vertebral tipping
4. Hourglass compressions resulting from degenerative joint disease of the articular processes and annular hypertrophy
5. Disease of the ligamentum flavum and vertebral arch

75. What causes dogs to develop cervical spondylomyelopathy?

The precise etiology of this syndrome is unknown, but is speculated to be multifactorial. Genetic, nutritional, and environmental factors, as well as trauma, have all been incriminated.

76. Is this disease associated with any particular dog breeds?

Young, male Great Danes and middle-age to geriatric Doberman Pinschers are the two frequently described breeds, but any large or giant breed of dog can be affected.

77. Do Great Danes and Dobermans typically have specific pathologic manifestations of the disease?

Yes. Young Great Danes usually have dorsal spinal cord compression resulting from malformation of the caudal cervical vertebrae. The C5, C6, and C7 vertebrae can be affected, although C6 is reportedly the most common. The clinical signs in older Dobermans are most often the result of ventral spinal cord compression from chronic degenerative disease of the caudal cervical discs (Fig. 5-4). Of interest is that Bassett Hounds may also present with clinical signs consistent with cervical spondylomyelopathy, which is usually attributed to stenosis of the cervical spinal canal in the C2-C3 area.

78. What are the clinical signs of cervical spondylomyelopathy?

The signs are extremely variable and depend on the nature, location, number, temporal onset, and severity of the lesions present. Slowly progressive pelvic limb ataxia and paraparesis often precede the development of thoracic limb deficits by weeks to months. Segmental spinal reflexes in the pelvic limbs are reflective of an upper motor neuron lesion, and a crossed extensor reflex

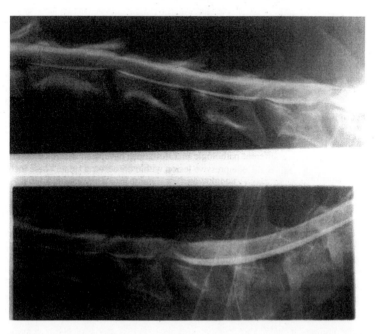

Figure 5-4.   Lateral myelographic views obtained from a Doberman with cervical spondylomyelopathy. Note the spinal cord compression at C6-C7, which is a typical lesion and location for cervical spondylomyelopathy in this breed.

may be apparent. Discrete cervical pain may or may not be present, but animals will often resent manipulation of the neck region. The thoracic limb girdle musculature may be atrophied, and animals may have a shortened, "tin-soldier"–like thoracic limb gait. Some dogs may develop severe, acute tetraparesis after minor trauma.

79. What diagnostic tests are recommended?

Diagnostic imaging studies are required for diagnosis. Plain cervical radiographs can reveal changes consistent with degenerative joint disease of the articular processes, IVDD, osseous vertebral malformations, and vertebral tipping, or the results may be normal. Myelography, CT, and MRI have all been used successfully to define the nature and location of disease in dogs with cervical spondylomyelopathy, and are crucial if surgical intervention is being considered.

80. Does conservative medical therapy have a role in the management of cervical spondylomyelopathy?

Yes, clinical signs will often improve significantly after a period of strict confinement and administration of nonsteroidal antiinflammatory drugs or antiinflammatory doses of corticosteroids. Some dogs with mild to moderate clinical signs can be maintained in clinical remission for extended periods with appropriate medical therapy. In general, however, owners should be advised that the clinical course of the disease is relentlessly progressive in the vast majority of dogs, and that chronic medical treatment does not significantly alter the adverse effects of protracted spinal cord compression.

81. What surgical options are available for dogs with cervical spondylomyelopathy?

There is no single surgical technique that can adequately address all of the potential pathologic alterations that can be present in dogs with cervical spondylomyelopathy. Several surgical techniques have been described that are designed to decompress the spinal cord and stabilize affected vertebrae. The technique used is largely dependent on the number, location, and type of lesions present and personal preference and experience of the surgeon. Surgical intervention is beneficial in most dogs but can be associated with deterioration in neurologic status (usually transient), prolonged recovery times, and severe postoperative complications. Clients considering surgery should be educated regarding the significant emotional, financial, and temporal commitments that will likely be required to provide adequate supportive care to a large or giant breed dog during the convalescent period.

82. Are there any clinical prognostic indicators in dogs with cervical spondylomyelopathy?

The prognosis is generally poor in the absence of treatment. Previously cited negative prognostic indicators include chronic clinical course of disease, the presence of severe neurologic dysfunction, and multilevel spinal cord compression. There is also the possibility that dogs that have recovered from surgery can experience clinical deterioration months to years later because of the development of a new compressive lesion adjacent to the previous surgical site, which is often referred to as the *domino effect.*

Degenerative Myelopathy

83. What is degenerative myelopathy (DM)?

DM is an insidiously progressive neurodegenerative thoracolumbar myelopathic disease of dogs.

84. What are the neuropathologic features of DM?

Pathologic findings include demyelination, reactive gliosis, and axonal degeneration that occur throughout the spinal cord. Lesions are more pronounced in thoracic spinal cord segments, with the most severe changes noted in dorsolateral and ventromedial funiculi.

85. What is the cause of DM?
The definitive etiologic trigger that initiates the degenerative changes in the spinal cord seen in dogs with DM is as of yet unknown. Expert opinions suggest that DM is an autoimmune disorder or may represent a degenerative process that occurs as a result of ischemic damage from chronic Type II disc disease.

86. Are their certain breeds of dogs that have a high incidence of DM?
Yes. German and Belgian Shepherds, Old English Sheepdogs, Weimaraners, and Rhodesian Ridgebacks are the primary breeds reported to have DM.

87. What is the clinical presentation of a typical dog with DM?
Middle-age (>5 years) to older dogs are usually affected, with a predisposition for males. Clinical signs are referable to a T3-L3 lesion and most often consist of slowly progressive pelvic limb ataxia and paresis. Pelvic limb neurologic deficits can be asymmetric. The toenails of the pelvic limbs are frequently worn or traumatized, and pelvic limb muscular atrophy can be marked in advanced cases. Segmental spinal reflexes in the pelvic limbs are normal to exaggerated. In some dogs, the patellar reflex may appear depressed, which is due to an afferent lesion resulting from degeneration of the dorsal root ganglia. A distinguishing clinical feature of degenerative myelopathy is that spinal hyperpathia is not present. Dogs typically maintain urinary and fecal continence. The thoracic limbs can become affected in the terminal stages of the disease process.

88. How is DM diagnosed?
Definitive diagnosis requires pathologic examination of spinal cord tissue. A tentative antemortem diagnosis requires exclusion of all other causes of transverse thoracolumbar myelopathy. Survey spinal radiographs frequently reveal incidental, unrelated degenerative changes such as spondylosis deformans. Abnormalities are not noted during myelography. With the increasing usage of spinal MR imaging in clinical neurology, dogs with histories and clinical examination findings consistent with DM are being observed to have multilevel Type II disc protrusions.

89. What is the typical clinical course of the disease?
As DM is an invariably progressive disorder of large breeds, most dogs develop nonambulatory paraparesis within 6 to 12 months of diagnosis, which often precipitates euthanasia.

90. Have any treatments been shown to be beneficial for dogs with DM?
There are no controlled scientific studies evaluating the therapeutic efficacy of any agent for the treatment of DM. The information available regarding treatment largely stems from expert opinion and clinical experience. Many neurologists recommend a combination of controlled exercise, dietary modification, vitamin supplementation, and medication with aminocaproic acid or N-acetylcysteine.

Lumbosacral Stenosis

91. What is lumbosacral stenosis?
Lumbosacral stenosis is a generic term used to describe compression, inflammation, ischemia, or destruction of the nerve roots or vasculature of the cauda equina that occurs as a result of developmental vertebral canal anomalies or acquired proliferation of lumbosacral soft tissue or osseous structures.

92. Are their other names for lumbosacral stenosis?
Lumbosacral stenosis has been called lumbosacral malformation, lumbosacral disease, or lumbosacral spondylomyelopathy.

93. Name two pathophysiologic factors that may contribute to the development of lumbosacral stenosis.
1. Congenital narrowing of the vertebral canal
2. Alteration in normal lumbosacral kinetics—degenerative changes in supporting soft-tissue structures such as the L7-S1 disc may result in lumbosacral instability. As a result, ligamentous, joint capsule, and osseous proliferation may occur as the body attempts to stabilize the abnormal vertebral segment

94. What types of dogs are affected by lumbosacral stenosis?
Medium- to large-breed, male, middle-age dogs are typically affected. Military working breeds have a high incidence of lumbosacral stenosis.

95. Name six historical complaints that are common in dogs with lumbosacral stenosis.
1. Reluctance to climb stairs, sit, exercise, work, or jump
2. Pelvic limb weakness/lameness
3. Caudal lumbar pain
4. Limp tail or tail weakness
5. Urinary or fecal incontinence
6. Paraesthesia of the limbs, tail, or perineum

96. What neurologic examination abnormalities are common in dogs with lumbosacral stenosis?
Neurologic abnormalities are referable to a cauda equina lesion (see Table 5-4) and include spinal hyperesthesia elicited on palpation of the lumbosacral space (percutaneous and on digital rectal examination), pelvic limb postural reaction deficits, paraparesis, neurogenic muscular atrophy of the hamstrings, and decreased perineal reflex and anal tone.

97. Provide five differential diagnoses for lumbosacral stenosis.
1. Canine hip dysplasia
2. Colonic, prostatic, or urethral inflammation or neoplasia
3. Discospondylitis
4. Gracilis myopathy
5. Perianal fistulas

98. What imaging techniques are effective for the diagnosis of lumbosacral stenosis?
1. Epidurography—sensitive in at least 75% of dogs
2. Discography—nearly 90% accurate in some studies
3. Myelography—successful in diagnosis in up to 75% of cases; results can be normal if the dural sac terminates cranial to the lumbosacral space
4. CT—very sensitive for detection of osseous abnormalities (Fig. 5-5)
5. MR—very sensitive and specific
6. Survey radiographs (Fig. 5-6)—lumbosacral abnormalities commonly noted (sacral osteochondrosis, transitional vertebrae, narrowing of L7-S1 disc space, subluxation of the sacrum, spondylosis deformans). Radiographic abnormalities are often seen in clinically normal dogs, and dogs with severe lumbosacral stenosis can have normal survey radiographs.

99. What dogs with lumbosacral stenosis are candidates for conservative treatment?
Conservative therapy is generally reserved for animals with their first episode of pain or intermittent bouts of spinal pain. Approximately 50% of dogs with lumbosacral stenosis that demonstrate clinical signs of pain only will respond to conservative treatment.

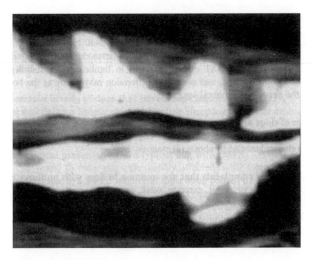

Figure 5-5. Sagittal CT scan from a German Shepherd dog with lumbosacral pain. Protrusion of the disc and spondylosis deformans are evident at L7-S1.

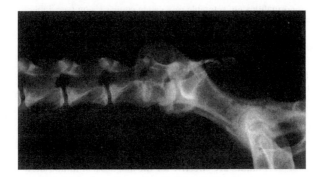

Figure 5-6. Lateral lumbosacral radiograph from a dog with lumbosacral stenosis. Notice the malformation of the L6-L7 vertebrae and endplate sclerosis and spondylosis deformans occurring at L7-S1.

100. When should I recommend surgical intervention in dogs with lumbosacral stenosis?

Surgical management should be a primary consideration in all dogs with moderate to severe neurologic deficits, severe pain, or pain that is unresponsive to conservative therapy.

101. What types of surgical procedures are used in the treatment of lumbosacral stenosis?

The exact surgical techniques used depend on the nature of the underlying compressive lesion. The most commonly used decompressive procedure is the dorsal laminectomy, which is often combined with discectomy, foraminotomy, or facetectomy. The dorsal laminectomy procedure can also be used in conjunction with various distraction and fusion techniques.

102. What is the prognosis for dogs with lumbosacral stenosis?

Generally, most pet dogs with mild to moderate neurologic deficits treated surgically have a good prognosis for functional recovery. The presence of chronic (>2 weeks' duration) urinary and fecal incontinence is a negative prognostic indicator in dogs with lumbosacral stenosis.

INFLAMMATORY AND INFECTIOUS DISEASES

Discospondylitis

103. What is discospondylitis?
Discospondylitis is a term that specifically denotes infection of the intervertebral disc and adjacent vertebral bodies. This condition has also been referred to as *intradiscal osteomyelitis.*

104. Are there certain infectious organisms that are frequently implicated in cases of discospondylitis?
Both bacterial and fungal organisms can cause discospondylitis. The most commonly incriminated bacterial species include *Staphylococcus, Streptococcus, Escherichia coli,* and *Brucella canis.* Fungal agents that have been reported to cause disease include *Aspergillus* and *Coccidioides immitis.*

105. How do these microbial agents establish infections in the disc?
Hematogenous spread from distant septic foci is the most frequently cited mode of infection. Infections of the oral cavity, genitourinary tract, integumentary system, and cardiac valves are often incriminated as point sources. Discospondylitis can also be a complication of penetrating trauma and spinal surgical procedures. In the western United States, discospondylitis can be a manifestation of the migration of inhaled plant awns. In these cases, discospondylitis results from the foreign material traveling through the thoracic cavity to become entrapped within the origins of the diaphragmatic crura along the ventral aspects of the L2-L4 vertebrae.

106. Provide the prototypical signalment of a dog with discospondylitis.
Discospondylitis is most often reported in young, male, large-breed dogs. The disease has been rarely documented in cats.

107. What is the most common clinical manifestation of neurologic dysfunction in dogs with discospondylitis?
Focal or multifocal spinal hyperpathia is the most commonly noted neurologic examination abnormality, although neurologic dysfunction is variable in severity and can range from pain to paralysis.

108. Are constitutional signs of illness frequently noted in dogs with discospondylitis?
Systemic signs of disease such as fever, weight loss, and inappetence are noted in approximately 30% of dogs. Therefore their absence should not preclude a diagnosis of discospondylitis.

109. What neuroanatomic sites are typically involved in dogs with discospondylitis?
The L7-S1 disc space is most frequently infected, with the T13-L1 and C6-C7 discs also being common sites. Any disc space can potentially be infected, and multifocal disease has been reportedly present in nearly 30% of dogs in some case studies.

110. What are the radiographic features of discospondylitis?
Abnormalities that may be seen on plain radiographs that are diagnostic for discospondylitis include irregular vertebral endplate margins, collapse of the disc space, and lysis of the endplates (Fig. 5-7). In chronic cases, the disc space may be widened secondary to extensive bone destruction, and there may be considerable osteosclerosis or bridging spondylosis. The development and resolution of radiographic lesions lags behind the clinical course of the disease. Thus radiographs may appear normal in the acute stages of infection and the radiographic appearance

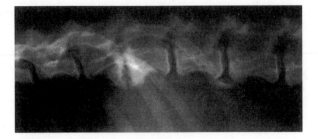

Figure 5-7.   Lateral thoracolumbar radiograph obtained from a dog with discospondylitis demonstrating the survey radiographic features of this disease at T13-L1.

of lesions may continue to deteriorate for several weeks in the face of appropriate antimicrobial therapy and despite clinical resolution of the disease.

111.   What other imaging modalities have been used to diagnose discospondylitis?

Myelography, CT (Fig. 5-8), and MR imaging have all been useful for the diagnosis of discospondylitis. These imaging techniques can reveal abnormalities specific for discospondylitis and are usually used in animals with clinical evidence of considerable neurologic disability, in which decompressive surgery is being considered. Radionuclide bone scanning using radiolabeled leukocytes has also been useful in demonstrating foci of infection prior to the appearance of radiographic lesions.

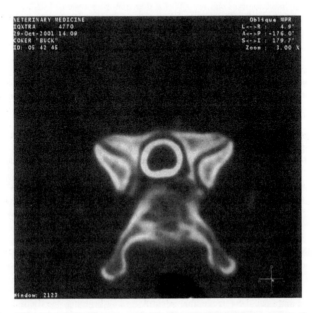

Figure 5-8.   Transverse CT/myelogram at C6-C7. Note the multiple lytic areas in the C6 endplate, consistent with discospondylitis.

112. Are their additional ancillary diagnostic tests that are recommended in cases of discospondylitis?

Performance of a complete blood cell count may reveal an inflammatory leukogram. Inflammatory sediment may be seen during urinalysis, in which case a urine culture is indicated. Confirmation of bacterial urinary tract infection by culture is possible in up to 50% of dogs with discospondylitis. In addition, blood cultures may be positive in nearly one half to two thirds of dogs with discospondylitis. Because of the potential public health risks and problematic treatment associated with brucellosis, serologic testing for this disease should be considered in all cases of discospondylitis. Percutaneous needle aspiration of infected disc spaces, which is most frequently performed with fluoroscopic guidance, may also provide samples for cytologic and microbiologic analysis.

113. What treatments are recommended for animals with discospondylitis?

Ideally, bactericidal antibiotics should be prescribed based on culture and sensitivity results obtained from blood, urine, affected disc spaces, or other septic tissue focus. In the absence of this type of information, the chosen antibiotic should be effective against staphylococcal organisms. First-generation cephalosporins are excellent empirical choices. Antibiotic treatment should be continued for 6 to 8 weeks. Analgesics and enforced cage confinement are also necessary adjuncts to antimicrobial therapy.

114. Under what circumstances is surgery indicated in animals with discospondylitis?

The following are the two main indications for surgery:
1. Exploration with the purpose of obtaining biopsy material for histopathologic and micro-biologic analysis
2. Therapeutic decompression in animals with severe neurologic deficits and diagnostic imaging evidence of compressive myelopathy or spinal instability.

Surgical exploration with diagnostic intent should be considered in animals that do not respond to appropriate initial therapy, and other means of obtaining samples for diagnostic confirmation have been unsuccessful.

115. What is the prognosis associated with discospondylitis?

Most dogs with discospondylitis will have a quick and favorable response to medical therapy, with dramatic clinical improvement usually being noticed within the first 3 to 10 days of treatment. Animals with substantial neurologic deficits have a more guarded prognosis, but can improve significantly with prompt and aggressive treatment. The dog with discospondylitis resulting from brucellosis presents a significant challenge considering the difficulties associated with treatment of this disease. Recurrence of discospondylitis is possible, and complete eradication of established infections can be problematic in immunocompromised animals.

Steroid Responsive Meningitis-Arteritis

116. What is steroid responsive meningitis-arteritis (SRMA)?

SRMA is a sterile inflammatory disease of the meninges and meningeal arteries of unknown etiology.

117. Are there other clinical syndromes that are similar to SRMA?

Yes, Beagle pain syndrome, necrotizing vasculitis, canine pain syndrome, canine juvenile polyarteritis, and polyarteritis are all recognized clinical entities that are similar to SRMA.

118. What are the neuropathologic features of SRMA?

The meninges and associated vasculature are affected in all areas of the CNS, but lesions are usually most severe in the cervical spinal cord. SRMA is characterized by a massive infiltration of the meninges by macrophages, plasma cells, lymphocytes, and polymorphonuclear cells. Periarteritis, hyaline degeneration, and fibrinoid necrosis of meningeal vessels are also apparent.

119. Are there certain breeds predisposed to SRMA?
Yes. Beagles, Boxers, and Bernese Mountain dogs (the three "Bs") are predisposed, but any breed of dog can be affected. Pointers have also been described as a breed at increased risk. SRMA typically affects young adult dogs younger than 2 years of age of either sex but can be seen in very young or geriatric animals.

120. What are the clinical manifestations of SRMA?
There are two clinical forms of SRMA. The first is referred to as the *acute typical form*. In this form of the disease, dogs classically present with fever, cervical hyperpathia, and a stilted gait with subtle or no additional neurologic deficits. The other form of SRMA is called the *atypical protracted form* and is characterized by more marked evidence of spinal cord dysfunction (e.g., ataxia and paresis), which may appear multifocal in nature.

121. Are there any readily available tests that are valuable in the diagnosis of SRMA?
Yes. An inflammatory leukogram is often present on complete blood cell count. CSF analysis is perhaps the most beneficial test for diagnostic confirmation. CSF obtained from dogs with SRMA will have an increased protein concentration and will have cytologic evidence of a marked neutrophilic pleocytosis in the acute typical form of the disease. The neutrophils are nondegenerate, and bacterial culture of CSF is negative. With the protracted form of the disease, CSF analysis will reveal a mixed or mononuclear pleocytosis of lesser magnitude. Dogs with SRMA have also been shown to have elevated serum and intrathecal concentrations of immunoglobulin A.

122. What are the primary differential diagnoses in a dog with clinical signs consistent with SRMA and a demonstrable suppurative pleocytosis in CSF?
Bacterial meningitis, granulomatous meningoencephalomyelitis, acute spinal cord trauma, and meningioma are all diseases that should be additional diagnostic considerations. All these can potentially affect young animals, cause a neutrophilic CSF pleocytosis, and can present similarly to SRMA.

123. How is SRMA treated?
Tapering immunosuppressive dosages of corticosteroids are the primary treatment. Long-term treatment with prednisone is often required to maintain remission, but is generally well tolerated. In the subset of animals in which remission cannot be obtained with prednisone alone, additional immunosuppressive drugs, most commonly azathioprine, can be beneficial.

124. Are there any negative prognostic indicators in dogs with SRMA?
Young dogs with the acute form of the SRMA have a good prognosis. One study has shown that dogs that have typical SRMA at an older age and that have high CSF immunoglobulin A concentrations often undergo more frequent clinical relapses, require longer periods of treatment, and have a less favorable prognosis. The prognosis associated with the protracted from of SRMA is guarded, with repeated clinical deterioration frequently occurring.

Neoplasms of the Spinal Cord and Vertebrae

125. How are neoplasms of the spinal cord and vertebrae classified?
Tumors affecting the spinal cord and column are usually classified as extradural, intradural/extramedullary, or intramedullary. Extradural neoplasms are most common and constitute approximately 50% of all spinal tumors.

126. What are the most common tumor types?
Table 5-5 summarizes some of the features of the spinal cord and vertebral neoplasms seen commonly. Primary tumors of bone are the most frequently diagnosed extradural neoplasms. Meningiomas are the most frequently seen primary spinal cord tumor.

Table 5-5 *Features of Common Neoplasms of the Spinal Cord and Vertebrae*

TISSUE OF ORIGIN	SPECIFIC TUMOR TYPE	LOCATION IN RELATION TO SPINAL CORD	DEFINING FEATURES	OPTIMAL TREATMENT
Vertebrae	Osteosarcoma	Extradural	Aggressive,	Surgery
	Osteochondroma	Extradural	lytic	Surgery
	Plasma cell tumor/myeloma	Extradural	vertebral lesions*	Chemotherapy, surgery
	Fibrosarcoma	Extradural		Surgery
Neural elements	Astrocytoma	Intramedullary	Within central	Radiation
	Ependymoma	Intramedullary	canal	Radiation ± surgery
Supporting structures	Meningioma	Intradural/ extramedullary	Cervical spinal cord	Surgery, radiation
	Nerve sheath tumor	Intradural/ extramedullary	common	Surgery
Other	Medulloep- ithelioma	Intradural/ extramedullary	T10-L2 location;	Surgery
	Lymphoma	Epidural; variable	young dogs; FeLV + cats; T-L location	Chemotherapy, radiation
Secondary (metastatic)	Mammary, prostatic carcinoma, transitional cell carcinoma	Extradural	Commonly affect vertebrae	Treat primary neoplasm,
	Hemangiosarcoma	Intramedullary		Adjunctive treatment

*Listed feature shared by all neoplasms in this group.

127. How do spinal tumors cause clinical signs?

Tumors of the spinal cord and vertebrae generally cause clinical signs by either invasion or destruction of neural elements or supporting structures of the spinal columns, or by compression of the spinal cord.

128. What diagnostic methods are recommended for these neoplasms?

Survey radiographs are very useful in the identification of primary and secondary osseous neoplasms affecting the vertebrae. Myelography also has the potential to localize and classify all types of neoplasms (Fig. 5-9). CT and MR (Fig. 5-10) imaging have revolutionized neuro-oncologic imaging of the spinal cord and provide information that is often crucial when surgery is being considered.

129. Are there any prognostic indicators available for animals with neoplasms of the spinal cord and vertebrae?

The prognosis is largely dependent on the location, histologic tumor type, severity of clinical signs, and potential for surgical resection. Animals with primary vertebral tumors and metastatic lesions generally have a poor prognosis. Extended periods of remission are possible with the multimodality treatment of some meningiomas and nerve sheath neoplasms that are amenable to surgical resection.

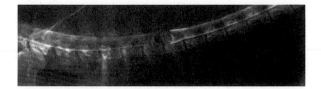

Figure 5-9.   Lateral thoracolumbar myelogram from a cat with chronic paraparesis. An intradural/ extramedullary lesion is evident at T3-T4. After surgical excision, the mass was determined to be a meningioma.

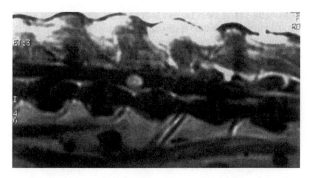

Figure 5-10.   Sagittal, postcontrast, T1-weighted MR image obtained from a dog with a metastatic hemangiosarcoma of the lumbar spinal cord, which appears as the ovoid, hyperintense lesion at L2-L3.

Acute Spinal Cord Trauma

130. What are the most common causes of spinal cord trauma?

Spinal cord trauma can be caused by both endogenous and exogenous disorders. The most frequently recognized causes of exogenous spinal trauma are the following:

1. Motor vehicular trauma
2. Penetrating missile injuries
3. Animal-animal encounters
4. High-rise syndrome (Fig. 5-11)
5. Malicious abuse

The most common disease causing endogenous acute spinal cord trauma is IVDD.

131. Are there any inciting factors that contribute to the severity of the spinal cord trauma?

Yes. When compressive types of spinal cord injury are referred to, the ultimate severity of the clinical degree of neurologic disability is related to the following four factors:

1. The velocity at which the compressive force is applied
2. The temporal duration of the compressive injury
3. The degree of spinal instability imparted by the inciting injury
4. The magnitude of mechanical deformation (e.g., degree of compromise to the transverse diameter) of the spinal cord.

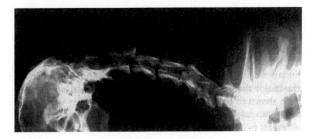

Figure 5-11. Lateral cervical radiograph obtained from a tetraplegic and dyspneic dog that fell approximately 3 m into an empty swimming pool. There is a subluxation of the C5 vertebra.

132. What pathophysiologic mechanisms are responsible for the clinical neurologic dysfunction seen in cases of acute spinal trauma?

Both primary and secondary effects play a role in the degree of neurologic dysfunction that results from traumatic spinal injuries. Primary injury refers to the disruption (laceration, contusion, concussion) of neural and glial spinal cord elements and associated vasculature that is a direct result of the trauma. Secondary spinal cord injury is a complex, self-perpetuating phenomenon that is initiated by the traumatic episode. Biochemical and ischemic derangements associated with secondary injury include production of free radicals, proinflammatory cytokines, and various vasoactive substances; accumulation of cytotoxic chemicals and excitatory neurotransmitters; and depletion of energy generating substrates. It is the ultimate intent of most medical treatments available for acute spinal cord injury to alter the progression of secondary spinal cord injury.

133. What are the primary treatment goals in animals with acute spinal cord trauma?

1. Prompt treatment of concurrent life-threatening injuries
2. Maintenance of normal mean systemic arterial blood pressure
3. Relief of spinal cord compression
4. Immobilization of an unstable spinal column
5. Eventually may require surgical realignment and stabilization
6. Medical treatment of secondary spinal injury (corticosteroids)
7. Provision of analgesia

134. What are the current recommendations regarding corticosteroid usage in acute spinal cord trauma?

The use of steroids for the treatment of acute spinal cord trauma is a controversial subject that is being intensely researched and debated. The only corticosteroid with demonstrable efficacy is methylprednisolone sodium succinate (MPSS). MPSS has a narrow therapeutic index, and ideally should be administered within 8 hours of the inciting injury for maximum benefit. MPSS dosing recommendations are as follows:

1. If the MPSS is administered within 3 hours of injury—30 mg/kg intravenous bolus followed by an infusion of 5.4 mg/kg/hr for 24 hours
2. If MPSS is administered within 3 to 8 hours after injury—30 mg/kg intravenous bolus followed by an infusion of 5.4 mg/kg/hr for 48 hours

Recently, the efficacy of this prolonged infusion technique has been questioned. Administration of MPSS outside of the 8-hour temporal window may actually be detrimental to the animal. These dosing schedules have been adopted from the human literature, and although they have been evaluated clinically in dogs, the ideal dosing regimen for MPSS has not yet been established.

Because of the potential for severe adverse effects (colonic perforation, pancreatitis, gastrointestinal hemorrhage) and questionable efficacy, dexamethasone is not recommended for the treatment of acute spinal cord injury.

135. What is the major theoretical benefit of MPSS use in acute spinal cord trauma?

MPSS has been shown to be an effective free radical scavenger when administered at high doses. Free radical associated lipid peroxidative cell membrane damage is one of the major pathophysiologic events in the secondary injury cascade.

136. Are there any predictors of spinal instability that can be obtained from a radiograph that may help identify animals requiring surgical stabilization?

Overt spinal instability can often be difficult to appreciate from a single radiographic projection. A three-compartment model has been proposed as a guide to predict which animals with spinal injuries may require surgical stabilization. If damage is noted to two or more compartments, the likelihood of spinal instability is high, and surgical intervention is warranted (Fig. 5-12). The three compartments are defined as follows:

1. Dorsal compartment—articular facets and joints, ligamentum flavum, dorsal vertebral arch and pedicle, spinous process, and interspinous ligaments
2. Middle compartment—dorsal annulus, dorsal vertebral body, and dorsal longitudinal ligament
3. Ventral compartment—ventral longitudinal ligament, annulus, and ventral vertebral body

VASCULAR DISORDERS

Ischemic Myelopathy

137. What is the cause of ischemic myelopathy?

Ischemic myelopathy generally refers to a clinical syndrome of spinal cord dysfunction resulting from ischemic necrosis of spinal cord white and gray matter, which occurs as a result of occlusion of the segmental spinal cord vascular supply. Ischemic myelopathy can result from any disease process that results in attenuation or obliteration of spinal cord vasculature, but the most commonly recognized cause of the syndrome seen in clinical medicine occurs secondary to occlusive vascular fibrocartilagenous emboli. For these reasons, the term *ischemic myelopathy* is often used synonymously with fibrocartilagenous embolic (FCE) myelopathy. Necropsy examinations of dogs and cats with FCE have identified the source of the vascular occlusion as fibrocartilage. This fibrocartilaginous substance, which has been noted in both spinal and

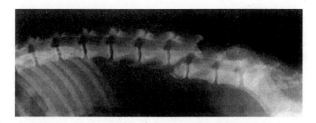

Figure 5-12.   Lateral lumbar radiograph obtained from a dog that was hit by a car. An L5 fracture and luxation is visible that demonstrates spinal instability resulting from damage to all three compartments of the spinal column.

meningeal arteries and veins, is biochemically and histologically similar to the fibrocartilage found in the nucleus pulposus of intervertebral discs.

138. How does fibrocartilage from the intervertebral disc occlude the spinal cord vasculature?

The precise pathophysiologic mechanism by which fibrocartilaginous emboli gain access to the spinal cord vascular supply is currently unknown. Several popular theories include the following:

1. Herniation of nucleus pulposus fragments into vertebral venous sinus system
2. Direct penetration of nucleus pulposus material into an artery
3. Disc herniation into vertebral marrow cavity with retrograde entrance into venous sinuses
4. Inflammatory neovascularization of degenerative discs with resultant embolization by way of injection of nuclear material into aberrant vasculature of the disc.

139. What historical findings should raise my clinical suspicion that ischemic myelopathy is present?

Ischemic myelopathy secondary to FCE has been reported in dogs and cats. Young to middle-age, large- and giant-breed dogs of both sexes are most commonly affected, although FCE has been reported with appreciable frequency in small-breed dogs, especially in the miniature Schnauzer and Shetland Sheepdog. Historically, animals with FCE typically have a peracute to acute onset of neurologic signs, unassociated with a traumatic episode. Many owners explain that the affected dog vocalized, as if in apparent pain, at the onset of disease, but does not otherwise appear painful. It is also often reported that the animal was exercising, usually in a routine manner, at the time the neurologic disability was first noticed.

140. Are there any neurologic examination findings that are pathognomonic for FCE?

Unfortunately not. Neurologic examination abnormalities vary tremendously from subtle deficits to paralysis with absent pain sensation. However, ischemic myelopathy resulting from FCE is classically described as an acute, nonpainful, nonprogressive, often asymmetrical myelopathic process, with the potential to affect any segments of the spinal cord.

141. How is a clinical diagnosis of ischemic myelopathy established?

Ischemic myelopathy is primarily a diagnosis of exclusion. Efforts should be made to rule out other causes of myelopathy.

142. Can animals with FCE have abnormalities detected during diagnostic evaluation?

Survey spinal radiographs are normal or reveal clinically insignificant changes such as spondylosis deformans. Cerebrospinal fluid analysis is often normal or reveals nonspecific abnormalities, most often consisting of an elevated protein concentration, mild pleocytosis, or xanthochromia. Myelographic studies are unremarkable or reveal an intramedullary pattern as a result of spinal cord edema. The performance of spinal magnetic resonance imaging is the best antemortem diagnostic test available, and can demonstrate spinal cord parenchymal changes consistent with infarction.

143. What treatments are available for the animal with ischemic myelopathy?

In the acute setting, animals may be treated medically with corticosteroids as for other types of spinal cord trauma. After the acute period, there are no specific treatments for embolic myelopathy secondary to FCE, only supportive. The principles and practice of good nursing and hygienic care should be followed to prevent decubitus and urinary tract complications. It has been reported that early initiation of a physical therapeutic regimen expedites functional recovery in some dogs.

144. Are there any clinical prognostic indicators in animals with FCE?

As is the case with most other myelopathies, animals that are lacking pain sensation for periods longer than 24 to 48 hours have usually sustained severe and permanent spinal cord damage. These animals have a poor prognosis for functional use of the affected limbs. Approximately 75% of dogs with reversible spinal cord damage associated with ischemic myelopathy will demonstrate significant clinical improvement within the first 2 to 3 weeks after the initial event. There is debate as to the validity of the negative prognostic significance of lower motor neuron signs in the limbs because of gray matter necrosis of the cervical or lumbar intumescences that has been cited in several publications. It has been shown that time required for functional recovery was not influenced by the neuroanatomic location of the lesion, involvement of an intumescence, or presence of intramedullary swelling on myelography.

Hemorrhagic Myelomalacia

145. What is hemorrhagic myelomalacia (HM)?

HM is a progressive ascending and descending ischemic and necrotic destruction of the spinal cord parenchyma that most often occurs as a result of endogenous or exogenous spinal cord trauma.

146. What pathophysiologic mechanisms result in HM?

The etiology and pathophysiologic mechanisms responsible for the initiation and perpetuation of this usually fatal event are not known. HM has also been referred to as *hematomyelia*.

147. What are the clinical signs of HM?

HM occurs most often as a result of acute, explosive Type I thoracolumbar disc herniations. Clinical indicators suggestive of HM include progression from an initially severe but focal myelopathic process to a diffuse spinal cord disease over several hours to a few days. In the case of an animal first presenting with signs of T3-L3 disease, lower motor neuron signs will develop in the pelvic limbs, anus, and urinary bladder as the disease descends the spinal cord. A cranially migrating level of cutaneous anesthesia and development of respiratory distress from intercostal and eventually diaphragmatic muscular paralysis characterize ascension of the disease. In addition to diaphragmatic failure, animals with HM involving the cervical spinal cord can develop bilateral Horner's syndrome. Animals with HM often appear to be in intractable pain, and many will develop pyrexia as the disease progresses.

148. How is HM diagnosed?

HM is most often made after recognition of the typical clinical signs in an animal with a known spinal cord injury. Performance of a durotomy during decompressive spinal surgery to allow for visual inspection of the spinal cord parenchyma has also been described as a means to diagnose HM.

149. Are there any radiographic abnormalities that are suggestive of HM?

Several myelographic imaging abnormalities have been described in animals with HM. These include contrast medium infiltration within the spinal cord parenchyma and spinal cord swelling.

150. Is treatment available for HM?

No. In most cases, HM is progressive and fatal within 36 to 48 hours of its onset because of respiratory failure. Humane euthanasia is often recommended in animals with impending complete respiratory paralysis resulting from cervical spinal cord involvement to avoid prolonged suffering. In cases in which HM does not progress to the cervical area, survival is possible, but animals are left with marked and permanent neurologic disability.

BIBLIOGRAPHY

Bagley RS, Gavin PR, Silver GM et al: Syringomyelia and hydromyelia in dogs and cats. *Comp Cont Educ Pract Vet* 22:471-479, 2000.

Beaver DP, Ellison GW, Lewis DD et al: Risk factors affecting the outcome of surgery for atlantoaxial subluxation in dogs: 46 cases (1978-1998). *J Am Vet Med Assoc* 216:1104-1109, 2000.

Bracken MB: Methylprednisolone and acute spinal cord injury. *Spine* 26:547-554, 2001.

Cauzinille L: Fibrocartilaginous embolism in dogs. *Vet Clin N Am Sm Anim Pract* 30:155-167, 2000.

Cizinauskas S, Jaggy A, Tipold A: Long-term treatment of dogs with steroid-responsive meningitis-arteritis: clinical, laboratory and therapeutic results. *J Sm Anim Pract* 41:295-301, 2000.

Coates JR: Intervertebral disc disease. *Vet Clin N Am Sm Anim Pract* 30:77-110, 2000.

Clemmons RM, Wheeler S, LeCouteur RA: How do I treat? Degenerative myelopathy. *Prog Vet Neurol* 6:71-72, 1995.

DeRisio L, Munana K, Murray M et al: Dorsal laminectomy for caudal cervical spondylomyelopathy: postoperative recovery and long-term follow up in 20 dogs. *Vet Surg* 31:418-427, 2002.

DeRisio L, Sharp NJH, Olby NJ et al: Predictors of outcome after dorsal laminectomy for degenerative lumbosacral stenosis in dogs: 69 cases (1987-1997). *J Am Vet Med Assoc* 219:624-628, 2001.

DeRisio L, Thomas WB, Sharp NJH: Degenerative lumbosacral stenosis. *Vet Clin N Am Sm Anim Pract* 30:111-132, 2000.

Fischer A, Mahaffey MB, Oliver JE: Fluoroscopically guided percutaneous disk aspiration in 10 dogs with diskospondylitis. *J Vet Int Med* 11:284-287, 1997.

Gandini G, Cizinauskas S, Lang J et al: Fibrocartilageous embolism in 75 dogs: clinical findings and factors influencing the recovery rate. *J Sm Anim Pract* 44:76-80, 2003.

Hurlbert JR: The role of steroids in acute spinal cord injury. *Spine* 26:539-546, 2001.

LeCouteur RA, Grandy JL: Diseases of the spinal cord. In Ettinger SJ, Feldman EC, editors: *Textbook of veterinary internal medicine* 5th ed., Philadelphia, 2000, WB Saunders Co.

Lipsitz RE, Chauvet AE et al: Magnetic resonance imaging features of cervical stenotic myelopathy in 21 dogs. *Vet Radiol Ultrasound* 42:20-27, 2001.

Lu D, Lamb CR, Targett MP: Results of myelography in seven dogs with myelomalacia. *Vet Radiol Ultrasound* 43:326-330, 2002.

Miller L, Tobias K: Dermoid sinuses: description, diagnosis, and treatment. *Comp Cont Educ Pract Vet* 25:295-299, 2003.

Olby N: Current concepts in the management of acute spinal cord injury. *J Vet Intern Med* 13:399-407, 1999.

Rusbridge C, MacSweeney JE, Davies JV et al: Syringohydromyelia in Cavalier King Charles spaniels. *J Am Anim Hosp Assoc* 36:34-41, 2000.

Scott HM, McKee WM: Laminectomy for 34 dogs with thoracolumbar disc disease and loss of deep pain perception. *J Small Anim Pract* 40:417-422, 1999.

Shamir MH, Tavor N, Aizenberg T: Radiographic findings during recovery from discospondylitis. *Vet Radiol Ultrasound* 42:496-503, 2001.

Skelly BJ, Franklin RJM: Recognition and diagnosis of lysosomal storage diseases in the cat and dog. *J Vet Intern Med* 16:133-141, 2002.

Thomas WB: Diskospondylitis and other vertebral infections. *Vet Clin N Am Sm Anim Pract* 30:169-182, 2000.

Section II
Cardiology
Section Editor: Jonathon A. Abbott

---

6. Acquired Valvular Disease
Jonathon A. Abbott

---

1. What diseases affect the cardiac valves in the dog?

Canine valvular disease most often takes the form of age-related degeneration, and, in fact, degenerative valvular disease is the most common acquired cardiac disease in the dog. This disorder is sometimes known as *myxomatous valvular degeneration,* and this term arguably most accurately describes its pathology. Some of the many synonyms include endocardiosis, chronic degenerative mitral valve disease, and, simply, chronic valve disease. Inflammatory valvular disease—infective endocarditis—is much less common, but is the only other important acquired valvular disease in the dog.

2. Describe the structure and function of the normal mitral valve apparatus.

The mitral valve apparatus consists of the mitral valve leaflets and the supporting structures: the left ventricular papillary muscles, chordae tendineae, and the mitral valve annulus. The mitral valve annulus is the fibrous ring that forms the left atrioventricular junction and the site at which the basilar aspect of the mitral leaflets are attached. There are two mitral valve leaflets. The septal, or anterior, leaflet has fibrous continuity with the aortic valve and forms the caudal boundary of the left ventricular outflow tract; the caudal or mural leaflet is more often referred to as the posterior mitral valve leaflet.

In a healthy animal, the leaflets are thin sheets of connective tissue covered by cardiac endothelium. The free edges of the leaflets are tethered by the chordae tendineae to the two left ventricular papillary muscles. These chords serve to anchor the mitral leaflets; during systole, they prevent prolapse of the leaflets into the left atrium. The function of the mitral valve is straightforward; it prevents the regurgitation of blood into the left atrium during ventricular systole and thus ensures that the force of ventricular contraction results only in useful flow into the aorta.

3. What is the histopathologic nature of degenerative valvular disease? What is the gross postmortem appearance?

Degenerative valvular disease is characterized by the accumulation of mucopolysaccharides within the spongiosa and fibrosa layers of the mitral leaflets; histologically, this lesion is known as myxomatous degeneration. Grossly, the leaflets are abnormally thick and have a nodular appearance. Lengthening of the chordae tendineae is also observed. Both atrioventricular valves can be affected; however, degenerative disease affecting the mitral valve is of greater clinical importance than degenerative tricuspid disease. Endocardiosis is a sterile degenerative process; inflammation or infection is not a feature.

4. What causes degenerative mitral valve disease?

Degenerative mitral valve disease (MVD) commonly affects chondrodystrophoid canine breeds that also have a high prevalence of collapsing trachea and intervertebral disc disease;

consequently, it has been suggested that MVD is but one manifestation of a more generalized connective tissue disorder. The cause of MVD is unknown, although a genetic basis is likely. MVD is common in certain breeds of dog; in the Cavalier King Charles Spaniel, the age at which MVD becomes clinically apparent has a heritable basis.

5.   What are the pathophysiologic consequences of MVD?

Distortion of the mitral valve leaflets prevents normal coaptation of the mitral valve leaflets; the consequence is mitral valve regurgitation. Lengthening and rupture of the mitral chordae tendineae predisposes to mitral valve prolapse, which can also contribute to mitral valve incompetence. Inadequate leaflet apposition allows a portion of the left ventricular stroke volume to be ejected backward into the left atrium. This regurgitant volume is augmented by the pulmonary venous return and then returns to the left ventricle during diastole. Incompetence of the mitral valve therefore imposes a volume overload on the left atrium and the left ventricle. Volume loading of the left heart is a stimulus for eccentric hypertrophy (hypertrophy accompanied by dilation).

Small volumes of mitral valve regurgitation (MR) are usually well tolerated, but two factors can potentially contribute to worsening of MR. Although the speed at which it does so is highly individual, MVD is generally progressive; ongoing alterations in valvular structure worsen mitral valve incompetence. Additionally, atrial/ventricular dilation itself distorts valvular anatomy and this further limits leaflet coaptation worsening MR. Systolic myocardial function of the left ventricle is not obviously affected by MR unless the valvular lesion is severe and longstanding. When substantial MR is present, the isovolumic phase of ventricular contraction does not take place because the ventricle can unload into the low-pressure reservoir provided by the left atrium. Therefore, myocardial oxygen demand is relatively low in the setting of MR; as a result, MR tends to be a lesion that is well tolerated at least in the sense that contractility can be preserved until late in the natural history of the disease. Longstanding, severe MR can, however, result in myocardial cell death, replacement fibrosis, and myocardial dysfunction that is known as *cardiomyopathy of overload*.

6.   What signalment is typical of animals that have MVD?

MVD is a degenerative disease that develops primarily in older dogs. Valvular lesions may develop in dogs of virtually any breed; however, the clinical consequences of MVD are observed almost exclusively in older dogs of the toy and small breeds.

The prevalence of MVD is not known with certainty, but it can be as high as 33% in dogs older than 10 years. It is the most common cardiac disease in the dog. Miniature and Toy Poodles, Pomeranians, Bichons Frises, Miniature Schnauzers, Dachshunds, Cavalier King Charles Spaniels, and mixed-breed dogs are commonly affected.

7.   What is distinctive about MVD that affects the Cavalier King Charles Spaniel?

Mitral valve disease in the Cavalier King Charles Spaniel is indistinguishable from MVD that affects other breeds. However, MVD in this breed is distinctive in that the disease becomes clinically evident at a relatively early age and in some individuals the disease is severe and rapidly progressive. In other breeds, clinical signs related to MVD are uncommon in dogs that are younger than about 8 years. In the Cavalier King Charles Spaniel, murmurs of mitral valve regurgitation are occasionally encountered in dogs as young as 2 and 3 years. Pedigree studies have demonstrated that the tendency to develop mitral valve lesions at an early age is heritable; the age of onset of MR in individual dogs can be approximately predicted by the age at which MR became evident in the parents.

8.   What are the clinical consequences of MVD?

It should be emphasized that murmurs resulting from MVD are more common than clinical signs related to the disease. Many animals have mild and only slowly progressive valvular lesions and ultimately succumb to extracardiac disease before the development of clinically consequential MR.

When MR is substantial, it imposes a volume overload on the left atrium and left ventricle. Elevated left atrial pressures are reflected back on the pulmonary venous circulation, potentially resulting in the development of pulmonary edema. The presence of cardiogenic pulmonary edema defines the clinical syndrome of left-sided congestive heart failure (CHF).

9.   What abnormalities are revealed by the animal's history?

Cough is the clinical sign that is most commonly associated with MVD. Respiratory distress is usually a feature of the history of those animals that have pulmonary edema. Other clinical signs such as syncope, ascites, weight loss, lethargy, and lack of appetite can also be observed.

10.   What causes cough in animals with MVD?

The cause of cough in dogs with MVD is multifactorial. Cough is an explosive, reflex-mediated exhalation, and the receptors that initiate this reflex are located primarily in the larger airways. Pulmonary edema can stimulate cough receptors, but generally does so when edema fluid floods the small airways; when pulmonary edema is the cause of cough, dyspnea is usually evident.

Compression of the left main stem bronchus by an enlarged left atrium is another potential cause of cough in dogs with MVD. Cough from bronchial compression resulting from left atrial enlargement seems to be unique to the animal population that has MVD. This might be partly explained by the high prevalence of concurrent primary airway diseases such as collapsing trachea in the dogs that commonly have MVD. The stimulation of juxtapulmonary receptors might also play a role in the pathogenesis of cough in some dogs with MVD. Stimulation of juxtapulmonary or J receptors by pulmonary venous distention results in reflex-mediated bronchoconstriction and increases in mucus production. Stimulation of J receptors might therefore contribute to cough in animals that have MVD but do not have pulmonary edema.

Regardless, it is important to recognize that animals with MVD can have a cough in the absence of CHF; this cough can be explained by cardiac disease, although in some cases concurrent primary respiratory tract disease plays a role.

11.   How is MVD detected on physical examination?

MVD becomes clinically apparent when it results in a cardiac murmur. Mitral valve regurgitation causes a systolic murmur that is usually heard best over the left cardiac apex. The correlation between murmur intensity and MR severity is imperfect; however, mild MR resulting from MVD generally results in a soft murmur, whereas severe MR usually results in a loud murmur. A soft murmur is typically evident early in the course of MVD; the murmur becomes louder as the animal ages and has progressively more severe MR. Mitral regurgitation continues as long as left ventricular pressure exceeds left atrial pressure; as a result, MR can persist beyond aortic valve closure and the murmur may therefore obscure the second heart sound. The murmur of moderate or severe MR has an intensity that typically changes little during the course of systole and is said to have a plateau-shaped configuration.

12.   What is a midsystolic click?

In some animals, a high-frequency midsystolic sound known as a click may precede the development of audible MR. Clicks are associated with mitral valve prolapse.

13.   Small-breed dogs with MR are often presented for the evaluation of cough; however, it can be difficult to determine whether heart disease or respiratory disease is the more important clinical problem. What history and physical findings are helpful in making this determination?

In small-breed dogs with MVD, heart disease or heart failure can explain cough; in some cases, however, the murmur of MR is incidental to the clinical presentation and the cough results from primary respiratory tract disease, such as collapsing trachea or chronic bronchitis. Although primary respiratory tract disease can certainly coexist, one of the two often dominates the clinical presentation.

A history of months or years of cough that occurs in the absence of dyspnea tends to support a diagnosis of airway disease. When MVD is sufficiently severe that it causes clinical signs, it is generally progressive. Therefore, untreated animals in which cardiac disease contributes importantly to cough tend to have a relatively short history; the clinical course often progresses to include dyspnea.

The body condition of the animal can provide useful clues. Animals that cough from heart disease or heart failure are often thin. Although exceptions certainly occur, obesity is more commonly associated with primary respiratory disease. The vital signs may also be useful. Healthy dogs often have a respiratory-associated arrhythmia that is evident on auscultation. In accordance with phasic variations in autonomic traffic, heart rate increases during inspiration and decreases during expiration. This respiratory sinus arrhythmia results primarily from fluctuations in vagal tone. When cardiac performance is impaired by severe MR, vagal discharge is inhibited and sympathetic tone becomes dominant. Thus in many animals with clinical signs related to cardiac disease, tachycardia develops and there is loss of physiologic, respiratory arrhythmia; the clinical finding of respiratory sinus arrhythmia is virtually incompatible with a diagnosis of heart failure. In contrast, many animals that cough mainly from primary respiratory disease have preserved and sometimes accentuated sinus arrhythmia.

In geriatric small-breed dogs, the absence of a cardiac murmur is generally an assurance that coughing results from primary respiratory tract disease. Soft murmurs resulting from MVD are seldom of clinical consequence. In contrast, animals that have clinical signs related to MVD almost always have loud cardiac murmurs.

It should be emphasized that these are guidelines only and exceptions do occur. Diagnostic studies, most particularly radiography, provide information that can help to solve the dilemma. As a general rule, however, respiratory disease is likely to be responsible for a chronic cough in an overweight dog with a soft murmur and preserved sinus arrhythmia. In contrast, heart disease, or even heart failure, is more likely responsible for cough in a thin animal with a loud murmur and tachycardia.

14. What radiographic findings are typical of MVD?

The appearance of the thoracic radiograph in animals with MVD is highly variable. Animals with mild MR may have a normal cardiac silhouette. Moderate or severe MR results in radiographic cardiomegaly that has a left-sided emphasis. Left ventricular enlargement typically accompanies left atrial enlargement, although the latter is more noticeable radiographically. Left atrial enlargement is evidenced by separation of the main stem bronchi and, in the lateral projection, loss of the "caudal waist" of the cardiac silhouette (Fig. 6-1). Engorgement of the pulmonary veins is sometimes observed in animals with elevated left atrial pressures, although this sign is inconsistent. The presence of pulmonary opacities in association with radiographic left atrial enlargement is diagnostic of CHF.

15. What methods are available to aid in the radiographic interpretation of heart size?

Assessment of radiographic heart size is largely subjective and accuracy of the determination is dependent on observer experience. The dogs that have MVD most commonly are small dogs that have a roughly cylindrical chest. This chest conformation can result in a misleadingly large cardiothoracic ratio in the lateral projection. These factors complicate the subjective assessment of thoracic radiographs and can cause the practitioner to conclude that cardiac enlargement is present when it is, in fact, not.

The vertebral heart sum is a useful method of cardiac mensuration and is a means by which to avoid some of the limitations of subjective radiographic assessment. Using the lateral radiographic projection, the ventrodorsal and craniocaudal dimensions of the cardiac silhouette

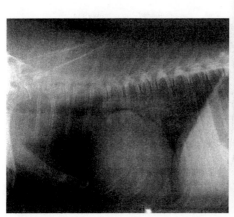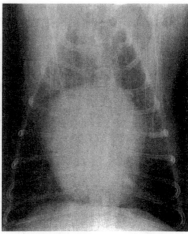

Figure 6-1. Lateral (*left*) and ventrodorsal (*right*) thoracic radiographs obtained from a 13-year-old male castrated Maltese dog. The cardiac silhouette is enlarged and there is evidence of left atrial enlargement. In the lateral projection, the trachea is elevated at the level of the carina, there is loss of the caudal waist, and the left atrium can be seen to compress the main stem bronchi. In the ventrodorsal projection, a bulge at the 3 o'clock position represents the enlarged left atrial appendage.

are measured and then summed using the "scale" provided by the thoracic vertebrae; the measurement is made from the fourth thoracic vertebra caudally (Fig. 6-2). Most normal dogs have a vertebral heart sum that is less than 10.5 vertebral units.

16. What echocardiographic abnormalities result from MR?

MR causes a volume overload of the left atrium and left ventricle. Volume loading results in eccentric hypertrophy, meaning dilation that is accompanied by an increase in myocardial mass; usually, the increase in wall thickness is proportional to the degree of dilation. When there is substantial MR, two-dimensional/M-mode echocardiography demonstrates left atrial and left ventricular dilation (Fig. 6-3). Often, the left ventricle and atrium enlarge to a similar degree. In some cases, the atrium is large when the ventricle is only mildly dilated; presumably, this results when the compliance of the left atrium is relatively greater than that of the ventricle.

When systolic myocardial function (contractility) is preserved, measurements of left ventricular performance such as fractional shortening usually reflect hyperdynamic wall motion. When substantial MR is present, the forces that oppose early systolic myocardial shortening are decreased; this is because it is relatively "easy" to eject blood into the low pressure reservoir that is provided by the left atrium. Therefore a high fractional shortening does not imply that contractility is greater than normal; it suggests only that cardiac loading conditions have been altered by the presence of MR.

Abnormalities of valve structure are commonly observed when MR results from MVD. The leaflets may be thicker than normal and have a verrucous appearance. Systolic prolapse of the leaflets beyond the plane of the mitral annulus can be observed (Fig. 6-4); this finding can result from a rupture or lengthening of chordae tendineae.

Variable degrees of right atrial/ventricular enlargement that reflect concurrent tricuspid valve involvement or the presence of pulmonary hypertension may also be observed.

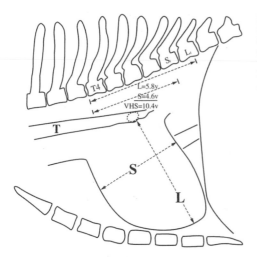

Figure 6-2. This schematic diagram illustrates the vertebral scale system for the radiographic measurement of canine heart size. *L,* long axis; *S,* short axis; *T,* trachea; *VHS,* vertebral heart sum. (Adapted from Buchanan JW, Bucheler JB: *J Am Vet Med Assoc* 206:194-199, 1995.)

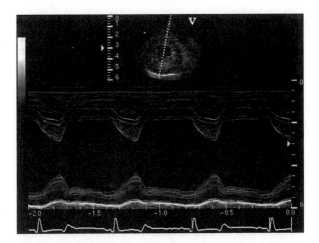

Figure 6-3. M-mode echocardiogram of the left ventricle obtained from a 10-year-old male Tibetan Terrier. M-mode echocardiography provides a one-dimensional view of the heart; the ordinate measures distance from the transducer to the abscissa, time. The two-dimensional image from which this M-mode was derived is shown in the inset. There is marked left ventricular dilation and hypertrophy. Left ventricular systolic performance is hyperdynamic.

17. What abnormalities are shown by Doppler echocardiography?

Doppler studies demonstrate the presence of disturbed flow within the left atrium during systole. MR is evident as a color-flow mosaic that extends a variable distance from the apposed mitral leaflets into the left atrium. Pulsed-wave Doppler interrogation of the left atrium reveals a high velocity, pansystolic jet; pulsed Doppler instruments cannot accurately describe high-velocity flow and directional ambiguity known because aliasing is usually observed (Fig. 6-5). Continuous-wave Doppler studies demonstrate a high-velocity jet directed away from the cardiac

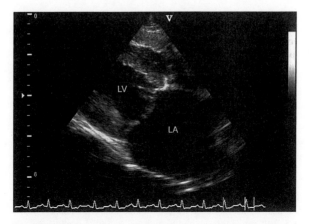

Figure 6-4. Systolic, right parasternal long axis echocardiographic image obtained from an 11-year-old male castrated Cavalier King Charles Spaniel. The left atrium (LA) is enlarged; prolapse of the mitral valve leaflets is evident. *LV,* Left ventricle.

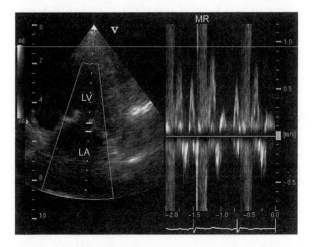

Figure 6-5. Pulsed-wave Doppler echocardiographic study (*right*) obtained from a 12-year-old female spayed Cocker Spaniel cross. The sample volume was placed in the left atrium; the two-dimensional echocardiographic image that was used to guide Doppler interrogation is shown (*left*). During systole, there is a high-velocity disturbed flow indicating mitral valve regurgitation; the second electrocardiographic complex is an atrial premature complex. *LA,* Left atrium; *LV,* left ventricle.

apex. The peak velocity of the jet is related to the instantaneous atrioventricular gradient; velocities approaching or exceeding 5 m/sec are typical.

18. How is the severity of MR assessed?

The severity of MR can be evaluated semiquantitatively or quantitatively by Doppler echocardiography. The area of the MR jet observed during color-flow Doppler mapping is one means of assessing MR severity that is attractive in its simplicity; however, factors that relate to both Doppler technology and the physics of blood flow limit the accuracy of this method. The density of the continuous-wave Doppler trace is roughly proportional to the regurgitant volume, and this index of MR severity is easy to obtain. Doppler echocardiography can also be used to quantify the regurgitant volume more precisely; the proximal flow convergence method and the use of velocity-time integrals can be used to calculate the regurgitant fraction. These methods are generally time-consuming and seldom used in clinical practice.

Surgical mitral valve repair is seldom performed in veterinary patients. Therefore, despite the availability of techniques that allow quantification of MR severity, it is may be of greater clinical importance to assess the *effects* of MR. The effect of MR can be assessed through the evaluation of heart size and by the determination of whether pulmonary edema is present. Thoracic radiographs alone are often adequate for this purpose although echocardiography is a useful adjunct.

19. What is the utility of echocardiography in the management of MVD?

Echocardiography can provide potentially useful information in all cases of MVD. However, in many cases the information is not essential. When an acquired, systolic apical murmur is heard in an elderly, small-breed dog, MVD is almost certainly the cause and echocardiographic confirmation of this suspicion is not necessary for case management.

Echocardiography is likely to be useful when it is uncertain from radiographic studies whether or not the heart is enlarged, when it is important to assess myocardial function, when pulmonary hypertension is suspected, and when there are historical or clinical findings that suggest that the cause of the animal's murmur is something other than MR.

20. What electrocardiographic abnormalities are associated with MVD?

In most affected animals, the electrocardiogram is normal. In some cases, electro-cardiographic patterns suggesting left atrial enlargement or left ventricular hypertrophy are observed. Sinus tachycardia is typical for animals that are in overt CHF. Pathologic arrhythmias are observed in some severely affected animals; often, the origin of these arrhythmias is supraventricular. Atrial premature complexes are common; the onset of atrial fibrillation usually reflects marked left atrial enlargement.

21. What diagnostic tests are indicated and when?

As in any disorder, the diagnostic approach is dictated by the animal's clinical status and the utility of the available diagnostic tests. When subclinical MR is first detected, thoracic radiographs are potentially useful. Therapy of animals with subclinical disease can probably be justified in some cases, and thoracic radiographs may provide prognostic information. The information provided by echocardiography is probably of greatest use in cases in which clinical signs result from MVD. Thoracic radiographs are essential in animals in which cough or dyspnea is part of the clinical presentation. Electrocardiography is indicated when pathologic arrhythmias are present or suspected.

22. Vasodilator drugs are often used in the management of MR; why is vasodilation beneficial?

When MR is present, the regurgitant volume depends on the size of the regurgitant orifice and the atrioventricular pressure difference. Except when the regurgitant orifice is "fixed," balanced vasodilation may alter the geometry of the ventricle so that the regurgitant volume decreases. A reduction in the atrioventricular pressure difference resulting from vasodilation may also contribute to the beneficial effect of vasodilation. In animals with moderate or severe MR, there is the potential for stroke volume to increase in response to vasodilation so that cardiac output is maintained or increases at lower arterial pressure. Blood pressure need not decrease markedly for a beneficial effect; it should be recognized that vasodilators are not indicated in animals with MR because those animals are hypertensive—they are not, unless they have concurrent disease—they are indicated because they favorably alter loading conditions.

23. What classes of vasodilators are used in the management of mitral valve disease?

The angiotensin-converting enzyme (ACE) inhibitors, which include enalapril, captopril, and benazepril, are drugs that inhibit the enzyme that converts angiotensin I to the active metabolite angiotensin II. Angiotensin II has numerous effects; it is a potent vasoconstrictor, but the release of angiotensin II also stimulates the secretion of aldosterone and augments the activity of the adrenergic nervous system. Thus the decrease in angiotensin II levels that accompanies ACE inhibition results not only in balanced vasodilation, but also diverse neuroendocrine effects.

Hydralazine is an arteriolar dilator that acts directly on vascular smooth muscle; the precise mechanism of action is unknown. The administration of hydralazine can result in a reflex-mediated increase in adrenergic nervous system activity with the potential clinical consequence of tachycardia. The notion that chronic activation of the adrenergic nervous system and the renin-angiotensin-aldosterone system (RAAS) contributes to the progressive nature of the heart failure state is now widely accepted. ACE inhibitors blunt these compensatory mechanisms, whereas hydralazine tends to augment them; it is primarily for this reason that ACE inhibitors have largely supplanted hydralazine as the vasodilator of first choice in animals with congestive heart failure resulting from MR. However, hydralazine may still have a role in animals that do not tolerate ACE inhibition or in animals with advanced CHF that is no longer responsive to diuretics and ACE inhibitors.

Similarly, the calcium channel antagonist amlodipine may have a role in the management of severe and chronic CHF resulting from MR. Nitrates, including nitroglycerin and nitroprusside, are used most often in the setting of acute or decompensated heart failure, although nitroglycerin is sometimes used in the chronic management of advanced CHF resulting from MR.

24. What is the role of medical therapy in subclinical (asymptomatic) MVD?

In the setting of MR, vasodilators can potentially decrease mitral valve regurgitation and therefore might slow the progression of associated cardiac enlargement. It has been suggested, although it is unproven, that ACE inhibitors might delay the onset of CHF in animals with subclinical MVD. However, it is likely that a therapeutic effect of these drugs requires activation of compensatory neuroendocrine mechanisms such as the adrenergic nervous system and the RAAS. Experimental studies demonstrate that RAAS activation is a feature of the heart failure state, and that pharmacologic suppression of the RAAS is beneficial. However, there may be differences between experimental models and spontaneous CHF observed in dogs. Interestingly, in one study, RAAS activation was not a feature of MVD in Cavalier King Charles Spaniels. Regardless, it seems unlikely that systemic RAAS is activated in animals that do not have substantial cardiac enlargement. Further, experimental and clinical studies suggest that the benefits of ACE inhibition are most evident in animals with myocardial disease. MVD is primarily a mechanical disease; many animals have overt CHF when systolic myocardial function is normal or only mildly diminished.

Hydralazine is a direct-acting vasodilator; although the favorable neuroendocrine effects that are associated with the ACE inhibitors have not been demonstrated for hydralazine, the latter is the more potent vasodilator. It may be that the mechanical vasodilatory property of hydralazine is of benefit to animals with MR resulting from MVD. The role of carvedilol, a relatively new beta-adrenergic antagonist with vasodilating properties, is yet to be assessed in animals with MVD.

Regardless, the role of medical therapy for subclinical (asymptomatic) MVD is uncertain. Published evidence that medical therapy slows the progression of MVD is lacking and a clinical trial that enrolled only Cavalier King Charles Spaniels provided evidence to the contrary. The results of a trial that included dogs with subclinical valvular disease irrespective of breed have not yet been published; the preliminary findings of that study suggest that ACE inhibition may have a modest benefit in this clinical scenario. On the basis of these data, it is difficult to justify treatment for dogs that have murmurs but not other clinical markers of disease. It is important to remember that the rate at which MR progresses is difficult to predict. Many animals with MVD never have morbidity related to heart disease and die of extracardiac disease long after the development of a murmur of MR. Still, because there is little evidence that carefully monitored therapy with these agents does harm, there may be a role for ACE inhibitors in subclinical animals with substantial cardiac enlargement resulting from MR.

25. What is the therapeutic approach to cough resulting from compression of the main stem bronchi by an enlarged left atrium?

The cough that develops in animals that have a large left atrium but do not have pulmonary edema probably has a multifactorial cause. Mechanical compression of the main stem bronchi is at least partly responsible for cough in some animals. However, concurrent primary respiratory tract disease and perhaps the presence of high pulmonary venous pressures are other factors that can contribute to cough related to MVD. Vasodilators such as ACE inhibitors or possibly hydralazine can be used in animals such as this; it is hoped that vasodilation will reduce regurgitant volume and therefore decrease left atrial pressure and, possibly, size. When cough persists despite the use of a vasodilator, it is important to consider the possibility that a concurrent, primary respiratory tract disease such as bronchitis is contributing to the pathogenesis of the cough. When this is the case, bronchodilators are sometimes helpful and, in the absence of pulmonary edema or infective respiratory disease, the use of antitussive agents can be considered. In general, the use of diuretics is avoided in animals that do not have radiographic evidence of pulmonary edema. However, a case might be made for diuretic use in animals with marked left atrial enlargement because these drugs tend to be quite effective in reducing cardiac size. Although preload reduction can have the undesirable consequence of RAAS activation, the decrease in ventricular size might potentially decrease regurgitant fraction.

26. What therapy is indicated for animals that have congestive heart failure resulting from MVD?

The results of a multicenter, double-blind, placebo-controlled trial attest to the efficacy of ACE inhibitors in CHF resulting from MVD; arguably, all animals with CHF resulting from MVD should receive an ACE inhibitor, provided the drug is tolerated. The concurrent use of diuretic agents is indicated when pulmonary edema results from MR. Furosemide is the diuretic used most commonly and the dose and dosage interval are tailored to relieve congestive signs without excessive reduction in ventricular filling pressures. An initial dose of 1 mg/kg orally every 12 hours is often adequate for animals receiving ACE inhibitors. Thus standard therapy for CHF from MVD consists of an ACE inhibitor together with a diuretic, usually furosemide. Digoxin is used concurrently in some cases.

27. Is digoxin useful in the management of MVD?

Digoxin has a modest inotropic effect that is mediated through an increase in intracellular calcium availability. Additionally, digoxin has important effects on the autonomic nervous system; specifically, it increases vagal discharge and this serves to slow the rate of sinus node discharge and atrioventricular nodal conduction velocity. The latter effect is commonly used to control the ventricular response rate of animals that have atrial fibrillation.

Increases in baroreceptor sensitivity are thought to be at least partly responsible for the therapeutic effect of digoxin in heart failure. The arterial baroreceptors are pressure-sensitive nerve endings located in the aorta and carotid arteries; stimulation of these receptors by increases in arterial pressure initiates a reflex arc that results in vagal discharge and inhibition of adrenergic tone. In heart failure, the sensitivity of the baroreceptors is diminished and this contributes to heightened and unopposed sympathetic tone. There is evidence that digoxin increases baroreceptor sensitivity and, in so doing, partially normalizes baroreceptor function, resulting in increased vagal discharge.

The use of digoxin in animals that have myocardial dysfunction (cardiomyopathy of overload) or atrial fibrillation as a complication of longstanding MR is almost universally accepted. However, overt CHF often results from MR when systolic myocardial function is apparently preserved; in these animals, the role of digoxin is debatable. Controlled studies of efficacy of digoxin in these animals are lacking. However, despite extensive evaluation of alternative agents, only digoxin, which is unique by virtue of its autonomic effects, has favorable long-term effects in humans. This suggests that the neuroendocrine effects of digoxin, which include normalization of baroreceptor function and reduction of renin levels, might be more important than the relatively weak inotropic effects of this drug. For this reason, some advocate the use of digoxin in all animals with moderate or severe CHF resulting from MR.

28. What medical therapy is indicated in cases of refractory or severe CHF?

When congestive signs are no longer controlled by standard therapy, or when the diuretic doses required to free the animal of congestive signs result in unacceptably low cardiac output, CHF can be considered to be refractory. Because of their proven efficacy, ACE inhibitors have become standard therapy for CHF resulting from MVD. However, these drugs are not potent vasodilators. For this reason, the use of hydralazine or possibly amlodipine in addition to ACE inhibitors can be considered for animals with refractory CHF resulting from severe MVD. This step should be undertaken with caution; monitoring of blood pressure is advisable because excessive vasodilation can result in dangerous hypotension.

The use of triple diuretic therapy—the administration of a potassium-sparing diuretic such as spironolactone and a thiazide in addition to furosemide—can also be considered for animals with severe or refractory CHF. Triple diuretic therapy uses the principle of sequential nephron blockade; each of the drugs act at functionally distinct sites of the nephron and this may help to overcome the development of resistance to single-agent diuresis. Additionally, the use of triple diuretic therapy can allow the use of lower doses of the component drugs, which may limit some of the adverse effects associated with aggressive diuresis. In addition to its diuretic effect, spironolactone may have favorable neurohumoral effects; this drug antagonizes the effect of aldosterone, a hormone that is implicated in the development of myocardial fibrosis.

29. Can MVD be treated surgically?

MVD is primarily a mechanical disorder and is well suited to surgical approaches that include mitral valve replacement and repair. Unfortunately, surgical exposure of the mitral valve apparatus requires cardiopulmonary bypass. Although this technique is successfully practiced at a few referral institutions, surgical therapy of MVD is in its infancy. The necessary expertise is not widely available and the costs associated with open heart surgery further limit the application of surgical approaches to this disease.

30. What can explain sudden clinical deterioration in animals with MVD?

It should be recognized that CHF in veterinary patients often has an apparently sudden onset. Many pet dogs are relatively sedentary; because of this, cardiac disease can progress unnoticed until a point when even minimal exertion results in severe dyspnea. Additionally, subtle changes in respiratory rate and character can be difficult for owners to recognize. These and possibly other factors delay recognition of CHF in animals until it is well advanced. However, animals with MVD are subject to catastrophes that can result in acute decompensation.

Rupture of a chorda tendineae is a relatively common acute complication of MVD; the severity of the resultant clinical signs is dependent on the functional importance of the ruptured chord and the compliance of the left atrium. Rupture of a first-order mitral chorda tendineae causes acute and severe mitral valve regurgitation and the resultant increase in left atrial pressure may result in fulminant pulmonary edema that is refractory to medical therapy. If a second-order chord ruptures in an animal with a compliant and capacious atrium, it may go undetected. In fact, ruptured chordae are sometimes found on postmortem examination of animals with MVD that succumb to extracardiac disease. Rupture of mitral chordae is most common in animals that have preexisting mitral valve regurgitation and associated cardiac enlargement. The result is clinical decompensation, the severity of which is determined by factors stated previously. Occasionally, rupture of a first-order mitral valve chorda is observed in animals that have only mild mitral valve disease. In these cases, the acute elevation in left atrial pressure is catastrophic and severe pulmonary edema results. This is one of the few clinical scenarios in veterinary medicine that results in truly acute heart failure; radiographically, the cardiac silhouette is only minimally enlarged in the presence of florid edema. Sometimes the pulmonary hypertension that develops subsequent to acute increases in left atrial pressure can result in right-sided CHF manifest clinically as ascites.

Rupture of the left atrium is an uncommon complication of MVD. Although surgical treatment of atrial rupture has been described, most often the result is death from tamponade. Rarely, rupture of the atrial septum results in an acquired atrial septal defect.

31. What is the cause of ascites in animals with degenerative valvular disease?
Although the effects of MR usually dominate the clinical presentation of animals with degenerative valvular disease, the tricuspid valve can also be affected. In some cases, tricuspid valve regurgitation results in right-sided CHF. In dogs, right-sided CHF is typically manifest as ascites. Pulmonary hypertension related to high left atrial pressures increases right ventricular afterload and this may contribute to the development of right-sided CHF in some animals.

BIBLIOGRAPHY

Buchanan JW: Chronic valvular disease (endocardiosis) in dogs. *Adv Vet Sci Comp Med* 21:75, 1979.
The COVE Study Group: Controlled clinical evaluation of enalapril in dogs with heart failure: results of the Cooperative Veterinary Enalapril Study Group. *J Vet Intern Med* 9:243, 1995.
The Digitalis Investigation Group: The effect of digoxin on mortality and morbidity in patients with heart failure. *N Engl J Med* 336:525-533, 1997.
Ettinger SJ, Benitz AM, Ericsson GF et al: Effects of enalapril maleate on survival of dogs with naturally acquired heart failure: the Long-Term Investigation of Veterinary Enalapril (LIVE) Study Group. *J Am Vet Med Assoc* 213:1573-1577, 1998.
Gheorghiade M, Pitt B: Digitalis Investigation Group (DIG) trial: a stimulus for further research. *Am Heart J* 134:3-12, 1997.
Haggstrom J, Hansson K, Kvart C et al: Effects of naturally acquired decompensated mitral valve regurgitation on the renin-angiotensin-aldosterone system and atrial natriuretic peptide concentration in dogs. *Am J Vet Res* 58:77-82, 1997.
Haggstrom J, Hansson K, Kvart C et al: Chronic valvular disease in the Cavalier King Charles Spaniel in Sweden. *Vet Rec* 131:549-553, 1992.
Hamlin RL: Pathophysiology of the failing heart. In Fox PR, Sisson D, Moise NS, editors: *Textbook of canine and feline cardiology: principles and clinical practice,* 2nd ed., Philadelphia, WB Saunders, 1999.
Keene BW, Rush JE: Therapy of heart failure. In Ettinger SJ, Feldman EC, editors: *Textbook of veterinary internal medicine,* 4th ed. Philadelphia, WB Saunders, 1993.
Kittleson MD: Myxomatous atrioventricular valvular degeneration. In Kittleson MD, Kiènle RD, editors: *Small animal cardiovascular medicine,* St Louis, Mosby, 1998.
O'Grady MR: Acquired valvular disease. In Ettinger SJ, Feldman EC, editors, *Textbook of veterinary internal medicine,* 4th ed., Philadelphia, WB Saunders, 1993.
Opie LH, Poole-Wilson PA, Sonnenblick EH et al: Angiotensin-converting enzyme inhibitors and conventional vasodilators. In Opie LH, editor, *Drugs for the heart,* 4th ed., Philadelphia, WB Saunders, 1997.
Sisson D, Kittleson MD: Management of heart failure: principles of treatment, therapeutic strategies and pharmacology. In Fox PR, Sisson D, Moise NS, editors, *Textbook of canine and feline cardiology: principles and clinical practice,* 2nd ed., Philadelphia, WB Saunders, 1999.

7. Pericardial Disease

Wendy A. Ware

1. What is the normal structure and function of the pericardium?

The pericardium is a double-layered sac that encases the heart and is attached to the great vessels at the heart base. It consists of an outer fibrous layer (parietal pericardium) and an inner serous membrane covering the heart (visceral pericardium or epicardium). A small amount of clear, serous fluid is normally present between these layers and acts to reduce friction. The pericardium limits acute distention of the heart and maintains normal cardiac position, geometry, and ventricular compliance. The pericardium also forms a barrier to inflammation or infection of surrounding structures.

2. What congenital pericardial malformations are of clinical concern?

Pericardioperitoneal diaphragmatic hernia (PPDH) is the most common pericardial malformation in dogs. Abnormal embryonic development (probably of the septum transversum) allows persistent communication between the pericardial and peritoneal cavities at the ventral midline. The pleural space is not involved. Other congenital defects such as umbilical hernia, sternal malformations, and cardiac anomalies may also be present. Males appear to be affected more frequently than females. Clinical signs are variable and result from herniation of abdominal contents into the pericardial space. Pericardial cysts are rare anomalies thought to originate from abnormal fetal mesenchymal tissue or from incarcerated omental or falciform fat from a small PPDH. Other congenital defects of the pericardium itself are extremely rare in dogs; most are discovered incidentally on postmortem examination. Both partial (usually on the left side) and complete absence of the pericardium have been reported.

3. How is PPDH diagnosed?

Clinical signs associated with PPDH usually develop within the first year or so of life but can appear at any age (cases have been diagnosed between 4 weeks and 15 years of age). Some animals never have clinical signs and are diagnosed fortuitously. Clinical signs are usually gastrointestinal or respiratory. Vomiting, diarrhea, anorexia, weight loss, abdominal pain, cough, dyspnea, and wheezing are most often reported; shock and collapse can also occur. The physical examination may indicate muffled heart sounds on one or both sides of the chest, displacement or attenuation of the apical precordial impulse, an "empty" feel on abdominal palpation (with herniation of many organs), and, rarely, signs of cardiac tamponade.

Thoracic radiography is often diagnostic or highly suggestive of PPDH. Characteristic findings include enlargement of the cardiac silhouette with dorsal tracheal displacement, overlap of the diaphragmic and caudal heart borders, and abnormal fat or gas densities within the cardiac silhouette. On lateral view, a pleural fold is usually evident extending between the caudal heart shadow and the diaphragm ventral to the caudal vena cava. Gas-filled loops of bowel crossing the diaphragm into the pericardial sac, a small liver, or few organs within the abdominal cavity may also be observed. Echocardiography is useful in confirming the diagnosis in animals in which the diagnosis is equivocal. A gastrointestinal barium series is diagnostic if stomach or intestines are in the pericardial cavity. Fluoroscopy, nonselective angiography (especially if only falciform fat or liver has herniated), celiography, or pneumopericardiography also have been used in diagnosis. Electrocardiographic changes are inconsistent; decreased amplitude complexes and axis deviations caused by cardiac position changes sometimes occur.

4.   What is the recommended treatment for PPDH?

In symptomatic animals, therapy involves surgical closure of the peritoneal-pericardial defect after returning viable organs to their normal location. The presence of other congenital abnormalities and the animal's clinical signs may influence the decision to operate. The prognosis in uncomplicated cases is excellent. Older animals without clinical signs may do well without surgery. Trauma to organs chronically adhered to the heart or pericardium during attempted repositioning is a potential concern in older animals.

5.   In what ways can a structurally normal pericardium become diseased?

The accumulation of excess or abnormal fluid (effusion) is the most common pericardial disorder. Constrictive pericardial disease is recognized occasionally in dogs.

6.   What types of fluid accumulate in the pericardium?

In dogs, most pericardial effusions are serosanguineous or sanguinous. The fluid usually appears dark red, with a packed cell volume of more than 7%, a specific gravity higher than 1.015, and a protein concentration between 3 and 6 g/dl. Mostly red blood cells are found on cytology, but reactive mesothelial, neoplastic, or other cells may be seen. The fluid does not clot unless the effusion resulted from very recent hemorrhage.

Transudates, modified transudates, and exudates are found occasionally. Pure transudates are clear, with a low cell count (less than 2500 cells/μl), specific gravity (less than 1.012), and protein content (less than 1 g/dl). Modified transudates may appear slightly cloudy or pink-tinged; cellularity is low but the specific gravity (1.015-1.030) and total protein concentration (2-5 g/dl) are higher than in a pure transudate. Exudates appear cloudy to opaque, or serofibrinous to serosanguineous. The white cell count (more than 15,000/μl), specific gravity (higher than 1.015), and protein concentration (more than 3 g/dl) are high. Cytologic findings are related to the cause.

7.   Most pericardial effusions in dogs are hemorrhagic. What are the typical causes?

Dogs older than 7 years are likely to have neoplastic hemorrhagic effusion. Hemangiosarcoma is by far the most common neoplasm causing hemorrhagic pericardial effusion. Hemorrhagic pericardial effusion also results from various heart base tumors and pericardial mesotheliomas. Hemangiosarcomas usually arise from the right atrial wall, especially in the auricular area. Chemodectoma, arising from chemoreceptor cells at the base of the aorta, is the most common heart base tumor. Other heart base tumors also can occur, including thyroid, parathyroid, lymphoid, or connective tissue neoplasms. Pericardial mesotheliomas are uncommon but have been reported.

Idiopathic (so-called benign) pericardial effusion has been described most frequently in medium-to-large breeds of dogs. The German Shepherd, Golden Retriever, Great Dane, and Saint Bernard may be predisposed. Although dogs of any age can be affected, most are 6 years old or younger. Evidence of mild inflammation is common and pericardial fibrosis can result with time.

Other causes of intrapericardial hemorrhage include left atrial rupture secondary to severe mitral insufficiency, coagulopathy (e.g., warfarin-type rodenticides), and penetrating trauma (including iatrogenic laceration of a coronary artery during pericardiocentesis).

8.   What conditions cause pericardial transudates and exudates?

Transudative effusions can be caused by congestive heart failure, pericardioperitoneal diaphragmatic hernia, hypoalbuminemia, pericardial cysts, or toxemias that increase vascular permeability (including uremia). Usually these conditions are associated with small volumes of pericardial effusion and cardiac tamponade is uncommon.

Exudates are rarely found in small animals. Pericarditis is unusual in association with systemic infections, but infectious pericarditis has been reported with actinomycosis, disseminated tuberculosis, *Pasteurella multocida* and other bacterial infections, coccidioidomycosis, and, rarely, systemic protozoal infections. Sterile exudative effusions have occurred with leptospirosis, canine distemper, and idiopathic benign pericardial effusion in dogs. Chronic uremia occasionally causes a sterile, serofibrinous, or hemorrhagic effusion in animals.

9. Does pericardial effusion always cause problems?

Unless intrapericardial fluid pressure rises to equal or exceed normal cardiac filling pressure, fluid accumulation within the pericardial space has little clinical consequence. When fluid accumulates slowly, the pericardium is able to distend and accommodate the increased volume while maintaining low intrapericardial pressure. As long as intrapericardial pressure is low, cardiac filling and output remain relatively normal. But, pericardial tissue is relatively non-compliant, so rapid fluid accumulation or large volume effusions cause intrapericardial pressure to rise quickly. Pericardial fibrosis and thickening further limit the compliance of this tissue. When intrapericardial pressure rises to and above normal atrial and venous pressures, cardiac filling is compromised. This is known as cardiac tamponade. Aside from the hemodynamic consequences of cardiac tamponade, very large pericardial effusions occasionally cause clinical signs from lung or tracheal compression (dyspnea and cough) or esophageal compression (dysphagia or regurgitation).

10. When is cardiac tamponade present?

Because the pericardium is relatively inelastic, there is a steep intrapericardial pressure-volume relationship when effusion accumulates quickly. Cardiac tamponade develops when intrapericardial pressure rises toward and exceeds cardiac diastolic pressure. This externally compresses the heart and progressively limits filling, causing cardiac output to fall. Eventually, diastolic pressures in all cardiac chambers and great veins equilibrate.

11. What are the consequences of cardiac tamponade?

Neurohumoral compensatory mechanisms of heart failure are activated when tamponade develops and cardiac output decreases. Signs of systemic venous congestion become especially prominent with time. Low cardiac output, arterial hypotension, and poor perfusion of other organs as well as the heart can ultimately lead to cardiogenic shock and death. The rate of pericardial fluid accumulation and the distensibility of the pericardial sac determine whether and how quickly cardiac tamponade develops. Rapid accumulation of even small volumes can markedly raise intrapericardial pressure, because the pericardium can stretch only slowly. The presence of a large volume of pericardial fluid implies a gradual process. Although cardiac contractility is not directly affected by pericardial effusion, reduced coronary perfusion during tamponade can impair both systolic and diastolic functions.

12. What clinical manifestations are characteristic of cardiac tamponade?

Clinical findings in animals with cardiac tamponade reflect poor cardiac output and right-sided (most commonly) congestive heart failure. Congestive failure arises from compensatory volume retention and the direct effects of impaired cardiac filling. Right-sided signs predominate because of the right heart's thinner walls and low pressures, although signs of biventricular failure may occur. Nonspecific clinical signs such as lethargy, weakness, poor exercise tolerance, or inappetence may be noted before obvious ascites develops. Rapid accumulation of even small volumes of fluid (50-100 ml) can cause acute tamponade, shock, and death. In such cases, pulmonary edema, jugular venous distention, and hypotension may be evident without signs of pleural and peritoneal effusions or radiographic cardiomegaly.

Historical findings of weakness, exercise intolerance, abdominal enlargement, tachypnea, syncope, and cough are typical. Significant loss of lean body mass occurs in some chronic cases. Jugular vein distention or positive hepatojugular reflux, hepatomegaly, ascites, labored respiration, and weakened femoral pulses are common physical examination findings. A palpable decrease in arterial pulse strength during inspiration (pulsus paradoxus) might be discernable in occasional cases. High sympathetic tone commonly produces sinus tachycardia, pale mucous membranes, and prolonged capillary refill time. The precordial impulse is palpably weak with a large pericardial fluid volume. Heart sounds are muffled in animals with moderate-to-large pericardial effusions. Lung sounds are muffled ventrally with pleural effusion. Although pericardial effusion does not cause a murmur, concurrent cardiac disease may do so. Fever may be associated with infectious pericarditis.

13. What is pulsus paradoxus?
Cardiac tamponade causes an exaggerated respiratory variation in arterial blood pressure called pulsus paradoxus. Inspiration reduces intrapericardial and right atrial pressures, thereby facilitating right heart filling and pulmonary blood flow. Simultaneously, left heart filling is reduced because more blood is held in the lungs and the interventricular septum bulges leftward from the inspiratory increase in right ventricular filling; consequently, left heart output and systemic arterial pressure decrease during inspiration. The variation in systolic arterial pressure is usually higher than 10 mm Hg in animals with cardiac tamponade and pulsus paradoxus.

14. What is the role of radiography in the diagnosis of pericardial disease?
Thoracic radiography is useful for detecting the enlarged cardiac silhouette resulting from pericardial fluid accumulation. Massive pericardial effusion causes the "classic" round, globoid-shaped cardiac shadow ("basketball heart") seen on both views. Other findings associated with tamponade include pleural effusion, caudal vena cava distension, hepatomegaly, and ascites. Pulmonary opacities compatible with edema and distended pulmonary veins are less frequently noted. Some heart base tumors cause deviation of the trachea or a soft-tissue mass effect. Metastatic lung lesions are common in dogs with hemangiosarcoma.

15. What is the role of echocardiography in the diagnosis of pericardial disease?
Echocardiography allows rapid detection of pericardial fluid noninvasively. It is therefore the diagnostic test of choice when available. Echocardiography is highly sensitive for detecting even small volumes of pericardial fluid. Because fluid is sonolucent, pericardial effusion appears as an echo-free space between the bright parietal pericardium and the epicardium (Fig. 7-1). Abnormal cardiac wall motion and chamber shape, as well as intrapericardial or intracardiac mass lesions, can also be imaged. The right ventricular and atrial walls are often well visualized and may appear hyperechoic because of the surrounding fluid. A complete two-dimensional echocardiographic examination is important to screen for mass lesions. All portions of the right atrium and auricle, right ventricle, ascending aorta, and pericardium itself should be carefully evaluated. The left cranial transducer position is especially useful for examining the right atrium and auricle. Better visualization of the heart base and mass lesions is generally obtained before pericardiocentesis is performed (Fig. 7-2). Transesophageal echocardiography is a sensitive technique for detecting intrapericardial mass lesions.
Diastolic compression or collapse of the right atrium and sometimes right ventricle is consistent with cardiac tamponade. It is important to remember that the volume of the effusion is not the main determinant of hemodynamic compromise, but rather how much increase in intrapericardial pressure it has caused.

16. How can I differentiate pleural effusion from pericardial effusion?
Identification of the parietal pericardium in relation to the echo-free fluid helps differentiate pleural from pericardial effusion. Most pericardial fluid accumulates near the cardiac apex, because the pericardium adheres more tightly to the heart base; there is usually little fluid behind the left atrium. Furthermore, evidence of collapsed lung lobes or pleural folds can often be seen within pleural effusion. Sometimes pleural effusion, a markedly enlarged left atrium, a dilated coronary sinus, or persistent left cranial vena cava can be confused with pericardial effusion. Careful scanning from several positions helps differentiate these conditions.

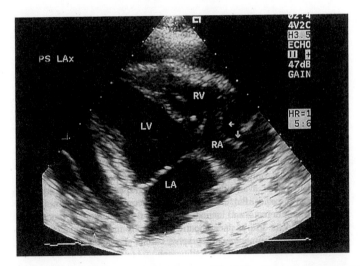

Figure 7-1. Two-dimensional echocardiogram from an older Golden Retriever with cardiac tamponade. Pericardial fluid surrounds the heart and collapse of the right atrial wall is apparent (*arrows*). Right ventricular size is also compromised. Right parasternal long axis view; *LA,* left atrium; *LV,* left ventricle; *RA,* right atrium; *RV,* right ventricle.

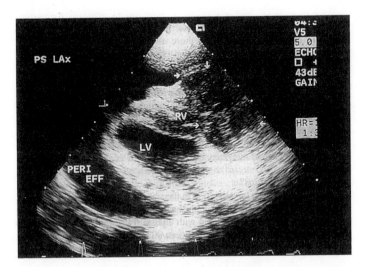

Figure 7-2. Echocardiogram from a 10-year-old Schnauzer/Poodle mix. A large volume of pericardial fluid (peri eff) is seen around the heart. A 3 × 4.5 cm tumor mass (*small arrows*) arising from the right atrium is seen adjacent and dorsal to the compressed right ventricle. *LV,* left ventricle; *RV,* right ventricle.

17. What if I do not have access to echocardiography?

In most cases, the presence of cardiac tamponade is strongly suggested by the clinical history and physical examination. Radiographic findings usually support the clinical suspicion. Suggestive electrocardiogram (ECG) findings may also be present. If the animal's condition appears stable and referral for echocardiography is feasible, then that can be pursued for definitive diagnosis. However, if the animal with suspected tamponade has severe signs, pericardiocentesis should be done immediately. If a catheter system is used for this, pneumopericardiography (see the following section) can be done after initial drainage if desired.

18. What other diagnostic techniques are available?

Other radiographic techniques are less commonly used. Fluoroscopy demonstrates diminished to absent motion of the cardiac shadow, because the heart is surrounded by fluid. Angiocardiography is used only rarely for the diagnosis of pericardial effusion and cardiac tumors because of the wide availability of echocardiography; however, it typically reveals increased endocardial-to-pericardial distance. Cardiac neoplasms can cause displacement of normal structures, filling defects, and angiographic vascular "blushing." Echocardiography has also essentially replaced the use of pneumopericardiography in the evaluation of animals with pericardial effusion. For pneumopericardiography, carbon dioxide or air is injected into the drained pericardial sac to outline the heart. Radiographs are taken from different orientations, but the left lateral and dorsoventral views are most helpful because they allow the injected gas to outline the right atrial and heart base areas, respectively, where tumors are most common.

Central venous pressure measurement may be useful in some cases, especially if jugular veins are difficult to assess or it is unclear whether right heart filling pressures are elevated. A central venous pressure above 10-12 cm H_2O is common with pericardial disease; normally central venous pressure is less than 8 cm H_2O.

19. Is a large, round cardiac silhouette on radiographs pathognomonic for pericardial effusion?

Although a large "globoid" cardiac silhouette is often seen, this totally round heart shape is not observed in many cases. Smaller volumes of pericardial fluid accumulation allow various cardiac contours to be identified, especially those associated with the atria. Conversely, other cardiac diseases besides large volume pericardial effusion can cause the cardiac silhouette to become very large and rounded, for example, dilated cardiomyopathy or tricuspid valve dysplasia.

20. Are there typical ECG changes that occur with pericardial disease?

Although there are no pathognomonic ECG findings, the following abnormalities are suggestive of pericardial effusion: diminished amplitude QRS complexes (less than 1 mV in dogs) and electrical alternans. ST segment elevation (suggesting an epicardial injury current) may accompany epicarditis. Sinus tachycardia is common in association with cardiac tamponade. Atrial or ventricular tachyarrhythmias may also occur.

21. What is electrical alternans?

Electrical alternans is a recurring alteration in the size of the QRS complex (or sometimes the T wave) with every other beat. It results from the heart physically swinging back and forth within the pericardium and is most often associated with a large volume of pericardial fluid. Electrical alternans may be most evident at heart rates between 90 and 140 beats/minute or in certain body positions (e.g., standing rather than lateral recumbency).

22. Because cardiac tamponade causes ascites and other signs of right heart failure, isn't treatment with furosemide, a vasodilator and digoxin appropriate?

It is important to differentiate cardiac tamponade from other causes of right-sided heart failure because the treatment is different. Diuretics and vasodilators, by reducing cardiac filling pressure, can further diminish cardiac output and exacerbate hypotension and shock. Digoxin and other positive inotropic drugs do not improve cardiac output or ameliorate the signs of tamponade, because the underlying pathophysiologic condition is impaired cardiac filling, not poor contractility. Pericardiocentesis is the therapeutic procedure of choice. It also provides diagnostic information. Signs of congestive heart failure usually resolve quickly after intrapericardial pressure is reduced by fluid removal. In some animals, a diuretic may be of limited value after pericardiocentesis. Pericardial effusions secondary to other diseases causing congestive heart failure, congenital malformations, or hypoalbuminemia do not usually cause tamponade and often resolve with management of the underlying condition.

23. What is the best initial treatment for cardiac tamponade?
PERICARDIOCENTESIS!

24. How can I safely drain the pericardial space?
Pericardiocentesis is a relatively safe procedure when carefully performed. Local anesthesia is used. Sedation may be helpful depending on the clinical status and temperament of the animal in order to prevent animal movement. An ECG monitor should be attached for the procedure, because needle/catheter contact with the heart commonly causes ventricular arrhythmias.

A variety of equipment can be used for pericardiocentesis. A butterfly needle or appropriately long hypodermic or spinal needle attached to extension tubing is adequate in emergency situations. A safer alternative, which reduces the risk of cardiopulmonary laceration during fluid aspiration, is an over-the-needle catheter system (e.g., Angiocath). An 18- to 20-gauge (1.5-2 inches long) size (depending on animal size) is easy to use as long as the needle-catheter unit is advanced well into the pericardial space so that the catheter is not deflected out of the pericardium as the needle is removed. Larger over-the-needle catheter systems (e.g. 12-16 gauge, 4 -6 inches long) allow for faster fluid removal in large dogs; a few additional small side holes can be precut (smoothly) near the tip of the catheter to facilitate flow. During initial catheter placement, extension tubing is attached to the needle stylet; after the catheter is advanced into the pericardial space and needle removed, the extension tubing is attached directly to the catheter. For all methods a three-way stopcock is placed between the tubing and a collection syringe.

25. How should the animal be positioned?
Pericardiocentesis is usually done from the right side of the chest to minimize risk of trauma to the lungs (by using the area of the cardiac notch) and major coronary vessels (which are located mostly on left). The animal is usually placed in left lateral or sternal recumbency to allow more stable restraint, especially if the animal is weak or excitable. Good success can also be had using an elevated echocardiography table with a large cutout; the animal is placed in right lateral recumbency and the tap is performed from underneath. The advantage with this method is that gravity pulls fluid down to the right side; but, if adequate space is not available for wide sterile skin preparation or needle/catheter manipulation, this approach is not advised. Echocardiogram guidance can be used, but is not necessary unless the effusion is of small volume or appears compartmentalized. Sometimes needle pericardiocentesis can be successfully performed on the standing animal, but the risk of injury is increased if the animal suddenly moves.

26. How do I perform the pericardial tap?
Shave and surgically prepare the skin over a wide area of the right precordium (from about the third to seventh intercostal spaces and from sternum to costochondral junction). Using sterile gloves and aseptic technique, locate the puncture site by palpating for where the cardiac impulse is strongest (usually between the fourth and sixth ribs just lateral to the sternum). Local anesthesia is necessary when using larger catheters and recommended for needle pericardiocentesis. Infiltrate 2% lidocaine (with sterile technique) at the skin puncture site, underlying intercostal muscles, and into the underlying pleura. A small stab incision is made in the skin to

allow catheter entry. Remember to avoid the intercostal vessels just caudal to each rib when entering the chest.

After the needle has penetrated the skin, the operator's assistant should gently apply negative pressure to the attached syringe as the operator slowly advances the needle toward the heart. It sometimes helps to aim the tip of the needle toward the animal's opposite shoulder. Be sure to observe the tubing so that fluid will be seen as soon as it is aspirated. Pleural fluid (usually straw colored) may enter the tubing first. The pericardium creates increased resistance to needle advancement and may produce a subtle scratching sensation. With gentle pressure, advance the needle through the pericardium; a loss of resistance may be noted with needle penetration and pericardial fluid (usually dark red) will appear in the tubing. If the needle contacts the heart, a scratching or tapping sensation is usually felt, the needle may move with the heartbeat, and ventricular premature complexes are usually provoked; the needle should be retracted slightly. Avoid excessive needle movement within the chest. If a catheter system is used, after the needle/stylet is well within the pericardial space advance the catheter, remove the stylet, and attach the extension tubing to the catheter. Remember to save initial fluid samples for cytology and microbiologic culture, then aspirate as much fluid as possible.

27. This fluid looks like blood—is it from inside the heart?

Pericardial effusion usually looks quite hemorrhagic and it may be disconcerting to see such dark, bloody fluid being aspirated from so near the heart. But, pericardial fluid can be differentiated from intracardiac blood in several ways. Unless there was very recent hemorrhage into the pericardium, the fluid will not clot. A few drops can be placed on the table or a few milliliters put into a serum (red top) tube to test this. If clotting does not occur, it is safe to continue aspirating. Additionally, the packed cell volume (PCV) of pericardial fluid is usually less than that of peripheral blood, and when spun in a hematocrit tube the supernatant is xanthochromic (yellow-tinged). Furthermore, as pericardial fluid is drained, the animal's ECG complexes increase in amplitude, tachycardia diminishes, and the animal often takes a deep breath and appears more comfortable.

28. What complications can occur from pericardiocentesis?

Complications of pericardiocentesis include ventricular tachyarrhythmias from direct myocardial injury or puncture; these are usually self-limiting when the needle is withdrawn. Coronary artery laceration with myocardial infarction or further bleeding into the pericardial space can occur but is uncommon especially when pericardiocentesis is done from the right side. Lung laceration causing pneumothorax or hemorrhage is also a potential complication during the procedure. In some cases, dissemination of infection or neoplastic cells into the pleural space may occur.

29. Can I tell from the pericardial fluid what the underlying cause is?

Pericardiocentesis usually yields a hemorrhagic effusion; less frequently, the fluid is suppurative or transudative. Samples should be submitted for cytologic analysis and saved for possible bacterial (or fungal) culture. However, differentiation of sanguinous neoplastic effusions from benign hemorrhagic pericarditis is usually impossible on the basis of cytology alone. Reactive mesothelial cells within the effusion may closely resemble neoplastic cells; furthermore, chemodectomas and hemangiosarcomas may not shed cells into the effusion.

Although neoplastic (and other noninflammatory) effusions tend to have a pH of 7.0 or greater and inflammatory effusions tend to have lower pH values, there appears to be too much overlap between these groups for pericardial fluid pH to be a reliable discriminator. If cytologic features suggest an infectious/inflammatory cause, the pericardial fluid should be cultured. Fungal titers (e.g., coccidioidomycosis) or other serologic tests may be helpful in some animals. It is not clear whether analysis of pericardial fluid for cardiac troponins or other substances will be useful in differentiating underlying causes.

30. How should a dog with idiopathic, "benign" pericardial effusion be managed after initial pericardiocentesis?

Dogs with idiopathic pericarditis are initially treated conservatively after pericardiocentesis. Medical therapy may consist of a glucocorticoid (e.g., prednisone, 1 mg/kg/day by mouth tapering over 2 to 4 weeks) after ruling out infectious causes by pericardial fluid culture or cytology. The efficacy of this in preventing recurrent idiopathic pericardial effusion is not known, however. Sometimes a 1- to 2-week course of antibiotic is also used.

Periodic reevaluation of these dogs using radiography or echocardiography is advised to detect recurrence. Apparent recovery occurs after one or two pericardial taps in about half of affected dogs. Cardiac tamponade recurs after a variable time (days to years) in other cases. Effusion that recurs after two or three pericardiocenteses and antiinflammatory therapy is treated by surgical subtotal pericardiectomy. Removal of the pericardium ventral to the phrenic nerves allows drainage to the larger absorptive surface of the pleural space. Creation of a pericardial window by thorascopic partial pericardiectomy or by percutaneous balloon pericardiotomy has been successful in some cases. The risks for adhesions/fibrosis leading to fluid reaccumulation with small pericardial openings are unclear.

31. For neoplastic pericardial effusions, what are the treatment options?

Neoplastic effusions are also initially drained to relieve cardiac tamponade. Therapy may involve attempted surgical resection or surgical biopsy, chemotherapy, or conservative therapy until episodes of cardiac tamponade become unmanageable. Surgical resection of hemangiosarcoma is often not possible because of the size and extent of the tumor, although small tumors involving only the tip of the right auricle have been successfully removed. If hemangiosarcoma is diagnosed or strongly suspected on the basis of clinicopathologic and echocardiographic findings, chemotherapy (e.g., doxorubicin, cyclophosphamide, with or without vincristine) may provide some palliation. Partial pericardiectomy (as discussed previously) may avert recurrence of tamponade. Metastatic dissemination throughout the thoracic cavity may be facilitated by this procedure, but this does not appear to affect survival time with hemangiosarcoma or mesothelioma. Prognosis is generally poor in dogs with hemangiosarcoma or mesothelioma.

Heart base tumors (e.g., chemodectoma) tend to be slow growing and locally invasive, with low metastatic potential. Partial pericardiectomy may prolong the life of affected dogs for months to years. Because of local invasion, complete surgical resection is rarely possible, but biopsy is indicated if chemotherapy is contemplated. Effusion resulting from myocardial lymphoma often responds to pericardiocentesis and chemotherapy.

32. What is constrictive pericardial disease?

Constrictive pericardial disease occurs when visceral or parietal pericardial thickening and scarring restrict ventricular diastolic filling. Fusion of the parietal and visceral pericardial layers can occur and obliterate the pericardial space, or the visceral layer (epicardium) alone can be involved. Sometimes a small amount of pericardial effusion is present (constrictive-effusive pericarditis). Histologically, there is usually increased fibrous connective tissue and variable amounts of inflammatory and reactive infiltrates. The etiology of constrictive pericardial disease is often unknown. Acute inflammation with fibrin deposition and perhaps varying degrees of pericardial effusion are thought to precede the development of constrictive disease. Specific causes identified in some dogs include recurrent idiopathic hemorrhagic effusion, infectious pericarditis (e.g., actinomycosis, mycobacteriosis, coccidioidomycoses), metallic foreign bodies in the pericardium, tumors, and idiopathic osseous metaplasia or fibrosis of the pericardium.

With advanced constrictive disease, ventricular filling is essentially limited to early diastole before ventricular expansion is abruptly curtailed. Any further ventricular filling is accomplished only at high venous pressures. Compromised filling reduces cardiac output. Compensatory mechanisms of heart failure cause fluid retention, tachycardia, and vasoconstriction.

33. How do I diagnose constrictive pericardial disease?

Diagnosis of constrictive pericardial disease can be difficult. Clinical signs of right-sided congestive heart failure predominate and abdominal distention (ascites), dyspnea or tachypnea, tiring, syncope, weakness, and weight loss are common owner complaints. Occasionally, there is a history of pericardial effusion. As with cardiac tamponade, ascites and jugular venous distinction are the most consistent clinical findings. Weakened femoral pulses and muffled heart sounds are also found. An audible, diastolic pericardial knock, resulting from the abrupt deceleration of ventricular filling in early diastole has been described, but has not been commonly identified in dogs. A systolic murmur or click, probably caused by concurrent valvular disease, or a diastolic gallop sound may be heard.

Radiographic findings include mild-to-moderate cardiomegaly, pleural effusion, and caudal vena cava distension. Reduced cardiac motion may be evident on fluoroscopy. Constrictive pericardial disease can produce subtle but suggestive echocardiographic changes, such as flattening of the left ventricular free wall in diastole and abnormal septal motion. The pericardium may appear thickened and intensely echogenic, but differentiation of this from normal pericardial echogenicity may be difficult. ECG abnormalities have included sinus tachycardia, P wave prolongation, and small QRS complexes.

Invasive hemodynamic studies are the most diagnostic. Central venous pressures of higher than 15 mm Hg and high mean atrial and diastolic ventricular pressures are common. The classic early diastolic dip in ventricular pressure, followed by a middiastolic plateau, is not consistently seen in dogs with constrictive pericardial disease, however. Angiocardiography can be normal or it may reveal atrial and vena caval enlargement, and increased endocardial-pericardial distance.

34. How is constrictive pericardial disease treated?

Constrictive pericardial disease is treated by surgical pericardiectomy. The procedure is more likely to be successful if the parietal pericardium is involved only. Visceral pericardial involvement requires epicardial stripping, which increases the difficulty and associated complications of surgery. Pulmonary thrombosis (sometimes massive) is reported to be a relatively common postoperative complication. Tachyarrhythmias are another complication of surgery. Moderate doses of a diuretic may be helpful in the postoperative period. The usefulness of angiotensin-converting enzyme inhibition is unclear, but positive inotropic and arteriolar vasodilating drugs are not indicated. Without surgical intervention the disease is progressive, and ultimately fatal.

BIBLIOGRAPHY

Aronsohn M: Cardiac hemangiosarcoma in the dog: a review of 38 cases, *J Am Vet Med Assoc* 187:922-926, 1985.
Aronsohn MG, Carpenter JL: Surgical treatment of idiopathic pericardial effusion in the dog: 25 cases (1978-1993), *J Am Anim Hosp Assoc* 35:521-525, 1999.
Aronson LR, Gregory CR: Infectious pericardial effusion in five dogs, *Vet Surg* 24:402-407, 1995.
Berg J: Pericardial disease and cardiac neoplasia, *Semin Vet Med Surg* 9:185-191, 1994.
Berry CR, Lombarde CW, Hager DA et al: Echocardiographic evaluation of cardiac tamponade in dogs before and after pericardiocentesis: four cases (1984-1986), *J Am Vet Med Assoc* 192:1597-1603, 1988.
Bouvy BM, Bjorling DE: Pericardial effusion in dogs and cats. Part I. Normal pericardium and causes and pathophysiology of pericardial effusion, *Compend Contin Educ* 13:417-424, 1991.
Bouvy BM, Bjorling DE: Pericardial effusion in dogs and cats. Part II. Diagnostic approach and treatment, *Compend Contin Educ* 13:633-641, 1991.
Brisson BA, Holmberg DL: Use of pericardial patch graft reconstruction of the right atrium for treatment of hemangiosarcoma in a dog, *J Am Vet Med Assoc* 218:723-725, 2001.
Closa JM, Font A, Mascort J: Pericardial mesothelioma in a dog: long term survival after pericardiectomy in combination with chemotherapy, *J Sm Anim Pract* 40:383-386, 1999.
Dunning D, Monnet E, Orton CE et al: Analysis of prognostic indicators for dogs with pericardial effusion: 46 cases (1985-1996), *J Am Vet Med Assoc* 212:1276-1280, 1998.

Edwards NJ: The diagnostic value of pericardial fluid pH determination, *J Am Anim Hosp Assoc* 32:63-67, 1996.

Fine DM, Tobias AH, Jacob KA: The pH of pericardial effusion does not reliably distinguish between idiopathic and neoplastic effusions [abstract], *J Vet Intern Med* 15:282, 2001.

Jackson J, Richter KP, Launer DP: Thorascopic partial pericardiectomy in 13 dogs. *J Vet Intern Med* 13:529-533, 1999.

Kerstetter KK, Krahwinkel DJ, Millis DL et al: Pericardiectomy in dogs: 22 cases (1978-1994), *J Am Vet Med Assoc* 211:736-740, 1997.

Miller MW, Sisson DD: Pericardial disorders. In Ettinger SJ, Feldman EC, editors, *Textbook of veterinary internal medicine*, ed 5, Philadelphia, 2000, WB Saunders.

Sidley JA, Atkins CE, Keene BW et al: Percutaneous balloon pericardiotomy as a treatment for recurrent pericardial effusion in 6 dogs, *J Vet Intern Med* 16:541-546, 2002.

Sisson D, Thomas WP, Ruehl WW et al: Diagnostic value of pericardial fluid analysis in the dog, *J Am Vet Med Assoc* 184:51-55, 1984.

Thomas WP, Reed JR, Bauer TG et al: Constrictive pericardial disease in the dog, *J Am Vet Med Assoc* 184:546-553, 1984.

Thomas WP, Reed JR, Gomez JA: Diagnostic pneumopericardiography in dogs with spontaneous pericardial effusion. *Vet Radiol* 25:2-16, 1984.

Thomas WP, Sisson D, Bauer TG et al: Detection of cardiac masses in dogs by two-dimensional echocardiography, *Vet Radiol* 25:65-72, 1984.

Vicari ED, Brown DC, Holt DE et al: Survival times of and prognostic indicators for dogs with heart base masses: 25 cases (1986-1999), *J Am Vet Med Assoc* 219:485-487, 2001.

Wallace J, Mullen HS, Lesser MB: A technique for surgical correction of peritoneal pericardial diaphragmatic hernia in dogs and cats, *J Am Anim Hosp Assoc* 28:503-510, 1992.

Ware WA, Hopper DL: Cardiac tumors in dogs: 1982-1995, *J Vet Intern Med* 13:95-103, 1999.

Wright KN, DeNovo RC, Patton CS et al: Effusive-constrictive pericardial disease secondary to osseous metaplasia of the pericardium in a dog, *J Am Vet Med Assoc* 209:2091-2095, 1996.

8. Management of Heart Failure

Jonathon A. Abbott

1. What is heart failure?

Heart failure is a syndrome in which cardiac dysfunction results in clinical signs associated with venous congestion or reduced cardiac output. It is important to recognize that heart *failure* results from heart disease and that practically any heart disease can result in heart failure. Though the distinction between low-output (forward) failure and congestive (backward) failure is artificial, heart failure in animals usually takes the form of congestive heart failure (CHF). The clinical signs are primarily the result of the development of abnormally high systemic or, more often, pulmonary venous pressures. Left-sided CHF is typically characterized by the presence of pulmonary congestion and edema. Right-sided CHF is manifested as body cavity effusions, usually ascites, or peripheral edema.

2. What cardiac diseases are most likely to cause an emergent presentation of CHF?

Most heart diseases in dogs are chronic; despite this, it is common for clinical signs to develop suddenly. The reasons for this are varied. Pets are largely sedentary, and, consequently, sub-clinical heart disease can progress until a minimum of stress or exertion provokes signs of cardiac dysfunction. Additionally, subtle changes in respiratory rate and character are difficult for pet owners to recognize. Regardless, it is common for chronic disorders such as degenerative mitral valve disease and canine dilated cardiomyopathy to result in clinical signs that are apparently sudden in onset and necessitate emergent management. Such a presentation might be best described as decompensation rather than acute heart failure. There are, however, a few examples of truly acute CHF in dogs. Rupture of a first-order mitral valve chorda tendinea can result in sudden elevations of left atrial pressure and acute, left-sided CHF. Similarly, destruction of the aortic or mitral valve by an aggressive infective lesion can also cause acute heart failure. Regardless of the precise pathogenesis, the sudden development of cough or dyspnea related to heart failure is an important veterinary emergency.

3.   What historical findings are associated with acute or decompensated CHF?
Respiratory distress related to pulmonary edema is the most consistent historical finding in severe CHF. Syncope, lack of appetite, cough, and depression may also be part of the animal's medical history. With the exception of cardiac tamponade, which is discussed in Chapter 7, the onset of right-sided CHF is in general more insidious and less often prompts urgent veterinary evaluation.

4.   What findings are expected on physical examination?
The physical examination reflects the effects of diminished cardiac performance and increases in ventricular filling pressures. Often, the disease that has resulted in heart failure is also apparent on physical examination. Tachycardia is a relatively consistent finding. It is important to recognize that the respiratory sinus arrhythmia that is common in healthy dogs results partly from vagal influence. Vagal discharge is inhibited in heart failure and, as a result, the finding of a respiratory-related arrhythmia is virtually incompatible with a diagnosis of overt CHF.
On physical examination, elevated ventricular filling pressures are manifested as dyspnea resulting from pulmonary edema or pleural effusion. Crackles are often audible when pulmonary edema is present, whereas significant pleural effusion may muffle heart and lung sounds.
Auscultatory findings may reflect the disease that is responsible for the heart failure state. Dogs with CHF resulting from degenerative mitral valve disease invariably have a systolic murmur of mitral valve regurgitation; most often, the murmur is loud. Dogs with dilated cardiomyopathy may have more subtle physical examination findings, although careful auscultation often reveals a soft murmur of functional mitral incompetence and/or a gallop rhythm.

5.   How is a diagnosis of left-sided CHF made?
The clinical signs of left-sided heart failure and primary respiratory tract disease are superficially similar. Because aggressive diuretic therapy can be lifesaving in CHF but harmful in the setting of respiratory tract disease, an accurate diagnosis is essential. A noninvasive diagnosis of left-sided CHF can be made radiographically; left atrial enlargement in the presence of pulmonary opacities compatible with edema is diagnostic (Fig. 8-1). Sometimes, the fragile clinical status of the animal is an impediment to careful radiographic examination and the risk-benefit ratio is in favor of empirical therapy. In these cases, a careful assessment of the history and physical examination findings is essential. Before empirical therapy, it is important to determine that a diagnosis of acute CHF is at least plausible.
A long history of cough and dyspnea suggests that primary respiratory tract disease is at least partly responsible for the clinical signs, because animals with overt CHF are unlikely to survive for months without treatment.
Heart failure results from heart disease; therefore it is important to consider whether it is likely that the animal has a cardiac disorder that could reasonably result in heart failure. The most common acquired heart diseases that result in left-sided CHF in dogs are dilated cardiomyopathy and degenerative mitral valve disease; the former most commonly affects middle aged, large-breed dogs, whereas the latter affects elderly, small-breed dogs. If CHF is present in an elderly small-breed dog, the murmur is usually loud. Conversely, it is extremely unlikely for an elderly small-breed dog to develop CHF in the absence of a murmur; in these cases, signs such as cough and dyspnea are almost always the result of respiratory tract disease. Dogs with dilated cardio-

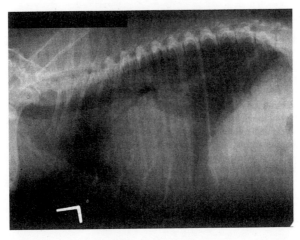

Figure 8-1. This lateral thoracic radiograph was obtained from a small-breed geriatric dog with congestive heart failure that resulted from degenerative mitral valve disease. The left atrium is enlarged, and there are pulmonary opacities that represent cardiogenic pulmonary edema.

myopathy may have relatively subtle auscultatory findings. In these instances, a soft murmur or a gallop rhythm may have great clinical importance.

6. What diagnostic studies are indicated when fulminant CHF is suspected?

Thoracic radiographs can provide a noninvasive diagnosis of left-sided CHF. When restraint for radiographic studies can be tolerated by the animal, thoracic radiographs guide the therapeutic approach. When available, echocardiography can provide useful information. Echocardiography cannot provide a diagnosis of CHF; however, echocardiography can be used to determine the cause of heart failure. Sometimes, a cursory echocardiographic examination can be performed using minimal restraint and this can be used to determine if the diagnosis of CHF is plausible.

7. What are the therapeutic goals in the management of acute or decompensated CHF?

The primary goals in the management of severe CHF are the restoration of normal ventilatory function and sometimes, augmentation of cardiac performance.

8. How do these goals differ from those in the management of chronic CHF?

The therapy of acute CHF is different from the therapy of chronic CHF in terms of method and intent. Evidence suggests that activation of compensatory neurohumoral mechanisms such as the adrenergic nervous system and the renin-angiotensin-aldosterone system play an important role in the progression of CHF; pharmacologic blunting of these mechanisms has been shown to improve long-term prognosis. For example, drug efficacy studies performed in people indicate that the long-term use of beta blockers has a cardioprotective effect despite the fact these drugs, at least acutely, can have a negative effect on cardiac performance. In contrast, the hemodynamic effect of therapy is of foremost importance in the management of acute CHF and specific therapeutic interventions can be classified based on their effect on the four primary determinants of cardiac output: preload, afterload, contractility, and heart rate.

9. How is preload manipulated in acute or decompensated CHF?

Preload is the force that distends the ventricle at end-diastole. It is approximated in the living animal by end-diastolic ventricular pressure or volume. Although end-diastolic left ventricular pressure can be estimated through the measurement of the pulmonary capillary wedge pressure, this is not routinely measured in small animals. However, the concept of preload and its pharmacologic manipulation is theoretically useful.

Cardiogenic pulmonary edema results when high mean atrial pressures are communicated to the pulmonary veins and capillaries. Diuretics cause animals to produce large volumes of urine; the administration of a powerful diuretic such as furosemide rapidly decreases intravascular volume and, therefore, preload. The consequent decrease in left atrial pressure alters the Starling forces at the level of the pulmonary capillary and facilitates the reabsorption of edema fluid.

Furosemide is a high-ceiling loop diuretic appropriate for use in the setting of fulminant CHF. Published furosemide doses vary widely and to a large extent the dose and dosing interval are dictated by clinical response. Intravenous doses in the range of 2 to 7 mg/kg in dogs are reasonable when faced with animals with fulminant CHF. The intravenous route is generally preferred when it can be obtained without imposing undue stress on the animal. Other diuretics such as the thiazides, spironolactone, and amiloride may have a role in the management of animals with chronic CHF; however, they have a weaker diuretic effect than does furosemide and see little use in the treatment of fulminant CHF.

10. How are nitrates used in the management of acute or decompensated CHF?

Nitrates such as nitroglycerin (NG) may have beneficial effects in severe CHF. These drugs cause dilation of capacitance veins and specific arterial beds through the release of nitric oxide. The clinical efficacy of NG in small animals is uncertain; however, based on what is known of its pharmacology, the administration of NG would be expected to decrease thoracic blood volume and therefore preload, limiting the accumulation of pulmonary edema.

The transdermal formulation of NG is used most often. Transdermal NG is available as a cream and as a controlled-dose adhesive patch. The former allows somewhat greater flexibility of dosing. In dogs, the dose is adjusted based on body weight; smaller dogs may receive $\frac{1}{4}$ inch of NG and large dogs as much as 1 inch. NG is commonly applied to the interior of the pinnae, although more central sites such as the inguinal area might lead to more rapid and reliable absorption.

11. How else can excessive preload be reduced?

Although it is seldom used, phlebotomy is an alternative means of rapidly decreasing preload. It has the obvious disadvantage that it results not only in the loss of intravascular fluid, but also in a loss of blood cells and proteins.

12. How does preload reduction affect cardiac performance?

Preload is related to cardiac performance through the Frank-Starling law of the heart; a decrease in preload diminishes the force of ventricular contraction and therefore decreases stroke volume. As a result, preload reduction generally results in a decrease in cardiac output. However, a few factors likely mitigate this effect in some cases.

Animals with systolic heart failure, for example, from mitral valve regurgitation or dilated cardiomyopathy have large ventricles and, potentially, a "flat" Frank-Starling relationship. That being the case, preload can be reduced until pulmonary vein pressures are low enough to prevent edema formation with little effect on stroke volume. When mitral valve regurgitation is the main factor that limits stroke volume, a reduction in preload can decrease mitral annular dilation, reduce valvular regurgitation, and conceivably increase stroke volume.

In general, preload reduction can be expected to have a negative effect on cardiac performance but this effect is buffered by a large ventricular volume. Animals that have dyspnea because of respiratory disease are likely to have normal or decreased ventricular filling pressures and therefore tolerate aggressive diuresis poorly.

13. How is afterload manipulated in systolic failure?

Resistance is the quantity that determines the amount of blood that flows through a vascular bed when subject to a given pressure. In a sense, resistance is a measure of how difficult it is to force blood through the vessels. Resistance is dependent on a number of factors, but the most important of these is vessel diameter because this factor is subject to physiologic influences and manipulation by vasodilating drugs.

Vascular resistance is an important determinant of blood pressure and therefore afterload. However, afterload is best approximated by wall stress, which is related not only to blood pressure, but also to ventricular diameter and wall thickness. If ventricular dilation is not offset by hypertrophy, afterload is increased even if blood pressure is normal. This is the case in animals with dilated cardiomyopathy; the dilated, thin-walled ventricle functions at a mechanical disadvantage because afterload is high even if blood pressure is normal.

In CHF, increases in adrenergic tone and vasoactive hormones such as angiotensin II result in vasoconstriction. In the short term, this has the favorable effect of maintaining systemic blood pressure when cardiac output is low. However, in animals with dilated, thin-walled ventricles, systolic wall stress (afterload) is elevated; this increase in afterload comes at the price of an increase in myocardial oxygen demand. When systolic myocardial failure is present, there is a mismatch between contractility and afterload. Judicious vasodilation reduces afterload, which permits an increase in stroke volume. When mitral valve regurgitation is the cause of CHF, there is an analogous mismatch between vascular resistance and the resistance imposed by the regurgitant orifice; the compensatory increase in vascular resistance is a factor that limits stroke volume.

Vasodilators are not indicated in systolic failure because systemic hypertension is present; rather, they are effective because they decrease vascular resistance and allow stroke volume to increase. The favorable effect of vasodilation is one of degree; excessive vasodilation results in hypotension in animals with systolic failure as it does in normal individuals.

14. What parenteral agent can be used to reduce afterload or vascular resistance in systolic failure?

Nitroprusside is a balanced vasodilator that has a pronounced effect on the systemic arterioles. Metabolism of nitroprusside is rapid and results in the release of cyanide and nitric oxide; the latter possesses vasodilatory properties. The agent is infused intravenously at a rate of 1 to 10 µg/kg/min. Nitroprusside is a potent vasodilator and should be used only in carefully monitored circumstances. Measurement of systemic blood pressure is recommended and the dose should be titrated based on serial blood pressure measurements and indices of peripheral perfusion. Cyanide toxicosis is a potential adverse effect associated with the use of this drug and it is suggested that the use of nitroprusside be limited to periods of less than 48 hours.

15. Are oral vasodilators useful in acute or decompensated CHF?

Angiotensin-converting enzyme (ACE) inhibitors are the oral vasodilators used most commonly in the management of CHF. However, the efficacy of these drugs has been demonstrated in chronic heart failure, not in the setting of acute cardiac decompensation. In fact, ACE inhibitors are not potent vasodilators and it is possible that many of the benefits of ACE inhibition are realized only after long-term use; further, these benefits are likely to result as much from reduced neuroendocrine activation as from the mechanical effect of vasodilation. In contrast, hydralazine is a potent vasodilator. Although the neuroendocrine activation that is associated with hydralazine administration is probably of lesser concern in fulminant CHF, the potency of hydralazine may represent a liability as this drug can cause clinically important hypotension.

The use of all oral vasodilators is problematic in that it can be difficult to titrate an oral drug according to effect and gastrointestinal absorption may be unpredictable in the critically ill animal. Vasodilators must always be administered with caution in animals with fulminant CHF.

16. Are inotropic drugs indicated in fulminant CHF?

When CHF is caused by dilated cardiomyopathy, the use of inotropic agents has an intuitive appeal. However, the role of inotropic support, at least for management of people with advanced heart failure, has recently been reevaluated. Inotropic therapy is certainly indicated for animals with severe heart failure that are hypotensive or that have prerenal azotemia. The value of inotropic support in less severely affected animals is uncertain.

17. Compare and contrast the available positive inotropes.

Positive inotropes act by increasing the availability of calcium within the sarcomere or by increasing the calcium sensitivity of the contractile apparatus. The positive inotropes that are used in the management of decompensated CHF fall into one of three pharmacologic categories. The digitalis glycosides include digoxin and digitoxin. The phosphodiesterase inhibitors that are used as positive inotropes are the bipyridine derivatives amrinone and milrinone. The other clinically useful inotropes are catecholamines or synthetic analogues of these hormones. Dopamine, dobutamine, and epinephrine fit in this category.

Digoxin can be administered intravenously or orally. The cardiac glycosides bind to and inhibit the Na/K pump of the cardiomyocyte. The resulting change in cellular tonicity increases intracellular calcium concentration that, in turn, increases the inotropic state. The digitalis glycosides also have autonomic effects that are likely favorable in the setting of CHF. However, the glycosides are relatively weak inotropes and the therapeutic index of these agents is low. They may be indicated in the chronic therapy of CHF, but have a limited role in the critical care setting.

Amrinone and milrinone are potent positive inotropes that also exert a vasodilatory effect. The action of these agents is mediated through inhibition of phosphodiesterase, an enzyme that catalyzes the breakdown of cAMP, an intracellular second messenger that has many effects, including elevation of the intracellular calcium concentration. Inhibition of phosphodiesterase results in an increase in cAMP. Clinical trials in people have not shown inotropes, other than possibly digitalis, to have a beneficial effect when given for extended periods. Consequently, these drugs are not available for oral administration and they must be administered by intravenous infusion. The increase in intracellular calcium concentration is potentially arrhythmogenic and electrocardiographic monitoring is recommended during administration.

Dobutamine and other catecholamine derivatives or analogues stimulate adrenergic receptors. These drugs must be administered by intravenous infusion. Dobutamine is a relatively selective agonist of beta-adrenergic receptors. In contrast, dopamine is referred to as a "flexible molecule" and can stimulate beta-adrenergic receptors, dopaminergic receptors, and alpha-adrenergic receptors. It should be noted that all catecholamine analogues lose receptor specificity at higher doses, causing alpha receptor–mediated vasoconstriction. It is therefore possible to increase peripheral vascular resistance to the animal's detriment using these drugs. The administration of dobutamine results in greater increases in stroke volume relative to increase in heart rate and for this and other reasons is superior to dopamine. Electrocardiographic monitoring is recommended during infusion of adrenergic agonists.

18. How is heart rate manipulated in severe CHF?

Tachycardia develops in most dogs with severe CHF. Partly, this results from the compensatory adrenergic nervous system activation that is a feature of heart failure. However, anxiety associated with the uncomfortable sensation of breathlessness likely contributes to the development of tachycardia and resolution of pulmonary edema is often accompanied by a return of the heart rate to normal or near normal. When CHF is present, pharmacologic control of physiologic tachycardia is rarely, if ever, indicated.

19. What is the role of oxygen supplementation?

The administration of supplemental oxygen is indicated when CHF is the cause of dyspnea. Animals with CHF are fragile and every effort should be made to limit stress and anxiety. An oxygen cage is a convenient method by which to increase the fraction of inspired oxygen; when tolerated, alternative methods include the use of a nasal cannula or face mask.

20. Should anxious animals with CHF be sedated?

Anxiety may increase respiratory rate and unnecessarily increase the work of breathing. Cautious sedation should therefore be considered for anxious animals with CHF. Morphine has an established role in the management of severe CHF in people and dogs. This drug reduces anxiety and as a favorable ancillary effect it results in venodilation; the latter serves to reduce pulmonary vein pressures facilitating the reabsorption of edema fluid. Morphine should be used cautiously because high doses result in central respiratory depression and can therefore worsen hypoxemia. Low doses of acepromazine, a phenothiazine that shares with morphine the potentially beneficial effect of vasodilation, can be considered as an alternative to opiates.

21. What about fluid therapy?

Except when a vehicle is required for the administration of medications, intravenous (IV) fluids should not be administered to animals with overt, left-sided CHF. In other, noncardiac causes of circulatory failure, the administration of IV fluids expands intravascular volume, increases preload, and, through the Frank-Starling law of the heart, improves cardiac performance. However, animals have cardiogenic pulmonary edema because of elevations in venous pressures; in a sense, preload is maximal and excessive. Therefore, when cardiogenic pulmonary edema is present, the administration of IV fluid is certain to worsen congestive signs and unlikely to provide the beneficial effects of increased cardiac output and renal blood flow expected in noncardiac disease. The cautious administration of IV or subcutaneous fluids can be considered for anorexic or dehydrated animals that have recovered from a bout of cardiogenic edema.

22. Does empirical therapy have a role? What response is expected when CHF is the cause of dyspnea?

In some animals with severe dyspnea, the risk associated with restraint for diagnostic evaluation cannot be justified and empiric therapy is reasonable. When physical and historical findings suggest a diagnosis of fulminant CHF, parenteral furosemide is administered with careful monitoring of clinical response. When cardiogenic pulmonary edema is the cause of dyspnea, the response to brisk diuresis is usually prompt and dramatic. Failure to respond to one or two doses of furosemide suggests that the presumptive diagnosis of CHF is incorrect, or possibly that the animal is refractory to conservative medical management. When response is poor, the risk-benefit ratio associated with diagnostic evaluation may shift so that physical or chemical restraint for diagnostic procedures can be justified. Prolonged and aggressive diuretic therapy can result in clinical deterioration in cases in which respiratory disease is actually responsible for clinical signs.

23. Suggest a protocol for the management of severe systolic failure.

- Supplemental oxygen
- Cage rest
- Morphine for anxious animals
- Furosemide (with or without nitroglycerin) administered based on clinical status and response

Most animals that are destined to survive an episode of acute, severe CHF are likely to do so with conservative therapy of this sort. In cases in which a definitive diagnosis of the disease responsible for CHF has been established, ancillary therapy might include: nitroprusside and, in some cases, concurrent dobutamine administration.

24. What monitoring is appropriate for an animal with acute or severe CHF?

Animals with CHF are fragile and the relative risk-benefit ratio of manipulation for diagnostic procedures must be carefully considered. Invasive monitoring including the placement of a Swan-Ganz catheter and an arterial cannula provides nearly complete hemodynamic information that can be used to modify therapy. However, complete instrumentation such as this requires intensive nursing care, is difficult to maintain, is expensive, and of uncertain benefit.

The use of indirect blood pressure measurement devices can provide useful information if the limitations of these techniques are recognized. Systemic blood pressure is a valuable measure because it is known that a mean perfusion pressure of about 60 mm Hg is necessary to maintain the viability of vital capillary beds in the brain and kidney. However, blood pressure is not a measure of flow and it is possible for blood pressure to be maintained at the expense of cardiac output. The measurement of central venous pressure can provide useful information and the technique is relatively easy. However, central venous pressure is a measure of right ventricular filling pressure; it does not provide information about pulmonary venous pressure when left ventricular dysfunction is present.

Despite the availability of numerous relatively elaborate monitoring techniques, most animals with severe CHF can be managed with careful attention to the vital signs. Monitoring of heart rate, respiratory rate and character, assessment of femoral arterial pulse, and observation of the mucous membranes provide invaluable information regarding response to therapy and short-term prognosis.

25. How does chronic CHF differ from acute (or decompensated) heart failure?

Unfortunately, the improvement in clinical status that accompanies elimination of pulmonary edema does not signal recovery from the syndrome of heart failure. The complex neuroendocrine responses that comprise the syndrome of CHF persist despite resolution of clinical signs. The term *overt CHF* is used to refer to animals that have clinical signs such as dyspnea or cough resulting from pulmonary edema. Animals with chronic heart failure have persistent cardiac dysfunction that has at some time resulted in signs of pulmonary or systemic congestion.

26. What is meant by neuroendocrine activation?

The compensatory response to diminished cardiac performance involves the activation of the adrenergic, or sympathetic, nervous system and the release of renin from the kidney. The former serves to provide inotropic and chronotropic support for the failing heart. Additionally, elevations in adrenergic tone result in vasoconstriction; this increases systemic vascular resistance, which allows maintenance of normal systemic blood pressure when cardiac output is low. Through an enzymatic cascade, the release of renin results in the elaboration of angiotensin II. Angiotensin II is not only a potent vasoconstrictor, it also induces the release of aldosterone and antidiuretic hormone and potentiates the activity of the adrenergic nervous system. Together, these effects result in vasoconstriction and contribute to the renal retention of salt and water. These responses observed in animals with cardiac dysfunction represent neuroendocrine activation. The results of clinical trials using people and animals suggest that the renin-angiotensin-aldosterone system (RAAS) and the adrenergic nervous system contribute to the progressive nature of CHF; from this, the concept of CHF as a neuroendocrine or neurohumoral syndrome has evolved.

27. How does the management of chronic heart failure differ from the management of acute or decompensated CHF?

Evidence suggests that the activation of compensatory mechanisms such as the adrenergic nervous system and the RAAS plays an important role in the progression of CHF; tempering these responses with drug therapy has been shown to improve long-term prognosis. In fact, drug efficacy studies performed in people demonstrate that long-term use of beta blockers has a cardioprotective effect despite the fact that these drugs can have a negative effect on cardiac performance in the short term. Thus the treatment of animals with chronic CHF is aimed not only at the elimination of clinical signs, but also at modifying the maladaptive compensatory responses associated with chronic cardiac dysfunction.

28. Why is the RAAS important in the management of chronic systolic failure?

The RAAS is activated when cardiac performance declines. Its endocrine products result in vasoconstriction and the renal retention of salt and water. In systolic failure, pharmacologic interference with this system through the use of ACE inhibitors results in vasodilation and a favorable decrease in afterload. ACE inhibitors were the first drugs subject to comparison with a placebo to demonstrate a favorable effect on mortality in people with CHF. Since that time, the efficacy of the ACE inhibitor enalapril has been shown in dogs with CHF from acquired valvular disease and dilated cardiomyopathy. That activation of the RAAS in heart failure has important implications was suggested by a therapeutic trial that compared a combination of hydralazine and isosorbide dinitrate with enalapril in people with CHF. Despite the fact that the hydralazine had the predicted beneficial effects on stroke volume, mortality was lower in the group receiving enalapril.

At least initially, the effects of the RAAS are likely to be positive; they help to maintain blood pressure and cardiac output. However, there is strong evidence that chronic activation of the RAAS contributes to the progressive nature of CHF. In people with CHF, markers of RAAS activation are associated with a poor prognosis but ACE inhibitors, which blunt the effect of the RAAS, reduce mortality. It is therefore likely that RAAS activation itself has a detrimental effect in chronic CHF.

29. If activation of the RAAS is "maladaptive," why is it tolerated by natural selection?

The RAAS and adrenergic nervous system have been preserved by evolution because they are well suited to the short-term maintenance of circulatory function. The neuroendocrine responses observed in heart failure are similar to those that result from acute hemorrhage. The effects of the RAAS and adrenergic nervous system are favorable when the cause of decreased cardiac performance is of short duration because vasoconstriction and sodium retention allow survival of acute circulatory embarrassment. Provided the cause of decreased cardiac performance resolves, homeostasis is restored and the compensatory mechanisms are again "turned off."

30. ACE inhibitors have demonstrated efficacy in the management of acquired valvular disease and dilated cardiomyopathy in dogs. Why are they thought to be superior to other vasodilators such as hydralazine?

Hydralazine is a more potent vasodilator than are the ACE inhibitors, and hydralazine is superior to the ACE inhibitors in terms of acute effects on cardiac performance. However, hydralazine results in reflex-mediated increases in adrenergic tone and activation of the RAAS, and this is probably the reason that clinical trials in people with CHF have demonstrated greater mortality reduction with the use of ACE inhibitors. That survival studies demonstrate the superiority of ACE inhibitors over a more potent and seemingly effective vasodilator underscores the importance of the RAAS in the pathogenesis of CHF. It should be recognized that the clinical trial that compared hydralazine with ACE inhibitors was performed in people who suffered from systolic myocardial dysfunction. Whether ACE inhibitors are in fact superior to hydralazine in animals with mitral valve disease is not known.

31. Do beta-adrenergic antagonists have a role in the management of systolic failure?

On a short-term basis, beta-adrenergic antagonists slow heart rate and decrease contractility. That these drugs might be beneficial to animals with systolic myocardial dysfunction is counterintuitive. However, recent clinical trials demonstrate that long-term use of beta blockers has favorable effects on morbidity and mortality in people with systolic myocardial dysfunction. The reason for the improvement in clinical status and reduction in mortality is not known; it is likely that beta blockers protect the heart from the toxic effect of persistently elevated adrenergic tone. Caution must be exercised in extrapolating this encouraging information to the treatment of animals with heart failure. Animals are generally presented for veterinary evaluation with advanced myocardial dysfunction; some of these animals may be critically dependent on elevated adrenergic tone in order to maintain cardiac output and blood pressure. When this is the case, the negatively inotropic effects of beta blockers can have catastrophic results.

32. Diuretics are a mainstay in the management of acute CHF; do they have a role in chronic CHF?

Diuretics most definitely have a role in the management of chronic CHF. The common acquired heart diseases in dogs result in progressive cardiac dysfunction and a persistent sodium-retaining state. While overly aggressive diuretic use can decrease cardiac performance and contribute to activation of the RAAS, most dogs with chronic CHF require lifelong diuretic therapy.

33. How is digoxin different from other positive inotropes?

Digoxin is a positive inotrope that has clinically important effects on the autonomic nervous system. The positive inotropic effect is mediated through increases in intracellular calcium concentration that result from paralysis of the cellular sodium-potassium pump. The autonomic effects of digoxin are diverse, but include increases in arterial baroreceptor sensitivity. In general, digoxin increases vagal tone and decreases sympathetic outflow; in so doing, digoxin slows the heart rate. Thus digoxin is unique among inotropes in that it slows the heart rate; this feature of digoxin may limit myocardial oxygen demand and partly explain the beneficial effects of this drug. On the basis of clinical studies performed in people, the long-term effects of digoxin are favorable; digoxin improves clinical status and decreases hospitalization because of worsening congestion. Although the effect of digoxin on mortality is neutral, this is in contrast to the negative effect on long-term survival that has been observed when other positive inotropes have been evaluated in people with heart failure. For this reason, it has been suggested that the beneficial effect of digoxin results not from inotropy but rather from the autonomic "sparing" effect of the drug.

34. What is pimobendan? Does it have a role in the management of canine heart failure?

Pimobendan is a drug that inhibits phosphodiesterase and, through an unknown mechanism, increases the calcium sensitivity of the contractile apparatus. These effects result in an increase in contractility and vasodilation placing pimobendan in a group of drugs known as "inodilators." A clinical trial compared pimobendan with placebo in Cocker Spaniels and Doberman Pinschers with heart failure from dilated cardiomyopathy. The sample size was relatively small, but the beneficial effect of pimobendan was quite pronounced in Doberman Pinschers. This drug is currently licensed in Europe, Canada, and Australia for the management of heart failure in dogs. Clinical evaluation in the United States is under way.

35. What about diet in CHF?

CHF is a clinical syndrome that is associated with renal retention of salt and water, and so dietary salt restriction has long been an aspect of its medical management. The availability of potent diuretics and ACE inhibitors has perhaps decreased the importance of dietary sodium manipulation. However, decreased salt intake has a preload-reducing effect and moderate salt restriction is reasonable for animals with chronic CHF.

36. Furosemide is the diuretic that is used most commonly in CHF; are any others important?

Evidence indicates that spironolactone, an aldosterone antagonist, decreases morbidity and mortality in human patients with CHF who are receiving a combination of an ACE inhibitor and loop diuretic. Interestingly, this favorable effect was evident at a dose of spironolactone that did not cause diuresis. This is probably explained by the extrarenal effects of aldosterone. Although this hormone stimulates the renal retention of sodium and water, it also promotes the development of myocardial fibrosis.

37. What is the prognosis?
Ultimately, the prognosis of animals with CHF is poor; unless the cause of heart failure can be identified and remedied, CHF is terminal and survival of 4 to 8 months is typical even with palliative medical therapy.

38. Is there anything new on the horizon for the treatment of heart failure?
In recent years, much attention has been directed toward the pharmacologic manipulation of the neuroendocrine responses that characterize CHF. The use of ACE inhibitors is well established, and, at least in people, beta-adrenergic blockade now plays an important role in the management of chronic heart failure. Blunting of other hormonal responses to impaired cardiac performance might also have promise.

Plasma levels of endothelin and arginine vasopressin are both elevated in the setting of heart failure. Endothelin is a potent endogenous vasoconstrictor. Arginine vasopressin, also known as antidiuretic hormone, is a vasoconstrictor that contributes to the renal retention of solute-free water. The clinical importance of these hormones in the pathogenesis of heart failure is not certain; however, it may be that agents that antagonize their effects would benefit animals with CHF. The preliminary results of clinical trials that examined the efficacy of endothelin antagonists in human patients with heart failure were not promising. Arginine vasopressin antagonists are in the investigational stage.

Atrial natriuretic peptide and related hormones, such as brain natriuretic peptide, are released in response to atrial and ventricular stretch; they contribute to vasodilation and renal sodium excretion. In a sense, they have effects that oppose those of RAAS and adrenergic nervous system. In CHF, the effect of the natriuretic peptides is overwhelmed by neuroendocrine responses that result in vasoconstriction and sodium retention. However, there might be a therapeutic role for agents that can increase the activity of these apparently "favorable" hormones. Antagonists of neutral endopeptidase, an enzyme that inactivates atrial natriuretic peptide and brain natriuretic peptide, have been used experimentally in canine heart failure and shown a promising effect.

CONTROVERSY

39. Are positive inotropes useful in the management of CHF?
In animals with chronic CHF resulting from dilated cardiomyopathy, it seems reasonable that an effective positive inotrope would improve cardiac performance and therefore reduce mortality. However, clinical trials conducted in people do not uphold this supposition. For example, the administration of milrinone, a potent positive inotrope, increased mortality in people with CHF from systolic myocardial dysfunction. Other positive inotropes including xamoterol and vesnarinone have had detrimental effects when administered over long periods to people with CHF. In fact, the only positive inotrope that has been shown to have positive long-term effects in people is digoxin, and it is possible that the favorable effects of this drug are related as much to its autonomic effects as its inotropic property. The reason that positive inotropes are potentially harmful is not known, but it might relate to metabolic cost of increased contractility. Inotropes generally increase myocardial oxygen demand, which may hasten the deterioration of cardiac function. However, the lesson from numerous clinical trials conducted in people is apparently clear: in the long term, inotropes other than digoxin are harmful and effective therapies for heart failure are ones that "spare the heart" by blunting the effects of neuroendocrine activation.

The extrapolation of conclusions drawn from studies of people to animals must always be undertaken with caution, however. Although the effect of milrinone on mortality in animals with CHF is not known, this drug has been shown to improve clinical signs in dogs with dilated cardiomyopathy. More recently, published evidence suggests that pimobendan decreases mortality in some dogs with CHF resulting from dilated cardiomyopathy. Why positive inotropes may have different effects in people and animals is unclear, although it might relate to severity of myocardial dysfunction that is observed in animals; dogs with dilated cardiomyopathy typically have advanced myocardial dysfunction. Perhaps in these cases it is more important to preserve cardiac performance than it is to "spare" the heart. Additionally, many dogs with CHF are euthanized before they die of progressive pump failure. Treatments that reliably improve clinical signs might cause owners to delay euthanasia, which could partly explain mortality reduction associated with the administration of positive inotropes such as pimobendan.

BIBLIOGRAPHY

Braunwald E, Colucci WS: Pathophysiology of heart failure. In Braunwald E, editor: *Heart disease: a textbook of cardiovascular medicine*, ed 4, Philadelphia, WB Saunders, 1997.

Cleland JGF, Bristow MR, Erdmann E et al: Beta-blocking agents in heart failure: should they be used and how? *Eur Heart J* 17:1629-1639, 1996.

Cody RJ: Hormonal alterations in heart failure. In Hosenpud JD, Greenberg BH, editors: *Congestive heart failure: pathophysiology, diagnosis, and approach to management*, ed 2, Philadelphia, 2000, Lippincott Williams & Wilkins.

The COVE Study Group: Controlled clinical evaluation of enalapril in dogs with heart failure: results of the Cooperative Veterinary Enalapril Study Group, *J Vet Intern Med* 9:243-252, 1995.

The Digitalis Investigation Group: The effect of digoxin on mortality and morbidity in patients with heart failure, *N Engl J Med* 336:525-533, 1997.

Gheorghiade M, Pitt B: Digitalis Investigation Group (DIG) trial: a stimulus for further research, *Am Heart J* 134:3-12, 1997.

Hamlin RL: Pathophysiology of the failing heart. In Fox PR, Sisson D, Moise NS, editors: *Textbook of canine and feline cardiology: principles and clinical practice*, ed 2, Philadelphia, 1999, WB Saunders.

Keene BW, Rush JE: Therapy of heart failure. In Ettinger SJ and Feldman EC, editors: *Textbook of veterinary internal medicine*, ed 4, Philadelphia, 1993, WB Saunders.

Kittleson MD: Management of heart failure. In Kittleson MD, Kienle RD, editors: *Small animal cardiovascular medicine*, St Louis, 1998, Mosby.

Kittleson MD: Pathophysiology of heart failure. In Kittleson MD, Kienle RD, editors: *Small animal cardiovascular medicine*, St Louis, 1998, Mosby.

Knight DH: Efficacy of inotropic support of the failing heart, *Vet Clin North Am Small Anim Pract* 21:879-904, 1991.

Luis Fuentes V, Kleeman R, Justus C et al: The effect of the novel inodilator pimobendan on heart failure status in cocker spaniels and dobermans with idiopathic dilated cardiomyopathy [abstract], *Proc Br Small Anim Vet Assoc Congress*, Birmingham, UK, 1998.

Nohria A, Lewis E, Stevenson LW: Medical management of advanced heart failure, *J Am Med Assoc* 287 628-640, 2002.

Packer M, Cohn JN, editor: Consensus recommendations for the management of chronic heart failure, *Am J Cardiol* 83:1A-38A, 1999.

Packer M, Bristow MR, Cohn JN et al: The effect of carvedilol on morbidity and mortality in patients with chronic heart failure, *N Engl J Med* 334:1349-1355, 1996.

Pitt B, Zannad F, Remme WJ et al: The effect of spironolactone on morbidity and mortality in patients with severe heart failure, *N Engl J Med* 341:709-717, 1999.

Sabbah HN, Shimoyama H, Kono T et al: Effects of long-term monotherapy with enalapril, metoprolol, and digoxin on the progression of left ventricular dysfunction and dilation in dogs with reduced ejection fraction, *Circulation* 89:2852-2859, 1994.

Sisson D, Kittleson MD: Management of heart failure: principles of treatment, therapeutic strategies and pharmacology. In Fox PR, Sisson D, Moise NS, editors: *Textbook of canine and feline cardiology: principles and clinical practice*, ed 2, Philadelphia, 1999, WB Saunders.

Ware WA, Keene BW: Outpatient management of chronic heart failure. In Bonagura JD, editor: *Kirk's current veterinary therapy XIII: small animal practice*, Philadelphia, 2000, WB Saunders.

9. Congenital Heart Disease

Jonathon A. Abbott

1. What is congenital heart disease (CHD)?

Congenital means present at birth. In canine medicine, congenital heart disease is essentially synonymous with cardiac malformation or "heart defect".

2. What causes congenital heart disease?

The cause of CHD is largely unknown. In occasional cases, teratogenic factors such as maternal infectious disease might play a role. However, distinct breed predispositions for the development of some malformations are recognized and in these cases, a genetic basis for CHD is suspected or has been established.

3. What is the evidence for a genetic cause for CHD?

CHD is most common in purebred dogs and many specific malformations have an obvious familial distribution. In some cases, breeding experiments have demonstrated that the malformation is genetically transmitted; on the basis of these studies, the mode of inheritance is known or suspected for some forms of CHD.

Interpretation of breed predisposition data must be undertaken with care. In some cases, apparent breed predispositions that do not take into account breed popularity have been reported in the literature. For example, German Shepherds have occasionally been reported to be at increased risk for patent ductus arteriosus (PDA) because they have been "overrepresented" in case series of dogs with PDA. However, the relatively high frequency with which PDA is diagnosed in German Shepherds, is partly due to the popularity of the breed. One way of overcoming the confounding influence of breed popularity is use of a statistic known as the odds ratio. Buchanan (see Bibliography), has reported odds ratios for heart disease in various breeds of dogs.

In a few cases, breeding experiments have demonstrated heritability of specific lesions. This is the case for subaortic stenosis in the Newfoundland, for PDA in Miniature Poodles, for pulmonic stenosis in Beagles, and for a spectrum of conotruncal defects in Keeshonden. In this last breed, it has recently been shown that conotruncal defects—meaning developmental abnormalities of ventricular outflow and the great vessels that include tetralogy of Fallot—are associated with a single genetic mutation.

4. What is the clinical relevance of breed predispositions in the management of CHD?

It is noteworthy that every published report of a breeding experiment in purebred dogs with CHD supports heritability of the malformation. So, despite the fact that a breed predisposition is not itself evidence of genetic transmission, it is probably appropriate to assume that all familial CHD in dogs has a genetic basis. It is therefore reasonable to advise against breeding any dog affected by CHD. A breed predisposition for development of a specific congenital cardiac malformation, even a very strong one, is not a substitute for a specific diagnosis. In some ways then, breed predispositions are most helpful to dog breeders and those who counsel them.

5. What are the clinical signs of CHD?

With few exceptions, animals with CHD have cardiac murmurs, and these are typically heard on auscultation, usually in a pup presented for routine evaluation and immunization. Of the few clinically consequential malformations that do not usually result in a heart murmur, most cause other clinical signs such as cyanosis, exercise intolerance, respiratory distress, or failure to thrive.

6. Of what value is the medical history in the evaluation of animals with CHD?

As in all areas of clinical veterinary medicine, a carefully elicited medical history can provide diagnostically useful information. However, most animals with CHD are free of clinical signs when the defect is first identified. Unfortunately, the absence of clinical signs is no assurance that the malformation lacks clinical importance. Therefore further diagnostic evaluation is recommended for all animals with physical findings that suggest CHD.

7. What procedures are used to diagnose CHD?

Not many years ago, cardiac catheterization was the primary procedure for antemortem diagnosis of CHD. Although angiographic and manometric data obtained from catheterization studies remain a gold standard of sorts, echocardiography has become widespread and has largely replaced diagnostic cardiac catheterization. More specifically, Doppler echocardiography, which provides information regarding the velocity, direction, and character of blood flow, allows noninvasive diagnosis of almost all forms of CHD. Other noninvasive procedures such as diagnostic radiography and electrocardiography generally provide ancillary information. A definitive diagnosis of CHD generally requires a complete Doppler echocardiographic study performed by a trained individual.

8. How is CHD treated?

Treatment of specific malformations is determined by the pathophysiology that results from the lesion. In general, CHD imposes an abnormal mechanical load—a pressure overload, volume overload, or both—on the malformed segments. Treatment is most appropriately mechanical and includes operative procedures that result in either palliation or definitive correction of the malformation. Some malformations such as PDA and some forms of pulmonic stenosis are amenable to surgical correction without cardiopulmonary bypass (CPB); unfortunately, however, CPB is required for definitive correction of most congenital cardiac lesions. Recently, interventional catheterization techniques have at least partly supplanted surgery in the management of CHD.

9. What is cardiopulmonary bypass (CPB)?

Cardiopulmonary bypass (CPB) is an extracardiac technique to circulate and oxygenate the blood. Because the heart is not included in the circuit—is bypassed—CPB allows a surgeon to perform open-heart procedures. The necessary instrumentation is relatively expensive and application of the technique requires considerable expertise. For these reasons, CPB is not widely practiced in veterinary surgery. A few institutions have programs that offer CPB in the surgical management of canine patients with congenital heart disease.

10. What is interventional cardiac catheterization?

Cardiac catheterization refers to manipulating catheters within the cardiovascular system. Most cardiac catheterization procedures are performed under fluoroscopic guidance. Angiographic, manometric, and oximetric data can be collected with this technique. Beginning in the 1960s pediatric cardiologists devised ways to use intravascular catheters to treat cardiovascular disease, and many of these so-called interventional cardiac catheterization techniques have been modified for clinical use in dogs. Balloon catheter dilation of pulmonic stenosis is widely practiced, and various techniques for transcatheter occlusion of a PDA have been described. The applicability of interventional techniques is somewhat limited by the availability of fluoroscopy and veterinarians with expertise in these techniques, but despite this, transcatheter intervention for CHD has become routine.

11. What forms of CHD are most common?

Patent ductus arteriosus (PDA), subvalvular aortic stenosis (SAS), pulmonic stenosis (PS), and ventricular septal defect (VSD) are the most common congenital malformations in the dog. Other lesions such as atrial septal defect, atrioventricular valve dysplasia, and various forms of cyanotic heart disease are relatively uncommon.

12. What causes PDA?

The ductus arteriosus, or arterial duct, is a blood vessel that forms during embryonic development and provides a communication between the systemic and pulmonary circulations. It arises from the proximal descending aorta and courses cranioventrally, where it joins the dorsal aspect of the main pulmonary artery. In utero the duct provides a means for fetal blood to skirt the pulmonary capillary bed. Although the precise mechanisms are incompletely understood, in mammals, postnatal increases in oxygen tension result in a prostaglandin cascade that causes contraction of the muscular layer of the ductus arteriosus and closure of the duct. The process begins immediately after birth and in most species is complete within 3 to 4 days. In some animals, closure of the duct does not occur or is incomplete, and the vessel is then known as a patent ductus arteriosus (PDA).

13. Trace the pattern of blood flow in a dog with a PDA; what are the pathophysiologic consequences of the PDA?

In a newborn with a PDA, if pulmonary vascular resistance falls appropriately after birth, blood can cross the duct from the high-pressure/high-resistance systemic circulation to enter the low-resistance pulmonary circulation. Therefore some of the blood pumped by the left ventricle into the aorta exits the aorta through the PDA and enters the main pulmonary artery. From here, the shunted aortic blood together with the systemic venous return is conveyed to the lungs and then, through the pulmonary veins, to the left atrium and ventricle. The volume of blood that is shunted from the aorta through the PDA to augment the pulmonary venous return increases the volume of blood entering the left atrium and subsequently the left ventricle. So, despite the fact that the shunt direction is "left-to-right", a PDA imposes a volume overload on the left atrium and left ventricle.

14. What is the pathogenesis of heart failure due to PDA?

When pulmonary vascular resistance is normal, the direction in which blood is shunted through a PDA is from left to right. The increase in pulmonary venous return results in left ventricular dilation and hypertrophy; the degree of cardiac enlargement is roughly proportional to the proportion of blood that is shunted through the PDA. The volume load on the left heart can cause diastolic pressures within the left ventricle to rise, and this pressure elevation is reflected back upon the pulmonary venous circulation. If pulmonary venous pressures become sufficiently high, fluid is forced out of the pulmonary capillaries and pulmonary edema results. Therefore left-sided congestive heart failure is a potential consequence of a left-to-right PDA.

15. What signalment is typical for dogs with PDA?

PDA is observed most commonly in small-breed dogs such as Miniature Poodles, Maltese, Bichon Frises, and Pomeranians. Females are affected more often than males, with a ratio of about 2.5 to 1. The lesion is usually detected early in life, often during the first routine veterinary visit. A typical signalment for a dog with a PDA would be a 3-month-old, female Pomeranian.

16. What findings are expected on auscultation?

A continuous murmur heard over the left craniodorsal aspect of the heart base is the auscultatory hallmark of a PDA. The murmur is often but not always loud and is usually relatively coarse; it peaks in intensity at or about the second heart sound and then fades during diastole.

This murmur is sometimes referred to as a *machinery* murmur. Continuous murmurs must be distinguished from to-and-fro or "bellows" murmurs, which consist of separate systolic and diastolic murmurs. In dogs, to-and-fro murmurs most commonly result from endocarditis of the aortic valve or ventricular septal defects that are complicated by aortic valve regurgitation.

Careful auscultation of the dog with a PDA may also reveal a systolic murmur over the left cardiac apex. This murmur is due to functional mitral valve regurgitation; that is, the cause is mitral valve regurgitation that results from distortion of the mitral apparatus associated with ventricular dilation, and not a structural abnormality of the mitral leaflets. In dogs with a large PDA, a third heart sound that reflects high transmitral flow rates and probably reduced ventricular compliance may result in a gallop rhythm.

17. How does a PDA affect the femoral arterial pulse?

In a dog with a PDA, the femoral arterial pulse is brisk or bounding, sometimes described as a "water-hammer" pulse. The amplitude or strength of the femoral arterial pulse reflects the difference between systolic and diastolic pressures, which is called the pulse pressure. With a PDA, the low-resistance pulmonary circulation provides a sink for diastolic "run-off". As a result, diastolic pressures tend to be abnormally low and the pulse pressure is wide.

18. What echocardiographic findings are associated with a PDA?

In animals with moderate or large PDAs (left-to-right shunts), dilation and hypertrophy of the left ventricle is evident echocardiographically (Fig. 9-1). Echocardiographic examination also demonstrates left atrial enlargement. Myocardial dysfunction, reflected in a large end-systolic ventricular dimension and often a low fractional shortening index, is sometimes evident. Direct visualization of the PDA is usually possible when the study is performed by an experienced echocardiographer. The PDA extends from the descending aorta to the bifurcation of the main pulmonary artery. It is best demonstrated by a cranial left parasternal image of the pulmonary artery bifurcation.

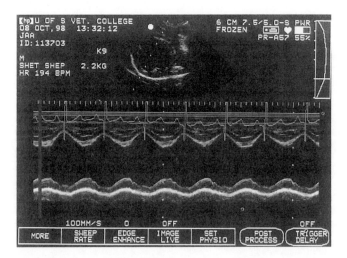

Figure 9-1. M-mode echocardiographic image obtained from an 8-week-old male Shetland Sheepdog. M-mode echocardiography provides a one-dimensional view of the heart; the ordinate measures distance from the transducer and the abscissa, time. The two-dimensional image from which this M-mode was derived is shown in the inset. The left ventricle is moderately dilated and systolic performance is normal.

Doppler flow studies are used to confirm that blood from a PDA flows into the main pulmonary artery. In animals with a PDA, this will be evident on color-flow Doppler studies as a diastolic color mosaic that originates near the pulmonary artery bifurcation and extends retrograde toward the pulmonic valve. In many cases, the jet extends beyond the pulmonic valve and results in mild pulmonic regurgitation. On spectral Doppler studies, continuously disturbed flow will be evident within the pulmonary artery (Fig. 9-2).

Additional findings detected by Doppler studies in a dog with a PDA include mitral valve regurgitation. When a substantial shunt is present, aortic flow velocities are often higher than normal. This does not necessarily reflect aortic obstruction but rather a larger left ventricular stroke volume.

19. Is echocardiography required for the diagnosis of PDA?

PDA is essentially a physical diagnosis. When a continuous murmur is present in a dog with a typical signalment, the cause is almost always a PDA. However, Doppler echocardiographic examination is recommended as a noninvasive means of confirming the diagnosis. The echocardiographic evaluation of systolic function may also provide prognostic information that can influence therapy (see Fig. 9-3). Additionally, echocardiography provides a noninvasive means of detecting concurrent cardiac defects that might have an impact on prognosis and management.

20. How is a PDA treated?

Traditionally, a PDA was treated by thoracotomy and surgical ligation of the duct. More recently, the interventional catheterization technique of transcatheter coil occlusion has been used as a minimally invasive alternative to surgery.

21. What is transcatheter ductal occlusion?

Recently, interventional cardiac catheterization techniques have been used in the management of animals with PDA. Various methods have been used, usually first in children and then in dogs. Most commonly, the ductus is occluded by the transcatheter placement of a thrombogenic coil

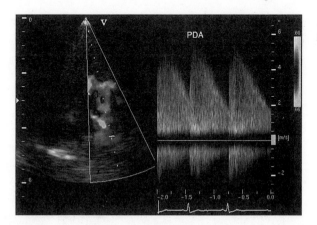

Figure 9-2. Continuous-wave Doppler echocardiographic study performed with the ultrasound beam directed through the patent duct of 16-month-old female Maltese dog. There is a high-velocity jet directed toward the transducer and into the main pulmonary artery. The signal is continuous, but the velocity peak occurs at about the T-wave of the electrocardiogram; this event corresponds to the second heart sound and the Doppler profile provides a graphic depiction of the dog's continuous murmur.

(e.g., Gianturco coils). Gianturco coils are available in various sizes and are supplied in straight, thin, tubular cartridges that facilitate their entry into cardiac catheters. The coils consist of metal with tufts of polyethylene terephthalate fiber (Dacron) that confer thrombogenicity; the coils have "structural memory" and when they are released from the cartridge or catheter, they form a predetermined number of loops.

Many variations of the basic technique for coil placement have been described. However, access to the PDA is commonly gained by a retrograde approach with the femoral artery. An appropriately sized catheter is placed by fluoroscopic guidance across the ductus. The coil or coils are then deployed through this catheter into the PDA (Fig. 9-3). When the procedure is successful, occlusion is rapid and complete.

22. What surgical techniques are used to treat a PDA?

Surgical techniques to treat a PDA involve ligation of the PDA through a left lateral thoracotomy incision. The conventional surgical approach to ductal ligation involves blunt dissection of the medial aspect of the PDA. Dissection is performed with forceps that are held parallel to the transverse plane of the ductus; the forceps are used to grasp the suture material, which is used to ligate and occlude the PDA.

Jackson and Henderson described an alternative surgical technique. Their method involves dissection of the medial aspect of the proximal aorta through a left lateral thoracotomy incision. A double length of suture material is placed around the ductus by manipulating a pair of blunt hemostats, one placed cranial and one caudal to the ductus. This technique requires less blunt dissection of the medial aspect of the DA and might therefore be safer.

23. What is the prognosis for animals with PDA? Do all dogs with PDA require treatment?

Uncorrected, the prognosis for most animals with a PDA is poor. Death due to left-sided CHF is high unless the defect is corrected. Given the high mortality rate associated with uncorrected PDA, it is important to recognize that, of all of the congenital cardiovascular malformations in the dog, PDA is the one most amenable to definitive repair. It must also be emphasized that, as with many other congenital cardiac defects in veterinary medicine, few animals with PDA have

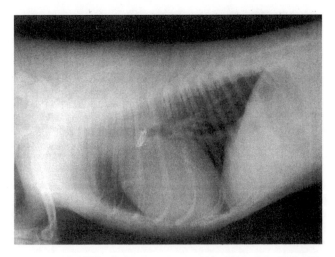

Figure 9-3.   Lateral thoracic radiograph obtained from a 16-month-old female Maltese dog. Two metallic coils have been placed in the ductus arteriosus.

clinical signs at the time of detection. This only serves to emphasize the importance of a definitive diagnosis in all cases of suspected congenital heart disease.

A small number of dogs have a shunt that is small enough that careful monitoring through serial echocardiographic studies can be considered as an alternative to occlusion or ligation of the duct. However, these cases are in the minority and repair is recommended for all but those that have a small shunt as assessed by a veterinarian with training in the evaluation of animals with congenital cardiac disease.

24. What is subvalvular aortic stenosis (SAS)?

Stenosis means narrowing. In the dog, congenital left ventricular outflow tract obstruction can result from valvular stenosis or, rarely, from supravalvular narrowing. However, aortic stenosis in dogs most commonly results from a subvalvular fibrous or fibrocartilaginous ring. This lesion is known as subvalvular or simply, subaortic, stenosis (SAS). It is one of the more common forms of CHD.

25. What is the pathophysiology associated with left ventricular outflow tract obstruction?

When obstruction is present, the left ventricle must generate abnormally high systolic pressures to maintain normal or subnormal pressures distal to the site of narrowing. A pressure difference (gradient) therefore develops across the outflow tract. SAS is an example of a pressure overload.

The pressure gradient, which can be measured directly during a cardiac catheterization procedure or estimated during a Doppler echocardiography study, is used as a clinical measure of stenosis severity. Gradients less than 40 mm Hg are considered to be mild and those greater than 80 or 100 mm Hg are severe; intermediate gradients are described as moderate.

26. What is the typical signalment and history of animals with SAS?

SAS is most common in large-breed dogs, including Golden Retrievers, Rottweilers, Boxers, Newfoundlands, and German Shepherds.

Clinical signs in puppies are uncommon; syncope and sudden death may be observed in young dogs with severe obstructions.

27. What abnormalities are detected on physical examination of animals with SAS?

Left ventricular outflow tract obstruction results in a systolic murmur that is generally heard best over the left heart base. When loud, the murmur tends to radiate to the right heart base and, occasionally, up the carotid arteries. In some cases, the murmur is heard best over the right heart base. It is important to recognize that SAS exhibits a broad spectrum of severity; some animals are mildly affected, and in these cases the physical findings are subtle. However, the intensity of the murmur generally correlates with the severity of obstruction, meaning that animals with severe SAS usually have loud murmurs. The arterial pulse is weak (hypokinetic) in severely affected dogs.

28. What is the diagnostic approach to SAS?

In animals with SAS, radiographic and electrocardiographic abnormalities are relatively inconsistent. Poststenotic dilation of the aorta is radiographically evident in many cases. Electrocardiographic studies may show left ventricular hypertrophy in some cases but in other cases the electrocardiogram is normal. As with other forms of CHD, Doppler echocardiography is the only definitive noninvasive study. Nevertheless, there is debate about the echocardiographic criteria that define mild SAS because structural abnormalities are not usually evident on echocardiograms in mildly affected individuals. In these cases, the diagnosis is based on Doppler characteristics of left ventricular ejection, including peak flow velocity. In cases of moderate or severe SAS, the diagnosis does not usually pose a challenge. In addition to structural abnormalities such as subvalvular narrowing and left ventricular hypertrophy (Fig. 9-4), peak Doppler-derived

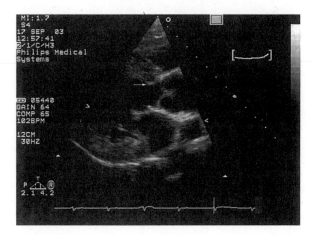

Figure 9-4.   This right parasternal long axis image was obtained from a young Rottweiler with severe subvalvular aortic stenosis. The subvalvular ring encircles the subvalvular outflow tract; in this image it is visible as echogenic ridges on the interventricular septum (*arrow*) and on the dorsal aspect of the septal mitral leaflet.

flow velocities are much greater than normal. The peak ejection velocity is used to estimate the pressure gradient, which is a prognostically useful measure of severity.

29. How is SAS treated?

Cardiopulmonary bypass is required for definitive surgical correction of SAS. However, recent data suggest that correction may not change the course of the disease. In one study, the incidence of sudden death was no lower in a cohort of dogs in whom SAS had been surgically treated than in an untreated control group. It is likely that transcatheter balloon dilation might be palliative in some cases. The value of medical therapy is uncertain. However, beta-blockade—because its effects decrease myocardial oxygen demand—may be helpful.

30. What is the prognosis for animals with SAS?

Many animals with mild obstruction suffer neither morbidity nor mortality. The development of congestive heart failure is relatively uncommon in dogs with SAS. Severe SAS most often results in syncope and sudden, presumably arrhythmic, death. Animals with SAS are predisposed to the development of bacterial endocarditis of the aortic valve, but this is probably not related to severity of the stenosis.

31. What are the gross pathologic characteristics of pulmonic stenosis in the dog?

Canine pulmonic stenosis (PS) is usually valvular, although subvalvular and supravalvular PS may occur. Most often, the valvular lesion is a form of dysplasia. The valve leaflets are thicker than normal and poorly mobile, and the annulus is often hypoplastic. Less commonly, valvular PS results from fusion of otherwise normal leaflets. In children, this form of PS is known as *simple* PS.

32. What is the pathophysiology of PS?

The disease process of PS is similar to that of left ventricular outflow tract obstruction. Because right ventricular outflow is abnormally decreased, the right ventricle must generate abnormally great systolic pressures to maintain normal or subnormal pressure and flow distal to the obstruction. A pressure gradient develops across the obstruction and the high-velocity, disturbed flow that results causes a cardiac murmur.

33. What physical findings are expected in animals with PS?
Animals with PS have a systolic murmur that is heard best over the left heart base. As in left ventricular outflow tract obstruction, the intensity of the murmur correlates roughly with the severity of obstruction. Thus severe PS usually results in a loud murmur.

34. What physical findings can be used to distinguish PS from SAS?
Both SAS and PS are characterized by systolic murmurs heard best over the left heart base. In general, murmurs resulting from SAS are more apt to radiate to the right base and murmurs caused by PS more often radiate ventrally, although this is not consistently true. Other features of the physical examination can be helpful. Dogs with severe SAS usually have a weak arterial pulse but in PS, the arterial pulse is more often normal. Though not strictly a physical finding, the signalment is sometimes helpful. Dogs with SAS are most often large, and there are strong breed predispositions that were noted earlier. PS is most often observed in relatively small dogs. Terriers, Miniature Schnauzers, and English Bulldogs are predisposed to the development of congenital PS.

35. How is PS treated?
Surgical techniques that can be performed without the use of CPB, including placement of a right ventricular outflow patch graft, have been described. However, most veterinary cardiologists recommend transcatheter balloon dilation as the first approach in the management of severely affected dogs. Briefly, an endhole catheter is fluoroscopically guided across the obstruction. A long guidewire—an exchange wire—is placed through this catheter, which is then removed. The guidewire provides a path along which the balloon catheter is advanced. Balloon catheters are available from various manufacturers in a variety of sizes. The specific length and diameter are determined by echocardiographic or angiographic data. Therapeutic balloon catheters are stiff and cannot be safely manipulated through the heart; for this reason the balloon catheter must only be passed over a preplaced exchange wire. When the balloon has been advanced to the level of the obstruction it is inflated several times with a combination of saline and radiographic contrast material. When the response is favorable, a waist or hourglass configuration is briefly visible but disappears at full inflation. The procedure results in more than 50% reduction in gradient in about 75% of animals. It is likely that the response to the procedure is primarily dependent on the pathologic nature of the stenosis. Animals with simple PS and a normal valve annulus usually respond favorably. Cases of dysplasia respond in a more variable fashion.

36. What is distinctive about PS in English Bulldogs?
Many English Bulldogs with PS have an associated anomaly of the coronary vessels such that a single right coronary artery gives rise to a left coronary artery that courses cranial to the right ventricular outflow. This anomaly precludes the use of surgical patch-graft procedures because the coronary artery is inevitably severed. Balloon dilation of affected animals is also problematic, and avulsion of the coronary artery has been reported as a consequence of this technique.

37. What is a ventricular septal defect (VSD)?
A ventricular septal defect (VSD) is a deficiency of the interventricular septum that creates a communication between the ventricles. Traumatic acquired ventricular septal defects are occasionally observed in people but have not been reported in animals. Failure of embryonic septal components to fuse or hypoplasia/agenesis of septal components is the presumed cause of most ventricular septal defects.

38. What is the anatomy of VSDs in small animals?

Most VSDs in small animals are located in the dorsal aspect of the interventricular septum. Because they affect the membranous part of the septum they are known as membranous (or perimembranous) VSDs. The defect is typically subaortic with a right ventricular orifice that is immediately ventral to the septal tricuspid valve leaflet.

39. What is a typical signalment for VSD in dogs?

VSDs are most commonly identified in young dogs, but there is no known sex predisposition. A few purebred dogs, including the English Bulldog and the English Springer Spaniel, are more likely to have a congenital VSD than dogs in the general veterinary hospital population.

40. What are the pathophysiologic consequences of a VSD? How does the presence of a VSD alter blood flow?

If the VSD is the only cardiac lesion and pulmonary vascular resistance is normal, then a portion of the left ventricular stroke volume enters the pulmonary circulation. The shunted blood augments the right ventricular output and is conveyed to the lungs. From the lungs, the enlarged pulmonary blood volume returns to the left atrium and left ventricle via the pulmonary veins. Thus a left-to-right VSD results in a volume load on the left atrium and left ventricle.

41. What determines the shunt fraction or size of the shunt?

When a VSD is the only cardiac lesion, the size and direction of the shunt is determined by (1) the size of the defect and (2) the relationship between pulmonary and systemic resistance.

The size of the defect can be classified in relation to the size of the aorta. If the area of the VSD is less than 40% of that of the aortic orifice, the defect is said to be small. Large defects are as large, or larger, than the aortic orifice, and moderately sized VSDs are between 40% and 100% of the size of the aortic orifice and are considered intermediate. Small VSDs are said to be restrictive; that is, the pressure difference between the left ventricle, which normally generates a high pressure, and the right ventricle, in which the systolic pressure is relatively low, is preserved. When the VSD is of moderate size, there is some "spillover" of pressure into the right ventricle. If the VSD is large, the pressures within the left and right ventricles equilibrate and the direction and size of the shunt depend entirely on the relationship between pulmonary and systemic vascular resistance.

42. What is the effect of concurrent cardiac anomalies?

Concurrent cardiac anomalies may affect intraventricular pressures and volumes, which can alter the clinical importance of the VSD. In dogs, two specific associated lesions are important to consider: (1) pulmonic stenosis, which increases the resistance to right ventricular emptying and therefore raises right ventricular pressure and (2) aortic valve incompetence, which can develop as a consequence of poor structural support of the aortic annulus related to the presence of a subaortic VSD.

Pulmonic stenosis, if severe, can result in a right-to-left shunt and, even if the VSD is small, this can result in hypoxemia and weakness. Aortic valve regurgitation imposes a volume load on the left ventricle. Aortic regurgitation tends to be poorly tolerated and the development of severe aortic regurgitation can have an impact on the prognosis in a dog with a small VSD that would be otherwise well tolerated.

43. What is the usual outcome for animals with VSD?

The clinical outcome depends upon variables that affect shunt size and direction. If the VSD is large, left-sided, or even biventricular, congestive heart failure develops early in life. Most VSDs in small animals are small and are well tolerated; in this case, the prognosis depends largely on whether concurrent defects are present.

44. What findings are expected on cardiac auscultation?

A VSD results in a systolic, plateau-shaped murmur; the pressure difference between the ventricles during diastole is insufficient to generate audible blood flow. The intensity of the murmur is inversely proportional to the size of the defect; small, restrictive defects, which are common, result in loud systolic murmurs that are often accompanied by a precordial thrill. Larger defects result in softer murmurs; if the VSD is as large as the aorta, the shunt may not result in a murmur at all. The point of maximal intensity of the murmur is variable and depends on the anatomy of the defect. However, most VSDs in dogs and cats have a right ventricular orifice that is immediately ventral to the septal tricuspid valve leaflet; thus, the murmur is typically heard best over the right cardiac apex.

In addition to the murmur generated by the shunt through the VSD, an additional murmur of "functional" pulmonic stenosis is occasionally heard.

45. What is functional pulmonic stenosis?

This murmur results when the shunt volume is large enough to substantially increase pulmonary artery flow velocity. When a left-to-right VSD is present, more blood than is normal passes through the pulmonary valve. The duration of systole remains about the same and therefore, the enlarged right ventricular stroke volume must be ejected at high velocity. If the velocity of blood flow is sufficiently high that flow becomes disturbed, a murmur may result. This murmur is usually of low intensity, is systolic, has a crescendo-decrescendo configuration, and is heard best over the left cardiac base. This murmur can develop in the absence of pulmonic valve disease; thus it is known as a murmur of functional pulmonic stenosis. When the VSD is large, this flow murmur might be the only auscultatory evidence of the defect.

46. What abnormalities are detected on echocardiographic examination?

Often, the VSD can be seen directly; usually, the defect is subaortic and directed toward the ventral aspect of the septal tricuspid valve leaflet. Caution must be exercised; the membranous part of the interventricular septal defect is thin, and so it often has the spurious appearance of a septal defect ("septal dropout").

Doppler echocardiographic examination is required for definitive, noninvasive diagnosis of a VSD. Shunting through the defect can be demonstrated by color-flow Doppler mapping. Spectral Doppler studies confirm the direction and velocity of the shunt (Fig. 9-5). The velocity of the jet is related to the pressure difference between the two ventricles. When continuous-wave Doppler studies are performed with a right parasternal transducer position, a positive velocity signal with a peak velocity greater than 5 m/sec is recorded when the beam is aligned with the jet arising from a restrictive VSD.

Additional and related findings might include aortic valve regurgitation and, on occasion, other congenital anomalies such as pulmonic stenosis, atrial septal defect, or AV valve incompetence.

47. How is a VSD treated?

Small and restrictive VSDs are usually well tolerated and do not require treatment. When a large shunt or aortic valve regurgitation has contributed to substantial left ventricular enlargement, consideration can be given to surgical correction of the defect. Definitive repair of a VSD can only be performed with cardiopulmonary bypass, and this technique is only available at a few referral centers.

48. What is the prognosis for animals with a VSD?

The prognosis for animals with an isolated, restrictive VSD is good; these animals are likely to have a normal life span without treatment. Animals with clinically important aortic valve regurgitation may fare less well, because this lesion tends to be poorly tolerated. The onset of congestive heart failure indicates that the defect will be, unless it is corrected, fatal.

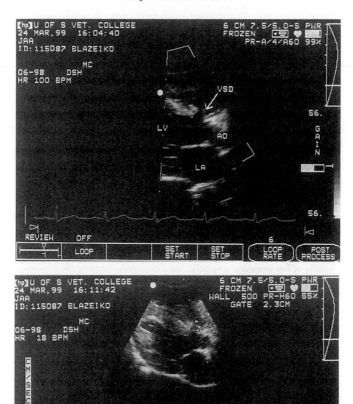

Figure 9-5. *Top,* Right parasternal long-axis echocardiographic image of the left ventricular outflow tract obtained from a 9-month-old castrated domestic shorthair cat. The subaortic ventricular septal defect (VSD) is labeled. *LV,* left ventricle; *LA,* left atrium; *AO,* aorta. *Bottom,* Pulsed-wave Doppler study performed with the sample volume placed adjacent to the right ventricular orifice of the VSD. A systolic, high velocity jet is evident; the spectral breadth of the signal is high, indicating disturbed flow.

49. What is tricuspid valve dysplasia (TVD)?

TVD refers to abnormal development of the tricuspid valve. Usually TVD results in tricuspid valve regurgitation and imposes a volume overload on the right atrium and right ventricle. Rarely, TVD causes tricuspid stenosis. Although a generally uncommon malformation, TVD is relatively prevalent in Labrador Retrievers, and in that breed the prevalence of TVD has apparently been increasing over the last 20 years.

50. What are the pathophysiologic consequences of an atrial septal defect?

An atrial septal defect (ASD) provides a communication between the left and right atria. When the ASD is an isolated lesion, the shunt direction is from left to right. In contrast to a VSD, the shunt is proximal to the atrioventricular valve. Blood that crosses the septum during ventricular systole enters the right ventricle during the next diastole; the diastolic shunt enters the right ventricle directly. A left-to-right ASD therefore imposes a volume load on the right atrium and right ventricle. Secondary tricuspid valve regurgitation, myocardial dysfunction, and right-sided congestive heart failure are potential consequences.

51. What physical findings are typical of an ASD?

The shunt that results from the presence of an ASD is not audible. When a murmur is present, it is caused by high-velocity right ventricular ejection associated with functional pulmonic stenosis (described earlier in this chapter).

52. What is cyanotic congenital heart disease?

The term *cyanotic congenital heart disease* refers to malformations that result in venous blood mixing with arterial blood due to right-to-left shunting. The lesion and the shunt that result cause abnormally high pressures within the pulmonary arteries, the right ventricle, or the right atrium. Tetralogy of Fallot is the most common form of cyanotic congenital heart disease in the dog. Other malformations in this category include various forms of Eisenmenger's syndrome and severe pulmonic or tricuspid valve stenosis with a concurrent atrial-level shunt.

53. What clinical signs result from cyanotic CHD?

All types of cyanotic CHD can cause weakness due to hypoxemia. Cyanosis may be evident at rest or provoked by exertion. Chronic hypoxemia stimulates erythrocytosis (polycythemia) and may cause a hyperviscosity syndrome.

54. What is tetralogy of Fallot (TF)?

TF consists of a VSD, which is typically large, right ventricular outflow tract obstruction, and right ventricular hypertrophy. The VSD is immediately subjacent to the aortic valve, an arrangement that is described as "aortic over-ride" and this arrangement is the fourth component of the tetralogy. The severity of TF depends on the size of the VSD and the severity pulmonic stenosis. Most dogs with TF have a murmur that results from the pulmonic stenosis, although a few with very severe PS and high blood viscosity lack this physical finding. Clinical signs result from hypoxemia and secondary erythrocytosis.

55. What is Eisenmenger's syndrome?

Eisenmenger's syndrome consists of pulmonary vascular disease and high pulmonary vascular resistance as a consequence of a left-to-right shunt. Pulmonary vessels may respond to large shunts by developing medial hypertrophy. Potentially, narrowing of the cross-sectional area of the pulmonary vascular tree results, and this, in turn, increases pulmonary vascular resistance. If pulmonary vascular resistance exceeds systemic vascular resistance, it becomes, in effect, "easier" for pulmonary blood to cross over into the systemic circulation and a right-to-left shunt results. It should be recognized that this phenomenon is uncommon in dogs, and when it does occur it almost always appears before the dog reaches the age of 6 or 8 months. The concern that an uncorrected PDA (or VSD) might "reverse" when the dog reaches adulthood, as may occur in children, seems to be largely unfounded. Clinical signs associated with Eisenmenger's syndrome are caused by hypoxemia and hyperviscosity. In general, dogs with a right-to-left PDA or VSD do not have cardiac murmurs.

56. What is differential cyanosis?

Differential cyanosis is a condition that may be seen in animals with a right-to-left PDA. Because the shunt in these cases is distal to the origin of the trunk of the brachiocephalic artery, the cranial mucous membranes are pink, but the caudal mucous membranes are cyanotic.

57. How is cyanotic CHD treated?

TF can be treated surgically, although more often it is treated medically by periodic phlebotomy and sometimes beta-blockade. Eisenmenger's syndrome is not amenable to surgical therapy and phlebotomy is used to control clinical signs resulting from secondary erythrocytosis. Central cyanosis associated with pulmonic or tricuspid valve stenosis can sometimes be improved by transcatheter balloon dilation.

BIBLIOGRAPHY

Bonagura JD, Lehmkuhl LB. Congenital heart disease. In Fox PR, Sisson D, Moise NS, editors: *Textbook of canine and feline cardiology: principles and clinical practice,* Philadelphia, 1999, WB Saunders.

Brown WA. Ventricular septal defects in the English springer spaniel. In Bonagura JD, editor: *Current veterinary therapy XII: small animal practice,* Philadelphia, 1995, WB Saunders, pp 827-829.

Buchanan JW. Prevalence of cardiovascular disorders. In Fox PR, Sisson D, Moise NS, editors: *Textbook of canine and feline cardiology: principles and clinical practice*, Philadelphia, 1999, WB Saunders.

Famula TR, Siemens LM, Davidson AP et al: Evaluation of the genetic basis of tricuspid valve dysplasia in Labrador Retrievers, *Am J Vet Res* 63:816-820, 2002.

Fellows CG, Lerche P, King G, Tometzki A: Treatment of patent ductus arteriosus by placement of two intravascular embolisation coils in a puppy, *J Small Anim Pract* 39:196-199, 1998.

Fox PR, Bond BR, Sommer RJ: Nonsurgical transcatheter coil occlusion of patent ductus arteriosus in two dogs using a preformed nitinol snare delivery technique, *J Vet Intern Med* 12:182-185, 1998.

Kienle RD: Congenital pulmonic stenosis. In Kittleson MD, Kienle RD, editors: *Small animal cardiovascular medicine,* St. Louis, 1998, Mosby.

Kittleson MD: Patent ductus arteriosus. In Kittleson MD, Kienle RD, editors: *Small animal cardiovascular medicine,* St. Louis, 1998, Mosby.

Kittleson MD: Septal defects. In Kittleson MD, Kienle RD, editors: *Small animal cardiovascular medicine*, St. Louis, 1998, Mosby.

Miller MW: Interventional cardiology: Catheter occlusion of patent ductus arteriosus in dogs. In Bonagura JD, editor: *Kirk's current veterinary therapy XIII: small animal practice,* Philadelphia, 2000, WB Saunders.

Orton EC, Herndon GD, Boon JA et al: Influence of open surgical correction on intermediate-term outcome in dogs with subvalvular aortic stenosis: 44 cases (1991-1998), *J Am Vet Med Assoc* 216:364-367, 2000.

Patterson DF: Congenital defects of the cardiovascular system of dogs: studies in comparative cardiology, *Adv Vet Sci Comp Med* 20:1-37, 1976.

Patterson DF: Epidemiologic and genetic studies of congenital heart disease in the dog, *Circ Res* 23:171-202, 1968.

Patterson DF, Pexieder T, Schnarr WR et al: A single major-gene defect underlying cardiac conotruncal malformations interferes with myocardial growth during embryonic development: studies in the CTD line of keeshond dogs, *Am J Hum Genet* 52:388-397, 1993.

Patterson DF, Pyle RL, Buchanan JW et al: Hereditary patent ductus arteriosus and its sequelae in the dog, *Circ Res* 29:1-13, 1971.

10. Canine Myocardial Disease

Jonathon A. Abbott

1. What is cardiomyopathy?

Cardiomyopathy is a disease of heart muscle that is associated with cardiac dysfunction. In the past, this term was reserved for idiopathic or primary heart muscle diseases. More recently, a task force of the World Health Organization (WHO) adopted the definition just stated. This was prompted by the growth of knowledge that has blurred the distinction between idiopathic myocardial disease and what were previously known as specific heart muscle diseases. The current WHO scheme classifies cardiomyopathies based on pathophysiology and cause, when it is known. The following morphopathologic designations are accepted: dilated cardiomyopathy, restrictive cardiomyopathy, hypertrophic cardiomyopathy, arrhythmogenic right ventricular cardiomyopathy, and unclassified cardiomyopathy. Each of these basic types of heart muscle disease can be described as idiopathic or as a specific cardiomyopathy when the cause is known.

2. What is dilated cardiomyopathy (DCM)?

DCM is characterized by ventricular and atrial dilation that results from contractile dysfunction. Most often, left ventricular or biventricular dilation is present.

3. What is the pathogenesis of DCM?

Loss of systolic myocardial function—a decrease in contractility—causes ventricular hypokinesis and initiates a series of events that lead to progressive ventricular dilation. Systolic myocardial dysfunction can result from loss of cardiomyocytes due to necrosis or from functional disorders of the contractile apparatus. However, the hemodynamic consequences of impaired systolic myocardial function are generally the same regardless of the cause of myocardial dysfunction.

When stroke volume declines as a result of systolic myocardial dysfunction (decreased contractility), the end-systolic ventricular volume increases. During diastole, this elevated end-systolic volume augments pulmonary venous return and this contributes to ventricular dilation. In addition, activation of the renin-angiotensin-aldosterone system (RAAS) occurs as a consequence of diminished cardiac output. One effect of RAAS activation is the retention of salt and water, which serves to expand the intravascular volume. This increase in intravascular volume further increases preload and contributes to progressive ventricular dilation. Elevated ventricular filling pressures together with atrioventricular valve incompetence resulting from distortion of the valvular apparatus associated with ventricular enlargement cause atrial dilation.

4. What are the causes of dilated cardiomyopathy?

In a sense, DCM is an "end-stage heart disease" that represents the end result of virtually any insult to the myocardium. This insult could be a viral infection, a toxin, a metabolic derangement, or a nutritional deficiency. For example, taurine deficiency has been associated with the development of DCM in Cocker Spaniels. In some dogs, myocardial carnitine deficiency may play a role in the pathogenesis of DCM. In addition, antineoplastic agents such as doxorubicin can cause irreversible myocardial dysfunction. Attempts to define a precise genetic or viral cause of canine DCM have not yet been successful. However, the occurrence and distinctive clinical features of familial or breed-associated DCM suggest that there is a genetic basis for many forms of this disease. Although the results of pedigree analysis were not conclusive, it is probable that DCM affecting Great Danes is an X-linked recessive trait. A juvenile-onset form of DCM that has been observed in Portuguese Water Dogs seems to have an autosomal recessive mode of inheritance. Patterns of inheritance have not been reported for other forms of breed-associated DCM. However, the widespread occurrence of DCM in breeds such as the Irish Wolfhound, Newfoundland and Doberman Pinscher provide strong, indirect evidence for a genetic cause or at least, a genetic susceptibility to an as yet unidentified etiologic agent.

5.   What is a typical signalment for a dog with dilated cardiomyopathy?

Large and giant-breed dogs, including Doberman Pinschers, Great Danes, and Boxers, are most commonly affected. There is a predisposition for males, and dogs with DCM are often middle-aged or older. A 5-year-old male Doberman Pinscher is a typical signalment for DCM.

6.   Are there differences in presentation among the breeds commonly afflicted?

Although some clinical features are common to all canine patients with DCM, the presentation of DCM in specific breeds is somewhat distinctive. Interestingly, these breed-associated differences in clinical presentation might provide further support for the contention that DCM in purebred dogs has a genetic basis, since it suggests that the disorder is different in genetically distinct populations. This occurrence of breed-specific clinical features might not be anticipated if DCM were in fact a homogeneous disorder that affected large dogs.

7.   What is Boxer cardiomyopathy?

Cardiomyopathy in Boxers is characterized by a high incidence of ventricular tachyarrhythmias and sudden death. Harpster classified the manner of presentation of Boxers with cardiomyopathy. Boxers in category 1 have ventricular arrhythmias but do not have associated clinical signs. In category 2 the syndrome manifests as syncope that is presumably related to ventricular tachyarrhythmia. Category 3 is characterized by congestive heart failure (CHF) due to systolic myocardial dysfunction. Progression from one category to the next does not appear to be inevitable, and ventricular tachyarrhythmia in the absence of overt myocardial dysfunction is common in Boxers. The arrhythmogenic form of cardiomyopathy in Boxers has a genetic basis; recent data suggest that it is an autosomal dominant trait, at least in some cases. Because of a presumed genetic basis as well as the electrocardiographic and pathologic characteristics of some Boxers with this disorder, it has been suggested that Boxer cardiomyopathy might be more appropriately described as a form of arrhythmogenic right ventricular cardiomyopathy. Dilated cardiomyopathy as typically observed in other breeds—that is, congestive heart failure due to systolic myocardial dysfunction—is less common in Boxers than are ventricular arrhythmias and might represent a separate and distinct disorder.

8.   What typifies DCM in Doberman Pinschers?

There are some similarities between the characteristics of cardiomyopathy in boxers and that in Doberman Pinschers. The incidence of ventricular tachyarrhythmia in affected Dobermans is high, as is the incidence of sudden cardiac death. CHF in Doberman Pinschers with DCM is often associated with a short and rapidly progressive course. The subclinical phase of DCM in Doberman Pinschers is long and, perhaps in contrast to the situation with respect to Boxers, arrhythmias and congestive heart failure appear to be manifestations of a single, progressive disorder. On the basis of pathologic studies, the disorder affects the left ventricle almost exclusively. Probably for this reason, signs of biventricular failure—pleural effusion and ascites in association with pulmonary edema—are relatively uncommon in this breed.

9.   What is occult DCM?

Studies performed in Doberman Pinschers demonstrate that DCM is a slowly progressive, insidious disorder. A long subclinical phase precedes the development of overt myocardial dysfunction; in some dogs, sudden death interrupts this progression. Working independently, O'Grady and Calvert have provided criteria that define subclinical or occult DCM in Doberman Pinschers. Quantitative echocardiographic findings that predict the development of overt myocardial dysfunction or sudden death have been reported. In some Doberman Pinschers, electrocardiographic abnormalities precede the development of myocardial dysfunction. The finding of more than 100 premature ventricular contractions (PVCs) in a 24-hour record of ambulatory electrocardiographic (Holter) monitoring also predicts the development of overt DCM in Dobermans.

10. What about dilated cardiomyopathy in giant-breed dogs?

Irish Wolfhounds, Great Danes, and Newfoundland dogs with DCM may have pleural effusions as a manifestation of congestive failure more commonly than do other breeds. The prevalence of atrial fibrillation tends to be high in these breeds, although the prevalence might simply reflect their large stature; in general, the propensity to develop and sustain atrial fibrillation depends on cardiac size.

11. What is distinctive about DCM in Cocker Spaniels?

The Cocker Spaniel is the only small-breed dog that commonly has DCM. The syndrome in Cocker Spaniels is further distinguished by low plasma taurine concentrations in affected dogs. Some Cocker Spaniels with DCM also have myocardial carnitine deficiency.

Taurine is an amino acid; the precise function of this nutrient relative to cardiovascular function is not known. However, an association between nutritional taurine deficiency and feline dilated cardiomyopathy was discovered in 1987. Subsequent supplementation of commercial cat foods resulted in a radical decrease in the prevalence of feline dilated cardiomyopathy. Taurine is not an essential amino acid in the dog, and decreased intake alone does not explain low plasma taurine levels in this species; a metabolic defect, perhaps in the ability to synthesize taurine, might explain the low plasma levels in affected dogs.

The Multicenter Spaniel Trial (MUST) was a double-blind clinical trial that compared the effect of nutritional supplementation with taurine and carnitine to placebo in Cocker Spaniels with DCM. All Cocker Spaniels enrolled in the study had low plasma taurine levels. Improvement in echocardiographic parameters was observed in animals that were randomly assigned to receive taurine and carnitine. The investigators were unblinded after 4 months; taurine and carnitine supplementation was then initiated in animals that had received placebo. Ultimately, it was possible to withdraw cardiovascular drugs from all animals that received taurine and carnitine. The improvement in myocardial function was apparently sustained and many of the dogs included in the study ultimately died of extracardiac disease. The importance of carnitine deficiency was not determined. However, it can be stated that taurine deficiency is prevalent in Cocker Spaniels with DCM and that nutritional supplementation with taurine and carnitine is likely to result in substantial clinical improvement. When DCM is observed in Cocker Spaniels, it is advisable to evaluate the plasma taurine level. In dogs in whom this value is low, nutritional supplementation with taurine and possibly carnitine is recommended. If the plasma taurine level cannot be obtained, or a delay in obtaining the result is anticipated, empirical supplementation is suggested.

12. Is taurine status relevant in other breeds of dogs with dilated cardiomyopathy?

Clinical findings in a group of dogs with dilated cardiomyopathy and blood or plasma taurine deficiency were recently reported. All of these dogs had been fed a diet that consisted partly of lamb meal, rice, or both. Improved cardiac function was documented after nutritional taurine supplementation. Interestingly, the majority of dogs in this case series were of breeds not known to be predisposed to DCM. Based on this, evaluation of blood or plasma taurine concentration should be considered whenever DCM is observed in atypical breeds.

13. What prompts the owner of a dog with DCM to seek veterinary attention?

Animals with DCM are usually presented for evaluation of clinical signs related to CHF. The history and physical examination may reveal dyspnea, cough, abdominal distention due to the presence of ascites, and syncope. In addition, the owner of a dog with DCM may observe exercise intolerance, weight loss, depression, and lack of appetite.

14. The physical findings in dilated cardiomyopathy often suggest the diagnosis. What might be expected on auscultation?

Animals with DCM often have CHF at the time of presentation. Consequently, tachycardia is commonly present and an arrhythmia may be evident on auscultation. Often, but not invariably, there is a murmur due to functional AV valve incompetence that results from distortion of the AV valve apparatus. The murmur is systolic, usually soft, and heard best over the left cardiac apex.

In some affected dogs, audibility of the third heart sound results in a gallop rhythm. Rapid deceleration of early diastolic transmitral flow is the hemodynamic event associated with the occurrence of an S_3 gallop. The rapid deceleration of early diastolic flow is probably related to the presence of a large end-systolic volume, high atrial pressures, and reduced ventricular compliance. In the presence of an audible third heart sound, pulmonary crackles suggest pulmonary edema.

15. Describe the expected radiographic findings.

The cardiac silhouette is usually enlarged and most often there is radiographic evidence of left atrial enlargement. When the left atrium is enlarged, pulmonary opacities indicate the presence of pulmonary edema and CHF (Fig. 10-1). It should be noted that on plain chest radiographs the resolution of specific cardiac chambers is limited and the radiographic appearance of DCM is variable. Some affected Doberman pinschers, for example, have minimal radiographic evidence of cardiac enlargement. In some affected dogs of this breed there may be only straightening of

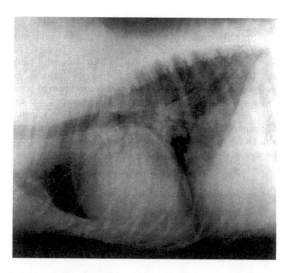

Figure 10-1.   Lateral thoracic radiograph in a 12-year-old male castrated Labrador Retriever cross with dilated cardiomyopathy. The cardiac silhouette is enlarged and there is evidence of left atrial enlargement. Cranially, there is the suggestion of pulmonary venous distention. Caudally, pulmonary vascular detail is poor, suggesting the presence of interstitial pulmonary edema.

the caudal border of the cardiac silhouette, indicating left atrial enlargement, and alveolar pulmonary infiltrates of edema.

16.　What abnormalities are detected on electrocardiographic examination?

In animals with DCM, the electrocardiogram (ECG) may reveal premature ventricular complexes, ventricular tachycardia, atrial premature complexes, atrial or junctional tachycardia, or atrial fibrillation. Sometimes there is evidence of ventricular hypertrophy, intraventricular conduction disturbances such as left bundle branch block, or evidence of left atrial enlargement. Broadening of the P wave beyond 40 ms suggests left atrial enlargement. The presence of concurrent P-wave notching may increase the specificity of P-wave broadening as a marker of left atrial enlargement.

17.　When is echocardiography indicated?

Echocardiography provides a noninvasive assessment of cardiac chamber dimensions and myocardial function. It is the means by which to obtain a definitive noninvasive diagnosis of DCM and should be considered in all animals in which myocardial disease is suspected.

18.　What are the echocardiographic characteristics of dilated cardiomyopathy?

In DCM, echocardiography demonstrates atrial and ventricular dilation with hypokinesis. Usually, there is left ventricular or biventricular dilation (Fig. 10-2). Fractional shortening (FS), an index of systolic myocardial function, is low in dogs with DCM; often, it is very low, in the range of 5% to 15%. Although it may progress rapidly, DCM usually develops gradually. Therefore diminished fractional shortening in the absence of ventricular and atrial dilation may be related to extracardiac disease, may be an artifact of the technique used for measurement, or might reflect the limits of biological variability; it is unlikely to explain signs of CHF. In DCM, the valves are structurally normal, although Doppler studies often demonstrate mitral and tricuspid valve regurgitation.

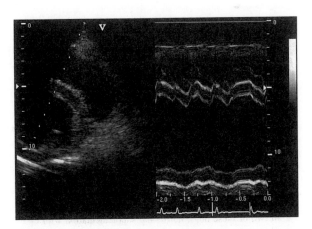

Figure 10-2.　M-mode echocardiogram of the left ventricle of a Doberman Pinscher with dilated cardiomyopathy. M-mode echocardiography provides a one-dimensional view of the heart; the ordinate measures distance from the transducer and the abscissa, time. The two-dimensional image from which this M-mode echocardiogram was derived is shown in the inset. The echocardiogram demonstrates moderate left ventricular dilation and hypokinesis. The cardiac rhythm is atrial fibrillation.

19. What medications are appropriate for the management of chronic CHF due to DCM?

A regimen that includes digoxin, an angiotensin-converting enzyme (ACE) inhibitor, and furosemide has become accepted for the management of CHF resulting from DCM. ACE inhibitors include captopril, enalapril, benazepril, and others. These drugs inhibit the enzyme that catalyzes the conversion of angiotensin I to angiotensin II. Angiotensin II is a vasoconstrictor that has numerous other effects that include modulation of the adrenergic nervous system, stimulation of antidiuretic hormone (ADH) and aldosterone release, and trophic effects on myocardium. The administration of enalapril to dogs with CHF due to DCM results in an improved quality of life and likely a favorable effect on mortality.

20. What is the role of digitalis in DCM?

Digitalis compounds have a positive inotropic effect and modulate the function of the adrenergic nervous system. They are unique in that they exert a positive inotropic effect while lowering heart rate and controlling the ventricular response rate in atrial fibrillation.

21. Furosemide is the diuretic that is used most commonly in dogs with CHF; are any others important?

The effect of diuresis on heart function is mechanical; reductions in intravascular volume decrease preload and limit the accumulation of edema. Furosemide is a potent loop diuretic that is widely used in the management of chronic CHF. There is evidence that spironolactone, an aldosterone antagonist, decreases morbidity and mortality in human patients with CHF who are receiving a combination of an ACE inhibitor and loop diuretic. Interestingly, this favorable effect was evident at a dose of spironolactone that did not cause diuresis. This is probably explained by the extrarenal effects of aldosterone. While this hormone stimulates the renal retention of sodium and water, it also promotes the development of myocardial fibrosis.

22. Should animals with subclinical or occult DCM be treated?

The efficacy of therapy for canine patients that have subclinical DCM has not been established. However, there is ample clinical evidence from studies of people in addition to experimental evidence to suggest that that the use of ACE inhibitors slows the progression of myocardial disease. Beta blockers may also have a role in the management of subclinical DCM. The use of these agents is consistent with the now accepted view that activation of the adrenergic nervous system and the RAAS contributes to the progressive nature of CHF. The use of an ACE inhibitor is reasonable when subclinical myocardial dysfunction has been demonstrated echocardiographically. Beta blockers may also have a role but the use of these drugs in animals with systolic myocardial dysfunction must be undertaken only with caution.

23. Does L-carnitine supplementation have a role in the management of DCM?

L-Carnitine is a quaternary amine that is synthesized from the amino acids lysine and methionine; the d-isomer of this compound is toxic, so only L-carnitine is discussed here. Carnitine plays an integral role in cardiac energy metabolism; it is required for the transfer of long chain fatty acids across the mitochondrial membrane. Additionally, carnitine functions as a metabolic "scavenger," esterifying toxic metabolites.

In 1991, Keene et al. documented myocardial carnitine deficiency in a family of Boxer dogs affected by DCM. In two of these dogs, nutritional supplementation with carnitine resulted in clinical and echocardiographic improvement that allowed the discontinuation of cardiovascular medications. Later, carnitine supplementation was stopped and myocardial dysfunction and signs of congestive heart failure returned. This work demonstrated that DCM in a family of Boxer dogs was the result of myocardial carnitine deficiency. Although myocardial free-carnitine deficiency was known to be prevalent in dogs with DCM, resolution of myocardial dysfunction had not been documented subsequent to the initial report. It is likely that in many dogs with DCM myocardial carnitine deficiency is simply a marker of another, yet to be discovered, metabolic defect.

The diagnosis of carnitine deficiency is difficult because of the complex disposition of this compound. Because carnitine is concentrated in the myocardium, plasma or serum carnitine levels do not necessarily reflect myocardial carnitine concentrations. Quantification of myocardial free– and esterified-carnitine levels can be performed on samples obtained by endomyocardial biopsy. However, the technique of endomyocardial biopsy is not widely practiced and the diagnosis of carnitine deficiency is generally a presumptive one that is made based on clinical response.

In most dogs with DCM, carnitine supplementation is unlikely to result in a cure; however, some dogs with DCM seem to improve clinically following administration of this neutraceutical. High doses (1-2 g orally 3 times/day for large-breed dogs) are generally recommended. The cost of carnitine is relatively high, although the use of a powdered form rather than tablets may reduce the cost. Because diarrhea is the only adverse effect possibly associated with the administration of carnitine, supplementation can be considered on an empiric basis when the financial burden can be borne by the pet owner.

24. How is atrial fibrillation (AF) managed in dogs with DCM?

Experimental studies show that a critical mass of atrial myocardium must be involved to support the arrhythmia of AF. Only a few breeds of dog are sufficiently large enough to have AF in the absence of cardiac disease. In dogs, AF usually signifies the presence of marked and possibly irreversible atrial enlargement (Fig. 10-3). Because DCM, the cause of AF, generally cannot be corrected in dogs, the value of attempting to convert to sinus rhythm has been questioned. Further, the risk of thromboembolism, which sometimes complicates AF in human beings, seems to be low in dogs. Therefore conversion to sinus rhythm is not generally attempted in dogs. Instead, treatment for AF in dogs with DCM is directed toward optimizing stroke volume and meeting myocardial oxygen demand by slowing the ventricular response rate.

25. What are the roles of calcium channel antagonists, beta blockers, and digitalis in AF caused by DCM?

Digoxin is used to control the ventricular response rate in dogs with AF associated with DCM. In some patients with DCM, the heart rate does not slow, even after control of congestive signs. In such cases, the cautious use of diltiazem, a calcium channel blocker, or a beta-adrenergic antagonist such as atenolol, carvedilol, or metoprolol, can be considered as adjunct therapy. Recent evidence obtained in clinical studies of human patients indicates that long-term use of beta-adrenergic antagonists in patients with CHF caused by systolic myocardial dysfunction has a beneficial effect on survival. For this reason, these agents may be preferred when it is necessary to use drugs in addition to digoxin to slow heart rate in dogs with AF associated with DCM; however, caution must be exercised, because drugs other than digoxin that slow heart rate are negative inotropes and beta blockers are potent in this regard.

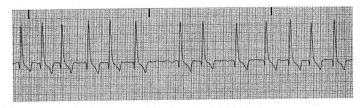

Figure 10-3. This electrocardiogram was recorded from a large-breed dog with dilated cardiomyopathy. The electrocardiographic diagnosis is atrial fibrillation—the rate is rapid, the rhythm is chaotically irregular, and evidence of organized atrial activation is lacking. (Paper speed 50 mm/sec, 1 mV = 1 cm)

26. What is pimobendan? Does it have a role in the management of canine dilated cardiomyopathy?

Pimobendan is a drug that inhibits phosphodiesterase and, through an unknown mechanism, increases the calcium sensitivity of the contractile apparatus. These effects result in an increase in contractility and vasodilation, which is why pimobendan and similar drugs are known as *inodilators.* A clinical trial compared pimobendan with placebo in Cocker Spaniels and Doberman Pinschers with heart failure due to dilated cardiomyopathy. The sample size was relatively small, but the beneficial effect of pimobendan was pronounced in Doberman Pinschers. This drug is currently licensed in Europe, Canada, and Australia for the management of heart failure in dogs. Clinical evaluation in the United States is underway.

27. What is the prognosis in DCM?

The prognosis when CHF results from DCM is generally poor. If the dog survives beyond the initial presentation, survival for 6 to 12 months and occasionally longer is possible with careful medical management. A few animals may respond favorably to supplementation with nutrients such as carnitine or taurine. A small number of animals with DCM seem to recover spontaneously. However, DCM in dogs is usually terminal.

28. What is hypertrophic cardiomyopathy? Do dogs have hypertrophic cardiomyopathy (HCM)?

HCM has been defined as hypertrophy of a nondilated ventricle that develops in the absence of other diseases that might result in myocardial growth. This disease has a genetic basis in people; in fact, more than 100 mutations of genes that code for sarcomeric proteins have been associated with human HCM. HCM is a relatively uncommon disorder in dogs, and relatively little is known of its cause, clinical presentation, or natural history.

29. How does the pathophysiologic process of HCM differ from that of DCM?

DCM results from impaired contractile function. In contrast, diastolic dysfunction is generally believed to be the principal pathophysiologic mechanism responsible for clinical signs associated with HCM. Diastolic function, which can be generally defined as the ability of the ventricle to fill at low pressure, plays a less-obvious role in cardiac performance compared with contractile performance. Diastolic function depends primarily on relaxation, the energy-dependent process by which the myocardium returns to its precontractile configuration, and the mechanical property of compliance. Compliance is the rate of change of pressure relative to volume; its reciprocal is stiffness. In animals with HCM, impaired myocardial relaxation results from myocardial ischemia associated with intramural narrowing of coronary vessels and perhaps, intrinsic diastolic myocardial abnormalities. Excessive hypertrophy reduces ventricular compliance. Together, slowed relaxation and increases in chamber stiffness alter the diastolic pressure-volume relationship of the ventricle so that diastolic pressures are abnormally high when ventricular volumes are normal or small.

Some animals with HCM have dynamic outflow tract obstruction that results from systolic anterior motion of the mitral valve (SAM). The precise causes of SAM have been debated. In general, SAM is observed when ventricular volumes are small, systolic performance is dynamic, and outflow resistance is reduced. Forces, perhaps drag related to ejection of the stroke volume, cause the mitral leaflets to move cranially and, potentially, to contact the interventricular septum during systole. This abnormal configuration of the mitral valve during systole has two primary consequences: left ventricular outflow tract obstruction and mitral valve regurgitation. The obstruction is said to be dynamic because it results not from a fixed anatomic obstacle but from abnormal movement of the mitral valve. The development of SAM is highly dependent on ventricular loading conditions and inotropic state; as a result, the phenomenon is labile. In general, increases in contractility, decreases in preload, and decreases in afterload may accentuate or provoke SAM. In some individuals, SAM is absent at rest but can be provoked pharmacologically or by stimuli that increase sympathetic tone.

30. What is the cause of canine HCM?

A genetic basis for HCM in humans has been established. Although the precise mechanism that results in inappropriate hypertrophy has yet to be conclusively determined, numerous mutations of genes that code for sarcomeric proteins have been associated with this disorder. On the basis of these findings, it is possible that canine HCM is a heritable disorder. However, differences between human and canine HCM have led some authors to suggest that alternate pathogenetic pathways might lead to ventricular hypertrophy. Most human patients with HCM have asymmetric left ventricular hypertrophy in which the interventricular septum is more prominently affected. In contrast, most canine patients with HCM have symmetric hypertrophy that affects the septum and left ventricular posterior wall more or less equally. Furthermore, a histologic hallmark of HCM, known as myofiber disarray, is lacking in most canine patients with this disease. Together, these observations suggest at least the possibility that the canine disorder represents a *secondary* hypertrophic response—perhaps resulting from dynamic outflow tract obstruction associated with mitral dysplasia or mild subvalvular aortic stenosis—as opposed to genetically determined, inappropriate myocardial growth. It is interesting that canine HCM is most often seen in breeds that frequently have subaortic stenosis.

31. How does canine HCM manifest clinically?

Canine HCM is generally recognized in young dogs, and it is possible that it is a congenital disorder. Most often, canine HCM becomes apparent when puppies with cardiac murmurs are subjected to echocardiographic scrutiny. In other cases, the disease is first identified during postmortem examination of dogs that died suddenly and unexpectedly. Although clinical and pathologic findings of congestive heart failure have been described in canine patients with HCM, signs such as cough and dyspnea appear to be uncommon.

32. What are the characteristics of the murmur heard in canine HCM?

Although left ventricular hypertrophy can distort the mitral valve apparatus and result in mitral valve regurgitation, it is generally only dogs with the "obstructive" form of HCM—those that have SAM—that have heart murmurs. The murmur associated with SAM is systolic and probably results from both mitral valve regurgitation and acceleration of ejection velocity resulting from dynamic obstruction. The lability of the pressure gradient and associated murmur is an important clinical feature; the intensity of the murmur may change markedly during the course of a single examination. In general, increases in contractility and decreases in preload and afterload increase the intensity of the murmur. In some affected individuals, the murmur is soft or even absent at rest but becomes loud with exercise or excitement.

33. What are the diagnostic findings in canine HCM?

Thoracic radiography and electrocardiography provide relatively little information about canine HCM. Hypertrophic cardiomyopathy is an echocardiographic diagnosis. In general, there is left ventricular hypertrophy, systolic performance as evaluated by fractional shortening is normal or greater than normal, and in some animals, the left atrium is enlarged. As discussed earlier, SAM is identified in most dogs with this disorder. Structural abnormalities other than those associated with hypertrophy or SAM are, by definition, lacking. It is important that disorders such as systemic hypertension, infiltrative disease, and aortic stenosis that might lead to left ventricular hypertrophy are excluded. It is important to note that hypovolemia can decrease the size of the ventricular lumen, causing an apparent hypertrophy.

34. How is subvalvular aortic stenosis (SAS) distinguished from canine HCM?

Most canine patients with HCM have left ventricular outflow tract obstruction due to SAM.

However, SAM occasionally complicates fixed outflow tract obstruction, making it difficult to distinguish between primary hypertrophy and hypertrophy resulting from SAS. When fixed obstruction is severe, narrowing of the outflow tract is often evident echocardiographically as a subvalvular ridge. In contrast, the left ventricular outflow tract of animals with HCM is structurally normal. Doppler-derived left ventricular outflow tract velocities are abnormally large in animals with fixed or dynamic obstruction. In general, SAM causes late-systolic acceleration of the outflow tract signal, which results in a relatively distinctive asymmetric velocity profile that has a dagger-type configuration. The gradient in SAM is highly labile and can sometimes be abolished by beta-adrenergic blockade or anesthesia. In contrast, the pressure gradient in SAS is, to a greater extent, "fixed." Animals with SAS are probably more likely to have aortic valve regurgitation and poststenotic dilation than are those with HCM. Despite these features, in many cases, it can be difficult to conclusively distinguish HCM from SAS. In fact, as alluded to earlier, there might be a genetic association between what appears to represent canine HCM and SAS/mitral valve dysplasia.

35. How is canine HCM treated?

Because canine HCM is uncommon, little is known about how to treat this disorder. Most affected animals do not have clinical signs of the disease and treatment has generally focused on the echocardiographically apparent feature of the disease, dynamic outflow tract obstruction. Beta-adrenergic antagonists are often effective at decreasing or abolishing the pressure gradient that develops in association with SAM. Whether this has a favorable effect on survival is not known. Witnessed sudden death in animals with canine HCM is often associated with exercise or excitement. For this reason, exercise restriction might improve prognosis and is unlikely to do harm. Though the development of congestive heart failure associated with canine HCM is uncommon, the use of furosemide perhaps in combination with beta-blockade seems reasonable if echocardiographic findings confirm that systolic function is preserved.

36. What is the prognosis in canine HCM?

If the natural history of canine HCM is similar to that of feline or human HCM, it is likely that there is a broad spectrum of severity. Some people with HCM remain asymptomatic through a normal life span, whereas others die suddenly and prematurely. Evidence has accumulated that the prognosis in affected persons is at least partly related to genetic factors in that some mutations are associated with a higher incidence of sudden death. In contrast to feline patients with HCM, dogs rarely have congestive heart failure or systemic embolism.

CONTROVERSY

37. Do beta-adrenergic antagonists have a role in the management of DCM?

Beta-adrenergic antagonists (beta blockers) reduce heart rate and decrease inotropic state. However, despite a pharmacodynamic profile that is apparently at odds with the pathophysiologic function of DCM, these agents have demonstrated efficacy in people with systolic myocardial dysfunction; when patients can tolerate long-term use of beta blockers, these drugs improve hemodynamics and clinical status and decrease mortality. The reason for this paradoxical favorable response is unknown; however, it is likely that beta blockers protect the heart from the cardiotoxic effect of prolonged elevations in sympathetic tone.

Caution must be used in applying these findings in human patients to the therapy of dogs with DCM. Dogs with DCM are often first seen for veterinary evaluation when myocardial dysfunction is advanced. It must be recognized that some animals with marked systolic dysfunction are critically dependent on elevations in sympathetic tone to maintain perfusion pressure and cardiac output. In these dogs, beta blockers are apt to be poorly tolerated. However, when suitable caution is exercised, there may be a role for beta blockers in some canine patients with DCM.

BIBLIOGRAPHY

Calvert CA, Chapman WL, Toal RL: Congestive cardiomyopathy in Doberman Pinscher dogs, *J Am Vet Med Assoc* 191:598-602, 1982.

Calvert CA, Hall G, Jacobs G et al: Clinical and pathologic findings in Doberman Pinschers with occult cardiomyopathy that died suddenly or developed congestive heart failure: 54 cases (1984-1991), *J Am Vet Med Assoc* 210:510-511, 1997.

Calvert CA, Jacobs G, Smith DD et al: Association between results of ambulatory electrocardiography and development of cardiomyopathy during long-term follow-up of Doberman Pinschers, *J Am Vet Med Assoc* 216:34-39, 2000.

Calvert CA, Meurs KM. CVT update: Doberman pinscher occult cardiomyopathy. In Bonagura JD, editor: *Kirk's current veterinary therapy XIII: small animal practice,* Philadelphia, 2000, WB Saunders.

Cleland JGF, Bristow MR, Erdmann E et al: Beta-blocking agents in heart failure: should they be used and how? *Eur Heart J* 17:1629-1639, 1996.

Cobb MA: Idiopathic dilated cardiomyopathy: advances in aetiology, pathogenesis and management, *J Small Anim Pract* 33:113-118, 1992.

The COVE Study Group: Controlled clinical evaluation of enalapril in dogs with heart failure: results of the Cooperative Veterinary Enalapril study group, *J Vet Intern Med* 9:243-252, 1995.

Ettinger SJ, Benitz AM, Ericsson GF et al: Effects of enalapril maleate on survival of dogs with naturally acquired heart failure: the Long-Term Investigation of Veterinary Enalapril (LIVE) Study Group, *J Am Vet Med Assoc* 213:1573-1577, 1998.

Fascetti AJ, Reed JR, Rogers QR et al: Taurine deficiency in dogs with dilated cardiomyopathy: 12 cases (1997-2001), *J Am Vet Med Assoc* 223:1137-1141, 2003.

Harpster NK: Boxer cardiomyopathy. In Kirk RW, editor: *Current veterinary therapy VIII: small animal practice,* Philadelphia, 1983, WB Saunders.

Keene BW, Panciera DP, Atkins CE et al: Myocardial L-caritine deficiency in a family of dogs with dilated cardiomyopathy, *J Am Vet Med Assoc* 198:647-650, 1991.

Kittleson MD: Primary myocardial disease leading to chronic myocardial failure (dilated cardiomyopathy and related diseases). In Kittleson MD, Kienle RD, editors: *Small animal cardiovascular medicine,* St. Louis, 1998, Mosby.

Kittleson MD: Taurine and carnitine responsive DCM in American Cocker spaniels. In Bonagura JD, editor: *Kirk's current veterinary therapy XIII: small animal practice,* Philadelphia, 2000, WB Saunders.

Kittleson MD, Keene B, Pion PD et al: Results of the multicenter spaniel trial (MUST): taurine- and carnitine-responsive dilated cardiomyopathy in American cocker spaniels with decreased plasma taurine concentration, *J Vet Intern Med* 11:204-211, 1997.

Meurs KM, Spier KV, Miller MV et al: Familial ventricular arrhythmias in boxers, *J Vet Intern Med* 13:437-439, 1999.

O'Grady MR, Horne R: Occult dilated cardiomyopathy: an echocardiographic and electrocardiographic study of 193 asymptomatic Doberman pinschers, *J Vet Intern Med* 6:112, 1992 (abstract).

Packer M, Bristow MR, Cohn JN et al: The effect of carvedilol on morbidity and mortality in patients with chronic heart failure, *N Engl J Med* 334:1349-1355, 1996.

Pitt B, Zannad F, Remme WJ et al: The effect of spironolactone on morbidity and mortality in patients with severe heart failure, *N Engl J Med* 341:709-717, 1999.

Richardson P, McKenna W, Bristow M et al: Report of the 1995 World Health Organization/International Society and Federation of Cardiology Task Force on the Definition and Classification of cardiomyopathies, *Circulation* 93:841-842, 1996.

Sabbah HN, Shimoyama H, Kono T et al: Effects of long-term monotherapy with enalapril, metoprolol, and digoxin on the progression of left ventricular dysfunction in patients with heart failure, *Circulation* 89:2852-2859, 1994.

Sisson D, O'Grady MR, Calvert CA: Myocardial diseases of dogs. In Fox PR, Sisson D, Moise NS, editors: *Textbook of canine and feline cardiology: principles and clinical practice,* Philadelphia, 1999, WB Saunders.

11. Infective Endocarditis

Clay A. Calvert and Michelle Wall

1. What is infective endocarditis?

Infective endocarditis (IE) is the infection of the endocardial surface of the heart by microbes. In more than 90% of human patients IE is the result of bacterial colonization of the heart valves and adjacent endocardium with associated tissue destruction.

2. Which valves are most often infected?

The valves of the high-pressure left ventricle, the aortic and mitral, are most often involved. Valve involvement is directly related to the force of blood on each valve.

- The aortic valve is the single most commonly affected valve, and in some cases both the aortic and mitral valves are infected. Approximately 90% of infections involve the aortic valve.
- The pulmonic and tricuspid valves are seldom infected.

3. Why are the heart valves almost exclusively infected rather than other endocardial surfaces?

The valves are naturally exposed to trauma during each cardiac cycle as they open and close, and this results in microscopic damage to the endothelium.

4. What is the incidence of IE in dogs and cats?

Infective endocarditis is rarely diagnosed in cats. Infective endocarditis is diagnosed in 5 to 10 dogs annually at some teaching hospitals. Bacteremia alone is more common than IE. The prevalence of IE is much lower than that of dilated cardiomyopathy and myxomatous mitral valve degeneration.

5. Are certain types of dogs more likely to acquire IE than others?

In general, bacteremia is more common in tropical and semitropical regions and in medium to large dogs. Some reports cite a 2:1 male preponderance, possibly because of chronic bacterial prostatitis. German Shepherds, Boxers, Golden Retrievers, Labrador Retrievers, and Rottweilers comprise a substantial proportion of affected dogs.

6. Have any predisposing factors been identified?

Procedures involving the gingiva, oropharynx, gastrointestinal tract, or infected tissues can cause bacteremia. Chronic infections, including pyodermas, abscesses, foreign body infections, bacterial gingivitis and stomatitis, perianal infections, prior surgery (especially extensive or protracted procedures), bone infections, and bacterial prostatitis, have been associated with IE.

7. Do congenital heart defects sometimes lead to IE?

Infective endocarditis is seldom associated with congenital heart disease in dogs, with the exception of subaortic stenosis (SAS). With SAS, turbulent, high-velocity blood flow in the left heart produces microtrauma on the valve leaflets and facilitates microbe colonization. Boxers, Rottweilers, and Golden Retrievers have relatively high incidences of both IE and SAS. No more than 10% of dogs with SAS have IE, and no more than 10% of dogs with bacterial endocarditis have SAS.

8. **Does immunosuppression predispose to IE?**
The use of corticosteroids has been associated with IE. Debilitation from cancer chemotherapy or any abnormality that impairs host defenses may predispose to IE.

9. **Other than corticosteroid use, can veterinary procedures or therapy cause IE?**
Bacteremia can develop as a result of indwelling intravenous and urinary catheters or any procedure involving the gingiva, oropharynx, or gastrointestinal tract. Furthermore, manipulation of infected tissue, causing increased interstitial pressure, can force bacteria into veins and lymphatic channels.
  - The body's defense mechanisms (macrophages in the liver and spleen and spleen and capillary neutrophils) are generally able to eradicate transient bacteremia.
  - Debilitated and immunosuppressed animals may have persistent bacteremia, and some of these will have IE.

10. **Should prophylactic antibiotic therapy be administered to dogs undergoing invasive procedures, dentistry, or surgery?**
There is little evidence to support a need for such an approach in normal dogs. Maintenance of oral hygiene is important. Dogs with congenital subaortic stenosis should receive antibiotics during dental treatment.
  - Ampicillin, penicillin, and amoxicillin are not good choices because coagulase-positive staphylococci, the most frequent pathogens in cases of IE, are usually resistant to these agents.
  - A first-generation cephalosporin, ticarcillin, or ticarcillin-clavulanate are better choices. One dose should be given during the procedure; therapy should not be initiated several days before the procedure.

11. **What are the most common bacteria involved in bacterial endocarditis?**
Coagulase-positive staphylococci and beta-hemolytic streptococci are most often isolated from blood or heart valves in cases of bacterial endocarditis. However, many different bacteria have been isolated, including *E. coli* and *Pseudomonas* spp. Recently *Bartonella* spp. have been implicated as a common cause of IE in dogs.

12. **Is endocarditis ever caused by fungi?**
Because of less frequent and less aggressive immunosuppressive treatments and the absence of prosthetic heart valve implantation in dogs as compared to human patients, the risk of fungal endocarditis in dogs is zero or nearly zero.

13. **Why use the term IE if only bacteria are involved?**
Occasionally IE is identified by echocardiography and blood cultures are negative. Results of polymerase chain reaction (PCR) analysis of blood cultures for *Bartonella* spp. have been positive in some of these dogs. *Bartonella, Brucella, Coxiella,* and *Chlamydia* may be causative agents in culture-negative cases.

14. **Does preexisting heart disease predispose to IE?**
Most dogs confirmed to have IE do not have known prior heart disease.
  - Other than subaortic stenosis, neither congenital heart defects nor myxomatous degeneration of the mitral valve are major risk factors. In fact, breeds with the highest incidence of myxomatous mitral valve degeneration have a very low incidence of IE.
  - Some bacteria, including some pathogenic staphylococci and streptococci, produce proteases that damage the endothelium and promote formation of platelet-fibrin meshes and deposition of red blood cells, predisposing to bacterial colonization of heart valves.

15. How can bacteremia be differentiated from IE?

Positive blood culture results, preferably more than one, are required for the diagnosis of bacteremia. Also, clinical signs and laboratory data consistent with bacteremia are important. Infective endocarditis is distinguished from bacteremia alone by the presence of endocardial bacterial colonization, which can be seen on echocardiography.

- A recent-onset cardiac murmur, especially if there is a diastolic component, indicates IE.
- Echocardiography greatly facilitates the diagnosis of IE.
  - An oscillating cardiac mass is typical of IE.
  - Aortic valve IE is easily identified.

16. Isn't it true that blood cultures are often unrewarding?

Blood cultures do lack sensitivity and specificity, but they should always be performed when an infective organism is suspected. The most common causes for negative blood culture results are the absence of bacteremia and inadequate sampling.

- Excluding the possibility of contamination, if one performs blood cultures on dogs without bacteremia, the results will be negative.
- When multiple blood samples (preferably three samples over a 24-hour period) of 7 to 10 ml each are obtained from dogs with a strong likelihood of bacteremia, positive results are often obtained. It is possible to collect these samples simultaneously from different venipuncture sites with results similar to those obtained by collecting the samples at different times over 24 hours.

17. What factors contribute to negative blood culture results in dogs that actually have bacteremia?

The primary factors contributing to negative results are the following

- Technique and diligence of the microbiology laboratory
- Low concentration of bacteria in the blood
- Prior antibiotic therapy
- Chronic IE with encapsulated vegetative lesions
- Inadequate sample volume (<7 ml) or too few samples obtained
- Intermittent shedding of organisms
- Failure to culture for, or the laboratory's inability to harvest, anaerobic organisms
- Infection by fastidious, slow-growing organisms
- Endogenous bactericidal factors (phagocytes and complement)
- Infection by *Bartonella*

18. How do we know that a bacterium isolated by blood culture is not a contaminant?

Strict attention to disinfection of the venipuncture site is critical. Sterile technique should be used when collecting blood samples.

- Isolating the same organism from multiple samples indicates that it is the pathogen.
- Isolating that same organism from a suspected site of infection, although seldom accomplished, is strong evidence that the organism is the cause of the infection.
- Isolating a nonpathogenic strain of bacteria (e.g., one known to be a skin commensal) from only one sample, or isolating different organisms from different samples, suggests contamination.
- Contamination is particularly likely when poor technique was used for sample acquisition.
- Contamination of the blood sample during transfer to the blood culture medium is also possible.

19. In dogs with suspected acute, severe bacteremia, should one allow 24 hours to pass so that three blood culture samples can be obtained prior to initiation of antibiotic therapy?

Clinical judgment is required. Studies in human patients found that the rates of positive results are similar when multiple samples are collected over 24 hours or at the same time from different sites. Alternatively, if the patient is receiving antibiotic therapy, collect the sample when the antibiotic is at trough concencentration. Using a blood culture vial that contains an antimicrobial absorbing resin can also increase the chances of isolating a microbe when antibiotics have been given.

20. Urine cultures are easier to obtain; can they be substituted for blood cultures?

Bacteria that cause bacteremia in dogs are often filtered into the urine and may be concentrated in the bladder.

- Urine cultures should not be substituted for blood cultures.
- However, because the urinary tract, including the prostate gland, can be the source of the bacteremia, in selected cases, urine and ejaculate should be cultured.

21. How useful is echocardiography in the diagnosis of IE?

The vegetative lesions of aortic valve IE are usually very easy to recognize during echocardiography.

- Vegetations on the mitral valve are more difficult to differentiate from myxomatous degeneration.
- Age, breed of the dog, and clinical signs can help distinguish IE from myxomatous degeneration.

22. What clinical signs are associated with IE?

Clinical signs associated with IE are often nonspecific and frequently extracardiac. All signs and symptoms of bacteremia, such as fever, trembling, myalgia, lameness, injected sclera, vomiting, diarrhea, and lethargy, can be associated with IE. Clinical signs of IE include the following:

- Heart murmur of recent onset
- Vague clinical signs such as lethargy and lack of appetite
- Lameness usually due to immune-mediated arthritis
- In some animals, dyspnea due to pulmonary edema caused by congestive heart failure

23. What are the characteristics of heart murmur in cases of IE?

Infection of any valve results in a systolic heart murmur of variable intensity.

- IE involving the aortic valve results in aortic valve regurgitation that produces a decrescendo diastolic murmur that is:
- Usually low intensity
- Heard best approximately midway on a line between the auscultation point for the tricuspid valve and the manubrium
- Often audible over the left heart base when the stethoscope head is held under the upper triceps
- Aortic regurgitation is strongly indicative of aortic valve IE.

24. Do the peripheral pulses change with IE?

The femoral pulses are usually normal in dogs with mitral valve endocarditis, but they may be weak in dogs with left-sided congestive heart failure. The femoral pulses of dogs with severe aortic valve IE are abnormal, which is indicative of the diagnosis.

- The volume overload associated with aortic regurgitation results in a high systolic pulse pressure and the rapid diastolic runoff back into the left ventricle causes a low diastolic pulse pressure.
- The characteristic pulse can be described as quick (short), hyperdynamic, and bounding.

25. Does the absence of fever rule out IE?

No! Chronic, low-grade bacterial infection may be associated with a normal body temperature and very few clinical signs. Fever is frequently absent at diagnosis because the bacterial load may be low as a result of previous therapy with the following:

- Antibiotics
- Steroids
- Nonsteroidal antiinflammatory drugs (NSAIDs).

26. How often is shifting leg lameness associated with IE?

Intermittent lameness, possibly involving multiple or "shifting" limbs, is common but not present in all cases.

- Lameness can be the result of septic arthritis (from emboli), but is usually the result of immune-complex arthritis. Synovial tissue may contain IgG, IgM, and complement.
- The clinical signs of primary immune-mediated arthritis and those of arthritis secondary to bacteremia and IE are identical.

27. What causes the immune-mediated complications of IE?

Circulating immune complexes are deposited along the glomerular basement membrane, on the synovium of joint capsules, and in the endothelium of vessels. This leads to the following:

- Glomerulonephritis
- Arthritis
- Vasculitis

28. What laboratory findings are typical of IE?

Abnormalities of the white blood cell differential (leukocyte) count, platelet count, serum chemistry profile, and results of urinalysis are common in dogs with IE.

- The white blood cell count often indicates the presence of inflammation.
- Chronic low-grade bacteremia may be associated with a normal white blood cell count or neutrophilia involving mature cells.
- Monocytosis is present in as many as 90% of dogs with IE.
- Mild to moderate thrombocytopenia (most commonly attributable to systemic vasculitis with immune or coagulatory consumption) is common.
- Low or low-normal levels of serum albumin, increased serum alkaline phosphatase activity, and low or low-normal concentration of serum glucose, alone or in combination, are associated with, but not exclusive to, bacteremia.
- Azotemia may be prerenal or caused by renal embolization and glomerulopathy.
- Proteinuria, pyuria, and bacteriuria are often detected in dogs with IE.

29. What are the sequelae to IE?

Most dogs with IE have left-sided congestive heart failure.

- Congestive heart failure is inevitable when IE involves the aortic valve.
- This condition is less common and is latent when IE involves the mitral valve.

Immune complex disease causes the following:

- Arthropathy
- Myositis
- Vasculitis
- Glomerulonephritis and renal failure
- Thrombotic disease
  - Spleen
  - Limbs
  - Myocardium

- Brain
- Kidneys

30. Is electrocardiography useful in the diagnosis of IE?

Premature ventricular contractions occur in most dogs (50% to 70% of documented cases) with IE, but they are not always detected on short recordings. Lethal ventricular tachycardia is rare. Chamber enlargement may be evident with chronic IE. If the aortic valve is involved, conduction abnormalities such as varying degrees of atrioventricular (AV) block or bundle branch blocks can be seen.

31. Is it more difficult to diagnose IE if sequelae are already present?

Although the presence of sequelae of IE should alert the veterinarian that IE may be the cause, the presence of renal failure or heart failure may distract attention from the underlying cause.
- Infective endocarditis is a polysystemic disease and may be difficult to differentiate from immune-mediated disease.
- Negative results of blood cultures can be misleading.

32. How can we really be certain that a dog has IE?

Ultrasound identification of an oscillating valvular mass is the best method to diagnose IE. Clinical and laboratory findings that point to this diagnosis include the following:
- Positive results of blood cultures
- Presence of a diastolic heart murmur
- Recent onset of a systolic heart murmur in a dog not prone to myxomatous degeneration
- Fever
- White blood cell count indicative of inflammation
- Presence of systemic emboli, and
- Arthropathy

33. Why is IE more difficult to eradicate than most bacterial infections?

The vegetative lesions of IE are composed of a platelet-thrombus-fibrin matrix that contains microbes.
- The pathogens are protected not only from neutrophils and macrophages, but also from antibiotics, which may fail to reach optimal concentrations within the vegetation.
- The bacteria are concentrated in this matrix and very few granulocytes are within the vegetation.
- Septic embolization to many organs and tissues, most notably the spleen and kidneys, establishes satellite infections that are difficult to eradicate.

34. What antibiotics are the best choice for treating IE?

Most infections are due to staphylococci or streptococci. On the basis of the general antibiotic sensitivity patterns of these commonly involved organisms, the following antibiotic regimens are likely to be effective:
- Cephalosporins, ticarcillin, ticarcillin-clavulanic acid, fluoroquinolones, clindamycin, and aminoglycosides are usually effective against coagulase-positive staphylococci.
- With the exception of the aminoglycosides and fluoroquinolones, these same antibiotics are usually effective against streptococci.
- The fluoroquinolones, aminoglycosides, and ticarcillin have good activity against a spectrum of Gram-negative organisms.
- A combination of ampicillin, a first-generation cephalosporin or ticarcillin, and an aminoglycoside provides excellent coverage.
- Another good combination is clindamycin plus a fluoroquinolone, the former providing excellent anaerobic activity.

35. Does the route of administration matter?

High serum concentrations must be achieved and maintained. Thus the intravenous route is superior to the oral route.

36. What about dosage?

Doses should be higher than those normally recommended for other conditions.

- High-dose therapy with ampicillin and ticarcillin seldom causes problems.
- High-dose therapy (20 mg/kg 3 times/day) with a first-generation cephalosporin is associated with an increased risk of vomiting, anaphylactoid reactions, blood dyscrasias, and nephrotoxicity.
- The parenteral dosage of enrofloxacin is 5 mg/kg every 12 hours or 10 mg/kg every 24 hours. The antibiotic dose must be diluted from a minimum of 1:1 to a maximum of 1:9 with a nonsaline-containing fluid, injected over a 10-minute period, and not injected into an intravenous line containing Ringer's or saline solution.
- The maximal systemic dosage of gentamicin is 6 mg/kg every 24 hours; for amikacin it is 15 mg/kg every 24 hours. These dosages must not be exceeded.
- Good hydration must be maintained.
- Administration of antibiotics for longer than 5 to 10 days is associated with a high risk of nephrotoxicity.
- Concurrent use of NSAIDS or furosemide predisposes to nephrotoxicity.
- Check the urine for granular casts; if present, they indicate impending renal compromise.

The antibiotic regimen should be adjusted, if necessary, based on the antibiogram (sensitivity pattern of a given bacterial or fungal strain to a specific antibiotic) results.

37. How long should therapy be continued?

Because of sanctuary sites on the heart valves, kidneys, bone/intervertebral disc, and septic emboli, treatment must be continued for at least 8 to 12 weeks.

- Intravenous therapy is continued as long as practical and at least until there is clinical and laboratory evidence of dramatic improvement.
- After intravenous treatment is completed, subcutaneous administration of antibiotics such as cephazolin, ticarcillin, or ticarcillin-clavulanate should be initiated and maintained for 3 to 6 weeks.
- Oral antibiotics should only be prescribed after laboratory and clinical signs have normalized and after at least 4 weeks of parenteral therapy.
- Bacteriostatic antibiotics should not be used.

38. What other therapeutic measures may be required?

Supportive therapy involves the following:

- Fluid, acid-base and electrolyte balance, and nutritional support (either parenteral or tube alimentation)
- Treatment of possible sources of infection such as wounds, abscesses, and stomatitis
- Removal and culture of any catheters that are indwelling at the time of diagnosis.

39. What if congestive heart failure develops?

Congestive heart failure almost always occurs within 3 months of the diagnosis of aortic valve IE, and it may be present at the time of diagnosis.

- Treatment of congestive heart failure includes administration of digoxin or pimobendan, an angiotensin-converting enzyme (ACE) inhibitor, a diuretic, spironolactone, a low-sodium diet, and severe restriction of activity.
- A potent afterload reducer, such as amlodipine or hydralazine, should be added after 2 weeks.
- Arteriolar dilation decreases systemic resistance.
- Mitral and aortic regurgitation volumes are decreased.

40. Is there any hope of long-term survival?

Dogs with the best chance for long-term survival with IE are those in whom the diagnosis is made early, the aortic valve is not involved, and the condition is treated aggressively.

- There is virtually 100% mortality, because of congestive heart failure, of all dogs with aortic valve IE that is not diagnosed early.
- Congestive heart failure can occur one or more years after the diagnosis of mitral valve IE.
- Administration of corticosteroids, late diagnosis, and inadequate antibiotic therapy all worsen the prognosis.
- Renal failure occasionally occurs as a consequence of IE.

41. Does heparin or aspirin reduce the severity of embolic complications?

In human patients with IE, heparin has not been shown to prevent embolization and increases the risk of hemorrhage. However, aspirin has been proved to reduce inflammation and embolic complications. In dogs a dosage of approximately 5 mg/kg orally every 24 hours is recommended.

42. Are infections that lead to IE always obvious or severe?

No, the initial infection that eventually leads to IE is often subtle and IE is usually not anticipated.

43. Can IE be prevented?

Yes, IE can be prevented, at least sometimes.

- Good principles of antibiotic therapy should be followed for all bacterial infections.
- Unnecessary use of corticosteroids can lead to IE.
- Castration will eliminate the prostate gland as a source of bacteremia.
- Maintenance of good oral hygiene is important.

BIBLIOGRAPHY

Calvert CA: Valvular bacterial endocarditis in the dog, *J Am Vet Med Assoc* 180:1080-1084, 1982.
Calvert CA, Greene CE, Hardie EM: Cardiovascular infections in dogs: epizootiology, clinical manifestations, and prognosis, *J Am Vet Med Assoc* 187:612-616, 1985.
Dow SW, Curtis CR, Jones RL et al: Bacterial culture of blood from critically ill dogs and cats: 100 cases (1985-1987), *J Am Vet Med Assoc* 195:113-117, 1989.
DeFrancesco TC: CVT Update: Infective endocarditis. In Kirk RW, Bonagura JD, editors: *Kirk's current veterinary therapy XIII: small animal practice,* Philadelphia, 2000, WB Saunders.
Sisson D, Thomas WP: Endocarditis of the aortic valve in the dog, *J Am Vet Med Assoc* 184:570-578, 1984.
Wall M, Calvert CA, Greene CE: Infective endocarditis in dogs, *Compendium* 24:614-625, 2003.

12. Canine Heartworm Disease

Clay A. Calvert and Laura Gaye Ridge

1. What is heartworm (HW) disease?

HW disease, or dirofilariasis, is the consequence of parasitic infection by a filarid nematode, *Dirofilaria immitis.* The dog is the primary host. Adult heartworms reside primarily within the pulmonary arteries but are occasionally found in the right atrium, right ventricle, or vena cava. The adult female worms release a larval form (L1) directly into the bloodstream; transmission of the infection is by mosquitoes, which are an obligatory intermediate host for the parasite.

2. What is the worldwide dissemination of *D. immitis* infection in dogs?

Mexico, Japan, South America, southern and southeastern Asia, Australia, Italy, and southern European countries are all endemic areas.

3. Are there any areas of the United States and Canada where the HW infection has not been detected?

HW infection is generally uncommon in Canada but has been reported in southern regions adjacent to Washington, Minnesota, New York, and lakes Huron, Ontario, and Erie. HW infection is rare in mountainous regions of the United States and in Alaska, Idaho, Montana, Wyoming, Nevada, Utah, Arizona, and the western parts of the Dakotas.

- A mobile public guarantees that infected dogs will be transported to nonendemic regions and, if the climate is suitable, infections will be established.
- Feral dogs and wild Canidae (principally coyotes and foxes) are reservoirs, making HW infection impossible to eradicate once introduced into a region.

4. What species other than dogs and cats are susceptible to *D. immitis* infections?

Other Canidae, sea lions, and ferrets are susceptible.

5. What does the term *occult* HW infection mean?

Occult HW infection refers to infections in which microfilariae are absent or present inconsistently in low numbers in serial venipuncture samples. Possible causes of occult HW infection include the following:

- There may be immune-mediated entrapment and destruction of microfilariae in the pulmonary microcirculation.
- Unisex infections can occur; these are more likely in nonendemic regions when the adult HW burden is low.
- The HW-preventative drugs Interceptor, Heartgard, ProHeart, Iverheart, and Revolution will stop microfilarial production and kill microfilariae over a period of 6 to 12 months.

6. Are all mosquitoes capable of transmitting infective *D. immitis* larvae?

Many (at least 60) species of mosquitoes can transmit the infection. *Culex* and *Aedes* spp. are the primary culprits in dogs, because they prefer to feed on dogs. *Culex pipiens* and perhaps other species prefer to feed on cats.

7. What are the microfilariae?

Microfilariae are the first-stage larvae (L1) that are produced by gravid female *D. immitis*.

- It is believed that microfilariae produce little or no disease and are a "dead end" for the parasite unless they are ingested by a mosquito.
- The L1 develop to the infective larval stage (L3) within the mosquito.

8. How long does it take for the Ll to develop to the infective (L3) stage within the mosquito?

The time varies with the ambient temperature. The maturation time is 30 to 130 days for ambient temperatures between 60° F and 64° F. At 80° F (27° C), 10 to 14 days are required for development from the L1 to L3 stage.

9. When can HW infection be transmitted?

Most HW infections are transmitted in the northern hemisphere during July and August. Even along the Gulf coast, transmission in December and January is uncommon.

10. How long after a dog is infected by L3 does it take for microfilariae to appear in the peripheral blood of the host?

Approximately 6 months is required.

11. Which stages of development are found in the pulmonary arteries?
The fifth-stage larvae (L5) develop 50 to 70 days after inoculation with L3 and reach the pulmonary arteries 70 to 110 days after L3 inoculation. Most are found in the caudal lobar pulmonary arteries because these vessels have the highest blood flow. The L5 grow and mature in the pulmonary arteries and are sexually mature 190 to 285 days after L3 inoculation. Thus the L5 (young adults) and adults are found in the pulmonary arteries.

12. Are adult HWs always present when microfilariae are detected?
Usually adult HWs are present, unless an adulticide treatment has been administered.
- It is uncommon (<1% of cases) for microfilariae to be present without adult worms in an untreated dog because the adult HW life span is longer.
- The true life span of adult HW is poorly documented, but microfilariae can live for 2 to 4 years.

13. Microfilariae are occasionally detected in puppies. What is the significance of this finding?
Microfilariae (L1) can be transmitted via the placenta to the fetus.
- If the puppy is younger than 7 months, the microfilariae cannot represent a patent HW infection.
- The microfilariae do little or no harm but the puppy serves as a reservoir for infection.
- If microfilariae are detected in a puppy that is at least 7 months of age, then an antigen test should be performed.

14. Is there any significance to the concentration of microfilariae in the peripheral blood?
The concentration of microfilariae detected in small samples of blood collected at various times varies throughout the day. Sometimes there are midday peaks but the periodicity is unpredictable.
- The concentration of microfilariae does not correlate strongly with the adult HW burden.
- The incidence of acute adverse reactions following the administration of Interceptor is increased when the microfilarial counts are high.

15. What actually causes the pulmonary artery disease associated with HW infection?
Sloughing of strips of endothelium occurs quickly after HW contact. Endothelin levels increase and platelets and leukocytes adhere to the damaged endothelium and growth factors are released. Multiplication and migration of smooth muscle cells and interstitial fibrosis result. There is villus hypertrophy characterized by protuberances consisting of smooth muscle covered by a healed endothelium. The healed endothelium of a villus may be damaged and then a secondary villus develops. Thickening of artery and arteriole walls leads to decreased blood flow, thromboembolism, and decreased compliance (relaxation) of the artery wall. Pulmonary hypertension can develop.

16. Do all dogs with HW infection have pulmonary hypertension?
Not all dogs have pulmonary hypertension, or at least it is mild in most cases.
- Some degree of pulmonary hypertension exists in most dogs with radiographic evidence of HW infection.
- Artery size apparent on radiographs does not necessarily correlate with the degree of hypertension.
- Two thirds of the pulmonary circulation must be obstructed before **severe** hypertension develops.
- The arterioles cannot dilate when severely diseased, and recruitment of collateral vessels does not occur because the vessels are already in use or are obstructed.
- Hypertension is exacerbated by exercise.

- There may be exercise-induced symptoms, including right-sided congestive heart failure and syncope.

17. Why is HW damage worse in some dogs than in others?

High adult HW burden (increased contact with endothelium) and immune-mediated responses cause severe damage. Longer duration of infection and higher levels of exercise also lead to more damage.

- Lobar arterial dilation, tortuosity, and obstruction tend to be more severe in dogs with HW disease that come from regions where HW disease is highly prevalent.
- Higher worm burden
- Higher incidence of immune-mediated occult infections
- Loss of pulmonary arterial compliance resulting from a thickening of the walls, fibrosis, embolism, and obstruction leads to pulmonary hypertension with the following results:
  - Right ventricular dilation and hypertrophy
  - Exercise intolerance
  - Syncope

18. When should dogs be tested for HW infection?

The recommendations for testing dogs for HW infection are as follows:

- Antigen testing should begin about 7 months after the end of the previous transmission season. This could be in April in northern states and June in the southern states and tropical regions.
- Young dogs should be tested 7 months after possible exposure.
- Annual antigen testing is recommended but is controversial and not necessary if an appropriate preventative program is maintained.
- An adult dog that is not or may not have been on an adequate HW preventative program should be tested 7 months after possible exposure.
- A microfilarial test is mandatory prior to initiating diethylcarbamazine prophylaxis.
- Antigen testing is advisable before initiating prophylaxis.

19. Is it really necessary to test annually?

It is well documented that client compliance with oral administration of HW preventative drugs is often poor. However, if Heartgard, Interceptor, Iverheart, or Revolution is given at least every 2 months, the likelihood of infection is small. Annual testing is recommended.

20. Has serologic (antigen) testing supplanted microfilarial detection as the preferred method of diagnosis?

Yes; however, a microfilarial test is mandatory before initiating diethylcarbamazine prophylaxis.

21. What is the best antigen test for the detection of HW infection?

There are numerous tests available and all are sensitive and specific. The two types of tests are the "stat" tests, which provide a quick answer while the client is at the clinic, and those more suitable for batching numerous samples to be run later in the day. Antigen tests are used for the following:

- Screening
- As part of the clinical evaluation of a dog with signs, radiographic findings, and laboratory findings consistent with HW infection
- Monitoring adulticide efficacy

22. False-positive test results are not supposed to happen, but they do. Why?

Theoretically, HW antigen tests have absolute specificity. The primary causes for false-positive results are cross-contamination and improper methods.

- Inadequate washing
- Excess time between test setup and test assessment
- Difficulty of interpreting weak reactions. HW antigen test kit manufacturers provide a confirmatory test service

23. Can false-negative test results occur?

Yes. There are several situations that can lead to a false-negative result, including the following:

- Only the female worm contributes to a positive result.
  - An all-male-worm infection will give a negative test result.
  - This is not truly a false-negative test result.
- Currently no test will detect early (up to 5 to 6 months after L3 inoculation) infections.
  - There is 100% sensitivity when three or more female worms 8 months old or older are present.
  - If only one female is present, negative results are possible.
  - The test kit or sample is not warmed to room temperature. Some newer test kits do not require refrigeration.

Dogs with few worms resulting from a recent infection are unlikely to have clinical signs and thus the false-negative test result is not really a problem as long as the dog is receiving prophylaxis.

- Prophylaxis will prevent superinfection.
- Heartgard will kill the few worms within 2 years.

24. What tests are used to detect circulating microfilariae and which are the best?

Microfilariae can be detected through examination of a direct blood smear. However, tests that concentrate the microfilaria are more sensitive.

- The modified Knott test uses centrifugation to concentrate microfilariae; the sediment is stained and examined microscopically.
- Filter tests rely on a small-pore filter to concentrate the microfilariae.
- Both the concentrating filter tests and modified Knott test are equally sensitive (75%).
- The direct blood smear, while quick and facilitating the identification of microfilariae *(D. immitis* compared with *Dipetalonema reconditum),* is at least 25% less sensitive than the concentration tests.
- Depending on the geographic region, 15% to 50% of all HW infections in dogs are not associated with circulating microfilariae if they are not receiving prophylaxis.
- The higher incidences of occult infections occur in highly endemic regions. It is estimated that in the southeastern United States 20% to 30% of all infections are occult, while in tropical areas the incidence may be as high as 50%.

25. Do we need to worry about a weakly positive HW antigen test in an asymptomatic dog?

A weakly positive antigen test indicates a low antigen burden, provided it is a true positive test result.

- Reevalute with a different test if the first test result is equivocal.
- It is difficult to differentiate between red blood cell (RBC) sedimentation and weak hemagglutination (Vetred). Repeat testing with a different method is recommended.
- The risk of symptomatic HW disease developing from a *recent* infection in such an animal is relatively low.
- The results of a Knott or filter test will probably be negative.
- Thoracic radiographs will probably appear normal or equivocal.

26. Should asymptomatic dogs with low-level antigenemia be treated?

The risk of serious adverse reactions in *recently acquired, low-worm-burden infections* treated with Immiticide is low. Because disease severity and rate of progression are usually limited, some clinicians initiate Heartgard prophylaxis to kill the adult worms over a period of about 24 months. This course is controversial.

- *Our recommendation is to treat with Immiticide.*

27. Are *D. reconditum* infections of any significance?

D. reconditum is a benign subcutaneous parasite commonly found in regions where *D. immitis* is endemic. The microfilariae of *D. reconditum* tend to be of lower concentration than those of *D. immitis,* can cause profound eosinophilia, and closely resemble those of *D. immitis* (Table 12-1).

- On a direct smear, the microfilariae of *D. reconditum* progress across the microscopic field while those of *D. immitis* tend to undulate in place without steady progression.
- *D. reconditum* have a more rounded or blunt "nose" and a hooked tail.
- Differentiation is best accomplished by measuring the organism's length and width.
- Neither Interceptor nor Heartgard kills the microfilariae of *D. reconditum.*
- The 50 μg/kg dose of ivermectin kills both the *D. immitis* and the *D. reconditum* microfilariae.

28. Can HW serologic tests be of value in determining the severity of infection?

Yes. All enzyme-linked immunosorbent assay (ELISA) antigen tests, but not immunochromatographic tests, provide a **crude** estimate of the HW burden. However, recent spontaneous death of worms will cause an antigen concentration spike. When an antigen concentration spike is due to a high worm burden, there will also be:

- More severe clinical signs
- The emergence of signs in an asymptomatic dog
- Increased likelihood of thromboembolic complications following Immiticide treatment.

Semiquantitation of the HW burden can be done by serial dilution (with phosphate-buffered saline) of the serum and determining to which titer (dilution) a positive result persists. A titer of more than 1:32 is associated with greater risk of thromboembolic disease. The severity of disease as determined by antigen level, the dog's history, and the results of the physical examination and thoracic radiography are used to select the appropriate therapy.

29. Are there any tests that can detect early infections?

A highly sensitive ELISA test that can detect infections as soon as 3 months after L3 inoculation may become available.

30. How is the severity of HW disease classified?

Dogs with class I HW infections are asymptomatic or have only occasional episodes of coughing. Dogs with class II infections have cough or mild exercise intolerance. Dogs with class

Table 12-1　*Differentiation of the Microfilariae of D. immitis from D. reconditum*

	D. IMMITIS	D. RECONDITUM
Filter test		
Length (μm)	235-285	215-240
Width (μm)	>6	<6
Knott test		
Length (μm)	>290	<275
Width (μm)	>6	<6

III infections have severe symptoms such as overt signs of congestive heart failure, syncope, and severe exercise intolerance (Table 12-2).

31. Which class of HW severity is most common?

In one study, approximately two thirds of the dogs had class II disease.

- Dogs with class II disease are typically about 5 years old compared with an average of 3 to 4 years for dogs with class I infection and approximately 7 to 8 years old for dogs with class III infections.
- In private practice, most infections are class I.

32. What determines why some dogs are more severely affected than others?

Worm burden, duration of infection, and the host immune response are factors that determine severity.

- Dogs with class I disease tend to be younger and have a lower serum antigen concentration than most dogs with class II disease.
- Dogs with class III infections are typically a little older but sometimes their serum antigen concentration is lower.
  - Presumably their worm burden was higher but some of the worms died (dead worms produce a severe reaction in the lungs).
- Dogs with class III disease sometimes have relatively few live worms and occasionally no worms on necropsy.

33. What clinical findings indicate pulmonary thromboembolism?

Cough, dyspnea, hemoptysis, fever, pulmonary crackles, a differential leukocyte count typical of inflammation, thrombocytopenia, hemoglobinuria, and patchy interstitial-alveolar pulmonary infiltrates (especially in the caudal lobes) are all associated with thromboembolism.

34. What clinical findings are associated with congestive heart failure due to HW disease?

The subset of dogs with class III disease and congestive heart failure exhibit the following:

- Ascites is present.
- Jugular vein distention/pulsation, hepatomegaly, coughing, dyspnea, exercise intolerance, and syncope are variably present.

Table 12-2 *Classification of Heartworm Disease in Dogs*

CLASS	SIGNS	RADIOGRAPHS
I	Absent-mild	Normal to slightly abnormal
II	Cough	Moderately abnormal
	Mild exercise intolerance	
	Mild weight loss	
III	Severe cough	Severely abnormal
	Exercise intolerance	
	Poor condition	
	Anemia	
	Ascites	
	Syncope	
	Dyspnea	
	Weight loss	

- Thoracic radiographs show severe enlargement and tortuosity of lobar arteries (best viewed on the dorsoventral projection).
- Electrocardiography (ECG) results often reflect right ventricular hypertrophy (deep S waves in leads I, II, V2, and V4).
- The ascitic fluid is a modified transudate with the following characteristics:
  - Specific gravity = 1.018-1.028
  - Protein concentration > 2.5 mg/dl
  - Moderate density of cells, mostly RBCs and lymphocytes

35. What is the appropriate minimum database that should be obtained prior to HW treatment?

Although this question has been debated for many years, with the advent of rapid, cost-effective laboratory services, in all infected dogs the following laboratory tests should be ordered:

- Complete blood count (CBC)
- Serum chemistry profile
- Urinalysis

36. Are thoracic radiographs necessary?

The single most useful test for determining the severity of HW infection is thoracic radiography.

- This component of the evaluation is the one most often omitted.
- Complications following adulticide administration can often be anticipated if thoracic radiographs are evaluated.

37. Not all the radiographic abnormalities associated with HW disease consist of arterial enlargement and tortuosity. What causes the alveolar changes commonly seen?

Small pulmonary arterioles are damaged by HW infection and these can leak fluid and inflammatory cells. This produces interstitial and alveolar infiltrates that are most concentrated in the caudal lung lobes adjacent to the lobar arteries. Extensive infiltrates sometimes develop.

- Most common and severe after adulticide therapy (3-30 days)
- Can occur before treatment, especially following exertion
- Immune-mediated occult infections in which an unusually severe allergic reaction occurs results in pulmonary infiltrates.

Heavy concentrations of eosinophils are found in the lungs and the radiographic pattern can resemble left-sided congestive heart failure (pulmonary edema), blastomycosis, and allergic pneumonitis unrelated to HW.

38. Are liver enzyme elevations common, and are they a contraindication to Immiticide administration?

Markedly increased levels of serum alkaline phosphatase (SAP) and alanine aminotransferase (ALT) are not common, nor are they predictive of Immiticide toxicity.

39. Is proteinuria an important abnormality?

Proteinuria is common with class III disease, but if mild (urine protein/creatine ratio < 3) and the serum albumin is normal, the best course of action is to eliminate the heartworms. The proteinuria is often due to the following:

- Immune complex glomerulonephritis
- Amyloidosis

Severe proteinuria, particularly with a mildly low or low normal albumin is cause for concern.

- An irreversible, progressive glomerulopathy may exist.
- Nonetheless, if the animal is otherwise a good candidate for treatment, then treat.

The nephrotic syndrome (ascites together with hypoalbuminemia and severe proteinuria) is indicative of a grave prognosis.

40. Is the ECG an important component of the clinical evaluation?
The ECG in most cases is normal, so it is not really important.
- Evidence of right ventricular hypertrophy is always indicative of class III (severe) HW infection. However, a thorough history and physical examination coupled with thoracic radiographs will identify such animals, and radiographs provide more information.
- Dogs with class III infections may have normal ECG findings.
- Atrial fibrillation can occur with class III infections when congestive heart failure is overt or imminent.

41. How valuable is echocardiography for HW detection or assessment of severity?
Most dogs with mild HW disease have normal "echo" results.
- Right ventricular dilation may be seen.
- Echocardiography may show two parallel, short, linear densities separated by a narrow lucent linear regionin the right heart, main pulmonary artery, and proximal lobar arteries when the HW burden is relatively high.
- Pulmonary hypertension can be detected and measured by spectral Doppler echocardiography when high-velocity tricuspid or pulmonic regurgitation is detected.

42. Should all HW-infected dogs be treated with the same adulticide protocol?
No. The standard Immiticide protocol is highly effective for class I HW disease.
- The alternative protocol is recommended for class III disease.
  - Increased risk of severe thromboembolic complications
  - Partial worm kill is safer
  - Many veterinarians use the alternate protocol for class I and class II infections also.

43. When is corticosteroid treatment appropriate for HW disease?
Antiinflammatory dosages of corticosteroids (1.0 mg/kg once daily of prednisolone *or* prednisone, for example) are indicated for the following
- Thromboembolism.
- Allergic pneumonitis associated with occult HW disease. The duration of treatment for this purpose is 3 to 5 days and adulticide therapy is then initiated.

Some clinicians routinely prescribe steroids following adulticide administration.
- They reduce the incidence of fever, coughing, and anorexia.
- Protracted corticosteroid administration promotes thromboembolism and causes reduced pulmonary arterial blood flow.

44. When is heparin indicated for HW disease?
Heparin (75 U/kg subcutaneously, 3 times/day) can be used for the most severe class III infections in an attempt to reduce pulmonary thromboembolism.
- It is administered for several days before, during, and for several weeks after adulticide treatment. It is coupled with severe exercise restriction.
- Heparin is also indicated for spontaneous or post-Immiticide hemoglobinuria and plummeting platelet counts associated with class III HW disease with pulmonary arterial fibrin and blood clot formation. Heparin reduces hemolysis and platelet consumption.

45. When is aspirin indicated for HW infection?
Aspirin is only indicated for the most severe class III infections. It is an alternative to the heparin protocol.

- Aspirin (5 to 7 mg/kg once daily) may help ameliorate the severity of pulmonary endothelial damage and reduce the severity of thromboembolism.
- Aspirin takes 1 week or longer to produce significant benefits and is therefore used prophylactically prior to, during, and following adulticide treatment, rather than as an acute treatment for thromboembolism.
- Aspirin can cause gastric bleeding and thus the hematocrit must be monitored and the animal should be observed for vomiting, anorexia, and melena.
- Aspirin is not indicated for class I and II HW disease.

46. Some veterinarians do not believe that it is necessary to treat asymptomatic HW infections. Is this position tenable?

If there are no signs and if radiographs reveal no or only equivocal abnormalities, then treatment does not have to be started immediately. However, the dog should be treated. Some argue that such dogs can be monitored for clinical signs and by radiographs, with treatment withheld until progressive disease is detected. Arguments against this approach are as follows:

- Client compliance is often poor and some dogs will be lost to follow-up.
- The risks associated with Immiticide treatment of asymptomatic dogs with minimal radiographic changes are small.

If a wait-and-see approach is chosen, prophylaxis should be prescribed. Heartgard will eradicate the adult worms within 24 months.

47. Should the "ancient" dog be treated?

Old dogs, especially those with concomitant disorders, are not always treated. Considerable clinical judgment is required and decisions are made on an individual basis.

48. Why not use Heartgard more often as an adulticide?

The success rate of Immiticide for animals with class I or II infection is high and adverse results are not usually severe when the proper protocol is followed and posttreatment confinement is enforced.

- There is little reason to deviate from the recommendations of the American Heartworm Society.
- The slow rate of kill produced by Heartgard might allow progressive pulmonary arterial changes and complications to develop before improvement begins.

49. Are there some young to middle-aged dogs that should not be treated for adult HW infection?

Young to middle-aged dogs that should not be treated include those who have

- The nephrotic syndrome
- Life-limiting comorbid disease not related to HW infection
- Overt right-sided congestive heart failure together with hepatic failure
- Severe renal failure.

Congestive heart failure (ascites) alone is not necessarily a contraindication to treatment, although the risk of treatment complications and mortality in these cases are higher than with class I and II HW disease alone (Table 12-3).

50. What is the difference between the standard and alternative or split Immiticide treatment protocols?

The standard protocol is one intramuscular (epaxial) injection, followed by a second injection on the opposite side 24 hours later. If an antigen test is positive 4 months later, the treatment is repeated. The alternative protocol consists of an initial injection followed in 4 to 6 weeks by two injections given 24 hours apart. If an antigen test is positive 4 to 6 months later, one or two more injections are administered 24 hours apart.

Table 12-3	*Standard and Alternate (Split) Immiticide Protocols*	
	STANDARD	ALTERNATE
Class	I	I, II, III
Dosage	2.5 mg/kg, IM	2.5 mg/kg, IM
Doses	2 (24 hr apart)	1
Site	Epaxial: L_3-L_5	Epaxial: L_3-L_5
Needle*	22 gauge	22 gauge
Follow-up	4 mo	4-6 wk
	Ag test	Immiticide: 2 doses 24 hr apart
	Repeat treatment if	4 mo: Ag test ‡
	Ag positive†	

*<15 kg, use $^3/_4$ inch; >15 kg, use 1 inch.
†Clinical judgment required.
‡Four months after the third dose.

51. How effective is the standard Immiticide protocol?

Approximately 75% of dogs will be antigen negative 4 months later. If the second set of injections is required, more than 95% of dogs will become antigen negative within 4 months.

52. If an antigen test is weakly positive 4 months after the first two injections, is it appropriate to wait 1 to 2 additional months and then repeat the test?

Yes.

53. Should all dogs with persistent low-grade antigenemia be retreated?

Clinical judgment is required.
- The decision is based on initial severity, degree of improvement, age, concomitant problems, any requirement of physical exertion by the dog, and the number of administered doses.
- After three or four doses, few worms will survive and the condition usually improves over a 3- to 6-month period.

Heartgard (prophylactic) administration will gradually kill the remaining worms.

54. How effective is the Immiticide alternative dosing regimen?

The first injection kills approximately 90% of the male worms and 15% to 20% of the females.
- Overall, 50% to 60% of the worms are killed by the first injection.
- An antigen test will be negative in 90% of the dogs 4 months after the third injection.

55. Isn't it true that some clinicians routinely use the alternative Immiticide protocol for all HW infections?

- Yes, the logic is that since the first two injections of the standard Immiticide kill most adult worms, the risk of pulmonary thromboembolic complications will be high, even with some class I infections.
- Graded worm kill reduces thromboembolic complications.
- Reports from private practitioners suggest that more severe thromboembolic complications occur following two injections of Immiticide than had been their experience with thiacetarsamide sodium.

56. Isn't it true that dogs become tolerant to organic arsenicals so that retreatment is not likely to cause problems?

Yes. Furthermore, once the worm burden is reduced, the risk of thromboembolism is reduced; in fact, thromboembolism is unlikely if no such problems were encountered with the first treatment.

57. Because young female worms are resistant, isn't it a waste of time to re-treat within a few months of the first treatment?

That might be true with thiacetarsamide, but worm resistance is less of a problem with Immiticide.

58. Are there any indications for surgical removal of heartworms?

Forceps removal of worms is the treatment of choice for the vena cava syndrome.
- Affected dogs have hundreds of worms in the vena cava and right heart.
- The procedure requires considerable expertise but can be highly effective and lifesaving.

Dogs with class III disease and echocardiographically confirmed high worm burden in the right heart and main pulmonary artery can be saved by the Ishihara technique, as follows.
- Under anesthesia and fluoroscopic guidance, a long, flexible Ishihara alligator forceps or horsehair-tipped probe is introduced via a jugular vein and repeatedly passed through the vena cava, heart, and pulmonary arteries; none to many worms may be retrieved per attempt.
- In experienced hands, many worms can be retrieved.
- The remaining worms can then be more safely killed by Immiticide.

59. How much of the pulmonary damage caused by HW disease is reversible?

Most dogs will experience significant improvement, even if a few worms persist.
- Even dogs with class III disease can be saved, although mortality is relatively high during the first month after administration of Immiticide.
- Recovery from a severe class III infection may never be enough to allow vigorous exertion, but function is adequate for many dogs that are pets.
- Some of the most severely affected dogs do not regain sufficient pulmonary function to survive with good quality of life.
- Some dogs whose treatment appears to be complete subsequently have progressive, severe pulmonary hypertension that leads to syncope or congestive heart failure months later.

60. What steps can be taken to minimize the risk of severe thromboembolic lung disease after treatment?

The first step is a good pretreatment evaluation so that high-risk dogs (those with class III disease) can be identified. The alternative protocol for dogs with class III infection is as follows.
- Severe restriction of activity for 4 to 6 weeks after treatment is imperative.
- Aspirin (5 to 7 mg/kg once daily) or heparin (75 U/kg 3 times/day subcutaneously) can be administered before, during, and for 3 to 4 weeks after treatment with a HW adulticide. This treatment is appropriate
  - For the most severely affected dogs only
  - Combined with strict confinement.
- Some veterinarians administer corticosteroids for 1 to 2 weeks after treatment:
  - Reduce the severity of inflammation, fever, and coughing
  - Promote coagulation and decreased pulmonary blood flow (this effect is not achieved with use for longer than 12 weeks).

61. How much toxicity is one likely to see after Immiticide treatment?

The therapeutic index is relatively low and the lungs are the most susceptible to overdosage.

- At 2.5 mg/kg, adverse effects are common but mild; they include the following:
- Lethargy
- Anorexia
- Fever
- Vomiting
- Tenderness at the injection site is common but of short duration.
  - It is due to drug leakage out of the needle tract.
  - Digital pressure should be applied during needle withdrawal and for 1 to 2 minutes thereafter.

62. Should dogs with congestive heart failure (ascites) be treated?

All dogs with class III disease should be evaluated carefully. Many can be treated successfully but mortality is greater than with class I and II infections.

- If the mucous membranes are gray or cyanotic, dyspnea is severe and constant, and the dog is anorexic, obviously unhappy, and in distress, death is the likely outcome.
- If the dog is eating, has at least pale pink mucous membranes, does not require oxygen supplementation, and looks reasonably happy, there is at least a 75% chance of survival.
- Strict cage confinement is necessary.
- An alternate Immiticide protocol should be instituted.
- Heparin or aspirin is an elective adjuvant.

63. What about diuretics and cardiac drugs for dogs with congestive heart failure?

Furosemide 1 to 2 mg/kg, 2 times/day, and a low-salt diet are recommended. Angiotensin-converting enzyme inhibitors such as enalapril may help, but should be initiated at a low dosage (0.25 mg/kg, once daily). The dosage is based on the dog's estimated lean weight. The dosage is increased after 5 to 7 days to 0.25 mg/kg, twice daily. The maximum dosage is 0.5 mg/kg twice daily.

- Hypotension is a potential complication of vasodilator use in dogs with right-sided congestive heart failure and fixed pulmonary arterial resistance.
- Digoxin is ineffective for cor pulmonale.
- Hydralazine and diltiazem should not be administered because they usually cause systemic hypotension in animals with class III disease.

64. Do corticosteroids reduce the efficacy of adulticide treatment?

The kill-rate of female worms was reduced in one study of thiacetarsamide efficacy in dogs administered prednisone. A negative impact of corticosteroids on Immiticide kill rates is unlikely.

65. What is the treatment recommendation if hemoglobinuria occurs with HW disease?

The recommended treatment is immediate, strict cage confinement and heparin (200 U/kg IV, followed by 75 U/kg subcutaneously 3 times/day).

- Oxygen therapy may be advisable.
- Hemoglobinuria is usually associated with class III disease.
- Thromboembolism is present.
- Oxygen is the only practical and effective way to dilate the pulmonary arteries.
- Short-term corticosteroid treatment (1.0 mg/kg once daily) may be of value.
- Treatment is continued until there is clinical, radiographic, and laboratory evidence of marked improvement (usually 3 to 5 days).

66. Is it necessary to kill microfilariae?

- Yes, but gradual kill as an aside to prophylaxis is acceptable.
- The risk, albeit low, of adverse reactions in all breeds is an argument against acute microfilaricide killing and in favor of slow kill with prophylaxis.

67. Is there a good reason to treat microfilariae?
The primary reason to treat is that a dog with persisting microfilariae serves as a reservoir for spreading HW infection.
- Eliminating microfilariae is important.
- Eliminating microfilariae within 1 month of Immiticide treatment is less important.

68. When should microfilaricide treatment be administered?
Treatment should be administered usually 4 weeks after the second (standard protocol) or third (alternate protocol) injection of Immiticide.

69. Is ivermectin (50 μg/kg) or Interceptor the preferred microfilaricide drug?
Both drugs are highly effective but neither are approved by the Food and Drug Administration (FDA) for this use.
- Either drug can be used for this purpose.
- Interceptor is the drug of choice.
- Prophylactic doses are adequate.
- This drug is associated with less risk of dosage error.

70. How effective is the Interceptor treatment for microfilariae?
Most (> 90%) microfilariae are killed by one dose of Interceptor. A microfilaria detection test is performed 4 weeks later, and if positive, the treatment can be repeated.

71. Is it necessary to repeat microfilaricide treatment?
Because most microfilariae are killed by the first dose, the rest can be killed over a period of 6 to 12 months simply by initiating monthly prophylaxis or ProHeart 6. A low level of microfilaremia is not likely to indicate that the dog is serving as a reservoir for the organisms.

72. Are adverse effects likely when Interceptor is given to dogs with microfilariae?
Whether there are adverse effects depends on the microfilarial concentration. Interceptor kills most of the microfilariae in less than 24 hours.
- If the count is high, acute vomiting, diarrhea, and a degree of circulatory collapse can occur.
- The overall incidence of adverse reactions is less than 10% and is usually restricted to vomiting, diarrhea, lethargy, and anorexia.
- Prednisone (1 mg/kg) given with Interceptor reduces the risk of reaction to almost zero.
- Most reactions begin within a few hours.
- It is recommended that the treatment be given in the morning and the dog discharged in the late afternoon.
- Occasionally, mild lethargy and anorexia develop the following day and persist for 1 to 2 days.

73. Is death possible?
Yes, but even severe reactions, if detected quickly, are treatable with IV fluids and soluble corticosteroid administered intravenously (IV).

74. Is there any advantage to one or another HW preventative drug?
In general, the monthly prophylactic drugs or injectable ProHeart have supplanted daily prophylaxis for the reason of convenience. All are highly effective and safe.

75. How long does it take for microfilariae to disappear from the blood after prophylaxis is begun?
They disappear in approximately 6 to 12 months with oral drugs and 1 month with ProHeart 6.

76. Is ProHeart 6 effective for longer than 6 months?
Yes. At a higher dosage it is effective for 1 year.

77. Which prophylactic is safest to administer to a dog with circulating microfilariae?
Heartgard, Revolution, and ProHeart 6 do not kill microfilariae quickly and therefore an acute reaction is rare. Interceptor is acutely microfilaricidal, and therefore some dogs (those with high concentrations) will experience an adverse reaction during the first 48 hours.

78. Should year-round prophylaxis be maintained?
Year-round prophylaxis is recommended because many owners are late or neglect to re-initiate prophylaxis at the start of a new mosquito season.
- In the southeastern United States, year-round prevention is maintained even though transmission is not likely during December and January.
- Prophylaxis should be year-round in Florida, the coastline of Texas, and other southeastern states, the Caribbean region, Hawaii, and tropical regions.
- It is customary in cooler climates to start as soon as mosquitoes appear and continue until 1 month after the first frost.
- ProHeart 12 would provide the highest likelihood of effective prevention. This medication is
  - Administered once per year
  - Coordinated with an annual wellness program
  - Not available in the United States

79. Can monthly preventatives be given bimonthly?
Alternate month administration is effective, but not recommended. The "reach back" effect is good, but not 100%, at 2-month intervals.

80. Do prophylactic drugs kill heartworms?
Both Heartgard and Interceptor, and presumably Iverheart, if given on a monthly basis starting 4 months or less after L3 infection and continued for 1 year, can prevent the development of persistent adult infection. Heartgard is most (approximately 98%) effective.

81. Are ProHeart 6 and Revolution as effective as Heartgard at terminating immature infections?
Probably not.

82. Do prophylactic drugs control other parasites?
Yes, at least with some products (Table 12-4).

83. Do monthly doses of Heartgard kill preexisting adult HW?
Adult worms can be gradually killed over a period of 24 months.

84. Are Interceptor, ProHeart 6, or Revolution as effective as Heartgard at killing adult heartworms?
Probably not.

85. Are Heartgard, Interceptor, Revolution, Iverheart, and ProHeart safe in Collies?
Yes.
- High-dose Ivermectin or Interceptor (4x preventative dosage) can cause serious toxicity in about one third of collies.
- The preventative dosages are not dangerous.

Table 12-4   Spectrum of Parasite Control for HW Preventative Products

DRUG	Mf	D. IMMITIS ADULT	L³-L⁵	ASCARIDS	WHIPWORMS	FLEAS	OTHER
Heartgard	Slow	Slow	+++				
Heartgard Plus	Slow	Slow	+++	T	A, U		
Interceptor	Rapid	?	+	T	A	±	
ProHeart 6	Slow	?	+				
Revolution	Slow	?	+		A	C	S, M, D
Iverheart	Slow	Slow	+++	T	A, U		

Mf, Microfilariae; *L*, larval stage; *U*, *Uncinaria stenocephala; A*, *Ancylostoma caninum, Ancylostoma braziliense; T, Toxocara canis, Toxascaris leonina; C*, controls hatching and molt of flea larvae, does not kill adult fleas; *M*, treatment and control of ear mites; *S*, treatment and control of *Sarcoptes scabiei; D*, control of *Dermacentor variabilis.*

- Toxic dosages produce varying (dose-related) severities of hypersalivation, mydriasis, blindness, ataxia, bradycardia, decreased respiration, coma, and death.

86. Is diethylcarbamazine (DEC) still an acceptable prophylactic drug?

Yes. At 5.5 mg/kg once daily, DEC is safe and highly effective. Extended parasite control is provided by the addition of oxybendazole (Filarabits Plus).

- A microfilarial test must be negative before treatment with DEC is initiated.
- The drug should be started at least 2 weeks before the mean daily temperature is above 57° F and continued until 2 months after the temperature drops below this level or after the first frost.
- Year-round treatment is recommended if the mean daily temperature is above 60° F for 9 months or more.
- Uncommonly, periportal hepatitis is associated with Filarabits Plus. Hepatitis is more likely with concomitant phenobarbital administration. If hepatitis occurs, it is potentially reversible.

87. Should all dogs be tested for antigens to HW before beginning prophylaxis with any product?

Yes, if exposure to HW could have occurred at least 7 months previously, the dog should be tested for antigens. If an antigen test is not performed first, and subsequently HW infection is confirmed, the following questions cannot be answered:

- Is it a drug prevention failure?
- Did an early infection already exist?

BIBLIOGRAPHY

Alkins C, Miller M: Is there a better way to administer heartworm adulticide therapy? *Vet Med* 310-317, 2003.
Calvert CA, Rawlings CA, McCall JW: Canine heartworm. In Fox PR, Sisson D, Moise NS, editors: *Textbook of canine and feline cardiology: principles and clinical practice,* ed 2, Philadelphia, 1999, WB Saunders.
Dillon R: Dirofilariasis in dogs and cats. In Ettinger SJ, Feldman SC, editors: *Textbook of veterinary internal medicine,* ed 5, Philadelphia, 2000, WB Saunders Co.
Ishihara K, Sasaki Y, Kitagawa H: Development of a flexible alligator forceps: a new instrument for removal of heart worms in the pulmonary arteries of dogs, *Jpn J Vet Sci* 48:989-995, 1986.
Jackson RE: Surgical treatment of heartworm disease, *J Am Vet Med Assoc* 154:383-388, 1969.
Knight DH: CVT Update: heartworm testing and prevention in dogs. In Bonagura JD, editor: *Kirk's current veterinary therapy XIII,* Philadelphia, 2000, WB Saunders Co.

McCall JW, McTeir TL, Supakomdej N et al: Clinical prophylactic activity of macrolides on young adult heartworms. In Soll MD, Knight FH, editors: *Proceedings of the Heartworm Symposium,* Batavia, IL, 1995, American Heartworm Society.

Miller MW, Keister MD, Tanner PA et al: Clinical efficacy of melarsomine dihydrochloride (RM340) and thiacetarsemide in dogs with moderate (Class 2) heartworm disease. In Soll MD, Knight DH, editors: *Proceedings of the Heartworm Symposium,* Batavia, IL, 1995, American Heartworm Society.

Vezzoni A, Genchi C: Reduction of post-adulticide thromboembolism complications with low dose heparin therapy. In Otto GF, editor: *Proceedings of the Heartworm Symposium,* Washington, DC, 1989, American Heartworm Society.

Section III
Pulmonary Disease
Section Editor: *Robert R. King*

13. Canine Rhinitis
Charles W. Brockus

1. What is rhinitis?

Rhinitis is inflammation of the nasal mucous membranes. Infiltrates of inflammatory cells, including neutrophils, lymphocytes, plasma cells, eosinophils, macrophages, and mast cells, occur in response to organisms, foreign bodies, parasites, allergens, and immune-mediated disorders.

2. What type of dogs most often present with rhinitis?

Nasal cavity anatomy varies significantly over the range of head shapes, from dolichocephalic to brachycephalic breeds. Mesocephalic and dolichocephalic breeds are the ones that most often present with nasal discharge. Brachycephalic breeds less frequently have rhinitis but they are more likely to have congenital malformations that predispose them to other respiratory diseases.

3. What are the clinical signs of rhinitis?

Nasal discharge is the most common clinical sign of rhinitis. This discharge can be unilateral or bilateral. Sneezing, head shaking, reverse sneezing, pawing at the mouth/nose, nasal stridor, or dyspnea may be present.

4. What types of nasal discharges are observed?

Discharges may be serous, mucoid, mucopurulent, or hemorrhagic. Because goblet cells are distributed throughout the respiratory epithelium of the nasal cavity, serous or mucoid discharges are more common; a mucopurulent discharge is typical with chronic rhinitis or may be a sign of secondary bacterial infection. It is important to establish that a nasal discharge is originating in the nasal cavity and not from lower portions of the respiratory tract; if the discharge is from the lower tract, examination limited to the nasal cavity will be unrewarding and potentially dangerous if it delays diagnosis of a serious condition such as congenital ciliary dysfunction or bronchopneumonia.

5. What diagnostic tests are typically performed first in a dog that presents with any form of rhinitis?

There are three phases of diagnostic testing.

Phase 1

A complete history and physical examination are essential in the initial evaluation of rhinitis. Placing a feather, cotton fibers, or other lightweight material in front of the nasal openings and watching for signs of airflow can be used to identify complete or partial nasal obstruction. Examination of the external nasal cavity and oral cavity, as much as possible, is a critical step. Obtaining specimens of the nasal discharge for cytologic examination is also helpful. Either a direct impression of the nasal discharge or a swab of the rostral nares may help identify nasal mites (*Pneumonyssoides caninum*). Microbiological cultures are unlikely to yield reliable information, are difficult to interpret, and can be expensive at this point. If the animal has recently received an antibiotic medication, however, bacteria may not be present. A complete blood count, biochemistry profile, and urinalysis are necessary when a specific cause cannot be identified from the initial examination.

6.   Can a therapeutic trial be initiated?

A therapeutic trial can be initiated if the client cannot afford additional diagnostic procedures or advanced diagnostic tests are not available. The trial therapy can be decided upon based on the results of a complete history (i.e., seasonal event, chronicity, etc.) and physical examination (oral examination) combined with the results of nasal discharge cytology. The effects of the trial therapy should be closely followed and the treatment adjusted based on the response.

Phase 2

A complete oral and nasal examination, including radiography, under anesthesia, is necessary to identify tooth root infections or fractures (periodontal probing), neoplasms, or foreign bodies. A dental mirror may help with examination of deep oral tissues. A rigid otoscope can be used for initial examination of the external nares and nasal area. Rhinoscopy, with a flexible endoscope, is an effective procedure to examine the mucosa and collect specimens of nasal tissues to culture for bacterial and fungal pathogens, if an infection is suspected. Another option is nasal flushing with sterile saline. Flushing saline from the pharyngeal region toward the nares will allow cellular material and debris to be collected on cotton gauze squares from which a specimen for culture can be taken. This procedure, which does not usually cause hemorrhage, is best performed after complete nasal examination but before tissue collection.

When tissue biopsy specimens are necessary they should be collected from both nasal passages. Taking a biopsy specimen from the nasal mucosa often causes hemorrhage because of the extreme vascularity of the submucosa, and the bleeding makes subsequent examination of the mucosa impossible. Therefore both nasal cavities must be examined completely before biopsy specimens are obtained. Cold saline infusion can be used to decrease the amount of bleeding during acquisition of biopsy specimens. When a "blind" biopsy is performed, it must be stressed that the biopsy instrument must not pass beyond the medial canthus of the eye, to avoid penetrating the cribiform plate during this procedure. Skull radiographs are critical to the success of this procedure, to measure distances for obtaining "blind" biopsies.

7.   What other tests are available to assist with the diagnosis of nasal cavity disease?

Phase 3

Computed tomography (CT) and magnetic resonance imaging (MRI) can be used to diagnose nasal cavity disease. CT and MRI are much more expensive than plain radiography; however, they offer a more complete assessment. CT and MRI may help localize lesions before rhinoscopy is performed but often cannot provide a definitive diagnosis. Previous trauma may have caused a sequestrum with a subsequent secondary bacterial infection. This may be identified on radiograph examination, CT, or MRI.

Rickettsial infections such as *Ehrlichia, Anaplasma*, Rocky Mountain spotted fever (RMSF), or *Bartonella* may cause rhinitis. Testing for these pathogens can be performed in any phase of the examination.

8.   Do biopsy results always provide definitive answers?

No, they do not always provide a definitive diagnosis. Cellular infiltrates may change with chronicity. Occasionally, different inflammatory cells may replace the initial cellular infiltrates and mask the initial inflammatory response. For example, a biopsy specimen from a dog with long-term allergic rhinitis may demonstrate lymphoplasmacytic inflammation due to the chronicity of the disorder. Also, biopsies in cases of infection, foreign body, or neoplastic disease may occasionally fail to help in reaching a definitive diagnosis because histologic changes may have occurred over the course of the disease. Therefore often a second series of biopsies is recommended if the initial diagnosis appears incorrect. It is important that both nasal passages are examined and undergo biopsy even if the nasal discharge is only unilateral.

9. Can rhinitis be cured?

Yes and no, depending if a definitive cause can be identified. Often, rhinitis is frustrating to manage, however, because a definitive diagnosis cannot be established and empiric treatment may be unsuccessful. This leaves the veterinarian and owner searching for an answer while the nasal discharge continues. Controlling the disorder may be a more reasonable goal than curing the disorder. Again, this depends on whether the cause of the rhinitis can be identified.

BIBLIOGRAPHY

Gartrell CL, O'Handley PA, Perry RL: Canine nasal disease – part II, *Compend Contin Educ Pract Vet* 17:539-547, 1995.
Johnson L: Rhinitis in dogs and cats (VET-329), Western States Conference Proceedings, Las Vegas, February 2004.
Johnson L: Sneezing and nasal discharge in the dog, ACVIM Proceedings, Minneapolis, June 2004.
Knotek Z, Fichtel T, Kohout P et al: Diseases of the nasal cavity in the dog, aetiology, symptomatology, diagnostics, *ACTA Vet BRNO* 70:73-82, 2001.
Kuehn NF: *Nasal discharge* (website): www.michvet.com.
Marks SL;. Diagnostics for nasal disease, Western States Conference Proceedings, Las Vegas, February 2003.
Venker-van Haagen AJ: Diseases of the nose and nasal sinuses. In Ettinger SJ, Feldman, EC, editors: *Textbook of veterinary internal medicine*, ed 6, St. Louis, 2005, Elsevier.

BACTERIAL RHINITIS

Charles W. Brockus

10. What clinical signs are present in dogs with bacterial rhinitis?

Typically, dogs with bacterial rhinitis have a mucopurulent discharge, and they may also sneeze or paw at the nose. Other signs include coughing, retching, constant swallowing, signs of pain in the nasal region, open-mouth breathing, noisy breathing, and/or ocular discharge. Depending on the chronicity and exact cause of the bacterial rhinitis, epistaxis may also be present if the infection has invaded the deeper mucosal membrane.

11. Is bacterial rhinitis common?

Rhinitis caused specifically by bacteria is rare. Secondary infection of the mucous membranes or turbinates in dogs with allergy (hypersensitivity), foreign bodies, neoplasms, immune disorders, oronasal fistula, boney sequestration, or colonization with fungal organisms is common.

12. What are the bacteria most often associated with primary bacterial rhinitis?

Pseudomonas aeruginosa, *Pasteurella multocida*, and *Staphylococcus* spp. are the bacteria that most frequently cause primary bacterial rhinitis. These bacteria have also been cultured from the respiratory tracts of animals without signs of clinical disease.

13. Should I culture the nasal discharge?

Culturing the external nasal discharge is neither a high-yield procedure nor a good prognostic test. However, microbiological culture of material from the deeper recesses of the nasal cavity may be helpful. Culture and sensitivity testing will help identify bacteria species present and their susceptibility to antibiotics. Even if the bacteria present are secondary to another disease, they can establish themselves and cause further damage. Also, culture and sensitivity testing of deep nasal tissue may be helpful when an infection does not respond to initial antibiotic therapy or to identify the causative organism for initial management.

14. What changes are observed on skull radiographs with bacterial rhinitis?

Abnormalities on skull radiographs of the nasal passages usually are limited to diffuse increase in opacity associated with mucinous material within the nasal cavity. However, osteolysis or turbinate destruction may also be seen. In more chronic cases bone destruction can occur but other causes, including fungal infection or neoplasia, must be eliminated.

15. How do I treat bacterial rhinitis?

Acute cases may resolve without antibiotics if a primary condition is identified and treated. Often a broad-spectrum antibiotic is used to treat bacterial rhinitis. Culture and sensitivity testing of deep tissues are helpful to identify the specific bacteria involved and to determine the most effective antibiotic. If a broad-spectrum antibiotic is used and the disease is non-responsive, culture and sensitivity testing are necessary. In this case one must be concerned that the bacterial infection is secondary to another condition. Treating secondary bacterial rhinitis with antibiotics can be helpful in reducing the volume and character of the nasal discharge, but resolution of clinical signs is problematic.

16. How long should I treat with antibiotics?

In mild cases a 7- to 10-day course of antibiotic therapy will be adequate. If the infection is chronic, with osteolysis or involving deep tissues, generally, long-term treatment is necessary and complete resolution of the nasal discharge may not be achieved.

17. What antibiotics are appropriate?

Because a chronic infection may have involved bone or cartilage, drugs with anaerobic activity, including clindamycin or amoxicillin (amoxicillin, amoxicillin/clavulanic acid), are often used. Clindamycin has good activity against Gram-positive and anaerobic bacteria and penetrates into deeper tissues. Metronidazole has also been used with success and has other beneficial qualities, including antiinflammatory and T-lymphocyte modulator activity. Azithromycin, doxycycline, enrofloxacin, and marbofloxacin also have been used with success.

18. What is the prognosis?

The prognosis in a case of primary bacterial rhinitis can be excellent, depending on the chronicity of the infection and the extent to which bone has become involved. The deeper infections associated with osteolysis can be much more difficult to treat. Secondary bacterial rhinitis has an excellent prognosis if the primary cause can be identified and treated effectively.

BIBLIOGRAPHY

Gartrell CL, O'Handley PA, Perry RL: Canine nasal disease – part II, *Compend Contin Educ Pract Vet* 17: 4:539-547, 1995.
Johnson L: Rhinitis in dogs and cats (VET-329), Western States Conference Proceedings, Las Vegas, February 2004.
Knotek Z, Fichtel T, Kohout P et al: Diseases of the nasal cavity in the dog, aetiology, symptomatology, diagnostics, *ACTA Vet BRNO* 70:73-82, 2001.
Marks SL. Diagnostics for nasal disease, Western States Conference Proceedings, Las Vegas, February 2003.
Venker-van Haagen AJ: Diseases of the nose and nasal sinuses. In Ettinger SJ, Feldman, EC, editors: *Textbook of veterinary internal medicine*, ed 6, St Louis, Elsevier.

MYCOTIC RHINITIS

John Crandell

19. How do dogs contract nasal aspergillosis?

Nasal aspergillosis is a common disease affecting dogs. It may be caused by infection with multiple species of *Aspergillus*, although the most common is *Aspergillus fumigatus* (Fig. 13-1).

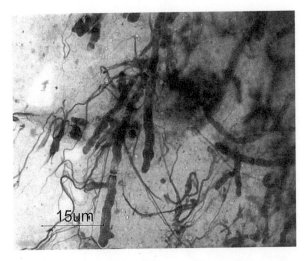

Figure 13-1.   Cytologic preparation of a nasal biopsy specimen from a dog with a nasal *Aspergillus* spp. infection.

Aspergillus spp. are saprophytic fungi that are ubiquitous in the environment and may be found in the soil, on household plants, around bird cages, and in house dust. Aspergillosis typically develops either as a localized sinonasal infection (more common) or as a disseminated disease. Aspergillosis typically results from inhalation and infection of the nasal passages and frontal sinuses. Although infection with *A. fumigatus* may occur as a primary infectious process, it should be recognized that it is typically considered an opportunistic pathogen and secondary infections resulting from preexisting nasal mucosal disease (e.g., foreign body, trauma, or neoplasia), prolonged antimicrobial therapy, or immune deficiencies can occur.

20. Are there any breeds or conformational characteristics of dogs that predispose to aspergillosis?
Young to middle-aged dolichocephalic dogs tend to be infected more readily than older and brachiocephalic breeds. German Shepherds, Rottweilers, and Labrador Retrievers are over-represented in reports of aspergillosis. Other than conformational structure, the authors know of no specific reason why aspergillosis seems to be more prevalent in Rottweilers and Labrador Retrievers. However, an abnormality of IgA production or regulation has been reported in German Shepherds that may predispose this breed to either nasal or disseminated aspergillosis.

21. I suspect a dog has nasal aspergillosis. What is the best way to diagnose the disease?
A diagnosis of nasal aspergillosis can be made using a combination of imaging modalities (e.g. computed tomography [CT], radiography), direct visualization of fungal plaques (Fig. 13-2), and identification of fungal hyphae on histologic examination. Of these modalities, direct visualization of a fungal plaque (typically located in the caudal aspect of the nasal passages or frontal sinuses), followed by histologic examination of a biopsy specimen, is the best way to diagnose fungal rhinitis. This typically requires rhinoscopic evaluation with a rigid arthroscope or flexible bronchoscope. Visualization may be attempted with an otoscope, although this only allows examination of the rostral nasal passages, which decreases the likelihood that fungal plaques in the deeper passages will be detected. Alternatively, more invasive procedures such as rhinotomy or sinusotomy may allow visualization and detection of fungal lesions. Direct

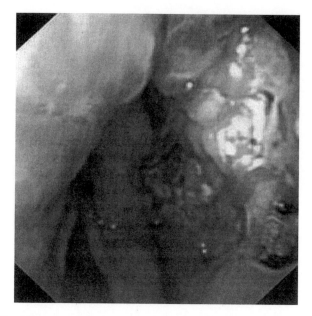

Figure 13-2. Rhinoscopic appearance of a fungal plaque caused by an *Aspergillus* spp. infection in a dog.

visualization of the fungal plaques is also beneficial in that it allows the clinician to thoroughly evaluate the animal for any underlying diseases that could lead to a secondary fungal infection. Radiographic and CT evaluation of the nasal passages and frontal sinuses may be beneficial in the diagnosis of sinonasal aspergillosis. However, imaging procedures should be performed before rhinoscopy to avoid artifactual changes induced by lavage and hemorrhage. Both imaging procedures will typically show evidence of soft tissue/fluid accumulation in the nasal passages and/or sinuses as well as turbinate destruction.

22. If I do not have access to rhinoscopy, can I still make the diagnosis of nasal aspergillosis?

Yes. In addition to clinical signs of sneezing, nasal discharge (copious, in the case of aspergillosis), nasal congestion or obstruction, and possibly epistaxis that can be seen with multiple nasal disorders, aspergillosis causes ulceration and depigmentation of the nares (Fig. 13-3). When rhinoscopy for direct fungal plaque visualization is unavailable, nasal lavage can be performed with a catheter placed either in the nares or retroflexed around the soft palate. Aggressive lavaging may dislodge fungal plaques that can then be collected by "straining" the outflowing lavage fluid through gauze. Tissue trapped in the gauze can then be examined histologically. Tissue may also be obtained by performing nasal lavage with reaming of the nasal cavity with a firm plastic tube, or by taking blind nasal pinch biopsies. However, all of these alternative techniques have the disadvantage that they do not involve direct visual assessment of the nasal passage and so limit the ability to adequately characterize the severity of the disease. A serum test for *Aspergillus* may be beneficial if the results are positive; the test has a sensitivity of approximately 69%. However, if the results are negative a fungal infection cannot be ruled out. Similarly, a serum culture for fungi may be used to aid in the diagnosis of aspergillosis, and

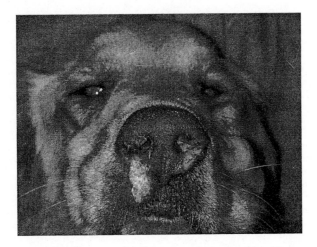

Figure 13-3. Nasal depigmentation and ulceration due to nasal aspergillosis in a dog.

culture results were positive in 62% of one series of dogs with aspergillosis, although negative results do not rule out the presence of *Aspergillus* spp.

23. How should I treat nasal aspergillosis?

Topical nasal antifungal infusion therapy is a relatively noninvasive technique with a reported success rate similar to that for frontal sinus trephination and catheter placement. The animal is placed under general anesthesia and intubated. Briefly, this technique involves placing a 24F Foley catheter dorsal to the junction of the hard and soft palate and inflating the cuff. Moistened laparotomy sponges are placed in the pharynx to absorb any infusion solution that might leak from around the catheter. Next, a 10F polypropylene catheter is placed in each dorsal nasal meatus and advanced to the level of the corresponding medial canthus. Optimally, these infusion catheters can be endoscopically guided to the level of the frontal sinus. Next, 12F Foley catheters are placed in each nostril and their cuffs are inflated to occlude the nasal passages. Each of the three Foley catheters should then be clamped off to prevent leakage of infusate through these catheters. The dog is then placed in the dorsal recumbent position and 50 ml of 1% clotrimazole is infused into each nostril slowly (over 1 hour). Every 15 minutes the dog's head is repositioned, to the right, left, or dorsal. After the infusion, the catheters and sponges are removed and any remaining solution is allowed to drain rostrally. The nasal infusion should be repeated every 2 to 3 weeks as necessary, depending on the clinical signs and evidence of fungal plaques on subsequent rhinoscopy. In studies of this procedure, a single infusion of 1% clotrimazole resulted in resolution of clinical signs in 65% of dogs and signs resolved in 87% of dogs following a second infusion. Similar success rates have been reported with infusion of either 1% or 2% enilconazole. However, a controlled study comparing intra-nasal infusion of clotrimazole versus enilconazole for the treatment of aspergillosis has not been performed.

Before performing topical infusion of an antifungal medication, the clinician should check for any signs of central nervous system (CNS) involvement, specifically loss of cribriform plate integrity. Ideally, a CT scan should be performed to look for damage or lysis of the cribriform plate. If bony destruction is noted in this area or CNS signs are observed, topical therapy should be avoided because contact of clotrimazole with intracranial structures can result in severe meningitis and encephalitis. If CNS signs or evidence of cribriform plate disease are detected, oral fluconazole therapy can be used in place of nasally infused medication.

24. Treatment with multiple infusions of either clotrimazole or enilconazole does not seem to be working. What next?

Nasal infusion of either clotrimazole or enilconazole is effective in treating nasal aspergillosis. However, a number of factors may lead to treatment failure. First, nasal infusion should only be performed *after* removing/debulking as much of the gross fungal plaques as possible. This can be performed by aggressively lavaging the nasal cavity with 0.9% saline prior to topical antifungal therapy. If a single fungal plaque is left in place, there may be a brief resolution of clinical signs but ultimately treatment failure is likely. It is also important that the infusion catheter be located in the caudal aspect of the nasal cavity or, if there is radiographic/CT evidence for frontal sinus involvement, in the frontal sinus. Placement of the infusion catheter in the frontal sinus can be performed rhinoscopically by an experienced endoscopist.

It is important to remember that *Aspergillus* spp. infection can be due to an underlying primary condition such as a foreign body or tumor. In these cases, clinical signs of sneezing and/or nasal discharge may persist despite resolution of the fungal infection. *Aspergillus* spp. infections can cause a severe destructive rhinitis that may cause a persistent mild nasal discharge even after clearance of the fungal infection. Additionally, secondary bacterial infections may develop as a result of turbinate and mucosal damage, and these infections can also contribute to persistent nasal discharge if not cleared. If these factors have been considered and multiple topical antifungal treatments have not been effective and there is rhinoscopic evidence of regrowth of fungal plaques, adjunctive oral antifungal therapy may be necessary. Oral ketoconazole (5 mg/kg twice daily) for 6 to 8 weeks may eliminate infection in approximately 50% of cases, without topical therapy. Oral itraconazole (5 mg/kg twice daily) for 60 to 90 days will cure approximately 60% to 70% of nasal aspergillosis infections in dogs. Either of these oral therapies, in conjunction with topical clotrimazole or enilconazole, may increase the success rate for elimination of infection. Alternatively, a rhinotomy and/or sinusotomy may be performed and, following turbinectomy, a povidone-iodine dressing can be placed and changed every 2 to 3 days until a healthy granulation bed forms.

BIBLIOGRAPHY

Davidson A: Coccidioidomycosis and aspergillosis. In Ettinger SJ, Feldman EC, editors: *Textbook of veterinary internal medicine,* ed 6, Philadelphia, 2005, Elsevier.

Davidson AP, Mathews KG: CVT update: therapy for nasal aspergillosis. In Bonagura JD, editor: *Kirk's current veterinary therapy,* ed 13, Philadelphia, 2000, WB Saunders.

Day MJ, Penhale WJ: An immunohistochemical study of canine disseminated aspergillosis, *Aust Vet J* 68: 383-386, 1991.

Legendre AM: Antimycotic drug therapy. In Bonagura JD, editor: *Kirk's current veterinary therapy,* ed 12, Philadelphia, 1995, WB Saunders.

Mathews KG, Davidson AP, Koblik PD et al: Comparison of topical administration of clotrimazole through surgically versus non-surgically placed catheters for treatment of nasal aspergillosis in dogs: 60 cases (1990-1996), *J Am Vet Med Assoc* 213:501-506, 1998.

McCullough SM, McKiernan BC, Grodsky BS: Endoscopically placed tubes for administration of enilconazole for treatment of nasal aspergillosis in dogs, *J Am Vet Med Assoc* 212:67-69, 1998.

Moore AH. Use of topical povidone-iodine dressings in the management of mycotic rhinitis in three dogs, *J Small Anim Pract* 44:326 2003.

Richardson EF, Matthes KG: Distribution of topical agents in the frontal sinuses and nasal cavity of dogs: comparison between current protocols for treatment of nasal aspergillosis and a new noninvasive technique, *Vet Surg* 24:476-483, 1995.

Sharp NJH, Sullivan M: Use of ketoconazole in treatment of canine nasal aspergillosis, *J Am Vet Med Assoc* 194:782-786; 1989.

Sharp NJH, Sullivan M, Harvey CE et al: Treatment of canine nasal aspergillosis with enilconazole, *J Vet Intern Med* 7:40-43; 1993.

Venker-van Haagen AJ: Diseases of the nose and nasal sinuses. In Ettinger SJ, Feldman EC, editors: *Textbook of veterinary internal medicine,* ed 6, Philadelphia, 2005, Elsevier.

Zonderland JL, Stork CK, Saunders JH et al: Intranasal infusion of enilconazole for treatment of sinonasal aspergillosis in dogs, *J Am Vet Med Assoc* 221:1421-1425, 2002.

ALLERGIC RHINITIS

Charles W. Brockus

25. What is allergic rhinitis (AR)?

In people, AR is called *hay fever.* This condition arises when an allergen is deposited onto the nasal mucous membrane, causing a hypersensitivity reaction. Examination of nasal tissues or secretions from patients with AR will reveal large numbers of eosinophils and few neutrophils. Initially, the discharge may be mild and brief. With repeated seasonal exposure, the discharge may become more profuse, start earlier in the season, and last longer.

26. What causes AR?

AR is an unusual disorder in dogs. It is caused by a type I hypersensitivity reaction to allergens inhaled by sensitized individuals, often those with seasonal allergies. Prolonged exposure to allergens may result in chronic nasal discharge, epithelial hyperplasia, and lymphoplasmacytic infiltration. As with any allergy, repeated exposure may lead to worsening and prolongation of clinical signs.

27. What are the clinical signs of AR?

The usual clinical signs are a serous nasal discharge that may become mucopurulent during specific "seasonal" exposures, unless exposure to the inciting agent/antigen occurs throughout the year, as with house dust or molds.

28. Are other conditions observed with AR?

Other allergic disorders such as atopic dermatitis and/or otitis externa may be present.

29. How is AR diagnosed?

The typical evaluation for AR (refer to phases 1 to 3, described earlier in this chapter) is similar to that for any nasal disorder. In cases of AR, histopathological or cytological examination of discharge/tissue specimens will reveal a majority of eosinophils with scattered neutrophils. After identification of the disorder as AR, with biopsy specimens, there are many options for treatment.

30. What is the prognosis for AR?

Even if the offending allergen cannot be identified, the prognosis for AR can be expected to be good. However, the extent of treatment necessary to achieve a response may vary, from simple measures such as limiting exposure to an allergen/irritant to topical treatment with a glucocorticoid medication to extensive hyposensitization testing and the addition of other medications to the treatment protocol.

31. How can I treat AR?

Effective treatment may take a significant period and numerous trials of various treatments, alone or in combination, to control this disease. Avoidance of the offending allergen is ideal; however, this is rarely possible.

Prednisolone, at an oral dosage of 0.25 to 1.0 mg/kg once daily or every other or every third day, may be effective during the allergy season. Recently, glucocorticoid nasal sprays (e.g., Nasacort, Flovent metered-dose inhaler, or Flonase spray) have been found to be helpful in managing AR in dogs, without the systemic side effects often seen with oral corticosteroid therapy. The problem with some of these medications that must be administered using metered-dose inhalers (MDIs) is adapting a muzzle chamber to the MDI so that the animal receives the appropriate measured dose of inhalant. This may take some time but the outcome is often successful.

Some common-sense, simple measures that may help are eliminating smoke, perfumes, carpet cleaners/fresheners, and incense from the house. Irritant inhalants may not cause AR but can exacerbate allergic reactions. Do not allow smoking near the dog. Wash all bedding in *hot* water to kill dust mites. Decrease dust by removing or reducing clutter in the living area. HEPA (high-efficiency particulate) filters or electrostatic air cleaners may help remove microscopic allergens.

Fish oils added to the diet have been used in conjunction with other treatments.

Intradermal skin testing can be helpful in identifying many allergens so that hyposensitization can be initiated. Hyposensitization (immunotherapy, desensitization) to the offending allergen based on in vitro and in vivo test results can be effective. This treatment is often used in human patients but it can be time-consuming and expensive, and there is a risk of anaphylactic reactions from hyposensitization injections.

Antihistamines (e.g., Claritin) may also be beneficial in reducing the amount of nasal discharge.

Mast cell stabilizers such as cromolyn sodium make mast cells in the airway less prone to releasing histamine and other substances in response to allergen exposure. Mast cell stabilizers only help to prevent nasal discharge; they will not relieve the clinical signs of AR. The stabilizer can be administered using a muzzle chamber. The stabilizer should be used regularly, starting 2 to 4 weeks before exposure to a seasonal allergen, if one has been identified. Cromolyn is available for administration using a metered-dose inhaler (MDI).

Piroxicam (0.3 mg/kg PO every day or every other day) has been used but it should *not* be administered concurrent with any form of steroid. In addition, piroxicam may cause gastrointestinal side affects.

Treatments to be considered in cases of suspected nasal mites include ivermectin 200 to 400 micrograms/kg SQ or PO, repeated in a week, a trial of 3 doses of milbemycin (1 mg/kg for each dose, 10 days apart), or fenbendazole 50 mg/kg for 2 weeks. It is important to note that ivermectin should be avoided in collies, border collies, collie crosses, and Australian shepherds.

Cyclosporin may be worth considering but has not been used extensively for this form of rhinitis and is expensive.

Treatments may be used in combination to control this form of rhinitis.

BIBLIOGRAPHY

Dowling PM: Inhalation therapy for coughing dogs and wheezing cats, Western Veterinary Conference, Las Vegas, February 2004.

Gartrell CL, O'Handley PA, Perry RL: Canine nasal disease – part II, *Compend Contin Educ Pract Vet* 17:539-547, 1995.

Johnson L: Rhinitis in dogs and cats (VET-329), Western States Conference Proceedings, Las Vegas, February 2004.

Johnson L: Sneezing and nasal discharge in the dog, ACVIM Proceedings, 2004.

Knotek Z, Fichtel T, Kohout P et al: Diseases of the nasal cavity in the dog, aetiology, symptomatology, diagnostics, *ACTA Vet BRNO* 70:73-82, 2001.

Marks SL. Diagnostics for nasal disease, Western States Conference Proceedings, Las Vegas, February 2003.

Venker-van Haagen AJ: Diseases of the nose and nasal sinuses. In Ettinger SJ, Feldman, EC, editors: *Textbook of veterinary internal medicine*, ed 6, St Louis, 2005, Elsevier.

LYMPHOPLASMACYTIC RHINITIS

Charles W. Brockus

32. What is lymphoplasmacytic rhinitis (LPR)?

This is a disease of unknown etiology that is characterized by prominent infiltration of the nasal mucosa and submucosa by mature lymphocytes and plasma cells, and occasionally neutrophils. LPR is usually considered to be idiopathic, similar to inflammatory bowel disease, because no definitive cause for LPR has yet been identified. LPR has been proposed to represent a primary immune-mediated process or a secondary chronic response to other nasal diseases, including fungal infection, foreign bodies, dental disease, neoplasia, or allergies. A solely immune-mediated mechanism for this disease is unlikely, based on the fact that the response to glucocorticoid therapy is often poor.

33. What causes LPR?

It appears that LPR can be a primary disease or due to another disorder (a secondary disease). LPR differs from type I hypersensitivity AR in that with LPR, infiltration of the nasal mucosa with significant numbers of eosinophils is not observed. LPR may represent a chronic form of AR, occurring when AR is not effectively treated. A wide variety of intranasal diseases (e.g., fungal infection, foreign body rhinitis, and neoplasia) often are associated with secondary lymphoplasmacytic inflammation. Also, some intranasal vaccines may cause a transient lymphoplasmacytic inflammation.

34. What are the clinical signs of LPR?

The most common clinical signs of LPR are unilateral or bilateral serous to mucoid to mucopurulent discharge with occasional hemorrhagic nasal discharge; sneezing; a dry, crusting discharge; decreased nasal airflow; increased lung sounds; coughing; ocular discharge; oral pain; and mild dyspnea have also been observed. Although signs of the disease may only appear unilaterally, the disease process may actually be bilateral.

35. What radiographic changes are observed?

Increased density of soft tissues (due to fluid accumulation), destruction of the turbinates, and sinus opacity have been seen on radiographs of dogs with LPR. The differential diagnosis of LPR is based on lack of evidence of neoplasia or a fungal infection on a CT scan (plain nasal radiographs do not provide sufficient resolution to rule out neoplasia or fungal infection) and negative findings for other conditions on the rhinoscopic examination.

36. What cell types are observed in biopsy specimens?

The most prominent cell types in biopsy specimens from dogs with LPR are mature lymphocytes, followed by plasma cells, both located within the mucosa and submucosa. Occasionally, neutrophils also are present. Some dogs have multifocal infiltrates and others diffuse infiltration; more severe clinical signs are associated with diffuse infiltration.

37. Are bacteria a secondary cause?

Very low to no growth of bacteria was observed in nasal cultures from cases of LPR.

38. Is any particular breed predisposed to LPR?

Large-breed dogs such as German shepherds and crosses, Labrador Retrievers, and Collies were over-represented in the most completely studied population reported upon.

39. What is the prognosis for LPR?

The prognosis for idiopathic LPR is guarded. LPR is not a life-threatening condition but responses to treatment have not been encouraging. Nevertheless, as the disease is studied more fully, and a specific cause can be identified, definitive and effective treatments may become available and the prognosis would improve.

40. How is LPR treated?

No treatment for LPR has been found that is universally effective. Antibiotics typically fail to affect resolution of clinical signs. Metronidazole has helped in some cases but the response to this medication may be associated with its antiinflammatory properties rather than its antimicrobial properties.

Corticosteroids appear to be the treatment of choice, but in many cases of idiopathic LPR they are ineffective. Prednisolone is often the first choice, at an oral dose of 1 to 2 mg/kg once daily for 2 weeks; once a response is seen, the dosage should be gradually tapered to the lowest amount required to maintain remission of clinical signs. Therapy is generally continued for many weeks, although an occasional dog may require treatment for a full year. Because aspergillosis or neoplasms may occasionally be associated with a lymphoplasmacytic infiltrate of the nasal mucosa, one must be certain that neither disease is present when initiating long-term corticosteroid therapy. Corticosteroid nasal sprays (e.g., Nasacort, Flovent metered-dose inhaler, or Flonase spray) can be tried for longer-term management of LPR if the response to systemic corticosteroid was positive. These nasally administered medications avoid the systemic side effects often seen with oral corticosteroid therapy. Animals with LPR often require more aggressive treatment than corticosteroids.

Some common-sense measures that can be taken include limiting or preventing the dog's exposure to any form of smoke, incense, perfumes, carpet cleaners/fresheners, or any other dusts or sprays.

Some clinicians have tried azathioprine, with varying success.

If nasal mites are suspected, ivermectin, 200 to 400 µg/kg SQ or PO, repeated in a week; or a trial of milbemycin (1 mg/kg for each of 3 doses, 10 days apart); or fenbendazole, 50 mg/kg for 2 weeks, may be tried. However, ivermectin should be avoided in Collie breeds/crosses, Border Collies, or Australian Shepherds.

Cyclosporin may be worth considering but has not been used extensively for this form of rhinitis and is expensive.

BIBLIOGRAPHY

Burgener DC, Slocombe RF, Zerbe CA: Lymphoplasmacytic rhinitis in five dogs, *J Am Anim Hosp Assoc* 23:565-568, 1987.
Gartrell CL, O'Handley PA, Perry RL: Canine nasal disease – part II, *Compend Contin Educ Pract Vet* 17:539-547, 1995.
Venker-van Haagen AJ: Diseases of the nose and nasal sinuses. In Ettinger SJ, Feldman, EC, editors: *Textbook of veterinary internal medicine,* ed 6, St Louis, 2005, Elsevier.
Windsor RC, Johnson LR, Herrgesell EJ et. Al: Idiopathic lymphoplasmacytic rhinitis in dogs: 37 cases (1997-2002), *J Am Vet Med Assoc* 224:1952-1957, 2004.

14. Conformational Disorders

Dawn D. Kingsbury

1.   Name some conformational disorders of the upper respiratory tract.

- **Nasal**: Cleft palate, stenotic nares, nasal dermoid sinus, primary ciliary dyskinesia, nasopharyngeal polyps
- **Palate, pharynx, and larynx**: Elongated soft palate, choanal atresia, nasopharyngeal polyps, cricopharyngeal achalasia, laryngeal hypoplasia, laryngeal collapse, laryngeal paralysis, everted laryngeal sacculi, laryngeal edema, subglottic stenosis

2.   Name some conformational disorders of the lower respiratory tract.

- **Trachea and bronchi:** Tracheal or bronchial compression due to lymphadenomegaly, thymic mass or branchial cyst, tracheal hypoplasia, primary ciliary dyskinesia, osteochondral dysplasia
- **Lung:** Pulmonary emphysema

- **Diaphragm:** Hernia (peritoneopericardial, pleuroperitoneal, hiatal)
- **Thoracic wall and sternum:** Rib abnormalities or fractures, which in the worst-case scenario result in a flail chest, pectus excavatum

3. Into what general categories can conformational disorders be classified?

Disorders can be classified by the presenting signs. The breathing pattern can help localize the disorder. An obstructed breathing pattern is found in cases of upper and lower airway disease, while a restricted pattern indicates disease in the thoracic wall, sternum, or diaphragm. Abnormal breath sounds are common in upper airway disease. Stertor (snore) is found in nasal or pharyngeal disease and stridor (wheeze) in laryngeal or lower airway disease. A voice change and inspiratory dyspnea are often noted in the history of dogs with laryngeal disease. Patients with disease in the lower airways may present with a cough, tachypnea, or varying degrees of respiratory distress.

Conformational changes may be congenital or acquired. Acquired disease may be secondary to physical characteristics such as negative intra-airway pressure generated during inspiration in brachiocephalic airway syndrome, inflammation or infection, nasopharyngeal polyps, or diaphragmatic hernia due to trauma. Changes may be structural or functional, static or dynamic. Having this knowledge helps determine what diagnostic tests are appropriate. For example, a direct examination of the larynx is needed to make a diagnosis of laryngeal paralysis; fluoroscopy or bronchoscopy may be needed to document tracheal or bronchial compression or obstruction due to lymphadenomegaly, which cannot be entirely ruled out by examination of static thoracic radiographs.

4. Name some breeds of dogs known to have predispositions for certain conformational disorders.

Brachycephalic breeds have their own syndrome—brachycephalic airway syndrome—and may be predisposed to pectus excavatum.

As a subset of the brachycephalics, English Bulldogs, Boston Terriers, and Boxers have a predisposition for tracheal hypoplasia.

The Chinese Shar-Pei has a risk similar to that of brachycephalic breeds of airway disease, specifically brachycephalic airway syndrome, and hiatal hernia.

Brachycephalic breeds, including Shih Tzus, Bulldogs, Pointers, and Swiss Sheepdogs, may inherit cleft palates.

Congenital laryngeal paralysis has been reported in Bouvier des Flanders, Bull Terriers, Dalmatians, Rottweilers, Siberian Huskies, and German Shepherds.

Many of these dogs will have other concurrent neurological abnormalities. Heritability has been proposed as the cause of these abnormalities in most cases.

A recent prospective study concluded that Labrador Retrievers and Rottweilers have a significantly higher risk for acquired laryngeal paralysis. Other large breeds including Irish Setters, Golden Retrievers, and Afghans, are also considered to be predisposed.

Bichon Frise, Border Collie, Bullmastiff, Chihuahua, Chinese Shar-Pei, Chow Chow, Dachshund, Dalmatian, Doberman Pinscher, English Springer Spaniel, English Pointer, English Setter, Golden Retriever, Gordon Setter, Miniature Poodle, Newfoundland, Old English Sheepdog, Rottweiler, and Staffordshire Bull Terrier are all breeds with reported cases of primary ciliary dyskinesia (PCD) or Kartagener's syndrome. With the exception of Newfoundlands, in which PCD shows an autosomal recessive pattern of heritability, sporadically reported cases do not represent specific breed predisposition for PCD. There is a rhinitis/bronchopneumonia syndrome in Irish Wolfhounds that is not PCD and is likely heritable.

5. Briefly describe a typical history for a dog with the following respiratory tract conformational disorders.

- **Cleft palate:** Pups may have drainage of milk from nares during or after nursing (nasal regurgitation) and rhinitis. Respiratory distress may be seen secondary to aspiration pneumonia.

- **Stenotic nares:** Brachycephalic breeds with stenotic nares will have intolerance to heat, exercise, and stress with inspiratory stertor and asphyxia. Early in the disease course, signs may be relieved by open-mouth breathing, but it is often part of brachycephalic airway syndrome, which incorporates other defects such as elongated soft palate, and leads to progressive, persistent signs.
- **Congenital laryngeal paralysis:** A young dog will present with inspiratory stridor and dyspnea that may be episodic but worsens with exercise.
- **Hypoplastic trachea:** At least half of the affected dogs have some degree of dyspnea; a quarter have stridor and/or coughing; an eighth have gagging and/or exercise intolerance, and a minority (~10%) have either more severe signs like syncope or may have no signs at all.
- **Primary ciliary dyskinesia:** Early in life, affected dogs will have a chronic recurring nasal discharge, coughing, sneezing, and abnormal respiratory sounds. Respiratory distress may accompany bouts of bronchopneumonia.
- **Pulmonary emphysema:** Respiratory distress can result if rupture of a bulla causes a pneumothorax, but often it is an incidental finding.

6. What is a "swimmer" puppy?

A swimmer puppy has an abnormal thoracic conformation (pectus excavatum) resulting from abnormal locomotion. Typically a puppy presents by 12 weeks of age for an inability to walk and moves around on its sternum by flailing its abducted limbs. Dorsal to ventral narrowing of the thorax develops and results in a flattened appearance. Often environmental factors such as hard slippery flooring contribute to an inability of the puppy to adduct its limbs and stand. Orthopedic abnormalities such as dislocation or subluxation of the shoulder, elbow, hip, or stifle should be ruled out. Correcting limb position and realigning joints (using hobbles to prevent abduction) typically eliminate the need for any thoracic splinting.

7. What is a nasal dermoid sinus cyst and how is it diagnosed?

Nasal dermoid sinus cysts are rare developmental defects related to abnormal ectoderm development in the pre-nasal space and may extend into the cranial vault. The typical presenting complaint is intermittent discharge from a small opening in the midline on the bridge of the nose at the junction between the nasal planum and the skin. Facial swelling and pain may also be noted in some dogs. Plain radiographs usually show no marked abnormality. However catheterization of the opening and positive contrast sinography under general anesthesia can confirm filling of a midline tract that passes caudally toward the nasal bones. Histopathologically, there are adnexal structures along a tract lined with stratified squamous epithelium.

8. What nonneoplastic differential diagnoses should be considered in a dog with nasopharyngeal disease?

Benign cystic masses associated with cystic Rathke's cleft and salivary retention (mucocele); foreign bodies, most commonly bones; nasopharyngeal stenosis (webbing); redundant mucosa; inflammatory polyps; lymphocytic/plasmacytic rhinitis; and fungal granulomas have all been reported as causes of non-neoplastic obstructive nasopharyngeal or laryngeal masses in the dog.

9. Describe cricopharyngeal achalasia.

This condition typically occurs in a young dog. The presenting complaint is a history of dysphagia; this results when the upper esophageal sphincter fails to open during swallowing and food is prevented from entering the proximal esophagus. There is often nasal regurgitation and aspiration pneumonia. Videofluoroscopic examination of a liquid barium swallow, documenting a significant delay in the opening and closing of the upper esophageal sphincter, helps point to the diagnosis.

10. What are some differential diagnoses for nodular airway disease in the dog?

Differential diagnoses include *Oslerus osleri* parasitism, nodular amyloidosis, eosinophilic granulomas, tracheal papillomatosis, tracheal neoplasia, and tracheobronchopathia osteochondroplastica.

11. Where are branchial cysts found?

Branchial cysts are rare anomalies that are due to failure of complete involution of the second branchial cleft in embryonic development. They occur as flocculent masses lined by epithelium that form anywhere along the branchial arches, which go on to form various parts of the head, neck, and thorax. Most commonly they are ventral cervical masses, but retropharyngeal and cranial mediastinal masses can occur.

12. What tests are needed to diagnose Kartagener's syndrome?

Kartagener's syndrome is comprised of the triad of situs inversus (transposition of the viscera), sinusitis, and bronchiectasis. The later two conditions are typically secondary to an immobility of the cilia (ciliary dyskinesia). Plain ventrodorsal thoracic and abdominal radiographs can show dextrocardia (location of the descending aorta on the right side of the spine) and location of the gastric fundus in the right cranial abdominal quadrant. There is typically a history of rhinosinusitis and on physical examination a nasal discharge will be evident. Bronchiectasis may be apparent on thoracic radiographs and can be confirmed with bronchoscopy. To identify the ciliary abnormalities, transmission electron microscopy is used. Additional tests are used to confirm the diagnosis and document any sequelae. Bronchopneumonia is often diagnosed based on cytologic examination of transtracheal washings or bronchoalveolar lavage fluid. Testicular aspirates show lack of sperm motility. Nuclear scintigraphy can demonstrate the absence of mucociliary clearance within the respiratory tree. Computed tomography may show hydrocephalus secondary to abnormal cilia.

13. How are cleft palates treated?

Cleft palates that are causing clinical signs such as rhinitis or aspiration pneumonia require surgical correction. If the mucosal edges of the defect are not hard to appose, a simple two-layer closure may be successful. Failure of this type of repair is usually due to excess tension at the surgical site. For larger soft palate defects, bilateral mucosal single-pedicle flaps (a flap of oral mucosa on one side and nasal mucosa on the opposite side) is recommended, with the flaps being overlapped and sutured with continuous, small-gauge absorbable sutures. This technique allows for complete mucosal covering of the defect and healing proceeds rapidly by primary intention. Large hard palate defects may require advancement of a palatal +/- buccal mucosal flap. For successful repair, care must be taken not to obliterate the flap's blood supply.

14. Describe the management of pectus excavatum.

Pectus excavatum should only be treated after progressive clinical signs (dyspnea) have been documented, because spontaneous resolution without intervention has been reported. Monitoring or judicious application of manual compression of the thorax by the pet owner may result in a puppy "outgrowing" a mild defect. In more severe cases, treatment depends on the dog's age at diagnosis; early recognition is key to noninvasive fixation. In dogs younger than 3 months of age, normalization of sternal conformation can be undertaken with an external U-shaped coaptation splint and sutures. The splint is made with moldable material (e.g., Orthoplast; Johnson and Johnson) contoured to the ventral thorax and padded. The cranial border should angle caudally so that the splint does not interfere with movement of the forelimbs. Circumferential sutures are passed percutaneously around the sternum with a tapered needle, carefully avoiding heart and lungs, passed through predrilled holes in the splint, and tied with sufficient tension to normalize conformation. Post-procedure radiographs are recommended to confirm correct conformation and rule out complications such as pneumothorax. Fixation for 1 to 2 weeks results in correction of the cosmetic defect and resolution of clinical signs. Dermatitis is not uncommon, but resolves with removal of the splint. Older dogs have decreased sternal and thoracic wall compliance and may require more invasive procedures such as partial sternectomy for definitive repair.

15. What differences are seen in responses to surgical versus medical management of flail chest?

In a recent retrospective study of 21 dogs, time spent in the hospital and ultimate outcome was not significantly different when the flail segment was stabilized or not stabilized. Treatment in all cases included pain control and administration of supplemental oxygen to manage the primary cause of respiratory dysfunction. In this case series, each case was managed on an individual basis;it will be interesting to see if a randomized, prospective study shows a similar lack of difference in outcome.

16. What distinguishes the various types of pulmonary cavitary lesions (cysts, blebs, and pneumatoceles)?

These lesions are distinguished by their histopathologic appearance:
- Bronchogenic cysts are airspaces lined by respiratory epithelium and represent poorly developed terminal bronchioles.
- Blebs are subpleural airspaces within the parenchyma that arise from the breakdown of alveolar septa.
- Pneumatoceles are large cavitary lesions that form in the lung parenchyma when necrotic tissue is replaced by air.

BIBLIOGRAPHY

Anderson DM, White RA: Nasal dermoid sinus cysts in the dog, *Vet Surg* 31:303-308, 2002.
Bailey TR, Holmberg DL, Yager JA: Nasal dermoid sinus in an American cocker spaniel, *Can Vet J* 42: 213-215, 2001.
Boudrieau RJ, Fossum TW, Hartsfield SM et al: Pectus excavatum in dogs and cats, *Compend Contin Educ Pract Vet* 12:341-355, 1990.
Braund KG, Shores A, Cochrane S et al: Laryngeal paralysis-polyneuropathy complex in young Dalmatians, *Am J Vet Res* 55:534-542, 1994.
Broome C, Burbidge HM, Pfeiffer DU: Prevalence of laryngeal paresis in dogs undergoing general anaesthesia, *Aust Vet J* 78:769-772, 2000.
Burrow RD: A nasal dermoid sinus in an English bull terrier, *J Small Anim Pract* 45:572-574, 2004.
Clercx C, Peeters D, Beths T et al: Use of ciliogenesis in the diagnosis of primary ciliary dyskinesia in a dog, *J Am Vet Med Assoc* 217:1681-1685, 2001.
Clercx C, Reichler I, Peeters D et al: hinitis/Bronchopneumonia syndrome in Irish Wolfhound, *J Vet Intern Med* 17:843-849, 2003.
Coyne BE, Fingland RB: Hpoplasia of the trachea in dogs: 103 cases (1974-1990), *J Am Vet Med Assoc* 201:768-772, 1992.
De Scally M, Lobetti RG, Van Wilpe E: Primary ciliary dyskinesia in a Staffordshire bull terrier, *J S Afr Vet Assoc* 75:150-152, 2004.
Foodman MS, Giger U, Stebbins K et al: Kartagener's syndrome in an old miniature poodle, *J Small Anim Pract* 30:96-100, 1989.
Griffiths LG, Sullivan M: Bilateral overlapping mucosal single-pedicle flaps for correction of soft palate defects, *J Am Anim Hosp Assoc* 37:183-186, 2001.
Harvey CE: Inherited and congenital airway conditions, *J Small Anim Pract* 30:184-187, 1989.
Holtsinger RH, Beale BS, Bellah JR et al: Spontaneoous pneumothorax in the dog: a retrospective analysis of 21 cases, *J Am Anim Hosp Assoc* 29:195-210, 1993.
Hong C, Crawford R: *Branchial cleft cyst,* Available at www.eMedicine.com, 2003.
Hoover JP, Howard-Martin MO, Bahr RJ: Chronic bronchitis, bronchiectasis, bronchiolitis, bronchiolitis obliterans, and bronchopneumonia in a Rottweiler with primary ciliary dyskinesia, *J Am Anim Hosp Assoc* 25:297-304, 1989.
Hunt GB, Perkins MC, Foster SF et al: Nasopharyngeal disorders of dogs and cats: a review and retrospective study, *Compend Contin Educ Pract Vet* 24:184-199, 2002.

Kipperman BS, Wong VJ, Plopper CG: Primary ciliary dyskinesia in a Gordon Setter, *J Am Anim Hosp Assoc* 28:375-379, 1992.

Koch DA, Arnold S, Madeleine Hubler M et al: Brachycephalic syndrome in dogs, *Compend Contin Educ Pract Vet* 25:48-55, 2003.

Ladlow J, Hardie RJ: Cricopharyngeal achalasia in dogs, *Compend Contin Educ Pract Vet* 22:750-755, 2000.

Luskin IR: Reconstruction of oral defects using mucogingival pedicle flaps, *Clin Tech Sm Anim Pract* 15:251-259, 2000.

Mahony OM, Knowles KE; Braund KG et al: Laryngeal paralysis-polyneuropathy complex in young Rottweilers, *J Vet Intern Med* 12:330-333, 1998.

Neil JA, Canapp SO, Cook CR et al: Kartagener's syndrome in a Dachshund dog, *J Am Anim Hosp Assoc* 38:45-49, 2002.

Olsen D, Renberg W, Perrett J et al: Clinical management of flail chest in dogs and cats: a retrospective study of 24 cases (1989-1999), *J Am Anim Hosp Assoc* 38:315-320, 2002.

Pollard RE, Marks SL, Davidson A et al: Quantitative videofluoroscopic evaluation of pharyngeal function in the dog, *Vet Radiol Ultrasound* 41:409-412, 2000.

Polizopoulou ZS, Koutinas AF, Papadopoulos GC et al: Juvenile laryngeal paralysis in three Siberian husky x Alaskan malamute puppies, *Vet Rec* 153:624-627, 2003.

Reichler IM, Hoerauf A, Guscetti F et al: Primary ciliary dyskinesia with situs inversus totalis, hydrocephalus internus and cardiac malformations in a dog, *J Small Anim Pract* 42:345-348, 2001.

Ridyard AE, Corcoran BM, Tasker S et al: Spontaneous laryngeal paralysis in four white-coated German shepherd dogs, *J Small Anim Pract* 41:558-561, 2000.

Sellon RK, Johnson JL, Leathers CW et al: Tracheobronchopathia osteochondroplastica in a dog, *J Vet Intern Med* 18:359-362, 2004.

Sivacolundhu RK, Read RA, Marchevsky AM: Hiatal hernia controversies—a review of pathophysiology and treatment options, *Aust Vet J* 80:48-53, 2002.

Sweet DC, Waters DJ: Role of surgery in the management of dogs with pathologic conditions of the thorax—part II, *Compend Contin Educ Pract Vet* 13:1671-1677, 1991.

Taboada J, Turnwald GH: The respiratory system, In Hoskins JD, editor, *Veterinary pediatrics,* ed 3, Philadelphia, 2001, WB Saunders, pp 80-102.

Warzee CC, Bellah JR, Richards D: Congenital unilateral cleft of the soft palate in six dogs, *J Small Anim Pract* 42:338-340, 2001.

Watson PJ, Herrtage ME, Peacock MA et al: Primary ciliary dyskinesia in Newfoundland dogs, *Vet Rec* 144:718-725, 1999.

15. Tumors of the Nasal and Paranasal Sinuses

Leslie E. Fox

1.   What are the most common tumors in the canine nasal cavity?

Most tumors in the nasal cavity of the dog are malignant. They typically originate from the epithelium lining the nasal and paranasal cavities. Adenocarcinomas are most frequent; while mesenchymal cell tumors (fibrosarcomas, chondrosarcomas, and osteosarcomas) are less frequently diagnosed. Unusual tumors are mast cell and transmissible venereal tumors.

2.   What is the signalment of dogs with nasal cancer?

On average, dogs with nasal cancer are about 10 years old, but nasal tumors have been reported in dogs younger than 1 year. Chondrosarcomas occur in younger dogs (mean, about 7 years old). Males may be more frequently affected. Dolichocephalic and mesocephalic breeds are at increased risk compared to brachycephalic (short-nosed) breeds, possibly because in dolichocephalic breeds more of the nasal turbinate surface is exposed to carcinogens. Living in urban areas and exposure to flea sprays, by-products of indoor kerosene/coal-burning heating units, and second hand tobacco smoke are associated with an increased risk of developing nasal neoplasms.

3.   What clinical signs are exhibited by dogs with nasal/paranasal sinus cancer?

The most common presenting clinical signs are epistaxis, unilateral or bilateral nasal discharge, airflow obstruction, stridor, facial deformity, and sneezing. Less frequent findings include dyspnea, coughing, weight loss, tonsillitis, exophthalmos, and reverse sneezing. These signs have often been present for 3 to 4 months prior to presentation to a veterinarian. The response to antimicrobial and/or corticosteroid therapy is often transient. Invasion of the cribriform plate causes neurologic abnormalities (seizures, paresis) and may be seen in dogs without any clinical evidence of nasal or paranasal sinus involvement. Paraneoplastic disorders are rare.

4.   What are the differential diagnoses for the most obvious clinical abnormalities of epistaxis and chronic nasal discharge?

The differential diagnoses for chronic nasal discharge include bacterial rhinitis; fungal rhinitis (aspergillosis, penicilliosis, rhinosporidiosis, cryptococcosis, and pythiosis); inflammatory disorders (lymphoplasmacytic or eosinophilic rhinitis); parasitic rhinitis (*Pneumonyssoides caninum*), foreign body (plant awn); abscess of a tooth root with drainage into the nasal cavity; and inflammatory polyp. Depending on the nature of the vessel destruction, epistaxis can occur alone or with a serous or mucopurulent nasal discharge. Nonrespiratory tract causes of epistaxis include disorders of primary hemostasis (von Willebrand's disease), immune-mediated thrombocytopenia, canine ehrlichiosis, coagulopathies, and vascular disorders (hypertension, hyperviscosity syndrome).

5.   How are nasal neoplasms differentiated from other nasal diseases?

The complete workup for a dog with a nasal discharge typically involves radiographs, computed tomography (CT), or magnetic resonance imaging (MRI) and biopsy (either blind or with rhinoscopy). Plain radiography will help confirm the presence of nasal/paranasal sinus disease but often does not help differentiate among infectious, inflammatory, and neoplastic diseases. Evaluation of nasal exudates obtained by swabbing or a saline solution flush is most often unrewarding. Aerobic culturing generally results in an abundant yield of normal bacterial flora or bacterial pathogens representing a secondary infection that accompanies the primary disease process. Fungal infections may be differentiated from neoplasia, bacterial infection, and allergic nasal disease with a combination of radiographic signs, rhinoscopic examination, and serologic examination. *Cryptococcus* organisms may be easily identified on cytologic examination of exudates; however, a cytologic diagnosis of nasal cancer from exudate examination alone is made infrequently. Fungal hyphae (*Aspergillus* spp.) may be observed in the exudates of healthy dogs. *Penicillium* and *Aspergillus* may be grown in cultures from healthy dogs or dogs with a variety of other nasal diseases. Unfortunately, fungal serology is only reliably useful for *Cryptococcus*.

Histopathologic examination of tissue from the nasal cavity is often the only way to differentiate between the varieties of nasal diseases, particularly nasal cancer. Few laboratory abnormalities are associated with the most common nasal tumors of dogs. On careful oral examination, palpation may reveal a mass in the pharynx or deviation of the hard palate or signs of dental disease may be noted in the maxillary arcade on the same side as the nasal discharge. Although thoracic metastasis at the time of presentation is uncommon, a suspicion of nasal or paranasal cancer warrants three-view thoracic radiographs to assess for metastasis.

6.   What is the best radiographic view for evaluating a suspected nasal tumor?

The most diagnostic skull radiographs are the open-mouth (dorsoventral or ventrodorsal intraoral) and the frontal sinus (rostrocaudal or "skyline") views (Figs. 15-1 and 15-2). Left and right lateral oblique views are also typically evaluated. Radiographs of diagnostic quality require general anesthesia to ensure immobility.

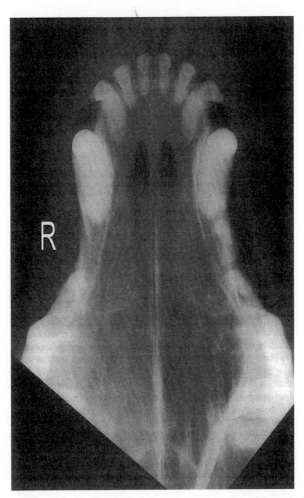

Figure 15-1. Open-mouth ventrodorsal radiograph of a dog with an adenocarcinoma in the nasal cavity on the right side. Increased opacity of soft tissues may be seen in the caudal area of the right nasal cavity. (Radiograph courtesy of the University of Florida.)

7. What plain radiographic findings are consistently associated with nasal tumors?

Unfortunately, tumor-related radiographic abnormalities are not always different from those caused by infectious/inflammatory disorders. Common findings include destruction of bone, increased nasal and frontal sinus densities, often consistent with a mass lesion, and septum deviation/destruction. A nasal neoplasm is more often associated with soft tissue opacities and loss of turbinate detail, usually predominantly in one cavity; deviation of the nasal septum; evidence of bone invasion (lysis); and soft tissue/fluid opacities within the frontal sinus on the affected side. In contrast, an inflammatory or infectious rhinitis is more likely to be associated with localized soft tissue opacities and increased foci of lucency. Frontal sinus involvement is not typical. Generally, fungal rhinitis is characterized by intense turbinate lysis (lucency) with minimal increased soft tissue opacity.

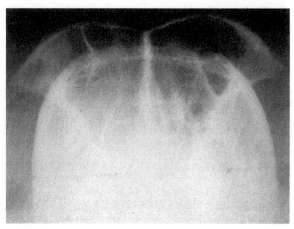

Figure 15-2.   Frontal sinus skyline view of a dog with an adenocarcinoma of the right nasal cavity. Increased opacity of the right frontal sinus is evident. (Radiograph courtesy of the University of Florida.)

8.   What does advanced imaging (CT or MRI) contribute to the diagnosis and treatment of nasal neoplasms?

Plain radiography is an adequate screening test to rule out some causes of epistaxis or nasal discharge; however, advanced imaging is needed to assess the disease more completely. CT with and without contrast/enhancement is more accurate for determining the extent of local tumor infiltration than is plain radiography (Fig. 15-3). Furthermore, the length of survival is related to the extent of tumor involvement based on CT findings for dogs treated with radiation therapy.

Dogs with neurologic abnormalities referable to the central nervous system should undergo CT and/or MRI to determine the extent of invasion into the calvarium. Unfortunately, as with plain radiography, there is no pattern of CT abnormalities consistently associated with nasal and paranasal sinus neoplasms. CT guidance of the biopsy instrument enhances tissue sampling accuracy. In general, soft tissue details are better imaged with MRI than with CT. MRI is superior to CT and plain radiography for demonstrating the extent of tumor invasion into the frontal and olfactory lobes. Because CT or MRI provides a better view of tumors than plain radiography, it is a prerequisite for radiation therapy. Computed tomography findings are used to calculate the radiation dose and the field for radiation treatments in most treatment centers. CT findings can help in estimating the extent of radiation damage to normal tissues, particularly the eye.

9.   What tests need to be performed before a tissue sample is obtained?

Before general anesthesia, a complete blood count (CBC) should be performed to assess for anemia or thrombocytopenia; a serum biochemical panel is needed to evaluate for adequate renal function, hepatocellular disease, serum protein concentration, and paraneoplastic hypercalcemia; and urinalysis should be performed to evaluate specific gravity (urine concentrating ability). Because nasal structures are highly vascular and hemostasis is often difficult during rhinoscopy, a coagulation screen should be performed (platelet count combined with either an activated clotting time or prothrombin/partial thromboplastin times). Determination of a normal buccal mucosal bleeding time to screen for von Willebrand's disease is warranted in high-risk dogs.

10.   What procedures are useful for obtaining cells or tissue needed to confirm a diagnosis of nasal tumor?

Procedures for obtaining diagnostic samples require general anesthesia. Complications caused

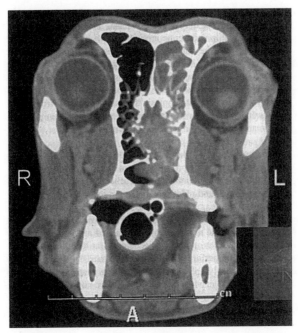

Figure 15-3.   Contrast-enhanced transverse computed tomography scan at the level of the caudal nasal cavity and rostral calvarium of a dog with a nasal adenocarcinoma. A large mass, visible in the left nasal cavity, has destroyed the turbinates and invaded the olfactory lobe and nasopharynx. The extent of tumor invasion into the brain would not be visible on radiographs. (CT image courtesy of Dr. E. Riedesel, Iowa State University.)

by hemorrhage (aspiration pneumonia, for example) can be avoided by packing the caudal pharynx with gauze and inflating the cuff of the endotracheal tube before obtaining biopsy samples. Serious complications are rare.

Blind transnasal core biopsy is very useful when the tumor cannot be visualized. Cytologic examination of a sample obtained by simple nasal flushing is seldom rewarding. Using abnormal radiographic or CT findings as a guide, a tissue core sample can be obtained via the external nares. A polypropylene tubular catheter case from an over-the-needle catheter cut at an angle and attached to a 20-ml syringe can be advanced into the tumor while gentle suction is applied. If the catheter is inserted beyond the medial canthus of the eye, then the biopsy instrument may perforate the cribriform plate. Alternatively, a 6 or 8 Fr urinary catheter or standard coring biopsy needle may be used to obtain tissue.

11. **Is it necessary to send a sample from a nasal mass suspected of being a tumor for microbial culture and antibiotic sensitivity testing?**
    Aerobic and anaerobic bacterial culture and antimicrobial sensitivity testing of a nasal mass suspected of being a tumor typically reveals growth of a variety of normal flora or bacterial pathogens secondary to tissue necrosis. If a diagnosis of nasal tumor is not certain, then initiation of fungal cultures is warranted. Unfortunately, growth of *Aspergillus* spp. or *Penicillium* spp. in culture is found in dogs with healthy and diseased nasal cavities.

12. How can a diagnosis of nasal neoplasm be made with rhinoscopy?

Direct visualization of the tumor may help guide tissue sampling. Using an approach through the mouth, retroflexing a flexible endoscope around the soft palate into the caudal nasal cavity usually allows visualization of the caudal nares and nasopharyngeal structures without obstruction by hemorrhage or exudate. Multiple pinch biopsies or brush samples may be obtained through the endoscope port. Likewise, a sufficiently small biopsy instrument may be passed beside the scope if a biopsy port is unavailable. Cytologic examination of direct tissue imprints on a glass slide more frequently suggest neoplasia than slides prepared from brush imprints. With brushings, only mucus and superficial mucosa overlying the mass are sampled, which can lead to a misdiagnosis of primary inflammation or lymphoplasmacytic rhinitis.

13. What do nasal neoplasms look like when viewed rhinoscopically?

A tumor typically appears as a mass protruding from the posterior choanae, but it can be easily obscured by blood and mucus. Lymphoma may diffusely affect the nasal cavity, causing the mucosa to appear thickened, rough, and reddened.

14. What kind of diagnostic tests are necessary for clinical staging to determine the extent of disease beyond the nasal cavity and immediately surrounding structures?

Although thoracic metastasis is uncommonly detected at the time of diagnosis, three-view thoracic radiographs should be performed. Because 10% to 20% of dogs with nasal neoplasms have early spread to the regional lymph nodes, fine-needle aspiration of the submandibular lymph nodes for cytology is warranted, even if the lymph nodes are normal or near normal in size.

15. How long do animals with nasal malignancies live if no therapy is attempted?

On average, clinical signs have been present for 3 to 4 months before a definitive diagnosis of nasal malignancy is made. Most dogs that are not treated are euthanized between 3 and 6 months after diagnosis because of symptoms due to progressive infiltration of the nasal cavity and surrounding bone. The most frequent sites of metastasis are regional lymph nodes, brain, and lung.

16. Is radiation therapy the standard of care for most dogs with nasal neoplasms?

The best treatment option for most dogs with nasal tumors is megavoltage radiation therapy. Most institutions have either a cobalt source radiation therapy unit or a linear accelerator, both of which produce megavoltage radiation sufficient for treating nasal tumors without surgical debulking. The median survival time of dogs with nasal tumors treated with megavoltage radiation is about 13 months, the mean survival time is 21 months, the estimated 1-year survival rate is about 60% and the 2-year survival rate is 20% to 25%. The effectiveness of radiation therapy for nasal tumors depends on the location and size (volume) and radiation-responsiveness of the tumor, as determined by the tumor histologic type and grade. It is not necessary to surgically reduce tumor size prior to therapy with megavoltage radiation; however, radiation therapy should be delayed 3 to 4 weeks after a surgical procedure to allow for adequate healing. Additionally, the dog must be able to safely undergo multiple anesthetic events (12 to 25 times depending on the protocol) and have an expected posttherapy longevity that will not be compromised by concurrent medical problems such as renal or cardiac insufficiency.

Advanced imaging with CT or MRI is essential for accurate treatment planning and predicting therapy-related adverse effects. CT is usually performed at the facility where the radiation therapy will be delivered. CT images are directly downloaded into a treatment-planning computer for use in determination of the radiation treatment dose and field. Linear accelerators equipped with a multileaf collimator are preferred because they allow the radiation field to be contoured to within a few millimeters of the shape of the tumor. Conformal therapy should decrease postradiation complications by avoiding radiation delivery to uninvolved nearby tissues such as the eye.

17. Could radiation therapy be used for palliation?

Palliative radiation therapy can be used to temporarily slow tumor growth and partially reduce tumor size. Three to five doses of radiation therapy, can help improve quality of life by decreasing epistaxis, relieving nasal obstruction, and decreasing bone pain, often at about a third to half the price of a full therapeutic course of radiation therapy. Palliative radiation therapy typically provides 3 to 4 months of improved quality of life before recurrence of clinical signs. In some cases, palliative radiation therapy may be repeated when clinical signs recur.

18. After the dog returns home from the radiation treatment facility, what evidence of radiation toxicity may be observed?

Most dogs experience some form of acute radiation toxicity, although generally not severe, and a few have late effects. Because of damage to the turbinates from the tumor itself and from radiation, most dogs with irradiated nasal cavities will have a mild, chronic nasal discharge for the remainder of their lives. Typically, it is serous or mucoid and not copious.

Acute toxicity usually begins during the course of radiation treatment and may continue for a variable number of weeks after the dog has completed therapy. Moist desquamation of the skin over the irradiated site (like a sunburn), rhinitis, and oral mucositis are likely. These changes are self-limiting and are managed by supportive care measures, including a combination of topical agents (Silvadene crème, vitamin E, aloe vera) and systemic analgesics consisting of anti-inflammatory doses of corticosteroids or nonsteroidal antiinflammatory drugs (NSAIDs). Good oral hygiene should be maintained, including frequently rinsing the mouth with a saline solution or tea. When the skin heals, alopecia, mild fibrosis, and a change in haircoat color or consistency may persist. Alopecia and altered haircoat color may be the only changes seen chronically. Although typically shielded from the radiation field, the eye can be adversely affected by repeated irradiation. Keratoconjunctivitis sicca, conjunctivitis, cornea damage, and, a year or more later, cataracts, may be observed. Keratoconjunctivitis is the most common problem involving the eye and may become permanent.

Late effects, for example, bilateral blindness and bone necrosis, may occur following higher radiation doses in dogs with longer survival times.

19. What role does surgery play in the management of nasal neoplasms?

Surgery has a limited role in the management of nasal neoplasms, because survival times are not improved compared to nonsurgical management. Similarly, surgery followed by megavoltage radiation therapy did not improve survival time compared with radiation therapy alone in all but one study, and in that study, the longer survival time was for dogs that had undergone tumor removal after radiation therapy (1.5 compared with 4 years). Rhinotomy may also be useful to obtain tissue for histologic examination, particularly when a firm mass is suspected of being a bony tumor.

20. Does chemotherapy have a role in the treatment of nasal neoplasms?

Chemotherapy alone has not been shown to be particularly useful in the definitive treatment of most nasal tumors. Systemic chemotherapy alone may be effective for a dog with a nasal lymphoma or a transmissible venereal tumor. In one study, palliative chemotherapy with cisplatin resulted in resolution of epistaxis within two doses in all dogs with nasal adenocarcinoma and no recurrence for up to 1 year. However, survival times were not improved. Radiation therapy along with chemotherapy would be expected to improve the overall response to therapy and survival times. Multimodality therapy will probably be the most effective treatment for control of nasal tumors.

21. Are NSAIDs potentially valuable for treatment of nasal neoplasms?

Increased expression of COX-2, an enzyme involved in the production of prostaglandins that play a role in tumor proliferation, angiogenesis, metastasis, and drug resistance, has been demonstrated in epithelial canine nasal tumors. The optimal dose and duration of treatment with a COX-2 inhibitor is unknown. Piroxicam has been used (0.3 mg/kg, by mouth, once a day), alone or in combination with chemotherapy. Piroxicam increases the renal toxicity of cisplatin and carboplatin in some animals.

22. What prognostic factors help predict the behavior of nasal tumors?

No prognostic factors have been consistently identified. Most dogs die or are euthanized because of progressive local tumor invasion. The prognostic value of histologic tumor examination is controversial. Median survival times for dogs with nasal adenocarcinoma without metastasis at the time of diagnosis are three times longer than dogs with metastatic lymph node and/or lung involvement. For dogs treated with radiation therapy, shorter survival times have been noted in older dogs (>10 years old) where tumor invasiveness has been demonstrated by regional lymph node metastasis, bone lysis, brain involvement or facial deformity. It is clear that in general, nasal neoplasms are detected so late in the course of the disease that effective management with any therapy is compromised by large tumor burden and local invasiveness.

BIBLIOGRAPHY

Adams WM, Bjorling DE, McAnulty JF: Outcome of accelerated radiotherapy alone or accelerated radiotherapy followed by exenteration of the nasal cavity in dogs with intranasal neoplasia: 53 cases (1990-2002), *J Am Vet Med Assoc* 227:936-941, 2005.

Adams WM, Miller PE, Vail DM et al: An accelerated technique for irradiation of malignant canine nasal and paranasal sinus tumors, *Vet Radiol Ultrasound* 39:475-481, 1998.

Bucowski JA, Wartenberg D, Goldschmidt M: Environmental causes for sinonasal cancers in pet dogs, and their usefulness as sentinels of indoor cancer risk, *J Toxicol Environ Health* 54:529-591, 1998.

Clercx C, Wallon J, Gilbert S et al: Imprint and brush cytology in the diagnosis of canine intranasal tumours, *J Small Anim Prac* 37:423-427, 1996.

Codner EC, Lurus AG, Miller JB et al: Comparison of computed tomography with radiography as a noninvasive diagnostic technique for chronic nasal disease in dogs, *J Am Vet Med Assoc* 202:1106-1110, 1993.

Fox LE, King RR: Cancers of the respiratory system, In Morrison WB, editor: *Cancer in dogs and cats,* Baltimore, 2004, Williams and Wilkins.

Gibbs C, Lane JG, Denny HR: Radiological features of intranasal lesions in the dog. A review of 100 cases, *J Small Anim Pract* 20:515-535, 1979.

Hahn KA, Knapp DW, Richardson RC et al: Clinical response of nasal adenocarcinoma to cisplatin chemotherapy in 11 dogs, *J Am Vet Med Assoc* 200:355-357, 1992.

Henry CJ, Brewer WG, Tyler JW et al: Survival in dogs with nasal adenocarcinoma: 64 cases (1981-1995), *J Vet Intern Med* 12:436-439, 1998.

LaDue TA, Dodge R, Page RL et al: Factors influencing survival after radiotherapy of nasal tumors in 130 dogs, *Vet Radiol Ultrasound* 40:312-317, 1999.

Love S, Barr A, Lucke VM, Lane JG: A catheter technique for biopsy of dogs with chronic nasal tumors, *J Small Anim Pract* 28:417-424, 1997.

McEntee MC: Neoplasms of the nasal cavity. In King LG, editor: *Textbook of respiratory diseases in dogs and cats,* Philadelphia, 2004, WB Saunders.

Morris JS, Dunn KJ, Dobson JM et al: Effects of radiotherapy alone and surgery and radiotherapy on survival of dogs with nasal tumors, *J Small Anim Pract* 35:567-573, 1994.

Morris SJ, Dunn KF, Dobson JM et al: Radiological assessment of severity of canine nasal tumours and relationship and relationship with survival, *J Small Anim Pract* 37:1-8, 1996.

Park RD, Beck ER, LeCouteur RA: Comparison of computed tomography and radiography for detecting changes induced by malignant nasal neoplasia in dogs, *J Am Vet Med Assoc* 201:1720-1724, 1992.

Reif JS, Bruns C, Lower KS: Cancer of the nasal cavity and paranasal sinuses and exposure to environmental tobacco smoke in pet dogs, *Am J Epidemiol* 147:488-492, 1998.

Smith MO, Turrel JM, Bailey CS et al: Neurologic abnormalities as the predominant signs of neoplasia of the nasal cavity in dogs and cats: seven cases (1973-1986), *J Am Vet Med Assoc* 195:242-245, 1989.

Spugnini EP, Thrall DE, Price S et al: Primary irradiation of canine intracranial masses, *Vet Radiol Ultrasound* 41:377-383, 2000.

Sullivan M, Lee R, Skae CA: The radiological features of sixty cases of intranasal neoplasia in the dog, *J Small Anim Pract* 28:575-586, 1987.

Theon AP, Madewell BR, Harb MF et al: Megavoltage irradiation of neoplasms of the nasal and paranasal cavities in 77 dogs, *J Am Vet Med Assoc* 202:1469-1475, 1993.

Thrall DE, Heidner GI, Novtney CA et al: Failure patterns following cobalt irradiation in dogs with nasal carcinoma, *Vet Radiol Ultrasound* 35:126-133, 1993.

Withrow SJ, Susaneck SJ, Macy DW et al: Aspiration and punch biopsy techniques for nasal tumors, *J An Anim Hosp Assoc* 21:551-554, 1985.

16. Upper Airway Disorders

Jo Ann Morrison

1.   Is there a typical signalment for a nasopharyngeal foreign body?
Foreign bodies are somewhat uncommon and most published reports have documented single cases. No common signalment has been identified. A table reviewing four reported cases is given (Table 16-1). Another report listed six cases of foreign bodies, including grass, cotton, gauze sponge, and a cocklebur. Individual patient descriptions were not available.

2.   What are the routes by which a dog can get a foreign body?
Several routes are possible: inhalation through the nares, vomiting, regurgitation, and oral penetration of the soft palate by a foreign object have all been reported. Congenital malformations could also predispose to a nasopharyngeal foreign body.

3.   What are the presenting complaints and physical exam findings?
Clinical symptoms are similar to those described for laryngitis and pharyngitis (e.g., sneezing, stertor). Signs may be acute if a foreign body ingestion or inhalation was witnessed. Dogs with nasopharyngeal foreign bodies are more commonly reported to have halitosis and purulent nasal discharge, especially if the foreign body has a more chronic duration. Also, clinical signs may be improved or relieved with opening the mouth. Alternatively, respirations and signs of stertor may be worsened with holding the mouth closed. In the nonsedated animal, oral examination may be grossly normal.

4.   What are the differential diagnoses for a nasopharyngeal foreign body?
Differentials, in addition to those listed for laryngitis/pharyngitis should include neoplasia, fungal granuloma (*Aspergillus* sp.), conformational abnormality, and parasitic infection with nasal mites or aberrant parasitic migration (*Cuterebra* spp.).

5.   What additional steps are taken in the diagnostic evaluation for a foreign object?
Disease should be localized to the nasopharynx on the basis of history, physical examination, and lack of substantial lesions elsewhere. Lateral skull radiographs have been used to demonstrate nasopharyngeal foreign objects in several cases. It is recommended that animals be placed under anesthesia for adequate radiographic studies. Anesthesia will also permit full nasopharyngeal evaluation. In a normal animal, radiographs of the skull do not show air in the oropharynx and the soft palate should be seen to extend from the hard palate to the epiglottis. Some breed variations do exist (brachycephalic breeds, for example). Radiographs may show a bone, mineral, or soft-tissue density foreign body in some cases. Also, other foreign material may be noted in the stomach. An air-filled esophagus may also be identified; however, interpretation is problematic as a gas-filled esophagus may normally develop while an animal is under anesthesia.

Table 16-1 Nasopharyngeal Foreign Bodies Retrieved from Four Dogs

AGE (YR)	BREED	DURATION OF SIGNS	FOREIGN BODY
1.5	Golden Retriever	2 weeks	Deer bone
1.4	Mixed breed	Several weeks	Chicken bone
9	Cocker Spaniel	10 days	Sand stone
5	Golden Retriever	Minutes	Pet fish

Computed tomography of the nasal passages and nasopharynx allows a detailed interpretation of this region and this technology is becoming more readily available. A complete evaluation of the nasopharynx should be obtained, including palpation of the soft palate. Some foreign bodies may be palpated dorsal to the soft palate. The caudal nasopharynx should be visualized with a flexible endoscope or dental mirror, as for laryngitis.

6. **How are foreign objects removed and what is the prognosis after removal?**
   After they are visualized, many foreign bodies can be manually removed with retraction into the oral cavity. Endoscopic retrieval, with grasping forceps, or a basket, may be used. Foreign objects may be digitally pushed from the area dorsal to the soft palate into the mouth. In some cases, flushing saline into the nares can expel a foreign object into the caudal nasopharynx, where it can then be more readily removed. Surgical excision through the palate or via rhinotomy may be required to remove some foreign bodies. After foreign material is removed, the area should be inspected again to ensure there is no retained material and to assess the health of the tissues. In most cases, the prognosis appears to be excellent, though no long-term studies have been performed. Long-term complications (stenotic changes) are possible from scar tissue formation.

BIBLIOGRAPHY

Coolman Br, Marretta SM, McKiernan BC et al: Choanal atresia and secondary nasopharyngeal stenosis in a dog. *J Am Anim Hosp Assoc* 34:497-501, 1998.
Laurendet H, Govendir M, Porges WL et al: Snoring and halitosis in a dog. *Aust Vet J* 76:250-251, 1998.
Papazoglou LG, Patsikas MN: What is your diagnosis? A radiopaque foreign body located in the nasopharynx. *J Small Anim Pract* 36:425-434, 1995.
Simpson AM, Harkin KR, Hoskinson JJ: Radiographic diagnosis: nasopharyngeal foreign body in a dog. *Vet Radiol Ultrasound* 41:326-328, 2000.
Tyler JW: Endoscopic retrieval of a large, nasopharyngeal foreign body. *J Am Anim Hosp Assoc* 33:512-516, 1997.
Venker-van Haagen AJ: Diseases of the throat. In Ettinger SJ, Feldman EC, editors: *Textbook of veterinary internal medicine,* 5th edition, 2000, Philadelphia, WB Saunders Co.
Willard MD, Radlinsky MA: Endoscopic examination of the choanae in dogs and cats: 118 cases (1988–1998). *J Am Vet Med Assoc* 215:1301-1305, 1999.

BRACHYCEPHALIC AIRWAY SYNDROME

Elizabeth Streeter

7. **What is the definition of brachycephalic airway syndrome?**
   Brachycephalic airway syndrome is a group of anatomical abnormalities normally seen in brachycephalic breeds. This group of anomalies typically includes stenotic nares, everted laryngeal saccules, elongated soft palate, and hypoplastic or collapsing trachea, and laryngeal collapse. These anomalies may occur singly, or animals may exhibit multiple problems.

8. What breeds are predisposed to brachycephalic airway syndrome?

Brachycephalic airway syndrome occurs in the chondrodysplastic breeds such as the English Bulldog, Pug, Boston Terrier, Pekingese, and Shih Tzu, among others. These breeds have been bred to have characteristics that contribute to their airway difficulties.

9. At what age are clinical signs associated with brachycephalic airway syndrome typically seen?

Signs of brachycephalic airway syndrome can occur at any age, but typically occur between 1 and 11 years of age. The severity of disease will increase with age. Older animals typically show signs of multiple aspects of the disorder.

10. What clinical signs are commonly seen in dogs with brachycephalic airway syndrome?

The clinical signs associated with brachycephalic airway syndrome are consistent with upper airway obstruction. Noisy breathing may be noted and may be more pronounced with exercise, obesity, or heat. Coughing and gagging may be noted. Signs of dyspnea or cyanosis may also be seen. Animals with brachycephalic airway syndrome may snore and have difficulty with sleep because of periods of asphyxia and upper airway obstruction. Owners may report exercise intolerance. Inspiratory stridor may be noted on physical examination.

11. What causes brachycephalic airway syndrome?

In certain chondrodysplastic breeds, as listed previously, early ankylosis of the bones of the skull leads to a shortened longitudinal axis of the skull. This shortening does not affect soft tissues of the head. The shortened skull with excessive soft tissue results in a decrease in airway size and lumen diameter. Animals with brachycephalic airway syndrome typically have stenotic nares, among other anatomic anomalies, resulting in a diminished airway. Also, an elongated soft palate may be found further contributing to the decreased opening of the upper airway. As the airway lumen narrows and pressure increases, other changes occur within the airway. Because of high pressures during inspiration, excess laryngeal tissue (everted laryngeal saccules) may be found, and eventually collapse of the airways (laryngeal and tracheal) may occur.

12. How is the diagnosis of brachycephalic airway syndrome made?

Diagnosis of brachycephalic airway syndrome is based on examination and identification of anomalies in a brachycephalic breed. Stenotic nares are easily visualized on physical examination. Little movement or flare of the wings of the nostrils is seen. In some cases, the nasal passage may be completely obstructed by the wings of the nostril. Sedation and laryngeal examination is necessary to examine the soft palate. An elongated soft palate will overlie the epiglottis and may be sucked into the glottis with inspiration. Everted laryngeal saccules, abnormalities of the tonsils, and laryngeal collapse may be seen at this time as well. Thoracic radiographs are necessary to evaluate lung parenchyma and evaluate diameter of the tracheal lumen. Fluoroscopy may be necessary to identify tracheal collapse.

13. What are the differential diagnoses for brachycephalic airway syndrome?

Any other cause of upper airway obstruction may cause signs similar to those of brachycephalic airway syndrome. These causes include masses, foreign body, laryngeal paralysis, and laryngeal collapse.

14. Is brachycephalic airway syndrome a progressive disease?

Brachycephalic airway syndrome is not necessarily progressive; however, clinical signs may worsen over time. Typically, initial anomalies, such as stenotic nares and elongated soft palate, will increase airway pressure during inspiration. This increase in pressures may lead to or exacerbate other problems, such as everted laryngeal saccules or upper airway irritation and edema. Eventually, this elevation in airway pressures will weaken laryngeal support muscles and lead to laryngeal collapse. Also, other factors, such as obesity, may exacerbate clinical signs.

15. What surgical treatments are available for brachycephalic airway syndrome?

Stenotic nares are the first anomaly to be addressed surgically. The surgical correction of stenotic nares involves a wedge resection of the nasal tissue to widen nasal passageways. Next, the soft palate and larynx are examined. Elongated soft palates may be surgically resected. This can be done using laser or by cutting excess tissue and suturing the incised edge. Everted laryngeal saccules are removed with long scissors. Laryngeal collapse is often difficult to treat surgically and is thought to be a result of high airway pressures. If treated early, repair of other anomalies may result in improvement in clinical signs. If no improvement is seen in animals with laryngeal collapse after addressing stenotic nares, elongated soft palate and everted laryngeal saccules, a permanent tracheostomy may be necessary to alleviate airway obstruction. Tracheal disease is much more difficult to address and surgical options may be limited. Tracheal collapse may be treated surgically with intraluminal stents or other types of prosthesis. These treatments are often associated with complications and reserved for end-stage disease not responsive to medical therapies.

16. What are preoperative and postoperative concerns for dogs with brachycephalic airway syndrome?

Animals with respiratory compromise require special attention in the preoperative and postoperative periods. Temporary tracheostomy may be considered to improve surgical access and provide a patent airway. One study documented poorer clinical recovery and increased complications in animals undergoing tracheostomy and recommended this be reserved for severely compromised animals. Supplemental oxygen should be provided, especially to severely affected animals. Anesthetic drugs should be selected that allow quick induction and recovery times to ensure ease of intubation. If there is concern about laryngeal function, drugs affecting this should be avoided to ensure adequate evaluation of laryngeal movement. Anticholinergics may be needed as premedication as many animals with upper airway disease have excessive vagal tone. Postoperatively, laryngeal edema and swelling may be of concern. Steroids at antiinflammatory doses may also be helpful. Also, animals should be closely monitored in the postoperative period for signs of upper airway obstruction and dyspnea. A patent airway should be maintained for as long as possible and the animal extubated only when fully awake. Temporary tracheostomy may be needed if worsening of airway obstruction does occur.

17. What is the prognosis for dogs affected with brachycephalic airway syndrome?

Prognosis is generally quite good for dogs treated at a young age. Older animals and animals with laryngeal collapse may have more questionable outcomes. Permanent tracheostomy may be needed in these animals to alleviate upper airway obstruction.

18. What postoperative complications are seen in brachycephalic airway dogs?

Brachycephalic dogs should be watched closely during the postoperative period for signs of upper airway obstruction and dyspnea. Coughing and gagging may result secondary to irritation of upper airway. Swelling may exacerbate signs of upper airway obstruction. Animals with tracheostomies may have pneumonia because of compromise of their natural protective mechanisms of the upper airway.

19. What medical therapies are available for management of dogs with brachycephalic airway syndrome?

Medical therapies are largely palliative and aimed at controlling clinical signs. These are not curative. Antitussives may be used to control signs of tracheal disease. Weight control may be of some benefit. Sedatives may be necessary to avoid excitement. Steroids, at antiinflammatory doses, may control swelling and edema of the upper airway. Avoiding heat and excessive exercise may also help to alleviate clinical signs.

20. What other diseases may occur concurrently with brachycephalic airway syndrome?

Dogs with signs of brachycephalic airway syndrome may have other problems related to their conformation. Corneal disease may be noted from exposure; these animals may be predisposed to proptosis. Skin fold dermatitis may also be seen. Dental abnormalities may be noted and other abnormalities, such as hydrocephalus, may be seen also related to breed.

BIBLIOGRAPHY

Davidson EB, Davis MS, Campbell GA et al: Evaluation of carbon dioxide laser and conventional incisional techniques for resection of soft palates in brachycephalic dogs. *J Am Vet Med Assoc* 219:776-781, 2001.
Heland CS: Surgery of the upper respiratory system. In Fossum TW editor: *Small animal surgery,* St Louis, 1997, Mosby.
Koch DA, Arnold S, Hubler M et al: Brachycephalic syndrome in dogs, *Compend Contin Educ Pract Vet* 25:48-55, 2003.

LARYNGEAL PARALYSIS

Elizabeth Streeter

21. What causes laryngeal paralysis?

Laryngeal paralysis is caused by disruption of nerve impulse transmission to the larynx. This interruption may be either from damage to the vagus or recurrent laryngeal nerves and may be either congenital or acquired. Lack of impulse conduction to laryngeal muscles results in the inability to abduct arytenoid cartilage and vocal folds. This then leads to upper airway obstruction.

Congenital causes of laryngeal paralysis are commonly seen in younger dogs (<1 year of age). An idiopathic acquired form also exists in older large-breed dogs. Other causes of acquired laryngeal paralysis include trauma, neuropathy, and iatrogenic nerve injury.

22. What breeds are commonly affected with laryngeal paralysis?

Laryngeal paralysis is commonly seen in older (>9 years old) large-breed dogs. The Labrador Retriever is the most common breed affected with the idiopathic acquired form; however, other large and giant breeds such as the Saint Bernard and Irish Setter may also be affected. Congenital laryngeal paralysis has been identified in several breeds including the Bouvier des Flandres, Siberian Husky, Bull Terrier, Dalmatian, and Rottweiler.

23. What are the clinical signs associated with laryngeal paralysis?

The clinical signs associated with laryngeal paralysis are dependent on the severity of the paralysis and whether one or both sides of the larynx are affected. The signs seen with laryngeal paralysis are due to upper airway obstruction. These signs are usually progressive over time and exacerbated with heat, anxiety, obesity, and exertion. Owners may report a change in bark and decreased exercise tolerance. Stridor will be noted on examination and periods of cyanosis and dyspnea may be observed. Coughing and gagging may also be noted. Other signs of neuropathy may be seen depending on the cause of the paralysis. Also, because of the inability to pant and exchange heat, dogs with laryngeal paralysis may be hyperthermic and may exhibit signs of heatstroke.

24. What diseases may occur concurrently with laryngeal paralysis?

Neuromuscular diseases may occur concurrently with laryngeal paralysis. Hypothyroidism has thought to be associated with laryngeal paralysis; however, this relationship is unclear, because some studies have shown this correlation is consequential rather than cause and effect.

Megaesophagus may also be seen concurrently in dogs with laryngeal paralysis. This is likely the result of the potential for neuropathy as the cause for the laryngeal dysfunction. Megaesophagus is important to identify in animals with laryngeal paralysis because it may contribute to an increased likelihood of complications such as aspiration pneumonia.

25. How is laryngeal paralysis diagnosed?

Laryngeal paralysis is diagnosed via upper airway examination under sedation or a light plane of anesthesia to visualize movement of the larynx. Paralysis may be unilateral or bilateral, although most animals with severe clinical signs have bilateral paralysis. A complete oral examination should be done at the time of diagnosis to identify any masses, swellings, or other abnormalities.

26. What anesthetic protocol may be used for laryngeal examination?

Care must be used in selecting an anesthetic protocol for laryngeal examination because many drugs interfere with normal motion of the arytenoid cartilage. Use of these drugs may result in a false-positive diagnosis. Adequate sedation must be given for relaxation of jaw tone and adequate visualization of the larynx. Several different protocols have been suggested. Ketamine, diazepam, and acepromazine, when combined with other drugs, have been shown to be the most suppressive of laryngeal function and are not recommended. Thiopental alone and acepromazine, combined with butorphanol and isoflurane via mask, appeared to be better alternatives according to one study. Other alternatives, such as propofol and thiopental, are also reported to provide good anesthetic depth with little affect on laryngeal function.

27. What is the role of doxapram in the diagnosis of laryngeal paralysis?

Doxapram is a central acting respiratory stimulant. Doxapram has been shown to be helpful in the diagnosis of laryngeal paralysis. A study evaluating the use of doxapram in diagnosis of laryngeal paralysis showed that normal dogs given doxapram showed increased respiratory rate, but no change in laryngeal function or glottal area size. Dogs with laryngeal paralysis, however, showed dramatic changes in glottal area size and paradoxic motion of the arytenoids. This vigorous laryngeal motion in some dogs with paralysis resulted in the need for intubation and emergent airway management.

28. What are the medical options for treatment of laryngeal paralysis?

Animals presenting in respiratory distress from laryngeal paralysis should have oxygen supplemented. Sedation may also be needed to alleviate anxiety from upper airway obstruction. Acepromazine (0.1 to 0.4 mg/kg) may be used. Intravenous access is essential for the laryngeal paralysis animal that presents in distress. If sedation, oxygen, and cooling are not adequate, intubation may be necessary to ensure a patent airway. Temporary tracheostomy in these cases may be necessary. Steroids have been suggested to decrease inflammation of the upper airway. Temperature should be monitored. Treatment for heatstroke and cooling may be indicated depending on the animal's condition.

29. How is surgery used to treat laryngeal paralysis?

There are many surgical corrections available for the larynx, and surgery is eventually needed in most cases of laryngeal paralysis. All surgical options involve opening of the airway and resolution of the obstruction. This may be accomplished by either removal of a portion of the vocal folds and arytenoid cartilage (ventriculocordectomy, partial arytenoidectomy) or by lateralization of the tissues (laryngeal tieback). There is debate as to the most effective or best procedure; the most commonly recommended surgical procedure is the unilateral arytenoid lateralization. A study done in 2001 compared the procedures and found unilateral treatment to be superior than bilateral. Also, this study documented fewer complications with unilateral arytenoid lateralization when compared with bilateral arytenoid lateralization or partial laryngectomy. Difficulties come when comparing individual surgical techniques, however, and the type of procedure chosen largely depends on surgeon preference and case criteria. Other types of surgical correction, such as castellated laryngofissure, are performed much less frequently and complications are more common.

30. What are complications associated with surgical correction of laryngeal paralysis?

Dogs with laryngeal paralysis may have several complications that develop after the procedure. Dogs are at risk for aspiration pneumonia. This risk is lifelong after the procedure is performed. Also, dogs may have recurrence of the airway obstruction and paralysis. Laryngeal webbing and scarring may also occur.

31. What is the long-term prognosis for dogs with laryngeal paralysis?

The long-term prognosis is good for dogs with laryngeal paralysis, assuming that surgery is successful and no complications are seen. Additional problems may arise, such as aspiration pneumonia and recurrence of the upper airway obstruction. These problems may occur at any time after surgery. Some dogs may initially do well with medical management for a time; however, because of the progressive nature of the disease, surgery is eventually required.

BIBLIOGRAPHY

Gross ME, Dodam JR, Pope ER et al.: A comparison of thiopental, propofol, and diazepam-ketamine anesthesia for evaluation of laryngeal function in dogs premedicated with butorphanol and glycopyrrolate. *J Am Anim Hosp Assoc* 38:503-506, 2002.
Jackson AM, Tobias K, Long et al: Effects of various anesthetic agents on laryngeal motion during laryngoscopy in normal dogs. *Vet Surg* 33:102-106, 2004.
MacPhail CM, Monnet E: Outcome and postoperative complications in dogs undergoing surgical treatment of laryngeal paralysis: 140 cases (1985-1998). *J Am Vet Med Assoc* 218:1949-1956, 2001.
Tobias KM, Jackson AM, Harvey RC: Efferyngeal paralysis. *Vet Anaesth Analg* 31:258-263, 2004.

17. Laryngeal Tumors

Leslie E. Fox

1. What are some of the most common tumors of the larynx in the dog?

Laryngeal tumors are rare. A wide variety of tumors have been reported in dogs; however, carcinomas and striated muscle tumors are most common.

2. What is a laryngeal oncocytoma?

An oncocytoma is a benign tumor presumed to be of epithelial origin with a characteristic ultrastructural cell morphology of abundant cytoplasm with enlarged, closely packed mitochondria. Although difficult to differentiate from poorly differentiated striated muscle cell tumors without immunohistochemistry, the distinction is clinically important because they may have a less aggressive biologic behavior.

3. What is the typical signalment for dogs with laryngeal tumors?

There is no breed or gender predilection for dogs with laryngeal tumors. Most dogs are about 7 years old and can be as young as 1 year old. Osteochondromas occur in growing dogs.

4. What typical clinical signs are associated with laryngeal tumors?

Clinical signs are often present for months before diagnosis. When clinical signs are present, dyspnea, voice change or loss, respiratory stridor/stertor, cough, and exercise intolerance are most frequent. Dysphagia, cyanosis, hemoptysis, sneezing, and ptyalism may also be noted. Clinical signs may have been present for months before diagnosis. The severity of the signs depends directly on the extent of airway obstruction.

5. What are the differential diagnoses for dogs with clinical signs referable to the larynx?

In appropriate breeds, elongated soft palate, epiglottic entrapment, and everted laryngeal saccules are seen often with secondary laryngeal mucosal edema. Laryngeal paralysis or collapse, mucosal edema from dyspnea, and excessive laryngeal scar tissue or webbing may be observed. Nonneoplastic masses found in the area of the larynx are laryngeal cyst, inflammatory polyp, granuloma, and pharyngeal salivary mucocele.

6. What diagnostic tests are most useful to evaluate the larynx?

The astute clinician may palpate a thickened larynx or mass dorsal to the larynx and anterior trachea, but, typically, a suspicion of laryngeal neoplasia is raised when increased soft-tissue density in the area of the larynx with or without calcification or distortion of larynx structures are observed on the lateral view of a survey radiograph. Evidence of local metastasis to regional lymph nodes may be seen. Thoracic plain radiography is useful to look for evidence of metastatic disease and changes that accompany upper chronic and severe upper airway obstruction, such as pulmonary edema or aspiration pneumonia. Clinicopathologic tests do not contribute to a diagnosis, but should be done before anesthesia and biopsy.

Direct visualization of the pharynx and larynx via light laryngoscopy is most helpful in differentiating various disorders of the larynx. A flexible fiberoptic endoscope is used to assess the distal larynx and trachea. Using ultrasound, a laryngeal mass may be hypoechoic or of mixed echogenicity with indistinct or distinct borders. Advanced imaging with computed tomography/magnetic resonance imaging allows the most accurate assessment of local invasion and regional lymph node status before surgical extirpation of the tumor.

Histopathologic diagnosis from a tissue sample is needed to definitively diagnose laryngeal tumors. Tissue biopsy under direct visualization of the larynx is often possible. Placement of a tracheostomy tube may be needed before biopsy if the airway is severely occluded. Corticosteroids administered in the perioperative period may help decrease laryngeal mucosal edema secondary to traumatic intubation and tissue manipulation. Careful extubation with an inflated endotracheal tube cuff in place will help prevent aspiration. Percutaneous ultrasound-guided fine needle aspiration is a safe and rewarding method to obtain a cellular sample for cytologic examination.

7. How are laryngeal neoplasms treated?

Surgical disease requires a thorough understanding of the anatomy and physiology of the larynx. Although tumor location often precludes complete surgical excision of the tumor, small or pedunculated lesions may be completely removed. Most tumors are advanced when detected, so partial laryngectomy may be all that is possible. Combined with conventional excision, carbon dioxide laser may be used to cut the cartilage and muscles of the larynx with decreased hemorrhage. Total laryngectomy has been tried with variable results. Airway and nutritional support may be necessary postoperatively.

Cobalt-60 teletherapy radiation has provided life extension in a few animals with radiosensitive tumors (typically, lymphoma, mast cell tumor, and some squamous cell carcinomas). Chemoresponsive tumors, such as lymphoma may be treated with a standard chemotherapy protocol. Ultimately, the most effective management of laryngeal tumors will probably be achieved with combination therapy such as surgical excision, radiation therapy, and chemotherapy given either before, during, or after local therapy.

8. What is the prognosis for dogs with laryngeal tumors?

The prognosis for a dog with a benign, completely resected tumor such as a rhabdomyoma is excellent. Because many malignant laryngeal tumors are quite locally invasive when discovered, the overall prognosis is poor and depends on size, histology, and local invasiveness. There are sporadic reports of prolonging life with a variety of combination treatments.

BIBLIOGRAPHY

Bjorling DE, McAnulty JA, Swainson S: Surgically treatable upper respiratory disorders. *Vet Clin North Am Small Anim Pract* 30:1227, 2000.
Block G, Clarke K, Salisbury SK et al: Total laryngectomy and permanent tracheostomy for the treatment of laryngeal rhabdomyosarcoma in a dog. *J Am Anim Hosp Assoc* 31:510-513, 1995.
Calderwood MB: Laryngeal oncocytoma in two dogs. *J Am Vet Med Assoc* 185:677-679, 1984.
Carlisle CH, Biery DN, Thrall DE: Tracheal and laryngeal tumors in the dogs and cat: literature review and additional 13 patients. *Vet Radiol* 31:229-235, 1991.
Clifford CA, Sorenmo KU: Tumors of the larynx and trachea. In King LG, editor, *Respiratory diseases in dogs and cats*, St Louis, 2004, Elsevier.
Holt TL, Mann FA: Soft tissue application of lasers. *Vet Clin North Am Small Anim Pract* 32:569-599, 2002.
Rudolf H, Brown P: Ultrasonography of laryngeal masses in six cats and one dog. *Vet Radiol Ultrasound* 39:430-434, 1998.
Saik JE, Toll SL, Diters RW et al: Canine and feline laryngeal neoplasia: a 10-year survey. *J Am Anim Hosp Assoc* 22:359-365, 1986.
Thrall DE, Dewhirst MW: Use of radiation and/or hyperthermia for the treatment of mast cell tumors and lymphosarcoma in dogs. *Vet Clin North Am Small Anim Pract* 15:835-843, 1985.
Venker-van Haagen AJ: Diseases of the larynx. *Vet Clin North Am Small Anim Pract* 22:1155-1172, 1992.

18. Tracheal Tumors

Leslie E. Fox

1. What are some of the most common tumors of the trachea in the dog?

Tumors of the trachea are rare and are typically malignant except for benign osteocartilaginous tumors associated with the tracheal rings in young dogs.

2. What is the typical signalment for dogs with tracheal tumors?

Dogs with tumors of the trachea are middle age to older with no gender or breed predilection. Dogs with osteochondromas are most often younger than 1 year old.

3. What are the typical clinical signs exhibited by dogs with tracheal tumors?

Because of partial airway occlusion, a progressive worsening of dyspnea, wheezing, coughing, and exaggerated expiratory effort are the most common clinical findings. Acute onset severe respiratory distress with cyanosis may be the primary presenting complaint.

4. What are the differential diagnoses for partial tracheal obstruction?

Polyps, abscess or granuloma, foreign body, vascular anomalies, collapsed tracheal rings from trauma, nodular amyloidosis, papillomatosis, and a granulomatous reaction to *Filaroides osleri*.

5. How are tracheal tumors diagnosed?

Auscultation of the trachea during physical examination may help identify the presence of a partial obstruction through localization of higher pitched airway sounds (wheezing or stridor) at the site of tracheal narrowing. Plain radiography may help delineate the location of the tumor; however, direct visualization of the mass with a bronchoscope is most useful. Histopathology of biopsy tissue samples obtained through the biopsy channel of the endoscope is usually sufficient to confirm a diagnosis.

6. Is plain radiography useful for the detection of tracheal masses?

Lateral cervical plain survey radiographs show either narrowing of the trachea or increased soft-tissue density.

7. What tests are needed for clinical staging?

To assess for general anesthesia and clinical staging, a complete blood cell count, serum biochemical panel, and urinalysis should be performed. Thoracic radiographs will allow evaluation for metastasis. If lymphoma is confirmed, additional clinical staging with abdominal plain survey radiography, abdominal ultrasonography, and bone marrow aspirate cytology is recommended.

8. What is the treatment for tracheal tumors?

Complete surgical excision should be curative for dogs with benign tumors such as rhabdomyoma or osteochondroma and may prolong the lives of some dogs with malignant tumors (rhabdomyosarcoma) without metastatic disease. Reported postsurgical survival is unknown, but information on a small number of cases gives a range of 3 to 12 months. The reader is referred to a description of surgical techniques used to extirpate the tumor while avoiding postoperative dehiscence, granuloma, and trachea lumen narrowing after tracheal ring resection. Twenty-five percent or up to 8 to 10 tracheal rings can be removed successfully. Antibiotics should be given perioperatively because bacteria from the lumen mucosa will contaminate the surgery site.

9. How valuable is radiation therapy in the treatment of tracheal tumors?

Radiation treatment may be used effectively for dogs with radiosensitive tumors such as lymphoma. Multidrug chemotherapy should be used in conjunction with local control with radiotherapy.

10. What is the prognosis for dogs with trachea tumors?

Too few cases of treated dogs with trachea tumors have been reported to make generalizations about survival times. The long-term prognosis is guarded and limited by aggressive behavior and the extent of local invasion and thus, resectability. Many dogs are euthanized at the time of diagnosis because of the poor prognosis; however, dogs with resectable benign tumors may be cured.

BIBLIOGRAPHY

Bjorling DE, McAnulty JA, Swainson S: Surgically treatable upper respiratory disorders. *Vet Clin North Am Small Anim Pract* 30:1227-1251, 2000.

Brown MR, Rogers KS: Primary tracheal tumors in dogs and cats. *Compend Contin Educ Pract Vet* 25:854-860, 2003.

Carlisle CH, Biery DN, Thrall DE: Literature review and 13 additional patients. *Vet Radiol* 32:639-643, 1991.

Clifford CA, Sorenmo KU: Tumors of the larynx and trachea. In King LG, editor. *Respiratory diseases in dogs and cats,* 2004, St Louis, Elsevier.

19. Large Airway Disorders

Jo Ann Morrison

1. What are common noninfectious disorders involving the canine trachea?

The most common disorders include the following:

- Tracheal collapse
- Hypoplastic trachea
- Tracheal trauma or laceration

2. What is the typical signalment, including breed predilection or heritability, for tracheal collapse?

Tracheal collapse is most commonly diagnosed in middle age (6-7 years), small, or toy breed dogs. Males and females appear to be affected with equal frequency. The most common breeds include the Yorkshire Terrier, Poodle, Pomeranian, Chihuahua, and Maltese. A genetic inheritance pattern has not been identified. However, histopathologic and ultrastructural evaluation of tissue from affected dogs has revealed tracheal cartilaginous rings that are hypocellular when compared with healthy dogs. The normal tracheal cartilage contains chondroitin sulfate, collagen, glycoproteins, glycosaminoglycans, and proteoglycans. Affected dogs show decreased levels of calcium, glycosaminoglycans, and chondroitin sulfate in tracheal rings. These deficiencies weaken and soften the cartilaginous tissue, allowing dynamic tracheal collapse with respirations. Some suspect that these cartilage defects may be inherited.

3. Are there any known causes for tracheal collapse?

As described previously, there may be an inherited or congenital weakness in the tracheal cartilaginous rings. There is also evidence that abnormal innervation to the trachealis muscle may play a role. Affected animals may be relatively asymptomatic, although careful questioning of the owner may reveal a prolonged history of mild signs, until a secondary or complicating factor arises. These are discussed in the following sections.

4. Are there different types of tracheal collapse?

There are two types of tracheal collapse: dorsoventral and lateral. Dorsoventral collapse is much more common, in which the dorsal tracheal membrane (which is often redundant) is drawn into the tracheal lumen with changes in intratracheal pressure with respiration. This type of collapse can occur in the cervical region, the intrathoracic region, and can extend to involve the mainstem bronchi. Cervical collapse is associated more with inspiration because of the resultant drop in intratracheal pressure. Intrathoracic collapse is more associated with expiration. This results from intrathoracic pressure exceeding airway opening pressure. Dorsoventral collapse can be graded on a scale of 1 to 4, as described in Table 19-1. The grade is assigned to the most severely affected portion. Lateral collapse of the trachea is uncommonly diagnosed. The few reported cases have been seen in association with other factors: a congenital malformation, secondary to tracheal surgery, or possibly after trauma.

5. What are the historical complaints with collapsing trachea?

The classic finding in tracheal collapse is an easily induced honking cough. There is typically an association with excitement, heat and humidity, swallowing when eating or drinking, and tracheal stimulation (pulling on a collar while walking). Signs are commonly exacerbated by exercise and by picking up or holding the animal.

Table 19-1   *Grades of Tracheal Collapse*

GRADE	TRACHEAL RING SHAPE	AIRWAY DIAMETER REDUCTION
I	Circular	25%
II	Partially flattened	50%
III	Nearly flat	75%
IV	Flat to dorsally inverted	≥90%

6.   What are the complicating factors that have been implicated?

Many cases of collapsing trachea have had a chronic cough that has worsened with time. The chronic cough will induce permanent airway injury. The mucosal surfaces of the airways are damaged, which leads to inflammation and hyperplasia of the mucous glands. The increased mucus production interferes with normal mucociliary clearance, leading to further airway compromise and coughing. The condition can then become self-perpetuating. It is also common to see an exacerbation of coughing following some "precipitating" event. Endotracheal intubation, obesity, respiratory infection, airway sensitivity (smoke inhalation or allergic disease), and cardiac disease have all been implicated. There is also a possible relationship with laryngeal paralysis, though this is less well defined.

7.   What is especially important in the physical exam and diagnostic workup?

Thoracic auscultation may be difficult because of concurrent upper airway noise, increased bronchial sounds, and obesity. Concurrent cardiac disease may be present and must be ruled out as a cause for coughing. Systolic murmurs, pulmonary edema, or cardiac arrhythmias may be detected. Hepatomegaly is commonly detected, in most cases from fat deposition; however, it may also be a sign of cardiac failure. Heartworm status should be ascertained. Thoracic radiographs are the initial imaging study performed. Both inspiratory and expiratory films of the entire tracheal length should be obtained. This may demonstrate dynamic tracheal collapse (84% of cases in one study). Radiographs may be difficult to interpret with an overlying esophagus, positioning, and motion. Radiographs should be carefully evaluated for signs of cardiac disease, pneumonia, or other airway disease. Lateral thoracic radiographs (Fig. 19-1) taken at the level of the thoracic inlet commonly demonstrate tracheal collapse in dogs with severe coughing on expiration. In cases where collapsing trachea is suspected but not seen on thoracic radiographs, other diagnostics may be employed. Fluoroscopy shows dynamic tracheal movement and is better able to demonstrate collapse of mainstem bronchi, which is difficult to appreciate on survey radiographs. In some cases, stimulating the animal to cough will help localize the area of collapse. Ultrasonographic techniques for evaluating tracheal collapse have also been described, though these may be difficult to perform because of the air interface within the trachea. The gold standard for diagnosing collapsing trachea is tracheobronchoscopy. This technique allows evaluation of the entire trachea and the mainstem bronchi. Deeper airways may also be evaluated, depending on the size of the dog. The degree of tracheal collapse is also most accurately determined with an endoscopic procedure. Samples may be obtained from the airways for cytologic evaluation and microbial or fungal culture. This is important to rule out concurrent airway disease or possible infectious processes. Owners should be warned that there is the potential for worsening of respiratory signs after this procedure.

8.   What are the current treatment recommendations for collapsing trachea?

Medical and environmental management are the initial treatments for this condition. *Environmental management* includes minimizing excitement; using a harness instead of a neck collar;

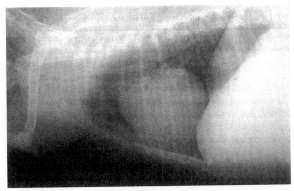

Figure 19-1. Lateral thoracic radiograph demonstrating significant tracheal collapse at the level of the thoracic inlet. (Radiograph courtesy of Dr. E. Riedesel, Iowa State University.)

avoiding dust and smoke in the air by cleaning or removing carpeting, using air purifiers, etc.; and minimizing time spent in hot and humid environments to reduce panting.

Medical management must include weight loss for an obese animal. There may be concurrent allergic airway disease (diagnosed via radiography and bronchoalveolar lavage cytology) that may be treated medically. Concurrent respiratory infections may be observed with tracheal collapse; however, the true incidence of this is unknown. There is not sufficient evidence to warrant empiric antibiotic therapy in dogs with tracheal collapse. Antitussive agents are employed in therapy for both acute and chronic cases. Narcotic agents are the most potent cough suppressants, but may be associated with sedation, constipation, and loss of appetite. The use of bronchodilators is controversial. These agents do not act on large airways. However, they may be effective at lowering intrathoracic pressure and improving small airway obstruction. Side effects of these medications include cardiovascular stimulation, tachycardia, arrhythmias, and central nervous system stimulation. Corticosteroids may be used on a short-term basis, primarily for laryngeal or tracheal inflammation or for chronic airway disease. The potential side effects (weight gain, sodium retention, panting) should be measured against the possible benefits. All medications should be tapered to the lowest effective dose to minimize side effects and possible drug interactions. The common medications used for the medical treatment of tracheal collapse are listed in Table 19-2. Recently, there was a report on the use of diphenoxylate/atropine (Lomotil) for collapsing trachea. Diphenoxylate has a narcotic, antitussive effect. Atropine has two effects: reduction in mucus secretion and bronchodilation. There have been no published studies documenting the efficacy of this therapy. Surgical options are available for animals with severe disease or animals that are unresponsive to medical management. These options include both intrathoracic and extrathoracic stenting procedures.

9. What is the prognosis for tracheal collapse?

The prognosis for tracheal collapse is guarded. Most animals will improve with medical and environmental management and can be maintained with an acceptable quality of life. Owners should be cautioned that complete resolution of signs is not typically achieved. If clinical signs have not improved within 2 weeks of initiating therapy, surgical options should be considered. There have been reports that dogs older than 6 years have a worse response to surgery. It has been suggested that animals should be evaluated as potential surgical candidates early in the disease before chronic airway changes have become permanent and the tracheal tissue has become irreversibly damaged. There is no definitive evidence to support that suggestion. Figure 19-2 shows a postoperative lateral thoracic radiograph after placement of intraluminal tracheal stents.

Table 19-2   *Pharmacologic Agents Used in the Treatment of Tracheal Collapse*

DRUG	DOSAGE	SIDE EFFECTS
Antitussives		Sedation, constipation
Hydrocodone	0.22 mg/kg PO q 6-12 h	
Butorphanol	0.5-1 mg/kg PO q 6-12 h	
Bronchodilators		Gastrointestinal upset, tachycardia, central nervous system stimulation
Theophylline	10-20 mg/kg PO q 12 h	
Terbutaline	0.625-5 mg/dog q 12 h (depending on size of dog)	
Albuterol	0.02-0.05 mg/kg PO q 12 h	
Antiinflammatories		Weight gain, polyuria, polydipsia, panting, immunosuppression
Prednisone	0.5-1 mg/kg PO q 12-24 h	

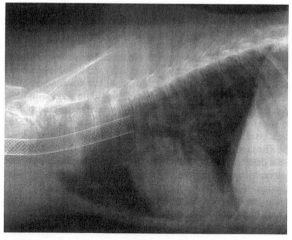

Figure 19-2.   A postoperative lateral thoracic radiograph, showing the placement of intraluminal tracheal stents. (Radiograph courtesy of Dr. E. Riedesel, Iowa State University.)

10. What is the definition of a hypoplastic trachea?

Tracheal hypoplasia results from inadequate growth of the tracheal rings. It is a congenital defect. However, the genetic defect has not been determined. The ends of the cartilaginous rings may be apposed or may overlap. The dorsal tracheal membrane may be absent. Hypoplastic trachea usually occurs concurrently with other components of the brachycephalic airway syndrome: elongated soft palate, stenotic nares, and everted laryngeal saccules.

11. Are there any breed predispositions to this condition?
Tracheal hypoplasia has been most commonly diagnosed in the English Bulldog (55% in one retrospective report) and the Boston Terrier (15% in the same report). There also appears to be an increased incidence in other brachycephalic breeds. Males have been more commonly diagnosed with the condition than females.

12. What are the presenting complaints and physical exam findings?
Some dogs with evidence of hypoplastic trachea may be clinically normal. This is especially true in the Bulldog breed. If signs are present, coughing, dyspnea, and stridor are most commonly reported. Hypoplastic trachea may be seen with other components of the brachycephalic syndrome (mentioned previously), cardiovascular abnormalities, and megaesophagus. These conditions may account for other clinical signs and physical exam findings: moist rales, productive cough, pneumonia, fever, regurgitation, syncope, and dysphagia.

13. How is the diagnosis of hypoplastic trachea made?
Two methods can be used to diagnose this condition and both are based on findings seen on lateral thoracic radiographs. Ideally, the radiographs should be obtained when the animal is as asymptomatic as possible, to reduce confounding variables. The first method compares the width of the tracheal lumen with the width of the third rib. The tracheal lumen is measured midway between the thoracic inlet and the carina. The third rib is measured at the end of the proximal one third of the rib. A hypoplastic trachea would be diagnosed if the width of the tracheal lumen is less than three times the width of the rib. The second method compares the diameter of the tracheal lumen with the thoracic inlet. The thoracic inlet is measured from the ventral aspect of the first thoracic vertebra to the manubrium. The tracheal lumen diameter is measured along that same line. Ratios have been determined for various types of dogs and are given in Table 19-3. It has been suggested that numeric values not be used as absolute cutoffs between normal and abnormal, because there are other factors that may be more significantly related to prognosis. It should be noted that these numbers do not correlate with the degree of respiratory distress. Figure 19-3 shows a lateral thoracic radiograph from a Boston Terrier with a hypoplastic trachea. The most objective way to diagnose hypoplastic trachea is histologic examination of the trachea.

14. What are the management and treatment options for hypoplastic trachea?
There is no treatment and no cure for hypoplastic trachea. However, there may be other, concurrent problems that require management: elongated soft palate or pneumonia, for example. There is evidence that these other problems may be more responsible for clinical signs than the hypoplastic trachea in affected animals. Concurrent problems, congenital or acquired, should be treated and resolved when possible. Emergency management of acute respiratory distress should consist of supplemental oxygen therapy, anti-inflammatories, and possibly bronchodilators (controversial, but may be of benefit if lower airways are involved) as with many cases of respiratory distress. Care should be taken if emergency intubation is considered because of the

Table 19-3   *Tracheal Lumen to Thoracic Inlet Diameter Ratios in Normal and Brachycephalic Dogs*

TRACHEAL LUMEN: THORACIC INLET DIAMETER	CANINE BREED
0.127:1	English Bulldog
0.160:1	Brachycephalic breeds (non-Bulldogs)
0.204:1	Nonbrachycephalic breeds

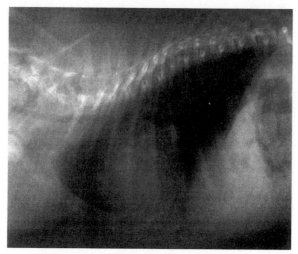

Figure 19-3. A lateral thoracic radiograph showing a hypoplastic trachea in a Boston Terrier. (Radiograph courtesy of Dr. E. Riedesel, Iowa State University.)

smaller than normal tracheal lumen. A clean, sanitary environment may reduce the possibility of pneumonia. Weight gain should be avoided. Affected animals should not be used for breeding.

15. What is the prognosis for dogs with hypoplastic trachea?

The initial prognosis should be guarded for dogs with hypoplastic trachea. However, if this is the only congenital defect present and no other complicating factors are identified, the prognosis may improve. Sixty percent of dogs in one study were considered clinically normal 6 months after diagnosis in one study. Young dogs may "outgrow" the condition. The degree of tracheal hypoplasia does not always correlate with clinical signs. Thus careful evaluation and thorough client education are necessary to successfully manage this condition.

16. What are the risk factors for tracheal laceration?

This is an uncommon condition; however, because most cases are the result of trauma, certain risk factors may predispose to this condition. Blunt trauma (hit by car, hunting accident) and dog fights have been identified as possible causes; therefore, larger, outdoor, male dogs may be predisposed. Also, iatrogenic trauma with jugular venipuncture has been associated with tracheal laceration, so animals that are fractious or difficult to restrain may be predisposed. Tracheal laceration may also be seen as a complication of a transtracheal wash procedure. There is also a report of tracheal perforation secondary to irritation of a suture knot from a previous ventral slot decompression at the C5-C6 intervertebral disc space. There have been several review articles on tracheal rupture in cats after endotracheal intubation and anesthetic malfunction, but iatrogenic tracheal trauma secondary to endotracheal intubation has not been reported in dogs.

17. What is the clinical presentation of a tracheal laceration?

Clinical signs are, in most cases, noted soon after perforation. In the case of a tracheal perforation resulting from suture reaction, respiratory signs were noted 8 weeks after surgery. Signs seen include subcutaneous emphysema and respiratory distress. Subcutaneous emphysema may be localized to the cervical region or may progress to generalized involvement of the entire body. Significant, generalized subcutaneous emphysema should alert the clinician to the possibility of a tracheal laceration. Respiratory distress may present including tachypnea, dyspnea, stridor, coughing, cyanosis, collapse, and shock.

18. How is a tracheal perforation identified?

Radiography should be the initial diagnostic test. Cervical and thoracic radiographs may reveal pneumomediastinum, subcutaneous emphysema, pneumothorax, and possibly pneumopericardium. Emphysema may also be seen in intramuscular and peritracheal tissues. Abdominal radiographs may show pneumoretroperitoneum. In some cases of intrathoracic tracheal trauma, the mucosal or serosal tissue may remain intact, preventing air leakage and subsequent pneumomediastinum. In those cases, inspiratory films may show a widening of trachea at the site of trauma, and expiratory films may show collapse of the trachea at the same location. Endoscopic evaluation of the airways may demonstrate the site and extent of the lesion, which is helpful for surgical planning, if indicated.

19. How do I manage a tracheal laceration?

Many cases of tracheal laceration will respond to conservative, medical management. If concurrent pneumothorax or hemothorax are present, thoracocentesis may be necessary if respiratory compromise is significant. Intermittent thoracocentesis or placement of thoracotomy tubes may be needed in some cases. Antimicrobial therapy may be instituted, ideally based on culture and sensitivity results, depending on the cause of the trauma (e.g., bite wounds). If there is generalized subcutaneous emphysema, aspiration of the air may be possible using a large-bore needle attached to a syringe. However, in most cases, this is unrewarding and does not reduce the amount of emphysema. Compression bandages around the site of emphysema may restrict breathing and worsen respiratory compromise. In all cases, if respiratory status worsens, or the animal decompensates, surgical exploration to identify the area of leakage is warranted.

BIBLIOGRAPHY

Binnington AG, Kreplin CA: An unusual lateral tracheal collapse in a dog. *Can Vet J* 18:190-192, 1977.
Bjorling D, McAnulty J, Swainson S: Surgically treatable upper respiratory disorders. *Vet Clin North Am Small Anim Pract* 30:1227-1251, 2000.
Buback JL, Boothe HW, Hobson HP: Surgical treatment of tracheal collapse in dogs: 90 cases (1983-1993). *J Am Vet Med Assoc* 208:380-384, 1996.
Clements DN, McGill S, Beths T et al: Tracheal perforation secondary to suture irritation in a dog following a ventral slot procedure. *J Small Anim Pract* 44:313-315, 2003.
Coyne BE, Fingland RB: Hypoplasia of the trachea in dogs: 103 cases (1974-1990). *J Am Vet Med Assoc* 201: 768-772, 1992.
Dallman MJ, McClure RC, Brown EM: Normal and collapsed trachea in the dog: scanning electron microscopy study. *Am J Vet Res* 46:2110-2115, 1985.
Dallman MJ, McClure RC, Brown EM: Histochemical study of normal and collapsed tracheas in dogs. *Am J Vet Res* 49:2117-2125, 1988.
Ettinger SJ, Kantrowitz B, Brayley K: Diseases of the trachea. In Ettinger SJ, Feldman EC, editors, *Textbook of veterinary internal medicine,* ed 5, Philadelphia, 2000, WB Saunders.
Hamaide A, Arnoczky SP, Ciarelli MJ et al: Effects of age and location on the biomechanical and biochemical properties of canine tracheal ring cartilage in dogs. *Am J Vet Res* 59:18-22, 1998.
Hardie EM, Spodnick GJ, Gilson SD et al: Tracheal rupture in cats: 16 cases (1983-1998). *J Am Vet Med Assoc* 214:508-512, 1999.
Hendricks JC: Recognition and treatment of congenital respiratory tract defects in brachycephalics. In Bonagura JD, editor: *Kirk's current veterinary therapy XII small animal practice,* Philadelphia, 1995, WB Saunders.
Herrtage ME, White RA: Management of tracheal collapse. In Bonagura JD, editor: *Kirk's current veterinary therapy XII small animal practice,* Philadelphia, 2000, WB Saunders.
Jerram RM, Fossum TW: Tracheal collapse in dogs. *Compend Contin Educ Pract Vet* 19:1049-1059, 1997.
Johnson L: Tracheal collapse, diagnosis and medical and surgical treatment. In Padrid P, editor: *The veterinary clinics of North America, small animal practice, respiratory medicine and surgery,* Philadelphia, 2000, WB Saunders.

Johnson LR, Fales WH: Clinical and microbiologic findings in dogs with bronchoscopically diagnosed tracheal collapse: 37 cases (1990-1995). *J Am Vet Med Assoc* 219:1247-1250, 2001.

Johnson LR, Krahwinkel DJ, McKiernan BC: Surgical management of atypical lateral tracheal collapse in a dog. *J Am Vet Med Assoc* 203:1693-1696, 1993.

Johnson LR, McKiernan BC: Diagnosis and medical management of tracheal collapse. *Semin Vet Med Surg* 10:101-108, 1995.

Mitchell SL, McCarthy R, Rudloff E et al: Tracheal rupture associated with intubation in cats: 20 cases (1996-1998). *J Am Vet Med Assoc* 216:1592-1595, 2000.

Puerto DA, Waddell LS: Brachycephalic airway syndrome. In Tilley LP, Smith FWK, editors: *The 5-minute veterinary consult, canine and feline*, ed 3, Philadelphia, 2004, Lippincott, Williams, and Wilkins.

Waddell LS, Puerto DA: Tracheal perforation. In Tilley LP, Smith FWK, editors: *The 5-minute veterinary consult, canine and feline*, ed 3, Philadelphia, 2004, Lippincott, Williams, and Wilkins.

White RA, Williams JM: Tracheal collapse—is there really a role for surgery? A survey of 100 cases. *J Small Anim Pract* 35:191-196, 1994.

20. Small Airway Disorders

Jo Ann Morrison

1.   What are common noninfectious disorders involving the canine bronchi?

The most common airway disorders of the bronchi are bronchitis, bronchiectasis, primary ciliary dyskinesia, bronchial mineralization, and bronchoesophageal fistula.

2.   How is bronchitis defined?

Bronchitis is defined as inflammation of the conducting airways. The inflammation is primarily neutrophilic, though eosinophilic inflammation may predominate. Macrophages, in various stages of activity, may also be present in the airways. As part of the definition, bronchitis results in a chronic, daily cough, lasting for at least 2 months, with no specific cause identified.

3.   What are the presenting complaints and initial clinical findings with bronchitis?

A chronic cough, sometimes lasting for years, is typical. The cough is generally nonproductive, though in some animals, the cough may terminate with gagging or retching. Because dogs cannot expectorate, the productivity of the cough is sometimes difficult to ascertain. Studies indicate that most dogs are bright, alert, responsive, and, other than the cough, normal on presentation. More severely affected animals may show exercise intolerance, syncope, or cyanosis. Physical examination demonstrates diffuse crackles and wheezes. There may be an end-expiratory push with prolonged expiration in more severely affected cases. Tracheal sensitivity may result in an easily induced cough on tracheal palpation. Sinus arrhythmias may be auscultated. Also, the heart rate may be in the normal range or even potentially decreased. This is in contrast to dogs that present in cardiac failure, in which the heart rates may be elevated in an attempt to maintain cardiac output. This is an important distinction to make, because both groups of dogs may present with a primary complaint of coughing.

4.   What should the diagnostic workup include?

The minimum database of complete blood count, serum chemistry, and urinalysis is helpful to exclude other causes of coughing. Heartworm serologic and fecal examinations should be included to rule out possible parasitic disease. Some cases of bronchitis will demonstrate a peripheral eosinophilia; polycythemia may be seen as a result of chronic hypoxia; serum alkaline phosphatase and alanine aminotransferase may be increased. Pulmonary function testing is becoming a more commonly used diagnostic tool. Arterial blood gas analysis may demonstrate hypoxemia (oxygen pressure less than 80 mm Hg at sea level). A concurrently elevated carbon dioxide pressure is associated with a poorer prognosis. Thoracic radiographs are an important part of the workup for bronchitis. They also are important for ruling out other differentials for coughing (e.g., congestive heart failure, neoplasia). Normal thoracic radiographs do *not* rule out the possibility of bronchitis. The most commonly reported changes on radiographs are a result of increased thickening of bronchial walls. These thickened walls are termed "tram lines" when viewed longitudinally and "doughnuts" when viewed in cross section. An increased interstitial pattern is also associated with bronchitis. However, one study found a similar frequency of interstitial patterns in dogs with bronchitis and normal controls. This same study showed only thickened bronchial walls and increased numbers of visible bronchial walls as significantly increased in dogs with bronchitis. Figure 20-1 shows a lateral thoracic radiograph of a dog with chronic bronchitis, demonstrating multiple "doughnuts" and prominent airway markings. Pulmonary hyperinflation and diaphragmatic flattening have been reported, though these are more common in cats. Bronchoscopy with bronchoalveolar lavage is considered the diagnostic test of choice for chronic bronchitis. It is recommended that this procedure be performed early in the course of the disease, when the animal's respiratory status is not severely compromised and anesthesia is still relatively safe. Bronchoscopic findings in affected airways include: erythema, mucus, nodular proliferation, irregular mucosa, and, potentially, dynamic airway collapse. Cytologic evaluation of airway secretions in dogs with active disease shows primarily neutrophilic inflammation. Other cell lines that may be present include eosinophils and macrophages. Curschmann's spirals also may be present. Samples should be obtained for culture and sensitivity, and it is recommended to perform a quantitative assessment of bacterial numbers. Cytologic samples should also be examined for intracellular bacteria or degenerate neutrophils to help determine the significance of possible infectious agents. It has been suggested that septic inflammation, single agent bacterial cultures, atypical bacterial resistance patterns, or acute clinical exacerbations (fever, inflammatory changes in the complete blood cell count, and radiographic evidence of pneumonia) may represent better evidence for a significant bacterial infection.

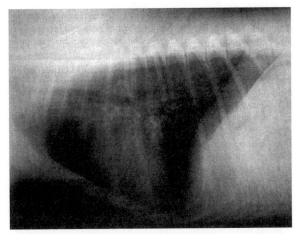

Figure 20-1. A lateral thoracic radiograph of a dog with chronic bronchitis, demonstrating multiple "doughnuts" and prominent airway markings. (Radiograph courtesy of Dr. E. Riedesel, Iowa State University.)

5.   Are there any risk factors for developing bronchitis?

Bronchitis historically was thought to be a disease limited to small-breed, terrier dogs. It is now known that medium and large-size dogs can also develop bronchitis. There may be an increased incidence in the Cocker Spaniel and West Highland White Terrier breeds. Obesity is a well-known risk factor. Chronic, inhaled airway irritants (smoke, allergens, and other airborne pollutants) are thought to play a role in the development of bronchitis, because it is a recurrent, low-grade infection. Periodontal disease and laryngeal disease may also play a role, allowing bacterial showering of the lower airways.

6.   Are the airway changes permanent?

After this condition develops, the airway changes may be progressive and the disease cannot be cured. Histologic examination of affected airways shows smooth muscle hypertrophy, goblet cell hyperplasia, lamina propria fibrosis, mucus gland hypertrophy, mucosal edema, epithelial erosion with loss of ciliated epithelium, and squamous metaplasia. Some aspects of the disease may be reversible, such as airway spasm or secondary bacterial infection.

7.   What is the treatment for chronic bronchitis?

Treatment is geared toward control of clinical signs and improvement in quality of life, not cure of the disease. Environmental factors should be addressed and potential airway irritants reduced or eliminated (e.g., smoke, dust, deodorizers). If the animal is overweight, a weight loss program should be instituted. If weight loss is difficult, evaluation for underlying endocrine disease should be performed (e.g., hypothyroidism, hyperadrenocorticism). Medical management generally involves antitussives, antiinflammatories, bronchodilators, and, potentially, antibiotics. Medications commonly prescribed for the treatment of chronic bronchitis is provided in Table 20-1. Antitussives are contraindicated when the cough is productive, because mucus retention can exacerbate airway inflammation and worsen disease progression. After inflammation is resolved and infection has been cleared, antitussives may be used. Sedation and constipation may be seen with these medications. The role of bronchoconstriction in chronic bronchitis is questionable. However, bronchodilators may have the beneficial effects of improving mucociliary clearance, improving diaphragmatic contractility, and allowing reduction in the dosage of glucocorticoids. Adverse effects include tachycardia, gastrointestinal upset, and excitability. Enrofloxacin, which may be a useful antibiotic for respiratory infections, impairs the metabolism of theophylline. This results in toxic levels of theophylline. Plasma levels of

Table 20-1   *Commonly Prescribed Medications for the Treatment of Chronic Bronchitis*

DRUG	ACTIVITY	DOSAGE (ALL DRUGS GIVEN ORALLY)
Bronchodilators		
Terbutaline	Beta agonist	1.25-5 mg/dog q 12 h
Theophylline	Methylxanthine derivative	20 mg/kg q 12 h (sustained release)
Albuterol	Beta agonist	0.02-0.05 mg/kg q 8-12 h
Antitussives		
Hydrocodone	Opiate agonist	0.22-1.0 mg/kg q 6-12 h
Butorphanol	Partial opiate agonist	0.55-1.0 mg/kg q 6-12 h
Codeine	Opiate agonist	1-2 mg/kg q 6-12 h
Antiinflammatories		
Prednisone	Glucocorticoid	0.5-1.0 mg/kg q 12-24 h for 5-7 days, then taper to alternate day dosing

theophylline may be measured through human laboratories; the peak goal range is 5-20 μg/ml. If these two medications are used simultaneously, the theophylline dose should be decreased by at least 30%. In some cases, generic alternatives for theophylline may be available. The bioavailability of some of these alternatives has been questionable, so generic substitutions should be avoided in most cases. Antibiotics are indicated with concurrent bacterial infection. Ideally, antibiotic choice is based on culture and sensitivity results. If culture results are not available, and there is sufficient evidence for a bacterial infection, a bactericidal antibiotic with gram negative spectrum and good penetration into respiratory tissues (e.g., fluoroquinolone, amoxicillin/clavulanic acid) should be chosen. There has been recent discussion about the use of inhalant therapy for dogs with chronic bronchitis. There has not been clinical evidence to support the use of inhalant therapy. Other medications that have been used in cats with feline asthma (cyproheptadine, cyclosporine) would not be expected to be of benefit in the treatment of dogs with chronic bronchitis.

8. Is the prognosis anything but guarded to poor?

The initial prognosis is guarded, but with aggressive identification and therapy, progression of the disease may be slow. It is important to educate clients that therapy does not offer a cure. Rather, the intent of therapy is to limit disease progression and slow the onset of complicating factors. Poorly controlled disease can result in airway fibrosis, pulmonary hypertension, cor pulmonale, and bronchiectasis and, when present, these factors worsen the prognosis.

9. What is the definition of bronchiectasis?

Bronchiectasis, a result of chronic airway inflammation, is the persistent, permanent dilation of bronchial walls. Suppuration is present and trapped mucus obstructs the airways. Recurrent pneumonia is common. The structural integrity of the airway walls is lost. These bronchi become irreversibly dilated secondary to traction from the surrounding pulmonary tissue. The normal epithelial ciliary mechanisms are also damaged, leading to ciliostasis. Ciliostasis, in combination with dilated airways, allows mucus retention which favors perpetual tissue damage because of bacterial colonization and chronic airway inflammation. The disease may be focal or diffuse.

10. How does the clinical presentation of bronchiectasis differ from chronic bronchitis?

Both diseases have a history of a chronic cough, though the cough associated with bronchiectasis may be more productive and moist than that of chronic bronchitis. Hemoptysis can occur. Concurrent bacterial infection and pneumonia are responsible for a portion of the pathologic changes seen with bronchiectasis, so these animals may have more signs of systemic illness: fever, inflammatory leukogram, hyperglobulinemia, or lethargy. There may be purulent nasal discharge if pneumonia is present.

11. Are there any breed predilections for bronchiectasis?

Certain breeds appear to be predisposed to the development of bronchiectasis. The American Cocker Spaniel is the most commonly affected breed. One retrospective study also found Miniature Poodles to be significantly overrepresented. In the same study, an increased risk for the development of bronchiectasis was noted in the West Highland White Terrier, Siberian Husky, and English Springer Spaniel. Young dogs are more commonly diagnosed when bronchiectasis is seen as part of the primary ciliary dyskinesia syndrome (discussed in the following section). Older dogs are more likely to develop bronchiectasis as a secondary condition. It may result from chronic pulmonary diseases or from physical trauma to the pulmonary parenchyma (smoke inhalation, radiation burn, previous pneumonia, airway obstruction, inhaled toxins).

12. What are the radiographic and bronchoscopic findings in bronchiectasis?

The most common radiographic finding in both canine and feline studies is cylindrical bronchiectasis. This is described as larger, thick-walled bronchi that are abnormally dilated with a loss of the normal tapering toward the periphery. The distended bronchi may project into consolidated lung lobes (Fig. 20-2). The abnormally thickened, dilated bronchial walls are easily seen bronchoscopically. Saccular bronchiectasis, which can be described as resembling a cluster of grapes, may also be seen, usually at the level of intermediate, mid-sized bronchi. The right cranial and middle lung lobes are the most commonly affected in dogs. This may represent the gravity-dependent position of those lung lobes, which allows easier bacterial colonization and reduced clearance of pulmonary secretions. Other radiographic lesions in dogs with bronchiectasis are frequently identified. Interstitial, bronchial, and alveolar pulmonary patterns, tracheal narrowing or tracheal distension, and pleural fibrosis have all been reported. Bronchoscopic lesions may be more striking with bronchiectasis, and bronchoscopy is the diagnostic test of choice. Large amounts of airway mucus, loss of normal airway tapering, mucosal hyperemia, and septic or suppurative inflammation are typically seen. Samples should be obtained for both aerobic and anaerobic cultures as the purulent environment may allow for the growth of anaerobic organisms. Mixed bacterial infections may be seen. *Streptococcus* spp., *Enterococcus* spp., *Staphylococcus* spp., *Escherichia coli*, *Pseudomonas aeruginosa*, *Pasteurella multocida*, *Mycoplasma* spp., *Klebsiella pneumonia*, *Lactobacillus* spp., *Micrococcus* spp., and *Burkholderia cepacia* have all been reported with bronchiectasis.

13. What are the treatment options and what is the prognosis for bronchiectasis?

Severely affected animals may require hospitalization, intravenous fluid support, supplemental oxygen and nebulization therapy, and aggressive (intravenous) antibiotic therapy. If culture and sensitivity results are not immediately available, broad-spectrum, empiric therapy should not be delayed. Coverage against gram-negative organisms should be included (aminoglycosides or fluoroquinolone). Long-term antibiotic therapy is commonly required (6 to 12 weeks) and lifelong therapy may be necessary. Bronchodilators are usually of minimal benefit. Cough suppressants should be avoided. If an animal has focal disease, surgical removal of the affected lung segment may provide long-term control of the disease. The prognosis is variable, because many dogs will have recurrent infections. Development of resistant bacterial strains, pulmonary hypertension, cor pulmonale, and systemic manifestations of disease (amyloidosis, glomerulone-

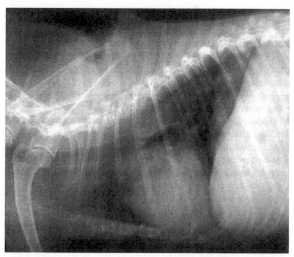

Figure 20-2. A lateral thoracic radiograph of a dog with bronchiectasis. The abnormally thickened, dilated bronchial walls are clearly visible. (Radiograph courtesy of Dr. E. Riedesel, Iowa State University.)

phritis) may all result from bronchiectasis. Animals with focal disease may have prolonged survival times after surgical removal of the affected lung. Even those animals with diffuse disease may have survival times of 16 months or more, with appropriate and aggressive therapy.

14. What is the definition and the prevalence of primary ciliary dyskinesia (PCD)?

Primary ciliary dyskinesia (PCD) is a congenital, inherited disorder characterized by physical abnormalities in respiratory cilia combined with asynchronous, uncoordinated ciliary movement. This leads to ineffectual mucociliary clearance in the respiratory tract. The normal respiratory cilia has a central pair of microtubules (central microtubule) surrounded by nine peripheral microtubular doublets (each doublet consisting of an A and B microtubule). The A microtubules are associated with dynein arms that slide between doublets during cilia motion. There are also nexin links to connect doublet pairs and radial spokes to provide anchorage. Coordinated movements of all of these components of the cilia allow for uniplanar, craniad movement of respiratory mucus. Specific lesions of the cilia seen in PCD include shortened or absent dynein arms, microtubular dislocation, defects in radial spokes and nexin links, and random and abnormal positioning of cilia. These defects cause abnormal ciliary motion, preventing normal movement and removal of respiratory mucus. PCD is a rare disease, thought to be inherited via an autosomal recessive pattern. It has been reported in several breeds: Bichon Frise, Border Collie, Bullmastiff, Chihuahua, Chow Chow, Dachshund, Dalmatian, Doberman, English Cocker Spaniel, English Setter, English Springer Spaniel, Golden Retriever, Gordon Setter, Miniature Poodle, Newfoundland, Norwegian Elkhound, Old English Sheepdog, Pointer, Rottweiler, Shar-Pei, and, most recently, the Staffordshire Bull Terrier. At this time, reported cases have only involved pure-bred dogs.

15. What other disorders are seen with PCD?

PCD results in chronic respiratory infections, pneumonia, bronchiectasis, rhinitis, and sinusitis. Other manifestations of PCD can be seen in any system with a ciliary component. Otitis media and hearing loss can be seen with auditory system involvement. Immotile, hypomotile sperm may be seen in male dogs. Hydrocephalus has been reported. There is also an association with neutrophil dysfunction and primary ciliary dyskinesia. Situs inversus has been reported in roughly 50% of canine cases of PCD. It has been suggested that dogs that present with chronic respiratory infections and situs inversus, in all likelihood, have PCD. There have also been reports of congenital cardiac malformations in canine cases of PCD.

16. How is the definitive diagnosis made?

The diagnostic evaluation should be initially performed as for any animal presenting with respiratory signs, as described previously for bronchitis and bronchiectasis. There should be a clinical suspicion for PCD in a young animal presenting with chronic respiratory signs since birth. Additional radiographic studies may show signs of situs inversus in animals with PCD. Of note, the most common bacterial isolates from airway cultures in PCD cases are *Pasteurella* and *Mycoplasma* spp. *Mycoplasma* spp. cultures require special handling and need to be specifically requested. Diagnosis of PCD is best made by demonstrating ultrastructural defects in cilia via electron microscopy. Specific defects need to be demonstrated in the majority of cilia and in cilia from different sites: nasal, bronchial, auricular, and spermatozoa. It should also be noted that some ultrastructural ciliary lesions may be secondary, or induced, by chronic inflammation or infection. These acquired lesions may appear similar to lesions seen with PCD. Electron microscopy has a limited availability and it is recommended to contact the nearest veterinary teaching hospital for testing options and sample collection requirements. Nuclear scintigraphic studies with technetium-99 macroaggregated albumin may demonstrate a reduction or absence of movement of the tracheal mucous blanket. This is strongly suggestive of PCD, but other factors may also reduce normal mucociliary clearance (smoke inhalation, *Mycoplasma* infection). Ciliogenesis, the process of culturing cilia obtained via biopsy, may be useful in confirming the diagnosis of PCD.

17. Is there a treatment for PCD and what is the prognosis?

As PCD is an inherited disorder; there is no cure. Treatment primarily centers on controlling respiratory infections. Appropriate antibiotic therapy, nebulization and coupage, supplemental oxygen therapy, and controlled exercise to facilitate respiration and induce coughing all play a role. Cough suppressants are absolutely contraindicated in this disease. Other manifestations of PCD (e.g., hydrocephalus, otitis) do not appear to be as clinically significant as respiratory symptoms. With aggressive therapy, some dogs may live with a relatively normal quality of life. However, acute bronchopneumonia may be fatal in some cases, and many owners elect euthanasia rather than lifelong disease management.

18. What causes bronchial mineralization?

Mineralization, or calcification, of soft tissue, is generally one of two types: dystrophic or metastatic. Dystrophic calcification occurs when the tissue has been previously injured, as in the case of a chronic inflammatory or infectious disease. As such, bronchial mineralization may be observed in cases of bronchiectasis or chronic bronchitis. When mineralization occurs in otherwise normal tissue, this is termed *metastatic calcification*. This is commonly associated with hypercalcemia or other disorders of calcium homeostasis and the lungs are a preferential site of calcium deposition. Hyperadrenocorticism is associated with pulmonary and interstitial mineralization, and there may also be mineralization in the airways. This is thought to represent a type of dystrophic calcification.

19. What is the clinical presentation of bronchial mineralization?

Mineralization of the bronchi may affect lung compliance, but has an unknown effect on gas exchange. Thus clinical signs are more likely to be related to the underlying disease process that led to airway mineralization, rather than the mineralization itself.

20. What should the diagnostic workup include?

Bronchial mineralization may be identified on survey thoracic radiographs. If noted, the clinician should initiate a search for an underlying disease. This workup may include minimum data base (complete blood cell count, serum chemistry, urinalysis), arterial blood gas analysis, ventilation:perfusion studies, adrenal axis testing for hyperadrenocorticism, or possibly bronchoscopy and bronchoalveolar lavage.

21. Are there any treatment options and what is the prognosis?

Mineralization is a permanent change. As such, there is no treatment to reverse the process. The prognosis is based on the underlying cause that may have led to bronchial mineralization.

22. Is bronchoesophageal fistula an acquired or congenital disease?

Bronchoesophageal fistula can be either an acquired or congenital disease. Both manifestations of this disease have been reported in dogs. Acquired disease may be noted in any age of animal and has been associated primarily with trauma and foreign bodies in the veterinary field. Congenital disease is typically diagnosed in younger animals, though signs may be quite mild, resulting in a delay in diagnosis. There has been a suggestion that Cairn Terriers may be overrepresented.

23. What are the presenting complaints with this condition?

Because there is a communication between the esophagus and the airway, signs are related to the introduction of water or food into the pulmonary system. Coughing, especially associated with eating or drinking, can be seen. Difficulty eating, recurrent pneumonia, and possibly hemoptysis may also be observed. Megaesophagus may also be associated with bronchoesophageal fistula and this may lead to signs of regurgitation.

24. How is the diagnosis made?
There should be a clinical suspicion for congenital disease when a young animal presents with chronic respiratory signs and thoracic radiographs demonstrate aspiration pneumonia, mega-esophagus, and focal soft-tissue densities in adjacent lung lobes. An esophageal diverticulum may also be present. Acquired disease should be suspected when there is a history of trauma or eso-phageal foreign body. Definitive diagnosis is made via contrast radiography with an esophagram or with fluoroscopy.

25. How is this treated and what is the prognosis?
The treatment for bronchoesophageal fistula is surgical resection of the fistula. Histopatho-logic evaluation of the resected tissue may assist in identifying a congenital lesion. In the human field, smooth muscle tissue and a lack of inflammatory cells are criteria used to diagnose con-genital fistulas. In some cases, lung lobectomy may also be necessary, especially if there are ex-tensive adhesions or abscesses. The prognosis appears to be good with successful therapy. In the few reported cases with concurrent megaesophagus, esophageal motility appeared to return to normal after surgical correction of the fistula.

BIBLIOGRAPHY

Basher AW, Hogan PM, Hanna PE et al: Surgical treatment of a congenital bronchoesophageal fistula in a dog. *J Am Vet Med Assoc* 199:479-482, 1991.
Berry CR, Hawkins EC, Hurley KJ et al: Frequency of pulmonary mineralization and hypoxemia in 21 dogs with pituitary-dependent hyperadrenocorticism. *J Vet Intern Med* 14:151-156, 2000.
Crager CS: Canine primary ciliary dyskinesia. *Compend Contin Educ Pract Vet* 14:1440-1445, 1992.
Edwards DF: Primary ciliary dyskinesia. In Tilley LP, Smith FWK, editors: *The 5-minute veterinary consult, canine and feline,* ed 3, Philadelphia, 2004, Lippincott, Williams, and Wilkins.
Hawkins EC, Basseches J, Berry CR et al: Demographic, clinical, and radiographic features of bronchiectasis in dogs: 316 cases (1988-2000). *J Am Vet Med Assoc* 223:1628-1635, 2003.
Johnson L: CVT update: canine chronic bronchitis. In Bonagura JD, editor: *Kirk's current veterinary therapy XIII small animal practice,* Philadelphia, 2000, WB Saunders.
Johnson L: Diseases of the bronchus. In Ettinger SJ, Feldman EC, editors: *Textbook of veterinary internal medicine,* ed 5, Philadelphia, 2000, WB Saunders.
Mantis P, Lamb CR, Boswood A: Assessment of the accuracy of thoracic radiography in the diagnosis of canine chronic bronchitis. *J Small Anim Pract* 39:518-520, 1998.
McKiernan BC: Chronic bronchitis (COPD). In Tilley LP, Smith FWK, editors: *The 5-minute veterinary consult, canine and feline,* ed 3, Philadelphia, 2004, Lippincott, Williams, and Wilkins.
McKiernan BC: Diagnosis and treatment of canine chronic bronchitis: twenty years of experience. *Vet Clin North Am Small Anim Pract* 30:1267-1278, 2000.
Morrison WB, Frank DE, Roth JA et al: Assessment of neutrophil function in dogs with primary ciliary dyskinesia. *J Am Vet Med Assoc* 191:425-430, 1987.
Padrid P: Diagnosis and therapy of canine chronic bronchitis. Proceedings of the World Small Animal Veterinary Association World Congress, Vancouver, July 2001.
Padrid P: Diagnosis and therapy of canine chronic bronchitis. In Bonagura JD, editor: *Kirk's current veterinary therapy XII small animal practice,* 1995, Philadelphia, WB Saunders.
Reichler IM, Hoerauf A, Guscetti F et al: Primary ciliary dyskinesia with situs inversus totalis, hydrocephalus internus and cardiac malformations in a dog. *J Small Anim Pract* 42:345-348, 2001.
van Ee RT, Dodd VM, Pope ER et al: Bronchoesophageal fistula and transient megaesophagus in a dog. *J Am Vet Med Assoc* 188:874-876, 1986.
Wheeldon EB, Pirie HM, Fisher EW et al: Chronic bronchitis in the dog. *Vet Rec* 94:466-471, 1974.

21. Parenchymal Disorders and Diseases

Elizabeth Streeter

1. What clinical signs are shown in dogs with pulmonary parenchymal disease?

Dogs with pulmonary parenchymal disease may have a variety of clinical signs ranging from mild to severe. Some animals may have subtle signs despite the presence of severe disease. Owners may report a cough or increased respiratory effort. With severe disease, open-mouthed breathing, cyanosis, and dyspnea may be seen. Other signs of systemic illness may also be noted, such as weight loss, anorexia, and lethargy.

2. What are some causes of pulmonary parenchymal disease?

There are several causes of pulmonary disease in dogs; individual diseases will be discussed in other sections of this book. Parenchymal disease may be caused by infection, such as bacterial, viral, or fungal pneumonia. Neoplasia can also affect the pulmonary parenchyma. Tumors may be either primary or metastatic. Traumatic events may lead to pulmonary contusions. Coagulopathy or thrombocytopenia may lead to pulmonary hemorrhage. Edema, either cardiogenic or noncardiogenic, may also result in impaired pulmonary function. Noncardiogenic edema may result from many causes such as head trauma, seizures, strangulation, and inhalation of smoke. Other causes of pulmonary parenchymal disease include parasitic diseases and hypersensitivities.

3. What diagnostic steps are important for diagnosis of pulmonary parenchymal disease?

The first step to diagnosis of pulmonary parenchyma disease is a thorough history and physical examination. Animals in respiratory distress may be intolerant of diagnostic procedures and the astute clinician should use their findings on history and exam to localize the disease to a specific area of the respiratory tract and institute therapy if appropriate. Thoracic radiographs, if tolerated by the dog, are extremely helpful in evaluation of the respiratory and cardiovascular systems. Thoracic radiographs should be evaluated for pulmonary masses, signs of edema, or other abnormalities. Cardiovascular structures should also be evaluated to rule out cardiogenic causes of respiratory difficulties. Baseline blood work, including complete blood cell counts, blood chemistries, and coagulation times, should be completed to evaluate for the presence of systemic illness and underlying conditions. These tests may suggest signs of infection or blood loss and may support a diagnosis. Additional evaluation of the thorax may be indicated because often radiographs may suggest disease but do not lend a diagnosis. Transtracheal wash or bronchoalveolar lavage may be beneficial. Thoracic ultrasound and transthoracic aspirate may also be helpful.

4. Is an arterial blood gas useful in diagnosis of pulmonary parenchymal disease?

An arterial blood gas is extremely beneficial in evaluation of the dog with pulmonary disease; however, the blood gas does not differentiate from causes of disease. The blood gas will allow evaluation of ventilation and gas exchange. Elevated carbon dioxide levels suggest hypoventilation and may indicate the need for mechanical ventilation. Decreased oxygen levels indicated the need for supplemental oxygen support. Repeated blood gas analysis may also be useful. Rechecking parameters may allow for evaluation of response to therapy.

5. What treatment options are available for an animal with pulmonary parenchymal disease?

The treatment options for animals with pulmonary parenchymal disease vary and depend largely on the cause of signs. Oxygen supplementation should be instituted in animals with hypoxemia. Antibiotics or antifungal medication may be warranted in cases of pneumonia. Chemotherapy may be warranted for neoplastic disease. In some diseases, such as traumatic pulmonary contusions, treatment is largely supportive; however, advanced therapies, such as mechanical ventilation may be needed if disease is severe. Cardiogenic causes of pulmonary disease should be treated as indicated based on the underlying disease. Diuretics may be indicated to treat pulmonary edema. The reader should consult other sections of this text for more details on treatment of individual diseases.

6.   How may cardiogenic diseases be differentiated from other types of pulmonary disease?
The differentiation between cardiogenic and noncardiogenic pulmonary disease can be quite difficult at times. In animals with cardiogenic disease, a complete physical examination may reveal distended jugular veins or a hepatojugular reflex. A heart murmur may be ausculted. Thoracic radiographs may also be useful in helping to differentiate cardiogenic and noncardiogenic causes. In cardiogenic diseases enlargement of cardiovascular structures may be noted. Pulmonary edema may be seen as well. Typically, the distribution of edema in cardiogenic failure can also help differentiate the cause of respiratory disease. Infiltrates from cardiogenic causes are typically distributed in a caudodorsal pattern, although some diseases may have variable patterns. These infiltrates may also be located in the perihilar region. Infiltrates from pneumonia typically are more cranioventrally distributed. Evaluation of protein content of edema fluid may also be of benefit. Fluid from cardiogenic causes is typically lower in protein content that fluid from noncardiogenic causes. Heart rate is usually elevated with heart failure.

7.   Outline the techniques and indications for oxygen therapy.
Initial evaluation of the dog in respiratory distress should involve some degree of oxygen supplementation. Oxygen supplementation may be provided via several routes, such as oxygen mask or hood, nasal, or intubation and mechanical ventilation. Each of these techniques has pros and cons, and the decision of which is preferred is dependent on the animal's condition and hospital resources. Oxygen mask and hood can provide variable amounts of supplemental oxygen, whereas oxygen cages and nasal catheters supply more reliable levels. For severely dyspneic animals that do not respond to routine methods of oxygen supplementation, intubation and mechanical ventilation may be needed. The need for oxygen therapy is best assessed with clinical data such as decreased oxygen saturation noted via pulse oximetry or hypoxemia noted on a blood gas. The dog's respiratory effort should also be considered when deciding whether oxygen supplementation is necessary. Some animals may maintain adequate oxygenation levels, but at the expense of an increase work of breathing. These animals may fatigue without supplementation and can acutely deteriorate.

8.   What other types of respiratory monitoring are useful in animals with pulmonary parenchymal disease?
Close monitoring of respiratory rates of any animal with pulmonary disease is essential. Animals should be frequently evaluated for signs of increasing respiratory rate and effort. Mucous membrane can be assessed for color; however, low oxygen saturation levels may be present before clinically detecting cyanosis. Pulse oximetry may be useful in assessing oxygen saturation. Levels lower than 92% should prompt the clinician to provide some source of oxygen supplementation. Arterial blood gas samples (as discussed previously) are also a useful indicator of oxygen status.

9.   Describe the typical radiographic appearance of animals with pulmonary parenchymal disease.
As discussed previously, cardiogenic causes of pulmonary infiltrates have a typical caudodorsal distribution with concentration in the perihilar areas. Abnormalities of the cardiovascular structures, such as enlargement of the cardiac silhouette, are also seen. Bacterial pneumonia typi-

cally involves a more cranioventral distribution, although appearance may vary. Fungal pneumonia and neoplastic diseases may have a nodular appearance. Noncardiogenic edema appears similar to that of cardiogenic causes; however, abnormalities of the cardiovascular structures are not seen. Traumatic pulmonary contusions and hemorrhage may have an irregular and patchy interstitial to alveolar pattern. Other atypical patterns can also be seen depending on the dog's disease state, onset of signs, and other variables. ·

BIBLIOGRAPHY

Forrester SD, Moon ML, Jacobson JD: Diagnostic evaluation of dogs and cats with respiratory distress. *Compend Contin Educ Pract Vet* 23:56-69, 2001.
Nelson OL, Sellon RK: Pulmonary parenchymal disease. In SJ Ettinger, EC Feldman, editors: *Textbook of veterinary internal medicine: diseases of the dog and cat,* St Louis, 2005, Elsevier Saunders.
Rozanski E, Chan DL: Approach to the patient with respiratory distress. *Vet Clin North Am Small Anim Pract* 35:307-317, 2005.

VIRAL DISEASES

Erin M. Portillo

10. What are the common viral causes of canine respiratory disease?
The primary causes of viral pneumonia in dogs are canine distemper virus (CDV), canine adenovirus type II (CAV-2), and parainfluenza virus type-II. Canine herpesvirus (CHV) can cause upper respiratory infection in adult dogs.

11. Which viruses are implicated in canine infectious tracheobronchitis?
Parainfluenza virus type-II is the most common, followed by CAV-2 and rarely canine adenovirus type I (CAV-1). Bacterial agents may also be involved concurrently, for example *Bordetella bronchiseptica, Mycoplasma,* and *Streptococcus* spp.

12. How are the respiratory viruses transmitted?
They are all transmitted by inhalation of respiratory droplets or contact with contaminated fomites. In addition, CHV can be transmitted by direct contact with both respiratory and genital secretions. These viral agents can be transmitted for up to 2 weeks after infection.

13. What are the clinical signs of viral pneumonia?
Most respiratory viral infections are asymptomatic or subclinical. Mild fever, oculonasal discharge, coughing and weight loss are common clinical findings. CDV generally causes a more severe illness than the other viral infections.

14. What other clinical symptoms may be seen with CDV?
Gastrointestinal signs such as vomiting and diarrhea can be seen. Neurologic signs such as myoclonus, seizures, and loss of vision have been noted. Additionally, hyperkeratosis of the footpad has been noted in chronic infections.

15. How is a viral respiratory infection diagnosed?
- A clinical diagnosis of canine infectious tracheobronchitis can be made on the basis of history of recent exposure, clinical signs of dry, hacking cough, and response to empiric therapy.
- Radiographic findings can vary but may be normal as with infectious tracheobronchitis, or may show a diffuse bronchointerstitial pattern as with viral pneumonia. There may be progression to an alveolar pattern if a secondary bacterial infection develops.
- A transtracheal wash or bronchoalveolar lavage may be performed. Harvested samples

should be submitted for both cytologic evaluation and culture. Respiratory epithelial and inflammatory cells can be evaluated for inclusion bodies. Eosinophilic nuclear inclusions may be detected with CDV infection, CAV-2 may show basophilic nuclear inclusions, and canine parainfluenza virus type II may show intracytoplasmic inclusions. These samples can also be submitted for virus isolation or immunofluorescence staining.

- Virus isolation can be performed on nasal, pharyngeal, or tracheal swabs. CHV can also be isolated from the genitalia and is usually only identified in the first 2 weeks of infection.
- Acute and convalescent serum neutralizing (CHV, CDV) or hemagglutinin inhibition (CAV-2) antibody titers may be measured. Documentation of a rising titer is not clinically applicable because of the short course of infection.
- Immunofluorescent techniques can be performed for CDV and CAV-2. These are often done on conjunctival, tonsillar, genital, or respiratory epithelium and can be performed on cytologic or biopsy specimens.

16. How are viral respiratory infections treated?

Supportive care is the mainstay of treatment for viral infections. This includes adequate hydration, housing the animal in a clean, warm environment, and occasionally administering bronchodilators or antitussives if there is not evidence of pneumonia. Because secondary bacterial infections are common, appropriate antibiotic therapy is often warranted. It is also important to isolate these animals and try to keep hospitalization to a minimum to prevent spread of these viruses to other animals.

17. What preventive measures can be taken in these cases?

Vaccination is the preventative measure against viral disease. There are vaccines against all of these viruses (except CHV) in both parenteral and intranasal routes of administration. Therefore, a good vaccination schedule, decreasing exposure of unvaccinated animals, and proper sanitation practices are all beneficial in prevention of disease and its spread.

18. Describe the new form of canine influenza.

Recently, a new canine influenza has been identified initially in the racing Greyhound populations in Florida. This virus has now spread to shelters, boarding kennels, and pet animals. Two forms of the disease have been identified. The first is a mild form in which dogs have a soft, moist cough that appears to be self-limiting and persists for several weeks. Most infected dogs have demonstrated this form. The second form is more severe in which the dogs have high fevers and display the clinical signs of pneumonia. This virus originated as an equine influenza that has infected dogs and has transformed to a new canine-specific influenza. Because this is a new virus, almost all dogs exposed become infected and about 80% show clinical signs, with most having the mild form.

19. How is the new canine influenza diagnosed?

Similar to the other viral diseases, serologic testing is an option ideally with both acute and convalescent samples. If the dog has died, samples of fresh lung tissue can be obtained for viral culture or polymerase chain reaction (PCR) testing.

20. What precautions should shelters/kennels/clinics take to prevent spread of disease?

Routine cleanliness and infectious disease precautions are important to controlling spread of disease. The influenza virus is killed by most disinfectants including quaternary ammonium compounds and diluted bleach. Animals with a suspected infection or a cough should be isolated from the other animals and caretakers should practice isolation protocols with thorough disinfection of cages and all instruments in contact with the animal.

BACTERIAL DISEASES

Robert R. King and Michelle A. Pressel

21. What is the normal flora of the lower respiratory tract?

Clinically healthy dogs normally have a low number of organisms (alpha-hemolytic streptococci, staphylococci, *B. bronchiseptica, Pasteurella multocida,* and *Klebsiella pneumoniae*) in the airways down to the first bronchial division. Microorganisms commonly cultured from the lower airways are identical to those identified from the upper airways in each individual animal. However, there is variation in what is cultured between dogs. By definition, evidence of inflammatory cells in the lower airways in addition to presence of large numbers of bacteria equate with a probable bacterial infection.

22. What is canine infectious tracheobronchitis and can it cause bronchopneumonia?

This is a highly contagious respiratory infection that is most commonly associated with a dry cough early in the pathogenesis of the disease. Owners often describe the cough as sounding like a goose honk. On physical examination, one can usually elicit a cough by palpating the trachea. *B. bronchiseptica* is the most commonly identified primary pathogen. It spreads through direct contact between dogs and through airborne contact leading to outbreaks in high-density situations (boarding kennels, dog shows). The incubation period is approximately 6 days and infection is typically self-limiting in adult dogs, although it can progress to pneumonia. *B. bronchiseptica* preferentially attaches to the cilia in the large airways in the lungs and produces a toxin that cause ciliostasis. This in turn leads to an increased the risk of secondary opportunistic infections that often result in a more severe pneumonia.

23. How do you treat respiratory infections caused by *B. bronchiseptica*?

Recommended antibiotics include trimethoprim-sulfonamide, amoxicillin-clavulanate, and doxycycline which have been shown to reduce the duration of the cough. Care should be taken when using doxycycline in young dogs as it can cause permanent yellow discoloration of the enamel in unerupted teeth. This is thought to be secondary to the formation of tetracycline-calcium phosphate complexes within the enamel and dentine. Activity and exercise can lead to paroxysmal coughing and should be limited. Antitussives (i.e., hydrocodone, butorphanol, dextromethorphan) are often helpful in reducing the cough cycle, but should be limited in their use because they reduce expectoration of accumulated airway secretions and increase the likelihood of secondary pneumonia. Therefore antitussives should be used to control *uncontrolled* paroxysmal coughing only. Occasional coughing is expected and is helpful in the removal of airway secretions. Infected dogs should be isolated for a minimum of 3 weeks to avoid exposing other dogs to the infection. However, some dogs can shed bacteria for up to 3 months. Dogs should be routinely vaccinated every 6 months or 5 days before potential exposure in high risk environments (i.e., boarding, dog shows) if not vaccinated within the previous 6 months.

24. How do bacteria enter the lower airways and then lead to bacterial pneumonia?

Bacteria gain access to the lower respiratory tract via the blood from extrapulmonary sources, by inhalation, and after aspiration of oropharyngeal flora. Predisposing factors include previous or concurrent viral infection, regurgitation, vomiting, neurologic abnormalities in mentation, various metabolic diseases (diabetes mellitus, hyperadrenocorticism), and immunosuppressive therapy (glucocorticoids, chemotherapy).

25. Does airway colonization always result in infection?

Colonization does not always equate with infection. Normally, bacteria are prevented from establishing residence in the lower airways by several defense mechanisms, which include filtration by the nasal turbinates, sneezing, coughing, and the mucociliary clearance system. When bacteria reach the distal airways and alveoli, the important factors related to the development of infection include (1) virulence of the bacteria, (2) adequacy of the host immune response, and (3) the number microorganisms introduced. The host immune response and effectiveness of the mucociliary clearance mechanism are probably most important in preventing bacterial colonization from proceeding to infection. Early clinical signs suggestive of infection include fever, malaise, inappetence, variable severity of dyspnea, coughing, and serous or mucopurulent nasal discharge.

26. What are the common pathogens that cause bacterial pneumonia?

P. multocida, *Escherichia coli*, *Streptococcal* spp., and less often *Klebsiella* spp., and *Staphylococcus* spp. are the organisms commonly associated with primary bacterial pneumonia. Most bacterial pneumonias occur subsequent to some predisposing cause or condition (i.e., stress, viral infection) and opportunistic bacteria are often isolated (*B. bronchiseptica*, *Mycoplasma* spp., and *Pseudomonas* spp.). Generally, a single organism is isolated, but mixed infections are also common with gram-negative infections predominating.

27. What predisposing factors lead to the development of bacterial pneumonia?

In healthy dogs, bacteria are normally cleared from the lower airways and alveoli by alveolar macrophages and, to some extent, neutrophils. A number of factors can lead to a breakdown in this defense system. The virulence of the bacteria plays an important role. Many bacterial species are able to adhere to the respiratory tissues through specific binding ligands or adhesions. Many of these same bacteria produce toxins that inhibit the mucociliary clearance or affect respiratory epithelial cell function. The mucociliary clearance system requires both functional cilia and the appropriate amount and viscosity of mucus. Changes in these properties can result in embedded bacteria remaining in the lower airways. Aspiration of gastric contents also predisposes to bacterial pneumonia. Dysphagia, laryngeal paralysis, megaesophagus, regurgitation, and vomiting all result in varying amounts of acid aspiration. Animals under anesthesia are also at risk of aspiration. A number of diseases or conditions provide a favorable environment for proliferation of gastrointestinal bacteria (gut stasis, acid-blocking drugs, periodontal disease), which can increase the bacterial counts in aspirated fluids.

28. What are common historic and clinical findings suggestive of bacterial pneumonia?

Dogs with bacterial pneumonia usually present with a history of a moist productive cough, malaise, anorexia, fever, dehydration, and possible dyspnea and nasal discharge. Lung auscultation reveals increased bronchial sounds, crackles, and wheezes. Aspiration pneumonia should be suspected in any animal that has recently under gone anesthesia, has been recumbent for extended periods, or has a history of regurgitation.

29. How is the diagnosis of bacterial pneumonia determined?

Bacterial pneumonia is considered a likely differential diagnosis based on the historical and physical examination findings, results of a complete blood count and evidence of pulmonary infiltrates on thoracic radiographs. A neutrophilia with or without a left shift is often found if the animal has not been treated with antibiotics. Serum biochemistries may demonstrate changes consistent with dehydration, but specific abnormalities are seldom found. Thoracic radiographs (Fig. 21-1) typically reveal an interstitial to alveolar pattern with air bronchograms often localized to the cranioventral lung fields. The right middle lung is commonly the case in cases of aspiration pneumonia because of the location of the airway leading to this lung lobe (rostral and ventral). Confirmatory diagnosis of bacterial pneumonia requires acquisition of uncontaminated fluid from the abnormal lung segments and the presence of intracellular bacteria and inflammatory cells. Several procedures can been used to acquire samples that are representative the disease process: (1) tracheal washing; (2) bronchoalveolar lavage; and (3) transthoracic fine needle lung aspiration.

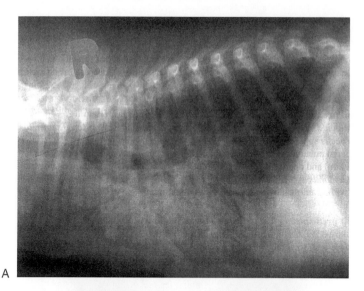

A

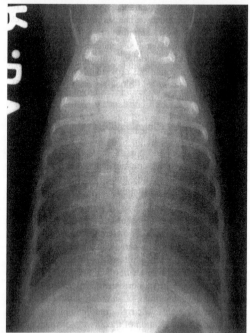

B

Figure 21-1. Thoracic radiographs from a dog showing increased pulmonary opacity involving the cranioventral two thirds of the lung (**A**). There are well-defined air bronchograms in the right cranial lobe, in the right middle lobe, and partial air bronchograms in the left cranial lobe (**B**). The severe bronchointerstitial and cranioventral alveolar lung patterns are consistent with diffuse pneumonia. (Radiograph courtesy of Dr. E. Riedsel, Iowa State University.)

30. What are the indications for transtracheal aspiration (washing)?

The procedure is indicated in animals with persistent coughing, wheezing, evidence of pulmonary parenchymal disease (this procedure seldom provides diagnostic material in these animals unless there is airway involvement), and the presence of radiographic patterns compatible with bronchopulmonary infiltration.

31. How much fluid (sterile saline) can be safely injected into the airway during the tracheal washing procedure?

Specific guidelines for the maximum total volume of instilled fluid have not been determined but 1.0 ml/kg body weight has been administered without causing signs of respiratory distress. It should be remembered that disease severity will vary with each animal and caution should be exercised in those with marked respiratory compromise.

32. What should be done with tracheal washing samples after collection?

Specimens of airway secretions recovered by tracheal washing should be rapidly processed for culture and cytologic examination. Delay may result in false-negative culture results. Material can be cultured for aerobic and anaerobic bacteria, mycoplasma, and fungal organisms. Aerobic bacteria predominate probably because oropharyngeal anaerobes are killed by ambient oxygen tension. Anaerobes are more likely to be present when aspiration pneumonia or pulmonary abscesses are present. Fungal species are uncommonly found unless the dog is immunosuppressed, receiving chronic antibiotic therapy, or has systemic mycosis.

33. How should tracheal washing samples be submitted to a laboratory for diagnostic purposes?

Samples should be separated into several containers (i.e., capped syringe or transport vial) for cytologic evaluation based on the preference of the diagnostic laboratory. Highly cellular samples should be placed in an EDTA (ethylenediamine tetraacetic acid) tube to prevent clot formation and clumping of cells. If cytologic evaluation cannot be done immediately, slides should be prepared to preserve cellular integrity (preferred method) or the sample should be refrigerated.

Most microbiology laboratories prefer to receive the actual tracheal wash fluid rather than a swab of the sample. If the sample cannot be plated within 3 hours, it should be placed in a vial containing transport media to prolong the viability of microorganisms and to prevent bacterial overgrowth. Samples placed in transport media can be kept at room temperature for up to 4 hours for isolation of aerobic bacteria, but should be refrigerated if they are to be kept beyond that time. Processing of the sample for anaerobic bacteria should be done within 10 minutes of collection if the sample is kept under anaerobic conditions (i.e., kept in a syringe with all the air expelled and capped with a rubber stopper) without transport media. *Mycoplasma* spp. and fungal agents require special culture procedures and it is recommended that the diagnostic laboratory be consulted before doing the tracheal washing procedure.

34. Should cytologic examination of the tracheal washing fluid be done before submitting the samples to the diagnostic laboratory?

Initially examining Diff Quik (Wright's) and Gram stains of air-dried smears of aspirated material will often provide helpful information in the assessment of the quality of samples to be submitted to the diagnostic laboratory. Aspirated airway secretions normally contain cellular elements and mucus. Large mononuclear cells predominate; neutrophils, eosinophils, small mononuclear cells, and ciliated epithelial cells account for 10% to 15% of the remaining cell types. Increase in neutrophil numbers suggests inflammatory or infectious conditions while eosinophil counts are elevated in allergic (hypersensitivity) and parasitic lung diseases. Lymphocyte counts may be increased or decreased in acute and chronic pulmonary diseases. Mucus hypersecretion and Curschmann spirals suggest chronic inflammatory disease. Organisms contained within phagocytic cells are generally pathogenic, with one species usually predominating.

Rational medical management can be made based on cytologic findings pending culture results. Variable types of bacteria suggest oropharyngeal contamination and the presence of squamous epithelial cells, often with *Simonsiella* spp. on their surface substantiate the suspicion (Fig. 21-2). Other elements such as parasite larvae, ova, or neoplastic cells are uncommon findings but, when present, establish a diagnosis.

35. How do sensitivity and specificity of tracheal washings compare with other available procedures for the diagnosis of pneumonia?

The sensitivity (recovery of organisms responsible for disease) and specificity (lack of contaminant organisms) of transtracheal aspiration in the diagnosis of bronchopneumonia has been addressed in a number of human studies, but infrequently in dogs. Tracheal washing is probably equal in sensitivity as compared with bronchoscopic procedures (combined cytologic and culture) and fine needle aspiration of the lung; however, it is less specific than combined bronchoscopic procedures and fine needle aspiration of the lung.

Although studies need to be done regarding sensitivity and specificity of tracheal washings in the diagnosis of pneumonia; it is easy to perform, inexpensive, and helpful in many cases of infectious and inflammatory tracheobronchial disease. Based on studies to date, tracheal washing should be considered the initial diagnostic procedure. More sensitive and specific procedures should be reserved when tracheal aspiration is not diagnostic, when complicated respiratory problems are encountered, or after unsuccessful resolution of a previously diagnosed bacterial pneumonia.

36. What are the potential complications or side effects of tracheal washing?

Mild transient hemoptysis, subcutaneous emphysema, pneumomediastinum, and severe hypoxemia have been reported in dogs. Other uncommon complications of tracheal washing include tracheal laceration, esophageal perforation, paratracheal infection, cardiac arrhythmias, and acute respiratory failure. Complications can be minimized if the procedure is done by experienced individuals on cooperative animals in whom the anatomic landmarks for the proce-

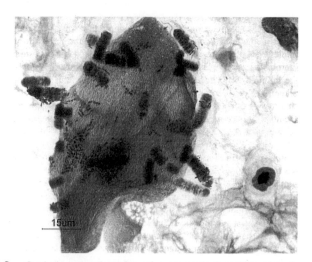

15µm

Figure 21-2. Cytologic preparation taken of a transtracheal washing taken from a dog with bronchopneumonia. Note the mixed population of bacteria and squamous epithelial cells typically found with upper airway contamination. (Cytologic preparation courtesy of Dr. Charles W. Brockus, Iowa State University.)

dure are easily identified. Before the procedure, abnormalities posing excess risk such as hypoxemia and coagulation defects should be assessed and corrected. Not unexpectedly, animals that are most susceptible to complications are most likely to benefit from the procedure.

37. What are the indications for bronchoscopic examination of the lung?

Indications for bronchoscopy include removal of foreign bodies, chronic coughing of undetermined origin, prior abnormal cytologic findings, unresolved pneumonia, hemoptysis, suction of obstructing secretions, and airway examination with culture, biopsy, lavage, or cytologic examination. It is also useful in the preoperative assessment of tentatively and definitively diagnosed conditions such as neoplasia, bronchiectasis, and lung abscesses where inspection of the entire respiratory tract for evidence of metastasis or progression of the disease may offer important information concerning the likelihood of successful resolution of the problem.

38. What are the potential complications or side effects associated with bronchoscopic procedures?

In general, bronchoscopy is considered safe with few complications. Reported problems include pneumothorax, hemorrhage, bronchospasm, and respiratory compromise in less than 1% of all bronchoscopic procedures. Deaths are uncommon. Arterial hypoxemia with a drop of 10 to 20 mm Hg in oxygen tension is common during bronchoscopy, and supplemental oxygen during the procedure is recommended for dogs with arterial oxygen tensions less than 60 mm Hg while breathing room air. Insertion of the flexible bronchoscope through an endotracheal tube can result in air flow resistance and it is recommended that endotracheal tube diameter be 3 mm greater than the bronchoscope insertion tube to minimize this potential problem. Despite reported complications, bronchoscopy is safe even in severely compromised animals provided that proper precautions are taken.

39. How can bronchoalveolar lavage analysis be used to diagnose bacterial pneumonia?

Bronchoalveolar lavage is done after placement of a flexible bronchoscope (or catheter) into the distal airways. Wedging the instrument or catheter will limit the region of lavage and result in better fluid recovery. Several instillations and subsequent withdrawals of 5 to 10 ml of sterile 0.9% saline are made. The total volume instilled varies with the animal's size (50 to 100 ml in medium to large dogs and 25 to 50 ml in small dogs). A recovery of 80% to 90% can be expected in normal animals, but fluid volume and color will be reduced or changed with smaller airway collapse secondary to inflammation, infection, and neoplasia. Total and differential nucleated cell counts can be determined in the recovered fluid and may be helpful in defining the cause of alveolar and interstitial infiltrates. Variations on the specifics of the lavage procedure (volume of instilled fluid and number of instillations) are common.

Recovered fluid also may be analyzed for microorganisms. Because the large airways are often inhabited by bacteria in health as well as disease, growth of bacteria from bronchoalveolar lavage fluid does not always indicate infection. Human studies have shown that bacterial counts in excess of 10^3 colonies per millimeter of recovered fluid are associated with pneumonia. Growth of more than 10 colonies per millimeter may represent infection, particularly in patients who have recently received antibiotics. One recent study involving 47 dogs showed that a bacterial count of 1.7×10 colonies per millimeter is representative of airway infection. Unfortunately, quantitative cultures are rarely done in veterinary medicine, so infection is usually "confirmed" if intracellular bacteria are identified cytologically in the absence of upper airway contamination.

Cases that pose a diagnostic dilemma are those with neutrophilic inflammation, no intracellular bacteria, and growth of organisms only following incubation of bronchoalveolar lavage fluid in enrichment media. These animals are often receiving antibiotics or have recently completed treatment. In these animals, an antibiotic trial or repeat bronchoscopic examination if clinical signs recur are considered rational options.

40. How is the protected catheter brush analysis used to diagnose bacterial pneumonia?

Bronchoscopic examination of the airways is used to visualize the area where infection is likely. The protected catheter brush system is used to obtain uncontaminated samples of airway fluid. Brush contamination is prevented by a disposable biodegradable plug that is not ejected until the catheter reaches the sampling area. The inner cannula is advanced, followed by the brush, and the sample is taken. The brush is retracted into the cannula and the entire device is withdrawn. Recovery of viable organisms is enhanced if cultures are made at the time of sample collection. Contamination rate protected catheter brush samples are low (less than 20%) and the likelihood of obtaining a culture of resident organisms in the distal airways is high (80%).

41. What are the indications for transthoracic fine needle lung aspiration?

Indications for transthoracic fine needle lung aspiration include identification of discrete lesions, confirmation of lung metastasis, evaluation of solitary pulmonary lesions, and obtaining material for microbiologic examination and culture.

42. How accurate is transthoracic fine needle lung aspiration in the diagnosis of bacterial pneumonia?

For identification of nontreated pulmonary infections, aspiration consistently yields the highest specificity (80% to 100%) and sensitivity (90% to 100%) of all available procedures, except for open lung biopsy. Missed diagnoses are usually from needle placement away from the lesion or sampling of peripheral inflammatory processes not representative of the entire lesion.

43. What are the potential complications or side effects of transthoracic fine needle lung aspiration?

Complications of transthoracic fine needle lung aspiration are common and potentially serious. Pneumothorax is most common and marked accumulations of air may require chest tube drainage. Less frequently encountered problems include hemoptysis, localized interstitial infiltrates adjacent to the puncture site and hemorrhagic pleural effusion. Deaths are rare. Using ultrathin (24- to 25-gauge) needle aspiration appears to produce fewer complications while maintaining similar diagnostic yields.

Patient selection is important, and screening for abnormalities of platelet count, clotting function, and arterial oxygen tension is essential. The value of this technique should always be weighed against the animal's ability to withstand transient pneumothorax or hemoptysis.

44. How is bacterial pneumonia treated?

Treatment of bacterial pneumonia consists of antibiotic therapy, maintaining hydration and the use of aerosolization along with supportive care. Antibiotic choice is based on culture and sensitivity. Empiric therapy is initially started by using a four-quadrant approach that covers for gram-negative and gram-positive aerobes and anaerobes. Common combinations include a fluoroquinolone or aminoglycosides and penicillin. Ideal penetration of antimicrobials into airways is seen with lipophilic and low-molecular-weight drugs. Drugs enter the bronchial secretions at a fraction of the serum concentrations in normal lungs. Increased penetration is seen in inflamed, pneumonic lungs. Choice of antibiotics can also be made based on cytologic analysis. Cocci are usually gram-positive bacteria and rods are more likely to be gram negative. Most secondary pneumonias are caused by either gram-negative or mixed bacteria. The choice of parenteral versus oral therapy is based on the severity of the disease process. Many animals will initially benefit from parenteral therapy, which can later be changed to oral therapy when the dog is eating well. Duration of antimicrobial therapy is based on the underlying cause. In general, it is recommended that therapy be continued 1 to 2 weeks beyond resolution of clinical and radiographic signs.

Maintaining hydration is also paramount to the success of treatment. Dehydration decreases the effectiveness of the mucociliary clearance mechanism because respiratory secretions are greater than 90% water. For this reason, most animals will initially benefit from intravenous fluid therapy. To specifically increase the hydration of the respiratory secretions, a nebulizer can be used to produce small particles (0.5 to 3.0 μm), which are then inhaled. Larger particles are ineffective because they do not penetrate the lower airways. Nebulization therapy is repeated two to four times daily for 20 minutes. After nebulization, the animal is encouraged to cough either by the chest coupage or by engaging in mild exercise. Overhydration is a potential complication because of damage to pulmonary vessels, and the dog must be watched closely for increasing respiratory rate and effort.

Supportive care includes the need for initial oxygen therapy in many dogs. This can be accomplished through an oxygen cage or nasal catheter. The use of antitussives and antihistamines is contraindicated because of their negative effect on the mucociliary clearance. The use of bronchodilators (i.e., methylxanthine) can be helpful to facilitate removal of exudates through nebulization and for their diaphragm sparing effects in dogs with increased respiratory effort. Nutrition is also important to maintain and can be accomplished through the use of parenteral feedings (i.e., partial or total parenteral nutrition) or feeding tubes (i.e., nasoesophageal, gastrotomy or jejunostomy tube). Each individual animal's needs and status must be assessed before choosing an appropriate feeding method.

BIBLIOGRAPHY

Angus JC, Jang SS, Hirsch DC: Microbiological study of transtracheal aspirates from dogs with suspected lower respiratory tract disease: 264 cases (1989-1995). *J Am Vet Med Assoc* 210:55-58, 1997.

Beachey EH, Courtney HS: Bacterial adherence of group A streptococci to mucosal surfaces. *Respiration* 55:33-40, 1989.

Bemis DA: Bordetella and mycoplasma respiratory infections in dogs and cats. *Vet Clin North Am Small Anim Pract* 22:1173-1186, 1992.

Bemis D, Appel M: Aerosol, parenteral, and oral antibiotic treatment of *Bordetella bronchiseptica* infections in dogs. *J Am Vet Med Assoc* 170:1082-1086, 1977.

Boucher RC: Human airway ion transport. Part two. *Am J Respir Crit Care Med* 150:581-593, 1994.

Brady CA: Bacterial pneumonia in dogs and cats. In King LG, editor: *Textbook of respiratory disease in dogs and cats,* St Louis, 2004, Saunders.

Brownlie SE: A retrospective study of diagnoses in 109 cases of canine lower respiratory disease. *J Small Anim Pract* 31:371-376, 1990.

Cole SG: Fine needle aspirates. In King LG, editor: *Textbook of respiratory disease in dogs and cats,* St Louis, 2004, Saunders.

Hawkins EC: Bronchoalveolar lavage. In King LG, editor: *Textbook of respiratory disease in dogs and cats,* St Louis, 2004, Saunders.

Hawkins EC: Diseases of the lower respiratory system. In Ettinger SJ, Feldman EC, editors: *Textbook of veterinary internal medicine,* ed 4, Philadelphia, 1995, Saunders.

Hirsh DC: Bacteriology of the lower respiratory tract. In Kirk RW, editor: *Current veterinary therapy IX,* Philadelphia, 1986, Saunders.

Jameson PH, King LA, Lappin MR et al: Comparison of clinical signs, diagnostic findings, organisms isolated, and clinical outcome in dogs with bacterial pneumonia: 93 cases (1986-1991). *J Am Vet Med Assoc* 206:206-209, 1995.

Johanson WG: Microbial adherence as a pathogenic factor in respiratory infections. In Sande MA, Hudson LD, Root RK, editors: *Respiratory infections,* New York, 1986, Churchill Livingstone.

Kuehn NF, Hess RS: Bronchoscopy. In King LG, editor: *Textbook of respiratory disease in dogs and cats,* St Louis, 2004, Saunders.

McKiernan BC, Smith AR, Kissil M: Bacterial isolates from the lower trachea of clinically healthy dogs. *J Am Anim Hosp Assoc* 20:139-142, 1984.

Niederman MS: The pathogenesis of airway colonization: lessons learned from the study of bacterial adherence. *Eur Respir J* 7:1737-1740, 1994.

Norris CR, Griffey SM, Samii V et al: Comparison of results of thoracic radiography, cytologic evaluation of bronchoalveolar lavage fluid, and histologic evaluation of lung specimens in dogs with respiratory tract disease: 16 cases (1996-2000). *J Am Vet Med Assoc* 218:1456-1461, 2001

Palmer LB: Bacterial colonization: pathogenesis and clinical significance. *Clin Chest Med* 8:455-466, 1987.

Peeters DE, McKiernan BC, Weisiger RM et al: Quantitative bacterial cultures and cytological examination of bronchoalveolar lavage specimens in dogs. *J Vet Intern Med* 14:534-541, 2000.

Reynolds HY: Normal and defective respiratory host defenses. In Pennington JE, editor: *Respiratory infections: diagnosis and management,* ed 3, New York, 1994, Raven Press.

Rose RM: The host defense network of the lungs: an overview. In Niederman MS, Sarosi GA, Glassroth J, editors: *Respiratory infections,* Philadelphia, 1994, Saunders.

Roudebush P: Infectious pneumonia. In Kirk RW, Bonagura JD, editors: *Current veterinary therapy XI,* Philadelphia, 1992, Saunders.

Salathe M, Wanner A: Nonspecific host defenses: mucociliary clearance and cough. In Niederman MS, Sarosi GA, Glassroth J, editors: *Respiratory infections,* Philadelphia, 1994, Saunders.

Souweine B, Veber B, Bedos JP et al: Diagnostic accuracy of protected specimen brush and bronchoalveolar lavage in nosocomial pneumonia: impact of previous antimicrobial treatments. *Crit Care Med* 26:236-244, 1998.

Syring RS: Tracheal washes. In King LG, editor: *Textbook of respiratory disease in dogs and cats,* St Louis, 2004, Saunders.

Thayer GW, Robinson SK: Bacterial bronchopneumonia in the dog: a review of 42 cases. *J Am Anim Hosp Assoc* 20:731-735, 1984.

Wilson R, Cole PJ: The effect of bacterial products on ciliary function. *Am Rev Respir Dis* 138:S49-S53, 1988.

Wynne JW, Ramphal R, Hood CI: Tracheal mucosal damage after aspiration. A scanning electron microscope study. *Am Rev Respir Dis* 124:728-732, 1981.

PARASITIC AND PROTOZOAL DISEASES

Catherine Kasai

45. What are the more common respiratory parasites?

- *Angiostrongylus vasorum* is a metastrongyloid nematode that lives in the pulmonary arteries. This parasite has been found in the eastern Canadian provinces, the United Kingdom, northern Europe, South America, and Uganda.
- *Capillaria aerophila* also known as *Eucoleus aerophilus* is a nematode that lives in the bronchial mucosa.
- *Crenosoma vulpis* is a lungworm that lives in the distal bronchial tree. This parasite can be found in the northeastern United States and the eastern provinces of Canada.
- *Filaroides hirthi* are small metastrongyloid nematode parasites that live in the terminal bronchioles and alveolar spaces.
- *Filaroides osleri* renamed *Oslerus osleri* is a lung worm usually found in dogs younger than 2 years of age. This parasite affects the trachea and the lining of the larger bronchi.
- *Paragonimus kellicotti* is a lung fluke (trematode) of the family Troglotrematidae. This trematode can be found in dogs in the Eastern United States around the Mississippi River, Great Lakes, and the Gulf of Mexico.
- *Pneumonyssoides caninum* are nonsarcoptiform mites. These mites live in the nasal and paranasal sinuses. They can be transmitted via direct contact from dog to dog.

This information is summarized in Table 21-1.

46. What clinical signs are seen with respiratory parasites that affect the trachea, bronchi, and lower airways?

Clinical signs include a chronic dry or moist productive cough, dyspnea, cyanosis, wheezing, respiratory distress, collapse, bleeding diatheses in the lungs, and exercise intolerance.

47. What is the life cycle of *A. vasorum*?

The female *A. vasorum* has its red intestines intertwined with its white ovaries and uterus which give it the appearance of a "barber pole." *A. vasorum* has a molluscan as its intermediate host. A molluscan ingests the L1 stage of the larvae and within the snail or slug, the larvae molts to the L3 stage. The dog ingests the molluscan and becomes infected with the L3 stage, which migrates to the host mesenteric lymph nodes. While in the lymph node, the L3 larvae molt into the immature adults and migrate to the right ventricle and pulmonary artery via the portal circulation. Females lay eggs which lodge in the terminal pulmonary arterioles and develop into stage 1 larvae. The

Table 21-1 *Respiratory Parasites, Sites of Infection, Distribution, and Mode of Transmission*

PARASITE	SITE OF INFECTION	GEOGRAPHIC DISTRIBUTION	TRANSMISSION
Angiostrongylus vasorum	Pulmonary vasculature	Eastern Canadian provinces, the United Kingdom, northern Europe, South America, and Uganda	Snails and slugs; transport hosts: frogs, lizards, birds, and rodents
Capillaria aerophila (Eucoleus aerophilus)	Lower respiratory tract	North America	Paratenic host: earthworms
Crenosoma vulpis	Lower respiratory tract	Worldwide	Snail
Filaroides osleri renamed *Oslerus osleri*	Upper respiratory tract, rarely the lower respiratory tract	Worldwide	Oral-oral, airway secretions-oral, fecal-oral contamination
Filaroides hirthi	Lower respiratory tract	North America	Fecal oral contamination
Paragonimus kellicotti	Lower respiratory tract	Eastern United States, around the Mississippi River, Great Lakes, and the Gulf of Mexico	Snail, crayfish, and crabs
Pneumonyssoides caninum	Upper respiratory tract	Worldwide	Dog to dog

larvae migrate into the alveoli then move up the bronchi to be coughed, swallowed, and excreted in the feces.

48. Describe the radiographic pattern seen on thoracic radiographs with *A. vasorum*.

The cardiac silhouette may have evidence of an enlarged right ventricle from the presence of *A. vasorum* in the right heart and pulmonary vessels. In the early stages of the disease, a multifocal or peripheral alveolar pattern can be visualized. This pattern is associated with pulmonary granulomas or hemorrhage caused by *A. vasorum*. As the infection progresses, an interstitial pattern is seen throughout the lung parenchyma, along with pleural fissure lines. Pneumothorax can also be seen.

49. How is *Capillaria aerophila* transmitted?

Dogs ingest eggs that have been passed by an infected host (canine or feline species). Eggs are produced by female parasites in the mucosal epithelium of the lungs of the dog. They are coughed up and swallowed by the dog and passed in feces. The eggs require 5 to 7 weeks in the soil to become infectious. Earthworms may act as the transport paratenic hosts.

50. Describe the clinical signs and radiographic changes seen with *Capillaria aerophila* infections.

Coughing and wheezing occur from bronchial inflammation. Thoracic radiographs show a bronchial pattern.

51. What radiographic distribution can be seen with dogs infected with *C. vulpis*?

Thoracic radiographs usually show a bronchointerstitial pattern. There is also enhanced definition in the hilus and shoulder regions of the bronchial walls. In animals with a productive cough, cardiomegaly and an interstitial lung pattern can be seen.

52. Which is the preferred diagnostic tool to isolate *F. hirthi* from feces?

The zinc-sulfate technique is 100 times more efficient than the Baermann apparatus in recovering larvae from feces.

53. What visual changes occur in the respiratory tract with *O. osleri* infections?

The nematode is found in fibrous nodules that project into the lumen of the trachea and the bronchi. As the nodules become larger, they may cause airway obstruction. A dry cough and possibly respiratory distress may be present in dogs with severe infections. The fibrous nodules can be seen during bronchoscopic examination of the airways.

54. What radiographic changes occur with *P. kellicotti* infections?

P. kellicotti infections cause irregular, nodular densities or focal areas of saccular bronchiolar dilation. Small air-filled cavities and cysts called pneumatocysts form within the lung parenchyma. They range from 20 to 30 mm in diameter and cyst walls are 2- to 4-mm thick. Radiographs may also show interstitial nodular densities or pneumothorax secondary to rupture of pneumatocysts.

55. What is the life cycle of *P. kellicotti*?

Eggs of *P. kellicotti* are shed in feces and may enter the water supply where they produce ciliated miracidium. The miracidium enter a snail host and undergo asexual multiplication to produce the cercarial stage. Cercariae leave the snail and invade crayfish where they become metacercariae. Crayfish containing metacercariae is ingested by a dog and the parasite enters the canine intestinal tract. After reaching the intestinal tract, the metacercariae move into the peritoneal cavity, migrate through the diaphragm, and enter the lungs. The flukes mature in the lungs and form cysts, where they produce eggs which are coughed up by the animal, swallowed, and passed in the feces.

56. What are the clinical signs of a *P. caninum* infection?

P. caninum live in the nasal and paranasal sinuses of the dog. Clinical signs include excessive lacrimation, orbital cellulitis, serous nasal discharge, facial pruritus, rhinitis, impaired ability to smell, sneezing, and reverse sneezing. Dogs may also present with inflammation of the upper respiratory tract, tonsillitis, and increased mucus in the maxillary and frontal sinuses.

57. How is *P. caninum* diagnosed?

Mites can be visualized in or around the external nares. The mites are pale yellow, oval, and 1.0 to 1.5 mm in length and all of the legs are in the anterior portion of the body. One can use a rhinoscope or otoscope to visualize the mites inside of the nasal cavity.

58. What intestinal parasites have pulmonary migration?

Ancylostoma caninum (hookworms), *Strongyloides stercoralis,* and *Toxocara canis* (roundworms) all migrate to the lungs. *A. caninum* enters through the dermis and migrates through the veins and lymphatic system to the alveoli and trachea. *S. stercoralis* migrates through the skin and is carried to the alveoli via blood vessels. The parasite migrates from the alveoli up to the trachea and is swallowed. Mature *S. stercoralis* migrate through the lower intestine or through the skin of the perianal area then back to the lungs of the dog. *T. canis* migrates via the portal circulation to the lungs, entering the alveoli and migrating up to the bronchioles, bronchi, and trachea.

59. How often are protozoan infections diagnosed in the respiratory tract of the dog?

Toxoplasma gondii and *Neospora caninum* usually do not have pneumonic manifestations. Pulmonary infections from toxoplasmosis are usually found in conjunction with distemper infections or in immunocompromised animals.

60. Which medications could be used to treat respiratory parasites?

See Table 21-2 for a summary of treatment recommendations.

Table 21-2 *Anthelminthic Treatments for Canine Respiratory Parasites*

DRUG	DOSE	PARASITE
Albendazole	50 mg/kg PO q 12 h for 5 days, repeat in 3 weeks	*Filaroides hirthi*
	25 to 50 mg/kg PO q 12 h for 14 days	*Paragonimus kellicott*
Fenbendazole	50 mg/kg PO q 24 h for 3 days	*Crenosoma vulpis, Toxocara canis*
	50 mg/kg PO q 24 h for 7 days	*Oslerus osleri*
	50 mg/kg PO q 24 h for 14 day	*Filaroides hirthi*
	25 to 50 mg/kg PO q 12 h for 14 days	*Paragonimus kellicotti, Capillaria aerophila (Eucoleus aerophilus)*
Ivermectin	0.4 mg/kg SC or PO	*Filaroides hirthi*
Levamisole	7.5 mg/kg PO q 24 h for 2 days followed by 10 mg/kg PO q 24 h on the next 2 days	*Angiostrongylus vasorum*
	7.5 mg/kg SC once, then repeat in 2 days	*C. vulpis*
Milbemycin oxime	0.5 to 1.0 mg/kg PO weekly for 3 weeks	*Pneumonyssoides caninum*
	0.5 mg/kg PO once	*C. vulpis*
	0.5 mg/kg PO once per week for 4 weeks	*Angiostrongylus vasorum*
Praziquantel	25 mg/kg PO q 8 h for 3 days	*P. kellicotti*

BIBLIOGRAPHY

Ah H., Chapman WL Jr: Extrapulmonary granulomatous lesions in canine Paragonimiasis, *Vet Parasit* 2:251-258, 1976.

Ballweber LB: Respiratory parasites (VET-308), Proceedings of the Western Veterinary Conference, Las Vegas, NV, February 2004.

Boag, AK, Lamb, CR, Chapman, PS et al: Radiographic findings in 16 dogs infected with *Angiostrongylus vasorum, Vet Rec* 154:426-430, 2004.

Boag AK, Murphy KF, Connolly DJ: Hypercalcaemia associated with Angiostrongylus vasorum in three dogs, *J Small Anim Pract* 46:79-84, 2005.

Bowman DD: Respiratory system parasites of the dog and cat (Part I): nasal mucosa and sinuses, and respiratory parenchyma. In Bowman DD, editor: *Companion and exotic animal parasitology,* Ithaca, NY, 2000, International Veterinary Information Service, document no. A0302.0400.

Bowman DD: Respiratory system parasites of the dog and cat (Part II): nasal mucosa and sinuses, and respiratory parenchyma. In Bowman DD, editor: *Companion and exotic animal parasitology,* Ithaca, NY, 2000, International Veterinary Information Service, document no. A0302.0400.

Chapman PS, Boag AK, Guitian J et al: *Angiostrongylus vasorum* infection in 23 dogs (1999-2002), *J Small Anim Pract* 45:435-440, 2004.

The Center for Food Security and Public Health: *Hookworms*, Ames, IA, 2005, Iowa State University.

Conboy G: Natural infections of *Crenosoma vulpis* and *Angiostrongylus vasorum* in dogs in Atlantic Canada and their treatment with milbemycin oxime, *Vet Rec* 155:16-18, 2004.

Dubey JP, Toussant EA, Miller TB et al: Experimental *Paragonimus kellicotti* infection in dogs, *Vet Parasit* 5:325-337, 1979.

Ettinger SJ, Feldman EC: *Textbook of veterinary internal medicine*, ed 6, St Louis, 2006, Elsevier.

Foreyt W: *Veterinary parasitology*, ed 3, 1994.

Plumb D: *Veterinary drug handbook*, ed 4, 2002.

Sherding R: Bronchopulmonary parasite infections. Proceedings of the World Small Animal Veterinary Association World Congress, 2001, Vancouver, B.C., Canada.

University of California at Davis. Strongyloides stercoralis (website): http://ucdnema.ucdavis.edu/imagemap/nemmap/Ent156html/nemas/strongyloidesstercoralis.

22. Pulmonary Thromboembolism

Erin M. Portillo

1. What is a pulmonary thromboembolism (PTE)?

A PTE occurs when a clot obstructs a pulmonary vessel. This can occur within the vessel itself (thrombus) or the clot can originate elsewhere and migrate to the pulmonary vasculature and become lodged (thromboembolism), therefore obstructing blood flow.

2. What is Virchow's triad?

Virchow's triad is composed of three elements that are risk factors for thrombosis. These include (1) vascular alteration or injury, (2) blood stasis or impairment of flow, and (3) hypercoagulability resulting from a defect in coagulation.

3. When should I be concerned about a PTE in my dogs?

In animals with one of the components of Virchow's triad, there should be concern. PTE has been associated with the following conditions: cardiac disease, protein-losing nephropathy, neoplasia, immune-mediated disease, hypercortisolism, diabetes mellitus, infectious disease, trauma, surgical procedures, necrotizing pancreatitis, and atherosclerosis. A recent study suggested that 60% of dogs diagnosed with thromboembolic disease had underlying protein-losing nephropathy or neoplasia.

Although these conditions are favorable for thrombosis, occurrence of a PTE is unpredictable and should be suspected if clinical signs become apparent.

4. Describe the pathophysiologic effects of PTE.

- A thromboembolic event to the pulmonary vasculature within a normal lung may be well tolerated because of significant reserve capacity. However, if there is cardiac or pulmonary compromise, clinically significant pulmonary or hemodynamic sequelae may ensue.
- The degree of vascular obstruction will dictate the severity of the consequences. A major problem is ventilation-perfusion (V/Q) mismatch. This is a ratio that expresses the difference between alveolar ventilation and alveolar blood flow. If perfusion is adequate to an area of lung that is inadequately ventilated or the reverse if there is inadequate flow to a well-ventilated lung then the result is a compromise in respiratory exchange. In a total

occlusion, which is rare, ventilation will continue despite absence of blood flow to the affected region.

- Arterial hypoxemia may follow partially the result of the V/Q mismatch. Cardiac disease resulting in decreased cardiac output or pulmonary disease resulting in diffusion impairment may also contribute to hypoxemia.
- Hyperventilation is a common consequence of hypoxemia, which, depending on the severity, can lead to hypocapnia. This may or may not be adequate to alleviate the hypoxemia.
- If the pulmonary arterial occlusion is complete, then the decreased blood flow to the type II pneumocytes, which make surfactants is compromised, resulting in depletion of surfactant, edema, and atelectasis. This can occur within 24 hours of the PTE event.
- Hemodynamic consequences also relate to the magnitude of the obstruction. There is a large reserve capacity of the pulmonary vasculature but after this is overloaded, pulmonary vascular resistance will increase and right ventricular afterload occurs. These are poor prognostic indicators because increased afterload leads to increased ventricular oxygen requirements; if these requirements are not met, ventricular failure and decreased cardiac output can occur.

5. What are the clinical signs associated with a PTE?

The signs of PTE are extremely variable and can range from a subclinical presentation to sudden severe dyspnea and death. The most common signs are a sudden onset of dyspnea, tachypnea, and depression. Other signs that can be associated with PTE are cyanosis, hemoptysis, coughing, and syncope. PTE should be suspected in any dog with acute onset of respiratory distress, especially without previous respiratory disease and in the presence of a hypercoagulable state or associated risk factors.

6. How is PTE diagnosed?

Diagnosis can be particularly challenging. First there must be a clinical suspicion based on history and clinical signs.

- Thoracic radiographs can be beneficial in identifying differentials (e.g., pneumothorax, pneumonia, pulmonary edema); however, up to 30% of thoracic radiographs with PTE can be normal. The most common radiographic findings are regional oligemia (hypovascular regions of the lungs) and pulmonary infiltrates.
- Arterial blood gas can be beneficial with common abnormalities of hypoxemia, hypocapnia and an elevated A-a gradient (see Question 7). Unfortunately, these are nonspecific tests and are not pathognomonic for PTE.
- Pulmonary scintigraphy, which is commonly used for diagnosis in humans, uses radiolabeled elements and a gamma camera to demonstrate the blood flow in the ventilated areas of the lung. A normal study result will eliminate PTE as the problem, but an abnormal study result is not specific to PTE and may be associated with decreased regional ventilation from other causes (e.g., pneumonia, edema). Unfortunately, this procedure is limited to a few select referral practices.
- Selective pulmonary angiography is the gold standard for diagnosing or ruling out PTE. It requires general anesthesia and is invasive. Contrast is injected in the pulmonary artery and it is therefore risky in a compromised animal. Nonselective angiography is a less invasive option, but results are much more difficult to interpret.
- Coagulation profiles and D-dimers are helpful in evaluating the status of the dog. D-dimer is an indication of fibrinolysis and requires plasmin action on the clot to be formed. It has been shown to be a sensitive indicator of thrombosis in humans and has recently been shown to be specific in dogs. It has been suggested that a negative D-dimer rules out PTE and a positive result suggests further that further diagnostic tests be indicated.

7. How do you calculate an A-a gradient?

A-a gradient = $PaO_2 - [(P_{atm} + PH_2O)FiO_2 - PaCO_2/RQ]$ P_{atm} = atmospheric or barometric pressure, PH_2O = water vapor pressure, FiO_2 = fraction of inspired oxygen, PaO_2 = partial pressure of oxygen in the arterial blood, $PaCO_2$ = partial pressure of carbon dioxide in the arterial blood, and RQ = respiratory quotient which is normally 0.8. The normal value for an A-a gradient is less than 15 mm Hg. A-a gradient calculations may be facilitated by a number of online calculators found on the World Wide Web (e.g., http://www-users.med.cornell.edu/~spon/picu/calc/aagrad.htm)

8. How is PTE treated?

- Treatment consists of supportive measures such as oxygen support, bronchodilators, and mechanical ventilation if needed.
- Optimize tissue perfusion to maximize tissue oxygen delivery. Adequate fluid therapy, positive inotropes, or vasopressors may all be used if needed.
- Prevent progression or reoccurrence of thrombi. Use of an anticoagulant such as heparin, low-molecular-weight heparin, or warfarin is considered routine. Heparin doses range from 50 to 250 U/kg every 6 to 12 hours; it is therefore necessary to titrate the heparin dose using the partial thromboplastin time or by measuring plasma heparin levels. Low-molecular-weight heparin has been replacing unfractionated heparin in human medicine because it works more consistently at specific doses, making monitoring unnecessary (unless the dog is in renal failure). More clinical studies need to be evaluated in veterinary patients. Warfarin is still the drug of choice in human patients for long-term therapy. In veterinary patients, this therapy can be difficult because close therapeutic monitoring and owner compliance are essential.
- Thrombolytics can be used to dissolve a PTE. They have been shown most effective on arterial thrombi and thrombi that have formed recently (within 14 days in humans). Streptokinase, urokinase, and tissue-type plasminogen activator have been shown to be effective in human and canine patients. There is limited veterinary experience with these agents. In humans, severe hemorrhage has limited its use in human medicine to patients with right ventricular dysfunction or who are hemodynamically unstable.
- Aspirin can also be used to inhibit platelet aggregation through inhibition of thromboxane. It is a relatively weak antiplatelet drug but could be combined with heparin or another anticoagulant. The canine dose is 0.5 mg/kg every 12 hours.
- Surgical removal of the clot or thrombectomy has been suggested in some animals, but success rates of this are undetermined.

BIBLIOGRAPHY

Guyton AC, Hall JE: Physical principles of gas exchange; diffusion of oxygen and carbon dioxide through the respiratory membrane. In *Textbook of medical physiology*, ed 10, Philadelphia, 2000, WB Saunders.
Hackner SG: Pulmonary thromboembolism. In King LG, editor: *Textbook of respiratory disease in dogs and cats*, St Louis, 2004, Saunders Elsevier.
Hackner SG: Pulmonary thromboembolism I: etiology, pathophysiology and diagnosis. Proceedings of the tenth annual International Veterinary Emergency and Critical Care Symposium, 2004, pp. 610-614.
Hackner SG: Pulmonary thromboembolism II: treatment and prevention. Proceedings of the tenth annual International Veterinary Emergency and Critical Care Symposium, 2004, pp. 615-620.
Nelson OL: Use of the D-dimer assay for diagnosing thromboembolic disease in the dog, *J Am Anim Hosp Assoc* 41:145-149, 2005.
Nelson OL, Andreasen C: The utility of plasma D-dimer to identify thromboembolic disease in the dog, *J Vet Intern Med* 17:830-834, 2003.
Rozanski EA, Rondeau MP: Respiratory pharmacotherapy in emergency and critical care medicine, *Vet Clin North Am Small Anim Pract* 32:1073-1086, 2002.
Silverstein D, Drobatz KJ: Clinical evaluation of the respiratory tract. In Ettinger SJ, editor: *Textbook of veterinary internal medicine*, ed 6, St. Louis, Elsevier Saunders.

23. Pleural Space Diseases

Robert R. King and Michelle A. Pressel

1. Describe the site of normal pleural fluid production and its constituents.

Normal pleural fluid is an ultrafiltrate of plasma secreted by the mesothelial cells. In dogs, the pleural fluid volume is small, about 0.1 to 0.2 ml/kg body weight. The pleural fluid protein concentration is 1.1 to 1.3 g/dl, whereas the total cell count is less than 3,000 cells/µl. The differential cell count includes mesothelial cells (70%), monocytes (28%), and lymphocytes (2%). Neutrophils are uncommonly present.

2. Describe the formation of normal pleural fluid and how it exits from the pleural space.

The main site of pleural fluid filtration is the parietal pleura. Fluid and solute filter from the parietal interstitium into the pleural cavity down a pressure gradient across the parietal pleura. Once formed, the pleural fluid drains into lymphatic stomata found along the dependant portions of the parietal pleura (mainly the diaphragmatic and mediastinal surfaces). Pleural fluid drainage is controlled, under normal conditions, by lymphatic drainage. No pulmonary lymphatics open or drain into the pleural space of dogs.

3. What are the common causes of the pleural effusion in dogs?

The most common causes of pleural effusions include diseases or disorders resulting in increased capillary hydrostatic pressure (right-sided heart failure, pericardial effusion, diaphragmatic hernia); decreased intravascular colloid osmotic pressure (hypoalbuminemia from chronic protein loss [renal disease] or lack of protein production [severe hepatic disease]); increased vascular capillary permeability (systemic inflammatory diseases, pneumonic processes); and decreased pleural fluid absorption or drainage as occurs secondary to pleural inflammation, neoplastic processes, or obstruction of the thoracic duct and draining lymph nodes.

4. What clinical signs are associated with significant accumulations of pleural fluid?

Clinical signs of pleural effusion vary depending on the volume of fluid, the rapidity of its accumulation and the underlying disease process. Mild pleural effusions are difficult to detect and many dogs show no clinical signs of illness. When pulmonary parenchymal disease is absent, signs of serious respiratory distress are usually not evident until 60 ml/kg body weight of pleural fluid has accumulated. In dogs with signs of pleural fluid accumulation, dyspnea (with or without cyanosis) may be observed as well as open-mouth breathing, orthopnea, tachypnea, and reduced tidal volumes. Physical examination findings depend on the primary disease process. In most dogs with pleural effusion, respiratory sounds are decreased, especially ventrally, with concomitant muffling of heart sounds. A percussible fluid line may also be noted with ventral hyporesonance. Other nonspecific signs include ascites, dehydration, depression, fever, lymphadenopathy, heart murmurs, arrhythmias, inappetence, pale mucous membranes, pulse deficits, and weight loss.

5. What routine diagnostic test is needed to confirm the presence of pleural effusion?

Thoracic radiographs are usually necessary to confirm the presence of a pleural effusion. Radiographically, the effusion can be classified as free or encapsulated. Free fluid moves within the pleural cavity and is most characteristic of transudative effusions. Encapsulated fluid is trapped by adhesions and is often associated with chronic exudative effusions, such as pyothorax.

The radiographic diagnosis of pleural effusion depends on finding one or more of the following radiographic signs: (1) the presence of interlobar fissure lines; (2) rounding of lung margins at the costophrenic angles; (3) separation of lung lobe borders away from the thoracic wall; (4) scalloping of the lung lobe margins dorsal to the sternum; (5) blurring of the cardiac silhouette; and (6) widening of the mediastinum. The radiographic views that are most helpful for recognizing small amounts (less than 100 ml) of pleural fluid are the lateral recumbent and ventrodorsal views. The earliest sign of pleural effusion is accumulation of fluid dorsal to the sternum in the lateral recumbent position, resulting in scalloping of the lung lobe borders as they retract from the thoracic walls. The ventrodorsal view is preferable to the dorsoventral view for dogs with small amounts of pleural fluid. Radiographs taken during expiration are also helpful when evaluating a dog with a small volume of pleural fluid because the volume of the lungs is less at this phase of breathing; therefore, the volume of effusion is relatively greater and is spread over a smaller area. Dramatic radiographic changes are associated with a large volume pleural effusion. Retraction and separation of the lung lobes from the thoracic wall should be present in all radiographic views. Thoracic width usually increases on the ventrodorsal and dorsoventral views. Lung lobes can collapse to half their original volumes. In the lateral and dorsoventral views, the heart, the mediastinum and the diaphragm may be totally obscured by fluid. Dorsal elevation of the trachea and caudal displacement of the liver and diaphragm are commonly present on the lateral view.

6. How does one obtain fluid or air from the pleural space to differentiate the various causes of pleural effusion?

Thoracocentesis is used as a diagnostic and therapeutic procedure. An area of the skin between the seventh and ninth intercostal space, just below the level of the costochondral junction is aseptically prepared and an 18- or 20-gauge needle attached to a three-way stopcock is introduced at the cranial rib border to avoid the intercostal vessels and nerve that traverse the caudal rib margin. The needle is advanced through the skin, subcutaneous tissues, and parietal pleural membrane. Constant negative pressure should be maintained on the syringe so that advancement of the needle is discontinued at the first sight of fluid. This will minimize the likelihood of damaging underlying lung tissue. In most cases, the volume of effusion is large enough that laceration of lung tissue is unlikely. In some instances, the effusion may be highly viscous (pyothorax and chylothorax) and difficult to aspirate. In these animals, chest tube placement may be necessary to completely evacuate the pleural space. Samples of the effusion should be collected for cytologic evaluation, determination of physical and biochemical characteristics, and aerobic, anaerobic, and fungal culture.

7. What are the physicochemical characteristics of pure and modified transudates?

Pure transudates are clear and have a low specific gravity (<1.018), low total protein content (<2.5 g/dl) and contain few cells (<1,000/μl). Small lymphocytes, well-preserved neutrophils, mesothelial cells, and monocytes are present. Disorders causing hypoproteinemia should be considered in the list of differential diagnoses.

Modified transudates have a total protein content of 2.5 to 3.5 g/dl and a total cell count between 500 and 10,000 cells/μl. Cell types are similar to transudates, but well-preserved neutrophils may be present in variable numbers depending on the degree of inflammation (as seen in resolving septic effusions or progression from a transudate to an exudate). Differential diagnoses are numerous and include neoplastic diseases (lymphoma, mesothelioma, thymoma), translocation of abdominal effusion (peritoneal dialysis, generalized abdominal inflammatory processes), selective causes of increased hydrostatic pressure (lung lobe torsion, diaphragmatic hernia, neoplasia), and causes of pleural or pulmonary vasculitis (systemic inflammation [sepsis, rickettsial infections], localized inflammation [pneumonia, pancreatitis]), immune-mediated diseases, and allergic or anaphylactic reactions (drug reactions, snake envenomation).

8. What are the physicochemical characteristics of hemorrhagic and sanguineous effusions?

Hemorrhagic effusions are characterized by packed cell volume, nucleated cell counts, and total protein content that are at least 25% of the peripheral blood. Platelets are not present unless bleeding has occurred 60 minutes before sampling. Erythrophagocytosis by macrophages is commonly seen. Sanguineous effusions have at least 5,000 to 6,000 red cells/µl. Differential diagnoses include trauma, coagulopathy, lung lobe torsion, diaphragmatic hernia, pulmonary infarction or abscesses, heartworm disease, and neoplasia.

9. What are the physiochemical characteristics of inflammatory and septic effusions (pyothorax)?

Inflammatory and septic effusions are characterized by large numbers of neutrophils. The fluid is cloudy and the color varies from red to brown to yellow. Total protein content is high (>3.0 g/dl) as well as the nucleated cell count (>5,000/µl). Septic effusions are differentiated from inflammatory effusions by the presence of intracellular bacterial (sometime fungal) organisms and degenerative neutrophils (Fig. 23-1). Anaerobic species alone or in combination with aerobes (multiple organism infections are the norm) are typically isolated from these exudative effusions. Common anaerobic bacteria include *Bacteroides* spp. and *Fusobacterium* spp. Gram-negative organisms *Actinomyces* spp., *Pasteurella* spp., and *Escherichia coli* are also common. Gram-positive bacteria (*Corynebacterium* spp., *Streptococcus* spp., and *Nocardia* spp.) are less often isolated. Nonseptic inflammatory effusions include those listed as causing modified transudates from chronic vasculitis. It should be remembered that the nonseptic inflammatory effusions can progress to septic effusions if the microorganism gain access to the effusion.

10. What are the physicochemical characteristics of chylous effusions?

Chylous effusions have the characteristics of modified transudates or exudates. They tend to be milky-white to opaque in appearance, although some will have a reddish color if repeated thoracocenteses have been done. Total protein content ranges from 2.0 to 6.5 g/dl. Lymphocytes

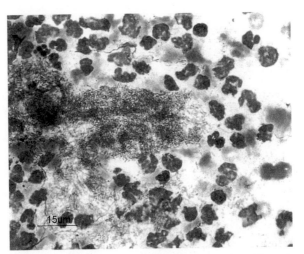

Figure 23-1. Cytologic preparation of a septic exudate from a dog with pyothorax. (Cytologic preparation courtesy of Dr. Charles W. Brockus, Iowa State University.)

are the major cell type; however, neutrophils may also be present (Fig. 23-2). Thoracic duct rupture resulting from trauma may occur, but more commonly recognized causes include mediastinal lymphoma, cardiomyopathy, heartworm disease, cranial vena cava thrombi, lung lobe torsion, and most commonly, unidentified (idiopathic) causes.

11. What is the common signalment of a dog suspected to have a pyothorax?
The mean age of affected dogs is 3.7 years old (range, 8 months to 13 years). Large-breed, male hunting dogs are overrepresented.

12. What are the common historical and physical examination findings in dogs with pyothorax?
Most cases occur in the fall and winter, when hunting and training take place. Predisposing conditions include superficial wound abscess (25%), pneumonia (12%), and migrating foreign bodies such as grass awns (10%). Physical examination findings attributable to pleural effusion include tachypnea (100%), dyspnea (89%), fever (87%), lethargy (77%), weight loss (65%), and cough (17%). Reluctance to lie down, decreased heart and lung sounds, dehydration, and abdominal breathing are commonly identified on examination.

13. What are the findings from thoracic radiography, hematologic analysis, and pleural fluid cytologic evaluation in dogs with pyothorax?
Studies of data from dogs with pyothorax demonstrate unilateral pleural effusion (43%), total blood leukocyte count of 20,000/µl (range, 10,000 to 33,000), and pleural fluid changes (total protein 4.3 g/dl [range, 2.9 to 5.9], total leukocyte count 149,000 cell/µl [range, 22,500 to 232,000], presence of bacteria in 38 of 38 dogs).

14. How do you make a definitive diagnosis of pyothorax?
Identification of organisms responsible for this infectious disease requires fluid aspiration either by thoracocentesis or tube thoracostomy. Fluid samples should be collected aseptically and submitted for both aerobic and anaerobic culture. Isolation of fungal organisms is uncommonly

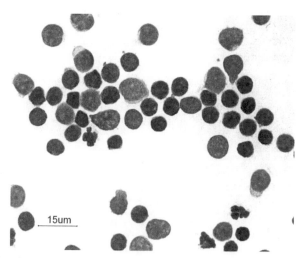

15um

Figure 23-2.   Cytologic preparation of pleural fluid from a dog with chylothorax. (Cytologic preparation courtesy of Dr. Charles W. Brockus, Iowa State University.)

reported, thus routine submission would not seem warranted. Cytologic evaluation of the recovered fluid should always be performed. The likelihood of infection can be determined from cytologic findings and initial antibiotic selections should be based on Gram stain results.

15. How should pyothorax be treated?

Pleural fluid drainage plus appropriate antibiotic therapy is essential for resolution of infection. Repeated thoracocenteses may be successful in some animals, but dogs will benefit the most from tube thoracostomy. Few studies in dogs have addressed differences in treatment outcomes with and without continuous chest tube drainage. Although the number of animals in these studies were relatively small (57 dogs in the former study and 22 dogs in the latter study), continuous chest tube drainage resulted in fewer hospital days (approximately 5.5 days) compared with intermittent chest tube drainage (8.3 days). Bilateral chest tubes may be required because of adhesions within the chest cavity or a complete mediastinum. The tube should extend within the chest as far cranial as possible, ideally along the ventral chest wall; however, migration of the tubes is common. Thoracic radiographs should be repeated after initial removal of the pleural effusion to assess proper placement of the chest tubes and to determine if an underlying disease process is present (e.g., lung lobe torsion, consolidation of multiple lung lobes) that might necessitate surgical intervention (Fig. 23-3). Thoracic radiographs should be repeated every 48 to 72 hours or more frequently if the animal shows signs of respiratory distress or fluid volume recovery terminated unexpectedly.

Antibiotic selection should be based on Gram stain results; however, historical data indicate that most gram-positive organisms are sensitive to ampicillin, gram-negative organisms are sensitive to enrofloxacin and obligate anaerobic organisms are sensitive to amoxicillin-clavulanic acid. Parenteral administration of selected antibiotics is recommended, particularly in animals with severe disease. After results of pleural fluid cultures are available, sensitivity patterns can be used to select more appropriate antibiotics.

Some authors have recommended thoracic lavage with 0.9% saline, lactated Ringer's solution, antibiotics, and fibrinolytics-anticoagulants. These reports all suggest an improved rate of resolution, although no controlled studies have been done to determine if shorter hospital stays occur for animals treated with any of these adjunctive therapies. Supportive therapy that has shown benefit includes conservative fluid administration to maintain hydration, pain management, and nutritional support.

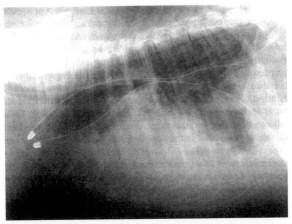

Figure 23-3.   A lateral thoracic radiograph taken after chest tube placement and removal of septic fluid from a dog with pyothorax. There is still fluid present in the ventral portion of the pleural space. (Radiograph courtesy of Dr. E. Riedesel, Iowa State University.)

Continuous suction of thoracostomy tubes is preferable, but it is not always possible. If continuous suction is not available, repeated fluid aspiration should be done every 2 to 4 hours for the first few days. This may require transfer of the dog to an emergency clinic if 24-hour care is not available. Fluid recovery volumes are initially large (1 to 2 L/day in large-breed dogs), but typically decrease after a few days if appropriate antibiotics have been selected and pleural fluid drainage has been successful. At this time, frequency of fluid drainage may be decreased to three to four times daily. Rationale for this decision should be based on serial reductions in daily fluid volumes and changes in the character of recovered fluid (absence of bacteria and progressive change in the fluid toward a modified transudate). Pleural fluid samples should be evaluated cytologically every 24 to 48 hours to help assess progression of disease.

16. What are the criteria for successful pleural space drainage?

Clinical status of the dog should show demonstrable improvement by 24 to 48 hours. Expected changes in the animal would include change in body temperature toward normal, resolution of respiratory distress, resolution of dehydration, improvement in attitude, and interest in eating. Thoracic radiographs should show partial to complete resolution of pulmonary infiltrates (if present on initial films) and complete pleural space drainage. Cytologic evaluation of the pleural fluid after 48 hours of therapy should demonstrate reduction or absence of bacteria and decreased total nucleated cell counts and protein content.

If these positive signs of clinical improvement and changes in pleural fluid volume and character have not occurred by 48 hours, the plan should be reassessed. This would include making certain that pleural fluid drainage is adequate and that placement of thoracostomy tubes is acceptable. Choice of antibiotics should be addressed, particularly if high numbers of bacteria are present in the effusion or if Gram stains reveal different bacterial staining characteristics.

17. What are the criteria for chest tube removal?

Removal of chest tubes should be possible when the following criteria are met: (1) thoracic radiographs show complete removal of fluid for at least 24 hours; (2) pleural fluid analysis is consistent with a sterile modified transudate; and (3) when pleural fluid production is less than 4 ml/kg/day.

18. When should surgical intervention be considered as a treatment option for pyothorax?

Some authors believe that pyothorax is a surgical disease and that resolution of the disease with medical therapy alone is rare. This is not true; many cases can be successfully managed with aggressive medical management using tube thoracostomy and continuous suction. The decision on a surgical option should be based on several factors. These include: (1) continued large volume of fluid production despite appropriate therapy; (2) persistence of large numbers of degenerative neutrophils rather than a reduction in their numbers and a change the cell population to nondegenerative forms; (3) continued presence of bacteria in the pleural fluid following appropriate therapy for at least 72 hours; (4) evidence of a disease process or finding on thoracic radiographs (or ultrasound evaluation) that suggests resolution of the pleural effusion is unlikely; and (5) lack of clinical improvement in the dog after 3 to 5 days.

19. What are common causes of a pneumothorax?

Blunt or penetrating trauma to the chest or abdomen is probably the most frequent cause of pneumothorax in dogs. Trauma to the esophagus via a sharp foreign body has also been associated with pneumothorax.

20. What is the difference between an open and closed pneumothorax?

An open pneumothorax occurs when external forces (bite wounds, gunshot) skin lacerations secondary to rib fractures or iatrogenic injuries (thoracocentesis, thoracotomy incisions) result in communication between the potential pleural space and the external environment. Blunt trauma can cause parenchymal lung damage with air leakage across the visceral (pulmonary) pleura into the potential pleural space. A tension pneumothorax results when a flap of skin or soft tissue acts as a one-way valve, allowing air to enter the pleural space during inspiration, but preventing its escape on expiration. This form of pneumothorax is rapidly progressive because increased pressure within the thorax compromises both respiration and venous return to the heart. This may lead to death if treatment is not provided in a timely manner.

21. What is a spontaneous pneumothorax?

A spontaneous or nontraumatic pneumothorax is a closed pneumothorax in which the lung is the source of the air leakage into the pleural space. Primary spontaneous pneumothorax is believed to be due to a collagen disorder leading to the formation of subpleural blebs and bullae. These bullae usually rupture and slowly leak air into the pleural space. Dogs presented with this condition typically show mild to moderate signs of respiratory distress and radiographic evidence of marked accumulation of air in the pleural space. Secondary spontaneous pneumothorax is associated with a number of pulmonary disorders and diseases (asthma, lung abscess, pulmonary neoplasia, parasitic lung disease, pneumonia, thromboembolism) in dogs. Cases usually occur in middle-age, deep-chested dogs.

22. When should a thoracostomy tube be used for continuous suction in a dog with pneumothorax?

Placement of a chest tube for continuous removal of air should be done in animals with recurrent pneumothorax. In general, it is recommended that a chest tube be placed after three consecutive thoracocentesis attempts have been unsuccessful in controlling recurrence.

23. What are the common causes and recommended treatment of hemothorax?

Trauma, coagulopathies (rodenticide toxicity), and neoplastic processes that erode through a major blood vessel are the most common causes of hemothorax. In most cases (excluding coagulation defects) the effusions are self-limiting.

Thoracocentesis is advisable if respiratory distress is present. Tube thoracostomy with continuous or intermittent drainage may be necessary if the effusion is large and recurrent. Coagulation abnormalities (based on coagulation studies) should be corrected with fresh whole blood or plasma. Vitamin K supplementation is required for dogs with coagulopathies from anticoagulant rodenticide intoxication. Treatment of hemorrhagic effusions resulting from neoplastic processes is dependent on several factors (type of neoplasm, anticipated prognosis, and the amount of effusion). In animals with advanced disease and poor short-term prognosis, therapeutic thoracocentesis may be a reasonable palliative option. Dogs with better prognoses may benefit from surgery and adjunctive chemotherapy.

24. What are the most common symptomatic treatments used to minimize chylous effusion accumulation?

Finding and treating the underlying cause of a chylous effusion is important as supportive measures are generally not sufficient to control the disease process. Symptomatic therapy includes (1) a low-fat diet may reduce the fat in the effusion and may help increase fluid absorption from the pleural space; (2) benzopyrene drugs such as Rutin may be beneficial in decreasing fluid accumulation in the pleural space (its mechanism of action is unclear, but macrophages may be stimulated to pick up lymphatic fluid more efficiently); and (3) intermittent thoracocentesis is usually necessary.

25. What is pseudochylous effusion and when does it occur?

Pseudochylous effusion is a term initially used to refer to cases of chylous effusion in which the thoracic duct was not ruptured. The term should be reserved for effusions in which the pleural fluid cholesterol concentration is greater than the serum cholesterol concentration and the pleural fluid triglyceride level is less than or equal to the serum triglyceride level. This is type of effusion is rare in dogs but has been associated with tuberculosis.

BIBLIOGRAPHY

Bauer T: Pyothorax, In Kirk RW, editor: *Current veterinary therapy IX,* Philadelphia, 1986, Saunders.
Brockman DJ, Puerto DA: Pneumomediastinum and pneumothorax. In King LG, editor: *Textbook of respiratory disease in dogs and cats,* St Louis, 2004, Saunders.
Campbell SL, Forrester SD, Johnston SA et al: Chylothorax associated with constrictive pericarditis in a dog, *J Am Vet Med Assoc* 206:1561-1564, 1995.
Forrester D, Troy G, Fossum T: Pleural effusions: pathophysiology and diagnostic consideration, *Compend Contin Educ Pract Vet* 10:121-136, 1988.
Fossum TW: Chylothorax. In King LG, editor: *Textbook of respiratory disease in dogs and cats,* St Louis, 2004, Saunders.
Fossum TW, Birchard SJ, Jacobs RM: Chylothorax in 34 dogs, *J Am Vet Med Assoc* 188:1315-1318, 1986.
Frendin J: Pyogranulomatous pleuritis with empyema in hunting dogs. *J Vet Med A* 44:167-178, 1997.
Hardie EM, Barsanti JA: Treatment of canine actinomycosis. *J Am Vet Med Assoc* 180:537-541, 1982.
Hodges CC, Fossum TW, Evering W: Evaluation of thoracic duct healing after experimental laceration and transaction, *Vet Surg* 22:431-435, 2003.
Holtsinger RH, Beale BS, Bellah JR et al: Spontaneous pneumothorax in the dog: a retrospective analysis of 21 cases, *J Am Anim Hosp Assoc* 29:195-210, 1993
Jang SS, Breher JE, Dabaco LA et al: Organisms isolated from dogs and cats with anaerobic infections and susceptibility to selected antimicrobial agents, *J Am Vet Med Assoc* 210:1610-1614, 1997.
McKiernan BC, Adams WM, Huse DC: Thoracic bite wounds and associated internal injury in 11 dogs and one cat, *J Am Vet Med Assoc* 8:959-964, 1984.
Miserocchi G, Agostoni E: Contents of the pleural space, *J Appl Physiol* 30:208-213, 1971.
Monnet E: Pyothorax. In King LG, editor: *Textbook of respiratory disease in dogs and cats,* St Louis, 2004, Saunders.
Negrini D, Venturoli D, Townsley MI et al: Permeability of parietal pleura to liquid and proteins, *J Appl Physiol* 76:627-633, 1994.
Orton EC: Pleural drainage. In Orton EC, editor: *Small animal thoracic surgery,* Malvern, Pa, 1995, Williams & Wilkins.
Padrid P: Canine and feline pleural disease, *Vet Clin North Am Small Anim Pract* 30:1295-1307, 2000.
Prittie J, Barton L: Hemothorax and sanguineous effusions, In King LG, editor: *Textbook of respiratory disease in dogs and cats,* St Louis, 2004, Saunders.
Robertson S, Stoddart M, Evans RJ et al: Thoracic empyema in the dog: a report of 22 cases, *J Small Anim Pract* 24:103-119, 1983.
Rooney MB, Monnet E: Medical and surgical treatment of pyothorax in dogs: 26 cases, *J Am Vet Med Assoc* 221:86-92, 2002.
Sanders NA, Slepper M: Pleural transudates and modified transudates. In King LG, editor: *Textbook of respiratory disease in dogs and cats,* St Louis, 2004, Saunders.
Silverstein DC: Pleural space disease. In King LG, editor: *Textbook of respiratory disease in dogs and cats,* St Louis, 2004, Saunders.
Turner WD, Breznock EM: Continuous suction drainage for management of canine pyothorax—a retrospective study, *J Am Anim Hosp Assoc* 24:485-494, 1988.
Valentine A, Smeak D, Allen D et al: Spontaneous pneumothorax in dogs, *Compend Contin Educ Pract Vet* 18:53-62, 1996.
Walker A, Jang SS, Hirsh DC: Bacteria associated with pyothorax of dogs and cats: 98 cases (1989-1998), *J Am Vet Med Assoc* 216:359-363, 2000.

24. Lower Respiratory Tract Tumors

Leslie E. Fox

1. What are the most common primary lung neoplasms in dogs?

Most lung tumors originate from the epithelium of the airways and alveolus. When classified by histologic pattern and cellular morphology, most lung tumors are adenocarcinomas (differentiated). Squamous cell carcinomas, anaplastic carcinomas, and sarcomas are less frequent, but more biologically aggressive. Benign tumors are rare. Occasionally, lymphoma, malignant histiocytosis, and lymphomatoid granulomatosis are found.

2. What is the typical signalment of dogs with primary lung tumors?

Typically, dogs with lung tumors are between 9 and 10 years old. Breed and gender preferences have not been consistently noted.

3. What clinical signs are most common in dogs with primary lung tumors?

Up to 56% of dogs with lung tumors have no clinical signs. A chronic, nonproductive cough that is unresponsive to antimicrobials and only temporarily responsive to corticosteroid therapy is most frequent. Systemic signs of inappetence and weight loss are frequent findings. Other less common signs are dyspnea, tachypnea, hemoptysis, and cyanosis. Lethargy, lameness, dysphagia, fever, cranial vena cava obstruction, diarrhea, ascites, and spontaneous pneumothorax are found infrequently.

4. Do we know what causes primary lung cancer?

Environmental chemical exposure is not well-documented in dogs, but airborne carcinogens are suspected causes of respiratory tract neoplasms. Second-hand smoke exposure increases the risk of lung cancer in brachycephalic breeds when compared with dolichocephalic breeds.

5. What is the typical radiographic location and appearance of lung neoplasms in dogs?

Lung neoplasms can be detected radiographically in almost any pattern. They can be solitary or disseminated, which includes multifocal or diffuse parenchymal patterns. The most typical are the solitary mass or diffuse interstitial patterns. Pleural effusion may be observed, and lobar consolidation is sometimes noted.

6. What other diseases can be confused with lung neoplasms?

Differential diagnoses for lung tumors can be generated from the radiographic lung pattern. Pneumonia, abscesses, fungal granulomas, lymphomatoid or eosinophilic pulmonary granulomatosis, hematomas, pulmonary thromboembolism, cysts, bullae, and primary and metastatic lung tumors can be seen radiographically as solitary or multifocal lung masses. Pneumonia, primary and metastatic lung neoplasms, hemorrhage, edema, fibrosis, and granulomatous diseases are observed in disseminated pulmonary patterns. Multicentric neoplasms involve the lung parenchyma simultaneously with other abnormalities including lymphoma, malignant histiocytosis/metastatic histiocytic sarcoma, and, rarely, mast cell tumor.

7. Can other imaging techniques be helpful in diagnosing lung neoplasms?

Detection of lung disease with plain survey radiography is limited to pulmonary masses larger than 3 to 5 mm in diameter. Computed tomography (CT) and magnetic resonance imaging provide additional information about the extent of the primary tumor's invasion into other thoracic structures such as the mediastinum and esophagus. It has been demonstrated that CT is more sensitive than plain thoracic radiography for detecting tracheobronchial lymphadenopathy. In one study, lymphadenopathy (with confirmed metastatic disease) was detectable with CT despite the finding of normal-size lymph nodes with plain survey films.

8. Where do lung tumors metastasize?

Metastasis can be vascular (by means of lymphatics or blood vessels) or alveolar (by local cell migration in the airways) or through the pleura. Local metastasis to structures in the thorax is more common than systemic spread. Regional lymph nodes (tracheobronchial and mediastinal) are more commonly affected than the pleura, pericardium, and heart. Dogs with locoregional metastasis may be presented for clinical signs referable to secondary invasion.

9. How is lung cancer diagnosed?

Solitary or multifocal masses seen with thoracic radiographs in an older dog raises the suspicion for primary or secondary lung neoplasms. Signs referable to the respiratory tract in an older dog should be investigated with thoracic radiography. Three view thoracic radiographs including left lateral, right lateral, and dorsal ventral or ventral dorsal views have been shown to improve detection of primary or metastatic lung tumors when compared with only two views. Aerated lung around the lesion helps demarcate the location, size, and shape of the mass. Although it is tempting and less costly to do only one lateral view, the heart, liver, pleural fluid, and atelectasis may obscure lung parenchymal masses.

Most solitary lung tumors are in the periphery of the lungs and are believed to originate from the small airways. Lymphomatoid granulomatosis can be considered an uncommon differential for most of the radiographic presentations common to dogs with primary lung tumors. It appears as a combination of mediastinal, sternal, or hilar lymphadenopathy, often with either diffuse alveolar-interstitial pulmonary infiltrate, interstitial-nodular infiltrate with large multifocal masses, or lobar consolidation. Pleural effusion is sometimes present. The radiographic appearance of dogs with malignant histiocytosis/metastatic histiocytic sarcoma is similar.

10. What is the initial diagnostic plan for suspected primary lung neoplasms?

Plain radiographs and fine-needle cellular aspiration may be all that is needed before therapeutic thoracotomy is performed. A complete blood cell count, serum biochemical panel, and urinalysis are indicated to rule out other diseases and suitability for general anesthesia. Screening for coagulation defects with determination of a platelet count with an activated clotting time or prothrombin/partial thromboplastin times is appropriate before needle aspiration. Abdominal radiography/ultrasound examination is useful to help assure that the pulmonary mass is not metastatic from an abdominal tumor.

11. Is thoracic ultrasonography useful in the diagnosis of lung tumors?

Thoracic ultrasound imaging is useful to localize lung lesions that are in contact with the thoracic wall and enables the sampling of pleural fluid. Ultrasound images of lung neoplasms are characterized by variable echogenicity and irregular borders. In the absence of vessels or a fluid-filled bronchus commonly observed with alveolar lung disease, pulmonary neoplasm is considered a likely diagnosis. Pleural effusion is readily seen and, because fluid improves resolution, soft-tissue lesions are enhanced, whereas pleural gas prevents visualization of solid structures in the lung.

Better diagnostic accuracy is achieved when needle placement for lesion aspiration is guided by ultrasound. Ultrasound guided fine-needle aspiration or tissue biopsy is most useful for lesions adjacent to the thoracic wall when little aerated lung is present between the mass and the thoracic wall to obscure visualization.

12. Are any routine laboratory tests helpful in distinguishing primary lung neoplasms from other pulmonary disorders?

There are no distinctive hematologic or biochemical abnormalities that support a diagnosis of primary pulmonary tumors. Normocytic, normochromic anemia may be present.

13. How do I obtain a sample for cytologic diagnosis?

Fine-needle cellular aspiration (blind or ultrasound-guided) is recommended even for dogs with diffuse pulmonary neoplasia. In most studies, it has been shown to be 80% to 90% successful in distinguishing a lung tumor from a nonmalignant cause and can be useful in identifying infectious agents as well. A specific cytologic diagnosis may be hindered by inflammation (nonseptic pyo- or pyogranulomatous inflammation) associated with lung neoplasms. Blind or guided fine-needle aspiration can be used to sample mass lesions and malignant pleural effusion. Pleural fluid obtained by percutaneous aspiration is often described as a modified transudate or exudate without evidence of neoplastic cells. Cytopathologic examination of tissue samples obtained by fine needle aspiration of the lung with a small-gauge (25 or 27 gauge, 1.5-inch needle on a 6-ml syringe is suggested) has been highly correlated with histopathologic examination of tissue obtained through thoracotomy. Cytopathologic diagnostic accuracy is improved with ultrasound guidance. Transthoracic fine needle aspiration is a minimally invasive procedure with rare to no adverse events reported after sampling. Many animals require no sedation or general anesthesia before a transthoracic fine needle aspiration.

When cutting core biopsy instruments are used to obtain a tissue sample (20 gauge Westcott needle, 18-20 gauge Menghini aspirate-biopsy needle [Tru-Cut]), complications are more frequent and potentially more severe. In one study, the overall diagnostic accuracy was 83%, but more than half of the animals had complications from the procedure. Asymptomatic pneumothorax was most common, and intrapulmonary hemorrhage, hemoptysis, and severe pneumothorax requiring removal of air were reported with rare deaths. Heavy sedation or general anesthesia is required. Transbronchial biopsy during bronchoscopic examination is seldom rewarding. Cytologic confirmation of neoplastic cells in fluid obtained from transtracheal wash or bronchoalveolar lavage is infrequently diagnostic, except in dogs with lymphoma.

Thoracotomy with lobectomy offers the opportunity for accurate histologic confirmation and is the also the treatment of choice for excisable tumors. Lymph node aspiration/biopsy can be obtained for clinical staging.

14. How useful is thoracoscopy and tissue biopsy?

Although the equipment necessary for thoracoscopy is expensive, it is minimally invasive with a rapid postoperative recovery. It is useful for lung and regional lymph node biopsies and lobectomy. Most intrathoracic structures of the left and right hemithorax are endoscopically visible and a sound knowledge of the anatomy of intrathoracic structures is a prerequisite for diagnostic and therapeutic thoracoscopy. Because cardiac output was decreased even at low intrathoracic pressures, insufflation-aided thoracoscopy should be used with caution and at the lowest possible insufflation pressure.

15. What information is required to clinically stage dogs with lung neoplasms?

Determining the extent of disease is important for prognosis. Thoracic radiographs along with a complete blood cell count and serum biochemical panel are the minimum tests for clinical staging, because the primary tumors, lymph node status, and presence of metastatic disease with or without concurrent illness can be assessed. The findings of palpably normal-size lymph nodes during thoracotomy or histologic metastasis-free lymph nodes have been demonstrated as predictors of longer survival when compared with dogs with enlarged or tumor-bearing lymph nodes. Dogs with a small (<2 cm diameter), solitary, or peripherally located mass have a better long-term outcome than dogs with large, multiple, or centrally located tumors.

16. What is the treatment of choice for dogs with lung neoplasms?

Surgical excision whenever possible is the standard treatment for solitary lung tumors. Tracheobronchial lymph nodes should be palpated and, whenever possible, histologically evaluated. Three-view thoracic radiographs give an evaluation of lung parenchyma, suggesting that radiographically visible tumor, whether solitary or multifocal, is potentially completely resectable with complete or partial lobectomy via thoracotomy. CT may more accurately determine the extent of disease. If all visible tumor is removed and regional lymph nodes are normal size, most dogs with adenocarcinomas have a median survival time of more than a year after surgery. Histologic evidence of tumor in regional lymph nodes is associated with shorter disease-free interval and survival.

17. Which chemotherapeutic agents are useful for lung neoplasms?

Chemotherapy is sometimes helpful for animals with unresectable or incompletely resected neoplasms. Anticancer drugs with activity against carcinomas may be effective in combination or as single-agent therapy such as cisplatin, carboplatin, doxorubicin, mitoxantrone, vindesine, cyclophosphamide, vincristine, and methotrexate.

Vinorelbine, a mitotic inhibitor (given at 15 mg/m^2, intravenous infusion over 5 minutes every 7 days) resulted in a partial response in a few dogs with either gross or microscopic evidence of bronchoalveolar carcinoma. Neutropenia was the dose-limiting toxicity.

Cyclooxygenase-2 is an inducible enzyme that is expressed by some neoplastic cells. Piroxicam is a nonsteroidal antiinflammatory used for antineoplastic effect on transitional cell carcinoma, squamous cell carcinoma, and mammary gland carcinoma. Suppressing the enzyme responsible for prostaglandin E_2 production indirectly decreases tumor proliferation, angiogenesis, and resistance to apoptosis. Dogs with either primary or secondary lung neoplasms may benefit from piroxicam (0.3 mg/kg, once per day by mouth).

18. Does radiation therapy have a role in the management of lung neoplasms?

Radiation therapy has been largely unproven in dogs with pulmonary neoplasms.

19. What prognostic factors are important for dogs with primary lung tumors?

One study reported 76 dogs with primary lung tumors treated with attempted complete surgical excision. Dogs with palpably small lymph nodes (intraoperatively), peripherally located tumors, solitary tumors, well-differentiated tumors (adenocarcinoma), and histologically negative lymph nodes were consistently found to have long remission and survival times. Although intraoperative lymph node size was the best single predictor of remission and survival times, radiographic evidence of lymph node enlargement may aid in identifying a potentially poor outcome before thoracotomy. After attempted complete surgical resection of the primary tumors, dogs with palpably enlarged lymph nodes had a median survival time of 2 months, when compared with a 1-year median survival time for dogs with normal-size lymph nodes.

In another study of 67 dogs, the median postoperative survival time was also about 1 year. The average survival for dogs treated with lung lobectomy for tumors less than 5 cm diameter was more than 1.6 years, whereas dogs with larger tumors survived 8 to 9 months. Factors associated with shorter remission and survival times were central location in the lung, presence of clinical signs at the time of diagnosis, histologic evidence of undifferentiated or squamous cell carcinomas, and high histologic grade. Dogs with well-differentiated carcinomas had a median time to disease progression of 16 months, whereas dogs with moderately differentiated tumors saw progression in about 6 months.

Many dogs with lymphoma have thoracic radiographic abnormalities consisting of thoracic lymphadenomegaly or pulmonary infiltrates. The presence of cranial mediastinal lymphadenomegaly was associated with shorter remission and survival times for dogs treated with chemotherapy, whereas the presence of pulmonary infiltrates was unrelated to remission/survival.

20. What paraneoplastic disorders are associated with primary lung neoplasms?

The most common paraneoplastic disorder is hypertrophic osteopathy, a disorder characterized by periosteal and connective tissue proliferation. Dogs with lung tumors may be presented for lameness only. Pain resulting from bone metastasis should be considered as a differential. Hypertrophic osteopathy progresses from the digits cranially. Some dogs may be asymptomatic; however, often, on physical examination, the limbs are thickened, edematous, warm, and painful to the touch. Recently, hypertrophic osteopathy related to pulmonary metastases of appendicular osteosarcoma was treated with pulmonary metastasectomy. Clinical signs (pain) associated with hypertrophic osteopathy resolved within 1 day after surgery and lasted more than 9 months. If the primary lung tumor is not resected, then corticosteroid or nonsteroidal antiinflammatory drug therapy can be used to decrease discomfort. Other paraneoplastic disorders include hypercalcemia, disseminated intravascular coagulation, and ectopic secretion of adrenocorticotropic hormone (ACTH) resulting in hyperadrenocorticism, generalized neuromyopathy, and fever.

21. What is lymphomatoid granulomatosis and is it a treatable disease?

Lymphomatoid granulomatosis behaves similarly to lymphoma (sometimes has an associated peripheral lymphadenopathy) and may be a form of atypical T-cell lymphoma. Because lymphomatoid granulomatosis has a better prognosis than other pulmonary disorders with the same radiographic appearance, every attempt should be made to obtain a cytologic/histologic diagnosis. It affects young to middle-age dogs, large-breed, and purebred dogs. Clinical signs of lymphomatoid granulomatosis are similar to those of respiratory neoplasms. Radiographic presentation is characterized by any of the patterns for primary or secondary lung tumors (nodular pulmonary masses, interstitial or alveolar infiltrates, lobar consolidation), usually with intrathoracic lymphadenopathy. Pleural effusion is sometimes present. Weight loss, ascites, mandibular lymphadenopathy, fever, gagging, choking, and vomiting are other reported nonrespiratory tract signs. Common clinicopathologic abnormalities are eosinophilia or basophilia. Other, more frequent causes of eosinophilia/basophilia associated with respiratory tract abnormalities are *Dirofilaria immitis* infection, respiratory tract parasitism, allergic airway disease, pulmonary fungal diseases, mast cell neoplasms, and occasionally lymphoma. It has been speculated that some of the abnormalities associated with lymphomatoid granulomatosis are related to heartworm disease.

Histologic evaluation is required to demonstrate angiocentric and angiodestructive pleomorphic infiltrates by an atypical lymphoid population because the clinical and radiographic findings of lymphomatoid granulomatosis are not different from the various presentations of lymphoma, primary and metastatic lung neoplasms, fungal and granulomatous disorders, and pulmonary infiltrates with eosinophilia. Cytologic diagnosis may be obscured by eosinophilic, basophilic, and neutrophilic inflammation.

Although chemotherapy is the treatment of choice for lymphomatoid granulomatosis, the most efficacious protocol is undetermined. Drugs used for the treatment of lymphoma (cyclophosphamide, prednisone, and vincristine, cytarabine) have been evaluated in only a few dogs with survival times of 4 days to 4 years.

22. What histiocytic diseases affect the lungs? Is effective therapy available?

Lung involvement in histiocytic diseases can be primary or secondary. The clinical presentation for dogs with pulmonary histiocytic disease is often cough, dyspnea, and tachypnea. Radiographically, an intrathoracic lymphadenopathy with or without a multinodular parenchymal pattern is most common and may include pleural effusion. Dogs with disseminated histiocytic diseases will typically have other clinical findings depending on the involved organs, which vary from nonpainful peripheral lymphadenopathy to seizures.

Two types of histiocytic disease affect the lungs and regional lymph nodes and may be confused with lymphoma. Histiocytic sarcomas occur as localized (or multifocal within one organ) lesions in predominantly in the skin and subcutis, spleen, and the soft tissue of long-bone joints. Histiocytic sarcoma is highly metastatic. Disseminated histiocytic sarcoma (also called malignant histiocytosis) will involve the spleen, lymph nodes, bone marrow, lung, and other organs. Unlike most dogs with primary lung neoplasms, dogs with disseminated histiocytic sarcoma typically have hematologic abnormalities (regenerative anemia or thrombocytopenia).

Because histiocytic sarcomas are highly metastatic to multiple organs and are often detected late in the course of the disease, they are difficult to distinguish from reactive histiocytic diseases that involve the similar organs, including the lung, and similar dog breeds. Distinguishing disseminated histiocytic sarcoma (malignant) from systemic histiocytosis (reactive) can be accomplished with immunohistochemistry and is important because the treatment and prognosis are quite different for each disease. If the primary presentation was for respiratory disease, a careful search for other evidence of malignant histiocytic organ infiltration may offer an opportunity to confirm the diagnosis without lung lesion aspiration or biopsy. Dogs with suspected reactive histiocytic disease should be carefully screened for infectious agents with bacterial cultures and special stains for organisms on paraffin-embedded tissues. Although chemotherapy protocols for lymphoma have been applied to dogs with disseminated histiocytic sarcoma, no effective therapy has been reported in the literature. Recently, in an unpublished study, lomustine (CCNU) was considered an active agent against histiocytic sarcoma in dogs with gross evidence of disease with a 50% response rate and overall median survival time of 4 months. Although reactive histiocytic diseases may wax and wane, immunosuppressive agents such as cyclosporine A may be needed to control systemic histiocytosis.

PULMONARY METASTATIC DISEASE OF DOGS

23. Which tumors frequently spread to the lungs?

Metastatic tumors are more common than primary lung tumors. Any carcinoma or sarcoma can metastasize to the small blood and lymphatic capillaries in the lungs; however, mammary gland tumors, osteosarcomas (other connective tissue sarcomas), oral melanomas, and hemangiosarcomas are most frequently found.

24. What clinical signs are most common in dogs with lung metastases?

Clinical signs of metastatic pulmonary disease are vague. Many dogs have no clinical signs referable to the respiratory tract. Much of the lung can be replaced by tumor (radiographically) and the dog may only be presented for signs indistinguishable from any metabolic disorder such as, weight loss, inappetence, and weakness. When present, respiratory complaints include cough, exercise intolerance, hemoptysis, tachypnea, and dyspnea.

25. How are pulmonary metastases distinguishable from primary lung neoplasms?

Most metastatic disease is presumptively diagnosed by finding lung lesions in concert with an aggressive-behaving tumor located somewhere else in the body (osteosarcoma, mammary gland carcinoma, hemangiosarcoma, oral melanoma). Primary lung tumors typically metastasize locally in the thorax first and then spread to distant sites. Histopathologic examination may help confirm the origin of the primary tumor.

26. How is pulmonary metastatic disease diagnosed?

Plain radiography underestimates the number of pulmonary metastases. CT is more sensitive and can detect smaller nodules and is the preferred imaging for metastasis screening in humans. magnetic resonance imaging may be more useful to delineate large masses from surrounding structures such as the mediastinum.

27. When pulmonary metastasis is suspected from evaluation of a survey radiograph and a primary tumor site cannot be readily identified, what other diseases should be considered?

Radiographic patterns of metastatic disease may not be different from other nodular respiratory diseases such as systemic fungal diseases (i.e., blastomycoses).

28. Does surgical resection of pulmonary metastatic nodules prolong life?

Identification of animals that might benefit from metastasectomy is based on features of the biologic behavior of the tumor and the response to previous therapy. Surgical resection of pulmonary metastasis in dogs with appendicular osteosarcoma treated with limb amputation and chemotherapy improved survival times in one study. Metastasectomy with the potential of complete resection is useful for dogs if they meet the criteria of fewer than three pulmonary nodules present on plain survey radiographs, tumor size has not doubled in a month, disease-free interval is longer than 300 days from the initial date of diagnosis, sufficient pulmonary parenchymal reserve, and no other evidence of metastatic disease.

29. Can systemic chemotherapy prolong survival when given after detection of pulmonary metastasis?

Doxorubicin has been shown to increase survival in dogs with pulmonary metastasis from mammary gland adenocarcinoma to a year. In a study of 45 dogs with appendicular osteosarcoma, sequential treatment with cisplatin, doxorubicin, and mitoxantrone chemotherapy was not effective for treatment of measurable metastatic disease in dogs. Diseases that arise in multiple sites simultaneously, such as lymphoma, which involves the lungs and other sites, can be treated effectively with combination chemotherapy protocols.

30. Is inhalation therapy helpful for control of pulmonary metastatic disease?

Therapeutic chemotherapy and cytokine immunotherapy delivered directly to the lungs via aerosol has resulted in complete and partial remission of pulmonary metastasis and increased survival times for dogs with a variety of histologic types.

31. How long does a dog live with pulmonary metastatic disease?

Dogs are generally euthanized within 3 months of diagnosis of parenchymal pulmonary metastasis; however, depending on the aggressiveness of the tumor and biologic behavior and morbidity, some dogs may not be euthanized for 6 to 8 months after metastasis is noted. Pulmonary metastasis is typically only associated with clinical signs when much of the parenchyma is involved or when a mass (lymph node or tumor) compresses the mainstem bronchi resulting in unrelenting cough. Most dogs with lymphoma have intrathoracic radiographic changes, some with pulmonary infiltrates. Only cranial mediastinal lymphadenomegaly was identified as having a negative impact on remission and survival times. Survival times should be commensurate with the chemotherapy protocol used.

BIBLIOGRAPHY

Affolter VK, Moore PF: Canine cutaneous and systemic histiocytosis: reactive histiocytosis of dermal dendritic cells. *Am J Dermatopathol* 22:40-48, 2000.

Affolter VK, Moore PF: Localized and disseminated histiocytic sarcoma of dendritic cell origin in dogs. *Vet Pathol* 39:74-83, 2002.

Baez JL, Sorenmo KU: Pulmonary and bronchial neoplasia, In King LG, editor: *Respiratory diseases in dogs and cats,* St Louis, 2004, Elsevier.

Barr FJ, Gibbs C, Brown PJ: The radiologic features of primary lung tumours in the dog: a review of 36 cases, *J Small Anim Pract* 27:493-505, 1986.

Berry CR, Moore PF, Thomas WP et al: Pulmonary lymphomatoid granulomatosis in seven dogs (1976-1987), *J Vet Int Med* 4:157-166, 1993.

Biller DS, Myer CW: Case examples demonstrating the clinical utility of obtaining both right and left lateral thoracic radiographs in small animals, *J Am Vet Med Assoc* 23:382-386, 1987.

Brodey RS: Hypertrophic osteoarthropathy in the dog: a clinicopathologic survey of 60 cases, *J Am Vet Med Assoc* 159:1242-1256, 1971.

Daly CM, Swalec-Tobias K, Tobias AH et al: Cardiopulmonary effects of intrathoracic insufflation in dogs, *J Am Anim Hosp Assoc* 38:515-520, 2002.

DeBerry JD, Norris CR, Sámii VF et al: Correlation between fine-needle aspiration cytopathology and histopathology of the lung in dogs and cats, *J Am Anim Hosp Assoc* 38:327-336, 2002.

De Rycke LM, Gielen IM, Polis I et al: Thoracoscopic anatomy of dogs positioned in lateral recumbency, *J Am Anim Hosp Assoc* 37:543-548, 2001.

Fitzgerald SK, Wolf DC, Carlton WW: Eight cases of canine lymphomatoid granulomatosis, *Vet Pathol* 28:241-245, 1991.

Fox LE, King RR: Cancers of the respiratory system. In Morrison WB, editor: *Cancer in dogs and cats,* 2004, Baltimore, Williams and Wilkins.

Hahn KA, Richardson RC, Knapp DW: Canine malignant mammary neoplasia: biological behavior, diagnosis, and treatment alternatives, *J Am Anim Hosp Assoc* 28:251-256, 1992.

Hawkins EC, Morrison WB, DeNicola DB et al: Cytologic analysis of bronchoalveolar lavage fluid from 47 dogs with multicentric malignant lymphoma, *J Am Vet Med Assoc* 203:1318-1425, 1993.

Johnson VS, Ramsey IK, Thompson H et al: Thoracic high-resolution computed tomography in the diagnosis of metastatic carcinoma, *J Small Anim Pract* 45:134-143, 2004.

Khannah C, Vail DM: Targeting the lung: preclinical and comparative evaluation of anticancer aerosols in dogs with naturally occurring cancers, *Curr Cancer Drug Targets* 3:265-273, 2003.

Kisseberth WC, MacEwen EG: Complications of cancer and its treatment. In Withrow SJ, MacEwen EG, editors: *Small animal clinical oncology,* ed 3, Philadelphia, 2001, WB Saunders.

Lang J, Wortman JA, Glickman LT et al: Sensitivity of radiographic detection of lung metastases in the dog, *Vet Radiol* 27:74-78, 1986.

Liptak JM, Monet E, Dernell WS et al: Pulmonary metastasectomy in the management of four dogs with hypertrophic osteopathy, *Vet Comp Oncol* 2:1-12, 2004.

Lora-Michiels M, Biller DS, Olsen D et al: The accessory lung lobe in thoracic disease: a case series and anatomical review, *J Am Anim Hosp Assoc* 39:452-458, 2003.

McNeil EA, Ogilvie GK, Powers BE et al: Evaluation of prognostic factors for dogs with primary lung tumors: 67 cases (1985-1992), *J Am Vet Med Assoc* 211:1422-1427, 1997.

Melhalf CJ, Leifer CE, Patnaik AM et al: Surgical treatment of primary pulmonary neoplasia in 15 dogs, *J Am Anim Hosp Assoc* 20:799-803, 1984.

Miles KG: A review of primary lung tumors in the dog and cat, *Vet Radiol Ultrasound* 29:122-128, 1989.

Miles KG, Lattimer JC, Jergens AE et al: A retrospective evaluation of the radiographic evidence of pulmonary metastatic disease on initial presentation in the dog, *Vet Radiol Ultrasound* 31:79-82, 1990.

O'Brien MG, Straw RC, Withrow SJ et al: Resection of pulmonary metastases in canine osteosarcoma: 36 cases (1983-1992), *Vet Surg* 22:105-109, 1993.

Ogilvie GK, Haschek WM, Withrow SJ et al: Classification of primary lung tumors in dogs: 210 cases (1975-1985), *J Am Vet Med Assoc* 195:106-108, 1989.

Ogilvie GK, Straw RC, Jameson VJ et al: Evaluation of single-agent chemotherapy for treatment of clinically evident osteosarcoma metastases in dogs: 45 cases (1987-1991), *J Am Vet Med Assoc* 202:304-306, 1993.

Ogilvie GK, Weigel RM, Haschek WM et al: Prognostic factors for tumor remission and survival in dogs after surgery for primary lung tumor: 76 cases (1975-1985), *J Am Vet Med Assoc* 195:109-112, 1989.

Ogilvie GK, Weigel RM, Haschek WM et al: Use of radiography in combination with computed tomography for the assessment of noncardiac thoracic disease in the dog and cat, *Vet Radiol Ultrasound* 46: 114-121, 2005.

Poirier VJ, Burgess KE, Adams WM et al: Toxicity, dosage, and efficacy of vinorelbine (Navelbine) in dogs with spontaneous neoplasia, *J Vet Int Med* 18:536-539, 2004.

Postorino NC, Wheeler SL, Park RD et al: A syndrome resembling lymphomatoid granulomatosis in the dog. *J Vet Int Med* 3:15-19, 1989.

Reichel JK, Wisner ER: Non-cardiac thoracic ultrasound in 75 feline and canine patients, *Vet Radiol Ultrasound* 41:154-162, 2000.

Reif JS, Dunn K, Ogilvie GK et al: Passive smoking and canine lung cancer risk, *Int J Epidemiol* 135:234-239, 1992.

Roudebush P, Green RA, Digilio KM: Percutaneous fine-needle aspiration biopsy of the lung in disseminated pulmonary disease, *J Am Anim Hosp Assoc* 17:109-116, 1981.

Schmidt ML, Rutteman GR, van Niel MH et al: Clinical and radiographic manifestations of canine malignant histiocytosis, *Vet Q* 15:117-120, 1993.

Shaiken LC, Evans SM, Goldschmidt MH: Radiographic findings in canine malignant histiocytosis, *Vet Radiol* 32:237-242, 1991.

Skorupski KA, Clifford CA, Paoloni MC et al: CCNU for the treatment of dogs with metastatic or disseminated histiocytic sarcoma. Proceedings of the twenty-third annual conference of the Veterinary Cancer Society, Madison, WI, 2003, p 36.

Smith KC, Day MJ, Shaw SC et al: Canine lymphomatoid granulomatosis and immunophenotypic analysis of three cases. *J Comp Pathol* 115:129-138, 1996.

Spugnini EP, Porrello A, Citro G et al: COX-2 overexpression in canine tumors: potential therapeutic targets in oncology, *Histol Histopathol* 20:1309-1312, 2005.

Stann SE, Bauer TG: Respiratory tract tumors, *Vet Clin North Am Small Animal Pract* 15:535-556, 1989.

Starrak GS, Berry CR, Page RL et al: Correlation between thoracic radiographic changes and remission/survival duration in 270 dogs with lymphosarcoma, *Vet Radiol Ultrasound* 38:411-418, 1997.

Stowalter JL, Lamb CR: Ultrasonography of noncardiac thoracic diseases in small animals, *J Am Vet Med Assoc* 195:514-520, 1989.

Suter PF, Carrig CB, O'Brien TR et al: Radiographic recognition of primary and metastatic pulmonary neoplasms of dogs and cats, *J Am Vet Radiol Soc* 15:3-25, 1974.

Teske E, Stokhof AA, van den Ingh TSGAM et al: Transthoracic needle aspiration biopsy of the lung in dogs with pulmonic diseases. *J Am Anim Hosp Assoc* 27:269-294, 1991.

Tidwell AS, Johnson KL: Computed tomography-guided percutaneous biopsy in the dog and cat: description of technique and preliminary evaluation in 14 patients, *Vet Radiol Ultrasound* 35:445-456, 1994.

Wisner ER, Pollard RE: Trends in veterinary cancer imaging. *Vet Comp Oncol* 2:49-74, 2004.

Withrow SJ: Lung cancer. In Withrow SJ, MacEwen EG, editors: *Small animal clinical oncology,* ed 3, Philadelphia, 2001, WB Saunders.

Wood EF, O'Brien RT, Young KM: Ultrasound-guided fine-needle aspiration of focal parenchymal lesions of the lung in dogs and cats. *J Vet Intern Med* 12:338-342, 1998.

Section IV
Endocrine Disease
Section Editor: David L. Panciera

25. Diabetes Mellitus
David L. Panciera

1. What is the cause of diabetes mellitus in the dog?

The cause in individual dogs is usually unknown and of little importance from a management standpoint, but it is important to note that most dogs with diabetes mellitus have an absolute deficiency of insulin caused by destruction of β-islet cells. Destruction of the islet cells is due to an autoimmune process in some dogs whereas other dogs presumably suffer islet cell destruction secondary to recurrent or chronic pancreatitis. Because either process leads to absolute deficiency of insulin, insulin administration is essential for management of diabetes mellitus in nearly all dogs. However, in some dogs diabetes mellitus results from insulin resistance secondary to hyperadrenocorticism or acromegaly, and treatment of the primary disorder may resolve the diabetes mellitus in these cases.

2. What clinical findings would be expected in a dog with diabetes mellitus?

Polyuria, polydipsia, polyphagia, and weight loss are the most common complaints in dogs found to have diabetes mellitus. Cataracts and blindness are sometimes the first problems noted by the dog's owner. Anorexia, vomiting, depression, and weakness are usually apparent in dogs with diabetes mellitus complicated by ketoacidosis. Common findings on the physical examination in such dogs include cataracts, hepatomegaly, and obesity. Rarely, peripheral neuropathy may result in weakness and hyporeflexia.

3. How is a diagnosis of diabetes mellitus confirmed?

Persistent fasting hyperglycemia and glycosuria in a dog with clinical signs of diabetes mellitus is adequate confirmation of the diagnosis. A blood glucose concentration above 250 to 300 mg/dl is diagnostic if clinical signs of diabetes are present.

4. What laboratory tests are appropriate, and what are the expected findings in a dog with newly diagnosed diabetes mellitus?

A complete blood count, serum biochemistries, urinalysis, and urine culture are recommended for initial evaluation of all dogs with newly diagnosed diabetes mellitus, in order to identify any concurrent illness or complications. The complete blood count is typically normal in dogs with uncomplicated diabetes. Serum biochemistries typically show, in addition to hyperglycemia, mild to moderate elevations of liver enzymes, hypercholesterolemia, and hypertriglyceridemia. Glycosuria is always found in dogs with diabetes mellitus, and ketonuria is present in more than 50% of diabetic dogs that do not have overt ketoacidosis. Urinary tract infections are common in dogs with diabetes, and because the urine sediment does not contain inflammatory cells in some cases, culturing urine for bacteria is recommended for all diabetic dogs.

5. **How should a dog with ketones in its urine but without other clinical evidence of diabetic ketoacidosis be treated?**

Ketonuria is a common finding at the time of diagnosis of diabetes mellitus. Unless there are clinical signs of diabetic ketoacidosis, no special treatment is indicated.

6. **What are the goals for treatment of diabetes mellitus in dogs?**

The goals are to reduce or eliminate clinical signs, prevent complications of diabetes mellitus, maintain euglycemia, and avoid hypoglycemia.

7. **What role does diet play in the management of diabetes mellitus in dogs?**

A high-fiber diet can be helpful in treating canine diabetes because it can minimize post-prandial increases in blood glucose and reduce insulin requirements in some cases. Diets high in simple carbohydrates, specifically semimoist foods, should be avoided. Feeding should coincide with insulin administration and/or peak insulin activity. If insulin is administered twice daily, the dog should be fed 50% of its daily caloric intake at the time of each injection. If insulin is administered once daily, 50% of the food should be fed at the time of injection and the balance 8 to 10 hours later.

8. **How does exercise affect management of diabetes in dogs?**

Exercise increases insulin delivery to and glucose utilization by the skeletal muscles, resulting in lowering of the blood glucose level. The blood glucose concentration can decrease rapidly and dramatically with exercise that is strenuous and prolonged, such as occurs with hunting. When strenuous exercise is planned, a reduction in the preexercise insulin dose to between 25% and 50% of normal is recommended, and a source of glucose should be available in case hypoglycemia occurs.

9. **Are oral hypoglycemic medications effective in dogs with diabetes mellitus?**

Oral hypoglycemic medications are not effective in diabetic dogs because most have negligible insulin secretion, so drugs that increase endogenous insulin secretion or cellular insulin sensitivity have inadequate treatment effects.

10. **What is the recommended protocol for initiating treatment for diabetes mellitus?**

The intermediate-acting insulins, lente insulins, and neutral protamine Hagedorn (NPH) insulins, are recommended for initial management of diabetes mellitus in dogs. The duration of action of lente insulin is slightly longer that of NPH insulin in some dogs. Although the structure of porcine insulin is identical to that of canine insulin, recombinant human insulin can be used successfully as well. Insulin analogues, such as glargine insulin, can be used in dogs, but advantages over other insulins have not been reported. The author currently recommends porcine lente insulin or human recombinant NPH insulin for initial treatment. Twice-daily administration of insulin provides better control than once-daily administration in most dogs, although once-daily insulin administration is effective in some dogs. Because insulin requirements vary considerably between individuals, a conservative initial dose of 0.5 U/kg is recommended. It is recommended that two to three blood samples be obtained 4 to 8 hours after the initial injection to evaluate for hypoglycemia. If hypoglycemia is not present, the dog is discharged to the owner after it has been ascertained that the owner has been thoroughly educated about the disease process, possible complications (cataracts, hypoglycemia), how to monitor the clinical response to insulin, and how to handle and administer insulin. An appointment to assess response to treatment is scheduled for approximately 1 week after discharge.

11. **What dose of insulin should be given if the dog does not eat at a normal feeding time?**

Because there are many reasons why a dog might not eat at a designated time, the insulin dosage should not be adjusted routinely based on failure to consume all of a single meal. However, if the owner notices signs that the dog is ill or food consumption is decreased for a subsequent meal, the dose of insulin should be reduced by 50%. The dose of insulin should not be skipped altogether unless hypoglycemia is suspected, because ketoacidosis may occur with the combination of lack of insulin, fasting, and possible concurrent illness.

12. How is the response to insulin treatment monitored?

A combination of clinical signs, physical examination findings, and blood glucose determinations is used to assess the response to treatment of diabetes in dogs. An observant owner is often able to assess the response to treatment by monitoring the dog's activity level, water consumption, urination, and strength. Assessments based on these observations have been shown to be similar in accuracy to assessments based on other measures. It is useful to have owners of diabetic dogs document their assessments on a standardized form, so they can provide a consistent and complete history of the dog's response to treatment. Stable or increasing body weight, improved quality of hair coat and skin, and improved muscle mass are indications of good control of blood glucose levels. Glucose curves are a very useful measure of how well the diabetes is controlled, but do have some limitations. Stress response or inappetance can invalidate the glucose curve and there is substantial variation from day to day in an individual dog, so the information gained from a glucose curve must be interpreted in light of other measures of glycemic control.

Follow-up visits are scheduled for the morning. For the initial follow-up visit, the owner is instructed to feed the dog as usual but to wait to administer the insulin injection until the office visit. At the visit, the owner administers insulin under observation by the veterinarian or technician, so that any problems with insulin handling and injection can be addressed. For subsequent follow-up visits, the owner is instructed to feed the dog and administer the insulin at home as usual prior to the appointment. A blood glucose curve is obtained by measuring blood glucose concentration every 2 hours for 8 to 12 hours after administration of insulin. Most handheld glucometers are sufficiently accurate for this purpose, and the stress of obtaining the sample can be minimized by using a lancet to collect capillary blood from the inner surface of the pinna. Some owners may be able to perform this procedure at home, but substantial training is necessary to ensure accurate results.

13. What role does monitoring urine glucose levels have in the management of diabetes mellitus in dogs?

Monitoring urine glucose levels can aid in identifying dogs with poorly controlled diabetes and may aid in detecting hypoglycemia before it becomes severe enough to cause symptoms, but it should not be used as the sole criterion for adjusting insulin dosage. Insulin-induced hyperglycemia (Somogyi phenomenon) can result in prolonged hyperglycemia following hypoglycemia subsequent to an insulin overdose. The resultant glycosuria will not be distinguishable from hyperglycemia associated with an insulin dose that is too low. If the insulin dosage is adjusted based on the presence of glycosuria, hypoglycemia may be worsened in dogs with insulin-induced hyperglycemia. A negative result of testing urine for glucose does not necessarily mean that the insulin dosage needs to be reduced, because when diabetes is well-controlled there should be little or no glucose in the urine.

14. What can be learned about blood glucose control by evaluating a glucose curve?

The blood glucose concentration at its nadir and the duration of effect of the insulin are the most important information that can be learned from a glucose curve. The nadir is the lowest glucose concentration obtained during the sampling and ideally should be between 100 and 150 mg/dl. If the nadir is below 80 to 100 mg/dl, the insulin dose should be reduced and if it is greater than 150 mg/dl the insulin dose should be increased. The amount by which the insulin dose should be altered depends on the degree to which the nadir varies from the ideal. If the nadir is higher than desired, an increase in the insulin dose by 1 to 3 units is indicated.

The duration of insulin effect is the time that the blood glucose concentration remains below 250 mg/dl. The optimal duration of effect for a dog receiving once-daily insulin injections is 22 to 26 hours, while the ideal duration with twice-daily dosing is 10 to 14 hours. If the duration of effect is inadequate, administration of a longer-acting insulin is necessary. If the duration of effect of insulin administered once daily is inadequate, administering that insulin twice daily is usually sufficient. When switching from once- to twice-daily insulin administration, the once-daily dose should be reduced by 25%. Lente insulin can be administered if NPH insulin is of insufficient duration. If lente insulin administered twice daily has too short a duration of effect, protamine zinc insulin (PZI) or ultralente insulin may be administered. About 1 week after a change in insulin dose or formulation, another assessment of clinical signs should be performed and a glucose curve should be obtained and the dosage of insulin should be adjusted if necessary, as just described.

15. Under what circumstances is it important to attempt "strict" control of blood glucose concentrations?

Dogs without cataracts or those with early cataracts but are still visual may benefit from treatment that maintains blood glucose concentrations between 80 and 100 mg/dl at the nadir and 150 to 200 mg/dl at the zenith. This "strict" degree of control may slow cataract formation and will, in most cases, resolve diabetic neuropathy. Because the risk of hypoglycemia is higher with stricter control of blood glucose, this degree of control is recommended primarily for dogs for whom preservation of vision is desired.

16. What might explain discrepancies between the clinical signs and glucose curve values?

Discrepancies are often due to improper storage or mixing of insulin, errors in insulin dosage or administration, use of the wrong insulin preparation, or an inappropriate feeding schedule. Such "owner-induced" problems should be ruled out first. Stress frequently causes an elevation of blood glucose concentration, so a glucose curve obtained while the dog is under stress may be invalid. If stress is thought to have had a significant effect on blood glucose values, greater reliance can be placed on clinical signs, urine glucose measurements, the results of at-home glucose monitoring, and measurement of serum fructosamine concentration. Fasting is probably the most important cause of low blood glucose concentration in a dog that is actually well controlled in the home environment. However, many dogs that become hypoglycemic at some point during the day will not show clinical signs of hypoglycemia that are recognized by the owner. The inherent variability in insulin absorption from subcutaneous injection sites can contribute to a discrepancy between the clinical response to insulin and values on a single glucose curve. It should be noted that glucose curves are imperfect measures of glycemic control. For this reason, clinicians should always attempt to correlate clinical signs with values on blood glucose curves, but perfect correlation should not be expected.

17. How accurately do serum fructosamine and glycosylated hemoglobin concentrations reflect control of diabetes mellitus?

All proteins undergo nonenzymatic glycation, the degree of which is dependent on the plasma glucose concentration over the life of the protein. Fructosamine consists of glycosylated plasma proteins, primarily albumin, that form for the duration that the protein is circulating (approximately 10 days for albumin), while hemoglobin is glycosylated over the lifespan of an erythrocyte (100-120 days). Transient elevations in blood glucose concentration have minimal impact on the concentrations of these glycosylated proteins, so theoretically, the concentrations of glycosylated proteins reflect the mean glucose concentration over the life spans of the proteins. Unfortunately there is considerable overlap in the ranges of fructosamine and glycosylated hemoglobin concentrations in well-controlled and in poorly controlled diabetics, which limits the usefulness of these values as measures of long-term glycemic control. In addition, glycated protein values provide no information about episodes of hypoglycemia. The fructosamine value is used more frequently in veterinary medicine as a measure of long-term glycemic control because tests to determine this value are readily available. Measurements of fructosamine concentration are useful when a valid glucose curve cannot be obtained but must be interpreted in light of other findings.

18. **What are some alternatives for evaluating glycemic control when a valid blood glucose curve cannot be obtained in the hospital because the animal becomes stressed during hospitalization?**

    Measurements of glycosylated hemoglobin and fructosamine, a careful history, and the physical examination all provide useful information about glycemic control. Measurements of urine glucose concentration are generally not recommended because they only detect hyperglycemia. Because hyperglycemia can be induced by insulin overdose (hypoglycemia induces release of counterregulatory hormones and that causes an increase in glucose concentration, resulting in the Somogyi phenomenon), glycosuria does not always indicate a need for an increase in the dosage of insulin.

    Another alternative to obtaining a glucose curve in the hospital is for the owner to obtain the glucose curve at home using a lancet device and a handheld glucometer. The lancet is used to puncture the pinnae, and when a droplet of blood forms, a glucometer strip is touched to the droplet. The blood is taken up by capillary action into the glucometer strip, and the glucose concentration is determined. With proper training, many owners are capable of obtaining glucose curves at home using this method.

19. **Are handheld glucometers accurate enough to use for monitoring blood glucose in diabetics?**

    The performance of a number of glucometers has been evaluated, and most have sufficient accuracy to be used to monitor blood glucose in diabetic dogs. Many instruments tend to underestimate the blood glucose concentration, with this effect becoming more apparent as the blood glucose increases. To estimate the size of the discrepancy, it is recommended that blood glucose be measured concurrently in several blood samples using the glucometer and a standard laboratory technique. Comparing the results over a range of values will allow users of the handheld glucometers to predict the discrepancy between the methods.

20. **What causes should be considered initially and what diagnostic approach should be taken when a diabetic dog is difficult to control?**

    The first step is to evaluate for owner-induced problems such as problems with insulin administration, insulin storage, insulin dosage, dispensation of the wrong type of insulin, feeding inappropriate foods or problems with the feeding schedule. The next step is evaluation for concurrent disease, particularly urinary tract infection (often clinically silent in diabetics). A thorough history and physical examination and basic laboratory studies (CBC, serum chemistry, urinalysis, and urine culture) are recommended, with further testing as appropriate based on the results of these initial tests.

    An 8- to 10-hour glucose curve should be obtained when diabetes is difficult to control. The glucose curve is useful for two reasons; first, it can confirm that the blood glucose level is poorly controlled, and second, it can demonstrate the duration of action of insulin and whether the dose is too high or too low. Insulin overdose can result in clinical signs similar to those of underdosing, because the counterregulatory response to hypoglycemia is marked hyperglycemia and glycosuria, leading to polyuria and polydipsia. Therefore it is crucial to obtain a blood glucose curve in every case. If the duration of action of insulin is shorter than 10 hours, the insulin preparation should be changed. Occasionally, poor absorption of insulin may cause an inadequate response, and administration of a different insulin preparation should be attempted if this is suspected.

21. What is the best approach to evaluating a dog that has developed insulin resistance?

Insulin resistance has been arbitrarily defined as inadequate control of blood glucose in a dog being administered insulin doses higher than 1.5 U/kg after ruling out owner-induced problems, short duration of action of insulin, insulin-induced hyperglycemia, and poor absorption. A careful history, including a drug history, should be obtained. Owners should be questioned specifically regarding treatment with progestins or corticosteroids, including topical and ophthalmic preparations, which can cause insulin resistance. Intact female dogs will have increased secretion of growth hormone in response to high levels of progesterone, such as occur with metestrus and for this reason, it is recommended that all female dogs with diabetes undergo ovariohysterectomy.

Concurrent disease is the most common cause of insulin resistance, so a thorough evaluation of the dog is necessary. Urinary tract infection, pancreatitis, and hyperadrenocorticism are perhaps the most common problems, but virtually any disease can cause insulin resistance. At a minimum, urinalysis and urine culture are indicated in most cases. Evaluation of adrenal function should be considered, particularly if there are clinical or laboratory signs of abnormal function such as a marked increase in serum alkaline phosphatase activity. The ACTH response test is preferred over the low-dose dexamethasone suppression test (LDDST) for evaluation of adrenal function because the former is less frequently affected by nonadrenal illness. Abdominal ultrasound should be considered if pyelonephritis, pancreatitis, hepatic disease, or another intraabdominal disorder is suspected. Thoracic radiographs to identify neoplasia or pulmonary infection should be performed if indicated by findings. Thyroid function should be evaluated in some cases as hypothyroidism causes insulin resistance. In rare cases, antiinsulin antibodies might cause insulin resistance.

22. What considerations should be given to the cause of hypoglycemia in a dog being treated for diabetes mellitus and how should insulin treatment be changed to avoid future problems?

Hypoglycemia as a consequence of insulin administration is a common problem in diabetic dogs. Owners should be well-educated regarding the signs of hypoglycemia. However, clinical signs of hypoglycemia are not always apparent, either because they occur when the animal is not observed or because the animal does not have a normal physiologic response to hypoglycemia. Predisposing factors for hypoglycemia in a dog with previously well-controlled diabetes mellitus include accidental overdose of insulin; fasting; excessive exercise; recent initiation of levothyroxine treatment for hypothyroidism; anesthesia and surgery; resolution of acute illness, especially hyperadrenocorticism, pancreatitis, or urinary tract infection; and resolution of a high-progesterone state.

Symptomatic hypoglycemia should be documented by measurement of blood glucose concentration. Treatment should be instituted as necessary, including feeding dog food, oral administration of a dextrose solution, or intravenous administration of dextrose and withholding insulin until persistent hyperglycemia is documented when the dog is no longer receiving glucose supplementation. It may require 48 hours or longer for the hypoglycemic effects of an insulin overdose to resolve. When insulin is restarted after such an episode, the starting dose is generally 50% of the previous dose if the hypoglycemia resulted in clinical signs. The blood glucose concentration should be measured every 2 hours for at least 8 hours after the first insulin dose is administered, to avoid recurrent hypoglycemia. Future dosage adjustments are made based on clinical signs and glucose curves. The dose reduction may be considerably less if hypoglycemia was asymptomatic and detected on a routine glucose curve.

DIABETIC KETOACIDOSIS

23. What factors play an important role in the development of diabetic ketoacidosis (DKA)?

Insulin resistance induced by counterregulatory hormones, fasting, a lack of insulin, and dehydration are necessary for development of DKA. Concurrent illness is often a factor in DKA because it causes insulin resistance and frequently anorexia. Severe hyperglycemia and ketone body production cause marked osmotic diuresis, which leads to dehydration and loss of sodium, potassium, and phosphate.

24. How is a diagnosis of DKA established?

Clinical signs of diabetes mellitus, including polydipsia, polyphagia, and weight loss, are usually present in a dog with DKA but are not always noted by the owner. Lethargy, anorexia, and vomiting are common in cases of DKA and may be related to the ketoacidosis or a concurrent illness (urinary tract infection, pancreatitis, hepatic or renal disease, neoplasia). Common findings on physical examination of a dog with DKA include thin body condition, dehydration, depression, hepatomegaly, tachypnea, and an acetone odor to the breath. The diagnosis of DKA is confirmed by finding ketonuria in a diabetic dog with compatible clinical signs. The presence of ketonuria without systemic illness (other than diabetes) is not diagnostic of DKA.

25. What laboratory studies are needed to evaluate DKA in a dog?

Because concurrent illness is common in dogs with DKA, the choice of laboratory studies should be directed by findings on the history and physical examination. A complete blood count, serum chemistry studies, urinalysis, and urine culture are indicated in the initial evaluation of all dogs with DKA. Abnormalities on the CBC are due primarily to concurrent diseases. Hyperglycemia, elevated liver enzymes, and hypercholesterolemia are likely in any dog with diabetes mellitus, whether or not DKA is present. Prerenal azotemia is often present in dehydrated dogs. Almost all dogs with DKA have deficiencies in potassium, sodium, and phosphate. These electrolyte deficiencies may initially be masked by dehydration and other factors and only become apparent after the start of treatment. Metabolic acidosis with a high anion gap is also present. Other abnormalities, such as elevated amylase and lipase levels, may be found depending on what concurrent illnesses are present. Glycosuria and ketonuria will be evident on urinalysis, and urinary tract infection is common although this will not always become apparent from examination of urine sediment, so urine culture is indicated in most cases.

26. How should the dehydration and electrolyte abnormalities common in dogs with diabetic ketoacidosis be treated?

The mainstays of treatment for DKA are intravenous (IV) fluid therapy and insulin administration. Both treatments, although essential to treat DKA, can promote hyponatremia, hypokalemia, and hypophosphatemia. The goals of IV fluid treatment are to replace volume deficits, improve tissue perfusion, replace electrolyte deficiencies, and lower the blood glucose concentration. The IV fluid of choice is 0.9% saline administered at a rate that corrects half the fluid deficits within the first 6 hours, and the remaining deficits over the next 18 hours in addition to supplying maintenance fluid requirements. Urine production should be monitored; an increase in production is to be expected within the first several hours. Failure to produce the expected volume of urine could indicate an underestimation of the magnitude of dehydration or oliguric renal failure. Because rehydration will decrease the plasma potassium concentration, potassium supplementation should be given if urine output is adequate within the first 4 hours. Ideally, the serum potassium level should be measured after 4 to 6 hours of treatment and the dose of supplemental potassium based on the results, but if serum potassium was not measured, 40 mEq of potassium chloride should be added to each liter of saline. If the serum potassium concentration is measured, the following guidelines can be used to determine the supplementation dose: serum potassium concentration less than 3.5 mEq/L, add supplement at a concentration of 20 mEq/L; potassium 3.0 to 3.5, add 30 mEq/L; potassium 2.5 to 3.0, add 40 mEq/L; 2.0-2.5, add 60 mEq/L; and potassium less than 2.0, add 80 mEq/L. The potassium supplementation rate should never exceed 0.5 mEq/kg/hour. Electrolytes should be monitored every 8 to 12 hours if possible, and potassium and sodium supplementation should be adjusted based on the results. If hypernatremia occurs, the saline infusion should be stopped and lactated Ringer's solution or 0.45% saline with 2.5% dextrose should be started.

Hypophosphatemia is a relatively common consequence of administering IV fluids and insulin to dogs with DKA. Severe hypophosphatemia (phosphate <1.0 mg/dl) can cause hemolysis, muscle weakness, respiratory depression, cardiac dysfunction, and decreased tissue delivery of oxygen. Phosphate should be supplemented when the serum phosphorus concentration is less than 1.0 to 1.5 mg/dl. Potassium phosphate should be administered at 0.01 to 0.03 mmol/kg of phosphate, which will also replace part of the potassium deficit. Potential side effects include hypocalcemia and soft tissue mineralization.

27. What is a safe and effective insulin administration regimen in a dog with DKA?

The goals of insulin administration are to gradually decrease the blood glucose concentration without inducing hypoglycemia, to halt ketone body formation and increase ketone metabolism, and to decrease lipolysis and protein catabolism. It is neither necessary nor desirable to reduce the blood glucose concentration to the normal range during management of DKA. A gradual reduction in blood glucose is desirable to prevent hypoglycemia and to reduce the likelihood of rapid decreases in plasma potassium and phosphate.

A low-dose intravenous infusion of regular insulin is probably the safest and most effective regimen for administration of insulin to a dog with DKA, provided appropriate monitoring can be provided. The recommended initial insulin dose is 2.2 U/kg over 24 hours (0.09 U/kg/hour) IV. The infusion solution is prepared by adding the daily dose of regular insulin (in units per kilogram) to 250 ml of 0.9% NaCl solution for IV infusion and administering the infusion at a rate of 10 ml/hour through an infusion pump. Before beginning the infusion, allow 50 ml of the infusate to flow through the IV administration set because insulin adheres to plastic. The blood glucose concentration should be monitored hourly and the insulin infusion rate adjusted based on these results. The goal is to maintain the blood glucose concentration between 200 and 300 mg/dl. When the blood glucose concentration reaches 250 mg/dl, and with each subsequent drop of 50 mg/dl, the infusion rate of the insulin solution should be decreased and the IV fluids being administered concurrently should be changed as follows:

Blood glucose concentration (mg/dl)	IV solution for rehydration and maintenance	Rate of infusion (IV solution with insulin dose added) (ml/hour)
>250	0.9% saline	10
200-250	0.45% saline, 2.5% dextrose	7
150-200	0.45% saline, 2.5% dextrose	5
100-150	0.45% saline, 5% dextrose	5
<100	0.45% saline, 5% dextrose	stop insulin infusion

Insulin treatment of DKA can also be accomplished by administering regular insulin intramuscularly (IM) at an initial dose of 0.2 U/kg, followed by hourly injections of 0.1 U/kg. Treatment is continued at that dose until the blood glucose concentration is less than 250 mg/dl (measured hourly prior to each treatment) or the glucose concentration is decreasing at the rate of more than 100 mg/dl/hour. When the blood glucose concentration becomes less than 250 mg/dl, start administering regular insulin, 0.1 to 0.4 U/kg IM every 4 to 6 hours. Blood glucose should be monitored at least every 2 hours and the dose and frequency of insulin injection adjusted to maintain a blood glucose concentration of 200 to 300 mg/dl. Dextrose should be added to the IV fluids to a final concentration of 5% dextrose when the blood glucose is less than 250 mg/dl with the rate adjusted to maintain the blood glucose at 200 to 300 mg/dl. Low-dose IM insulin treatment requires more procedural time than the IV protocol, making it more cumbersome in a busy clinic.

High-dose IM insulin is another option for treatment of DKA. Regular insulin, 0.25 to 0.5 U/kg is administered IM every 4 hours, and blood glucose is monitored every 2 to 4 hours. When the blood glucose drops below 250 mg/dl, 5% dextrose is administered at a rate of 60 ml/kg/hour, and the dosage of insulin is adjusted to maintain the blood glucose between 200 and 300 mg/dl. While this treatment may be simple, it carries a higher risk of hypoglycemia and hypokalemia because the glucose concentration may decrease more rapidly than is optimal.

28. Is it necessary to treat the acidosis associated with DKA by administering sodium bicarbonate?

The acidosis of DKA usually resolves during IV fluid therapy and insulin administration, making specific treatment of the acidosis with bicarbonate unnecessary in most cases. Administration of sodium bicarbonate should be reserved for dogs with a documented blood pH below 7.0 or a total CO_2 of less than 10 mEq/L. Side effects of sodium bicarbonate administration include worsening of hypokalemia, paradoxical central nervous system (CNS) acidosis, and reduced ketone body metabolism. If treatment is indicated, the dose of sodium bicarbonate (in milliequivalents per liter) is calculated as follows:

$$\text{Body weight (kg)} \times (24 - \text{patient bicarbonate in mEq/L}) \times 0.4 \times 0.25.$$

The factor 0.25 is included because only 25% of the bicarbonate deficit should be administered initially. Subsequent treatment is determined by blood gas analysis following bicarbonate treatment.

29. When can an intermediate or long-acting insulin be administered to a dog with ketoacidosis?

When the dog's condition has been stable for at least 24 hours and the dog is eating, regular insulin can be discontinued and an insulin preparation with a longer duration of action can be administered.

30. What is the prognosis for a dog with diabetic ketoacidosis?

When intensive treatment for DKA is provided, the prognosis is probably more closely related to any concurrent disease than to DKA itself. Therefore, aggressive diagnostic testing should be performed early in the course of treatment for DKA to diagnose underlying disorders. Overall, approximately 70% of dogs with DKA will survive.

26. Hypoadrenocorticism

David L. Panciera

1. What are the causes of hypoadrenocorticism?

The most common cause of hypoadrenocorticism is idiopathic destruction of the adrenal cortex. The resulting primary hypoadrenocorticism causes glucocorticoid and mineralocorticoid deficiencies. Primary hypoadrenocorticism can also develop secondary to excessive mitotane administration. Secondary hypoadrenocorticism, which causes a deficiency of glucocorticoid hormone production only, results from decreased secretion of adrenocorticotropic hormone (ACTH) and is most common following withdrawal of long-term glucocorticoid or progestin treatment. Atypical hypoadrenocorticism, an uncommon variant of idiopathic primary hypoadrenocorticism, occurs when only glucocorticoid secretion is impaired.

2. What are the common clinical signs of hypoadrenocorticism?

Hypoadrenocorticism is typically seen in young to middle-aged dogs, with a predisposition for females. In the acute form of hypoadrenocorticism (Addisonian or hypoadrenocortical crisis), weakness, dehydration, weak pulses, collapse, diarrhea, and shaking are often present. Weakness, dehydration, hypothermia, bradycardia, and melena are common physical examination findings.

Clinical signs of more chronic hypoadrenocorticism are weakness, dehydration, hypothermia, bradycardia, and melena, but in milder form than is seen with acute disease. Other findings in dogs with chronic hypoadrenocorticism include weight loss, polyuria, and polydipsia. Typically, the clinical signs follow a waxing and waning course. The dog may have a history of previous nondescript illness that responded to supportive treatment. The finding of bradycardia or a lower than expected heart rate in a dog with dehydration and weak pulses should lead to a suspicion of hyperkalemia.

3. What routine laboratory test abnormalities would be expected in a dog with hypoadrenocorticism?

Hyperkalemia and hyponatremia are present in almost all cases of primary hypoadrenocorticism. Hypochloremia is also usually present. Metabolic acidosis is common and may be severe. Elevated blood urea nitrogen (BUN), creatinine, and phosphorus concentrations are common and may be marked in cases of prerenal azotemia. Mild to moderate hypercalcemia is common. Hypoglycemia is fairly common and the blood glucose level may be low enough to cause clinical signs. Hypoproteinemia and hypoalbuminemia are frequent findings, particularly after rehydration. Mild nonregenerative anemia is the most common abnormality identified from the results of a complete blood count (CBC). Lymphocytosis and eosinophilia may be present in some cases, but often cell counts are normal. The absence of a stress leukogram in an ill dog is another laboratory finding suggestive of hypoadrenocorticism. Another important laboratory finding is a urine specific gravity that is lower (<1.030) than expected in a dog with dehydration and azotemia.

4. Is it possible for a dog without electrolyte abnormalities to have hypoadrenocorticism?

Dogs with atypical hypoadrenocorticism have glucocorticoid deficiency but not electrolyte abnormalities. Clinical signs in these cases include lethargy, weight loss, vomiting, diarrhea, melena, polyuria, polydipsia, regurgitation (due to megaesophagus), weakness, and collapse or seizures related to hypoglycemia; bradycardia is not present. Often these dogs have normal stress leukograms and no evidence of nonregenerative anemia, hypocholesterolemia, hypoalbuminemia, or hypoglycemia. A diagnosis of atypical hypoadrenocorticism requires a high index of suspicion and often is arrived at only after extensive testing fails to identify a primary gastrointestinal or systemic disorder.

5. What electrocardiographic abnormalities occur in dogs in acute hypoadrenocortical crisis?

Electrocardiographic (ECG) abnormalities in dogs with hyperkalemia include bradycardia, prolonged PR interval, evidence of atrial standstill (lack of visible P waves), prolonged QRS duration, high T-wave amplitude, low R-wave amplitude, and evidence of heart block. Atrial standstill and marked prolongation of QRS duration indicate severe hyperkalemia.

6. Why is it necessary to confirm a diagnosis of hypoadrenocorticism using an ACTH response test in a dog with compatible clinical signs, hyperkalemia, and hyponatremia?

A low sodium:potassium ratio (<23) can result from many causes, particularly renal failure; urinary tract obstruction or rupture; gastrointestinal disorders, including pancreatitis and intestinal parasitism; neoplasia; and pleural effusion. These disorders result in clinical signs and diagnostic test results similar to those seen in cases of hypoadrenocorticism. Treatment of hypoadrenocorticism requires lifelong mineralocorticoid and glucocorticoid supplementation, which is quite costly. Therefore an ACTH response test should be performed in all cases to confirm the diagnosis.

7. **Vomiting, diarrhea, lethargy, and dehydration can be due to many disorders; what should lead to the suspicion that they are due to hypoadrenocorticism?**

Absence of a stress leukogram in an ill dog and the presence of nonregenerative anemia, electrolyte and other serum chemistry abnormalities, and poorly concentrated urine all support a diagnosis of hypoadrenocorticism. Atypical hypoadrenocorticism is more difficult to diagnose. If routine diagnostic testing fails to identify a cause for a nonspecific illness, particularly one accompanied by any combination of vomiting, diarrhea, weight loss, hypoalbuminemia, hypocholesterolemia, and hypoglycemia, an ACTH response test should be performed.

8. **How is a diagnosis of hypoadrenocorticism confirmed?**

The diagnosis of hypoadrenocorticism is confirmed by finding a low plasma cortisol concentration at baseline and following the administration of ACTH (ACTH response test). The ACTH response test protocol is identical to that used for diagnosis of hyperadrenocorticism. Most dogs with hypoadrenocorticism have low plasma cortisol concentrations and no response to ACTH, although a few dogs will have a slight response. Dogs with iatrogenic hypoadrenocorticism resulting from withdrawal of long-term glucocorticoid administration will also have a suppressed response. The ACTH response test should be performed prior to glucocorticoid administration (unless dexamethasone is administered), because recent administration of most glucocorticoid agents, with the exception of dexamethasone, will cause a false elevation in cortisol concentration and thus a false-positive result on the ACTH response test.

9. **What is the most appropriate fluid therapy for a dog suspected of having hypoadrenocorticism?**

Intravenous (IV) administration of 0.9% saline at rate of 40 to 80 ml/kg/hour for the first 1 to 2 hours is recommended to replace the fluid deficit and to reduce plasma potassium concentrations by dilution and increasing urinary losses. Fluid therapy can then be continued at one to two times maintenance rates. Urine output should be monitored to ensure that the animal does not have oliguric renal failure and to identify animals at risk for overhydration.

10. **Is any specific treatment required to reduce the effects of the hyperkalemia?**

The plasma potassium concentration typically decreases rapidly during intravenous administration of saline. If hyperkalemia is severe and death due to cardiac arrhythmia seems eminent or if signs of hyperkalemia fail to respond rapidly to fluid therapy, the effects of hyperkalemia on the myocardium may be antagonized by administration of sodium bicarbonate to correct acidosis and enhance K^+ transport into cells; another choice is to administer calcium gluconate (10% solution; 0.5 to 1 ml/kg IV over 10 minutes). Alternatively, a combination of glucose and insulin can be administered. In this case, total doses of 0.5 U/kg regular insulin and 3 g of glucose/unit of insulin are divided in half; half of each dose should be given as a bolus and the remainder should be added to the intravenous fluid solution and administered over 6 hours.

11. **What hormone is most appropriate for a dog in adrenocortical crisis?**

Hydrocortisone is preferable because it has both mineralocorticoid and glucocorticoid activity. Hydrocortisone sodium succinate should be administered as a constant-rate infusion (0.3 mg/kg/hour IV) or in IV boluses of 2 mg/kg every 6 hours. Alternatively, prednisolone sodium succinate (1-2 mg/kg IV) or dexamethasone sodium phosphate (0.2-0.4 mg/kg IV) can be administered. Mineralocorticoid supplementation is generally reserved for dogs with a diagnosis of hypoadrenocorticism confirmed by an ACTH response test. Oral administration of glucocorticoid and mineralocorticoid hormones can be instituted on the first day of treatment in many cases.

12. **How should a dog with the chronic form of hypoadrenocorticism be treated initially?**

If a dog is not dehydrated and does not have severe electrolyte abnormalities, aggressive intravenous treatment is not necessary. These dogs can be managed as outpatients by oral administration of mineralocorticoid and glucocorticoid agents. All dogs should initially receive the glucocorticoid prednisone, 0.4 mg/kg daily. Then the prednisone dosage should be slowly tapered to the lowest dose that prevents signs of illness. These dogs should be monitored closely by their owners and reevaluated if improvement is not noted within 2 to 3 days of starting therapy or if signs worsen. Some dogs with chronic hypoadrenocorticism will require fluid therapy and parenteral glucocorticoid supplementation.

13. Is desoxycorticosterone pivalate (DOCP) better than fludrocortisone for long-term treatment of hypoadrenocorticism?

Either drug can be used successfully for chronic management of hypoadrenocorticism. The choice is often a matter of convenience and expense. Fludrocortisone acetate (Florinef) is administered orally at an initial dose of 0.01 mg/kg twice daily. Serum electrolyte concentrations are measured every 1 to 2 weeks and the dosage is adjusted based on the results. When the dose that maintains electrolyte concentrations within normal ranges is found, the serum chemistry should be rechecked every 3 to 4 months, because some dogs will require a higher dose to maintain the response to chronic treatment. Adding NaCl (0.1 g/kg/day) to the treatment regimen can be useful in reducing the dose of fludrocortisone, maintaining a serum sodium concentration in the normal range, and perhaps reducing the severity of polyuria and polydipsia, which can be a problem in some dogs receiving fludrocortisone.

Desoxycorticosterone pivalate (DOCP; Percorten-V) is a repositol form of mineralocorticoid that is slowly released over a period of about 3 to 4 weeks. The initial dose is 2.2 mg/kg administered intramuscularly (IM) or subcutaneously (SQ). Serum electrolyte and BUN concentrations should be measured 2, 3, and 4 weeks after the initial treatment until the appropriate dose and frequency of administration are determined. If electrolyte concentrations are abnormal 2 weeks after the initial treatment, the next dose should be adjusted (increased if hyperkalemia and hyponatremia are present and decreased if the opposite conditions are found) by about 10%. The electrolyte concentrations measured 3 and 4 weeks after beginning therapy provide information about the duration of treatment effects and thus are used to determine the frequency of medication administration. On average, DOCP should be administered every 25 days.

14. Is glucocorticoid supplementation necessary when fludrocortisone or desoxycorticosterone pivalate is used?

Not all dogs treated with fludrocortisone require glucocorticoid treatment in addition to the fludrocortisone; in dogs receiving fludrocortisone, the dosage of prednisone can be gradually tapered over a 6-week period and discontinued if signs of illness do not occur. DOCP does not have glucocorticoid activity, so all dogs being treated with this mineralocorticoid should also receive prednisone or another glucocorticoid medication. Prednisone should be administered at a dose of 0.4 to 0.6 mg/kg if an animal is ill, has surgery, or experiences another type of stress.

15. What is the recommended treatment for a dog with atypical hypoadrenocorticism?

Prednisone is the only treatment necessary in these cases. Prednisone should be administered at a dosage of 0.4 mg/kg daily. After 2 to 4 weeks the dosage may be reduced to 0.2 mg/kg, and if symptoms do not recur, the dosage may be decreased further after 2 to 4 weeks of treatment at the lower dosage.

27. Hyperadrenocorticism

David L. Panciera

1. What are the causes of hyperadrenocorticism?

Hyperadrenocorticism is a syndrome characterized by clinical and biochemical changes related to a state of glucocorticoid excess. It can be caused by an adrenocortical neoplasm (adrenal dependent hyperadrenocorticism [ADH]), by excessive production of adrenocorticotropic hormone (ACTH) by a pituitary tumor or pituitary hyperplasia (pituitary-dependent hyperadrenocorticism [PDH]), or as a result of glucocorticoid administration (iatrogenic). Adrenal tumors are found in 15% to 20% of cases and the remaining 80% to 85% of dogs with spontaneous hyperadrenocorticism have PDH.

2. What clinical signs are associated with hyperadrenocorticism?

A history of polyuria and polydipsia is reported in more than 75% of dogs with hyperadrenocorticism. Polyphagia is also frequently noted. Changes in the integument are common, and include bilaterally symmetrical alopecia, thin hair coat, slow hair regrowth after clipping, hyperpigmentation, thin skin, comedones, calcinosis cutis, and seborrhea. Dogs with hyperadrenocorticism are prone to recurrent pyoderma and *Malassezia* infection. An enlarged, pendulous abdomen also is common, occurring because of muscle weakness and hepatomegaly. Mild to moderate obesity with distribution of fat to the trunk also alters the dog's appearance. Weakness and lethargy are often noted. Excessive panting also occurs in some dogs.

3. What clinical signs would be associated with a pituitary macroadenoma?

Behavioral changes, dullness, pacing, ataxia, tetraparesis, circling, blindness, and seizures are the predominant clinical findings in addition to the typical signs of hyperadrenocorticism that are usually present.

4. What abnormalities of routine laboratory tests would be expected in a dog with hyperadrenocorticism?

Nonspecific findings on a complete blood count may include mild erythrocytosis and stress leukogram. An elevated serum alkaline phosphatase (ALP) activity is found in most dogs with hyperadrenocorticism. This is primarily the steroid isoenzyme and the degree of elevation may be marked. Serum alanine aminotransferase (ALT) activity may also be elevated, but this is a less consistent finding and the elevation is not as great as for ALP. Hypercholesterolemia and mild hyperglycemia are common. Urine specific gravity usually indicates isosthenuria or hyposthenuria. Proteinuria may be present secondary to glomerular leakage or infection.

5. Is it necessary to culture urine of dogs with hyperadrenocorticism if the urinalysis shows an inactive sediment?

Urinary tract infection is found in about 50% of dogs with hyperadrenocorticism, and most dogs do not have clinical signs associated with the infection. In addition, pyuria and bacteriuria are absent in about one third of infections associated with hyperadrenocorticism. These findings indicate that it is appropriate to culture the urine of all dogs with hyperadrenocorticism regardless of the results of urinalysis.

6. When should an adrenal function test be performed in a dog?

Most dogs with hyperadrenocorticism have multiple clinical signs of their disease and the decision to test these dogs is straightforward. Dogs with few clinical signs, (e.g., just polyuria/polydipsia [PU/PD] or serum enzyme abnormalities) may also be tested, although if the results indicate hyperadrenocorticism, the dog may not necessarily require treatment. Because false positive results on adrenal function tests occur with some frequency, it is important to consider the entire clinical picture when interpreting the test results.

7.   When should an adrenal function test *not* be performed?
Conditions other than primary adrenal disease can greatly affect the accuracy of adrenal function tests. More than half of dogs with a significant systemic illness will have a false-positive result on the low-dose dexamethasone suppression test (LDDST). The ACTH response test for hyperadrenocorticism is affected less frequently, but false-positive results are still common. Because it is rarely if ever necessary to make a diagnosis of hyperadrenocorticism on an emergency basis, adrenal function testing should be postponed until the illness can be resolved or stabilized for 2 to 4 weeks.

8.   What is the best test for diagnosis of hyperadrenocorticism in the dog?
There is no single best test for all situations. Overall, the low-dose dexamethasone suppression test (LDDST) is more sensitive than the ACTH response test and has the advantage of differentiating PDH from ADH in 25% to 50% of cases. On the other hand, the LDDST is more susceptible to the effects of conditions other than primary adrenal disease, so false-positive results are much more likely on the LDDST.

9.   What role does the urine cortisol:creatinine ratio play in the diagnosis of hyperadrenocorticism?
Urinary cortisol excretion is dependent on the average plasma cortisol concentration over the period of time that the urine was produced. Almost all dogs with hyperadrenocorticism have an elevated urine cortisol:creatinine ratio. However, this ratio is also elevated in many if not most dogs with conditions other than primary adrenal disease, so this test has low specificity despite its high sensitivity. Because the stress of a visit to the veterinary practice can elevate the dog's urine cortisol:creatinine ratio, urine samples for this test should be collected by the owner at home. Although it is not recommended for routine use, the urine cortisol:creatinine ratio can be a useful screening test in that a negative result makes hyperadrenocorticism unlikely.

10.   When is the ACTH response test preferred over the LDDST?
The advantages of the ACTH response test are that it is less often affected by nonadrenal illness, it can be performed more rapidly, it is diagnostic of iatrogenic hyperadrenocorticism, and it can be used to monitor the response to treatment with mitotane. Therefore the ACTH response test is preferred if an animal is suspected of having nonadrenal illness or has a history of recent corticosteroid administration. The ACTH response test is performed by obtaining blood samples to test for cortisol levels before and 1 hour after intravenous (IV) or intramuscular (IM) administration of 5 µg/kg (maximum dose of 250 µg) synthetic ACTH. The ACTH can be frozen and stored for 6 months, allowing for a number of tests to be performed using the same vial.

11.   When is the LDDST preferred over the ACTH response test?
The advantages of the LDDST is that it is more sensitive than the ACTH response test particularly in dogs with adrenal tumors, it can differentiate between PDH and ADH in up to 50% of dogs with hyperadrenocorticism, and it does not require ACTH. The LDDST is preferred by many as the primary screening test for diagnosis of hyperadrenocorticism.

12.   How is the LDDST performed and interpreted?
Blood samples for measurement of cortisol are collected before, 4 hours, and 8 hours after IV administration of dexamethasone, 0.01 mg/kg. The dexamethasone must be diluted to ensure

accurate dosing. The 8-hour post-dexamethasone cortisol concentration should be evaluated first, because this value indicates whether hyperadrenocorticism is present. Administration of dexamethasone to a dog without hyperadrenocorticism should result in a marked decrease in the cortisol concentration 8 hours after administration, but a normal level in dogs with hyperadrenocorticism, regardless of whether the origin is PDH or ADH. If the cortisol concentration is decreased (usually <1.0 µg/dl) in the 8-hour sample, no further blood tests are necessary; the dog does not have hyperadrenocorticism, based on the results of this test. If the cortisol concentration is more than 1.5 µg/dl in the 8-hour sample, the cortisol concentration in the 4-hour sample should be measured. A cortisol level in the expected range (<1.5 µg/dl) or less than 50% of the level in the baseline sample is diagnostic of PDH (minimal suppression would be expected with ADH).

13. **What additional testing can be performed in a dog suspected of hyperadrenocorticism but with ACTH response test or LDDST results that are not diagnostic for hyperadrenocorticism?**

    If only one of these screening tests was performed, it is usually most productive to perform the other test. If this second test is not diagnostic, the dog either does not have hyperadrenocorticism or has a mild form, or its adrenal glands are producing a noncortisol steroid hormone. If hyperadrenocorticism is still high on the list of possible diagnoses, it is recommended to measure progesterone, 17-hydroxyprogesterone, and/or androstenedione on samples collected using the standard ACTH response test protocol. Some dogs with PDH or ADH will secrete excessive amounts of these or other adrenal steroid hormones and have signs of hyperadrenocorticism without elevated cortisol concentrations.

14. **Is it necessary to differentiate between PDH and ADH?**

    Yes, because the treatment differs. Even if an owner is unwilling to pursue surgery as a treatment for an adrenal tumor, the medical management of PDH and ADH differ.

15. **How is pituitary-dependent hyperadrenocorticism (PDH) best differentiated from adrenal-dependent hyperadrenocorticism (ADH) due to an adrenal tumor?**

    Tests to differentiate PDH and ADH should only be performed if a diagnosis of hyperadrenocorticism has already been established. If the results of a LDDST were diagnostic of hyperadrenocorticism and showed suppression of cortisol consistent with PDH, no further testing is necessary.

    Although no method of discrimination is perfect, an abdominal ultrasound examination that clearly identifies both adrenal glands is an effective tool. In most cases of hyperadrenocorticism, both adrenal glands will be enlarged, usually with retention of the normal shape. In dogs with adrenal tumors, the gland with the tumor is enlarged, usually as a mass effect, while the contralateral gland is small or of normal size. Because nodular hyperplasia of the adrenal glands can sometimes mimic small neoplasms, and the adrenal glands are not always delineated adequately, ultrasound has some limitations. Ultrasound of the adrenal glands alone is not an effective method for diagnosing hyperadrenocorticism.

    A high-dose dexamethasone suppression test (HDDST) is effective in confirming PDH in about 75% of cases, specifically, those in which plasma cortisol concentration decreases in response to dexamethasone administration. The test is performed by obtaining blood samples before and 4 hours and 8 hours after administration of 0.1 mg/kg dexamethasone IV. Suppression is defined as a decrease from baseline of 50% or more in the plasma cortisol concentration in one or both of the 4 hour and 8 hour samples. Suppression is diagnostic of PDH. However, suppression fails to occur in approximately 25% of dogs with PDH and all dogs with adrenal tumors.

    Plasma ACTH concentration is expected to be normal or elevated (>40 pg/ml) in dogs with PDH and suppressed (<20 pg/ml) in dogs with adrenal tumors. Unfortunately, many samples fall in the nondiagnostic range. Careful sample handling is important. The sample should be collected in a plastic tube because ACTH adheres to glass. Then the sample should be centrifuged immediately after collection and stored frozen, or aprotinin, which inhibits degradation of ACTH, should be added; addition of aprotinin eliminates the need for special handling.

16. Should all dogs with hyperadrenocorticism be treated?

Dogs with few or mild clinical signs caused by PDH probably do not need to be treated. The risks and expense of treatment may outweigh the potential benefits in these cases. However, the owner should be made aware of the potential complications of untreated hyperadrenocorticism. Because of the potential for local invasion and metastasis of adrenal tumors, treatment of ADH is generally recommended.

17. What are the common complications of hyperadrenocorticism?

Urinary tract infections are one of the most common complications of hyperadrenocorticism and some dogs will have cystic calculi (usually calcium oxalate). Hypertension is also common but is often overlooked. Diabetes mellitus, thromboembolism, pancreatitis, systemic infections, congestive heart failure, and signs related to macroadenoma also occur.

18. What treatment is recommended for routine management of PDH?

Mitotane (o,p'DDD) is an adrenocorticolytic drug that selectively destroys the cortisol-producing layers of the adrenal cortex, usually sparing the zona glomerulosa that produces aldosterone. It can be used safely in most cases but side effects occur in about 25% of cases. Treatment involves an initial induction phase followed by the maintenance phase.

19. What is the protocol for the induction phase of mitotane treatment?

In the induction phase, mitotane 50 mg/kg is administered daily, divided into 2 or 3 doses and given with food. After treatment has continued for 7 days, or until water consumption returns to normal, the appetite abruptly decreases, or side effects, which include vomiting, anorexia, lethargy, diarrhea, weakness, and ataxia, occur. At this point, mitotane administration is stopped, and an ACTH response test is performed. Adequate control of the hyperadrenocorticism is indicated by a post-ACTH cortisol concentration in the normal *resting* range (1-4 µg/dl). If this goal is reached, maintenance treatment is begun. If the post-ACTH cortisol concentration is above 4 µg/dl, mitotane is administered at the initial dosage for an additional 2 to 7 days. The duration of treatment is dependent on the degree of suppression noted on the ACTH response test. This protocol of treatment and ACTH response testing is repeated until the target post-ACTH cortisol concentration of 1 to 4 µg/dl is reached.

20. What is the protocol for the maintenance phase of mitotane treatment?

Maintenance treatment is begun when adequate suppression of adrenocortical function has been accomplished by the induction phase of mitotane treatment. If the post-ACTH cortisol concentration is below 1 µg/dl, maintenance treatment should be delayed for 2 to 4 weeks. In the maintenance phase, mitotane 25 to 50 mg/kg is administered weekly, divided into 2 to 3 doses and given with food. The owner should be vigilant for side effects of the mitotane and should discontinue treatment and follow the suggestions for treatment if these are noted.

21. What treatment should be administered for side effects of mitotane?

The mitotane should be discontinued and prednisone (0.4 mg/kg by mouth [PO]) should be administered if side effects are noted. A supply of prednisone should be dispensed with mitotane during all phases of treatment so the owner has a ready supply if needed. If side effects of mitotane do not resolve within a few hours of prednisone administration, the dog should be evaluated and if needed, an injectable form of a glucocorticoid and intravenous fluids should be administered. Electrolyte levels should be evaluated to determine if mineralocorticoid activity has been affected. If hyperkalemia, hyponatremia, and a low plasma cortisol level occur without a response to ACTH, the hypoadrenocorticism is usually permanent and mineralocorticoid supplementation should be instituted.

22. How is mitotane treatment monitored?

Treatment is monitored by owner assessment of clinical signs and by periodic ACTH response testing. It is recommended that an ACTH response test be performed 1 month after initiating maintenance treatment and then every 6 months, or if clinical signs of hyperadrenocorticism are noted. If the post-ACTH cortisol concentration rises above 4 µg/dl, mitotane at the induction-phase dosage should be administered for 2 to 7 days. If the post-ACTH cortisol concentration is adequately suppressed after this treatment, maintenance therapy is reinstituted at a dosage approximately 25% to 50% higher than previously.

23. How often is it necessary to adjust the mitotane dosage?

About half the dogs treated with mitotane will have a recurrence of clinical signs of hyper-adrenocorticism or an elevated post-ACTH test cortisol level within 1 year of initiating treatment.

24. What is trilostane and how is it used in the treatment of hyperadrenocorticism?

Trilostane inhibits one of the enzymes responsible for synthesis of adrenal steroid hormones. It has been found to be an effective and relatively safe treatment for PDH and may be effective in treating ADH as well. Trilostane is administered once daily, 30 mg for dogs weighing less than 5 kg, 60 mg for dogs weighing 5 to 20 kg, and 120 mg for dogs weighing more than 20 kg. An initial dosage of 10 mg/kg once daily has been recommended but may be difficult to administer because the standard capsule size is 30 mg. It is recommended that ACTH response testing be performed every 2 to 4 weeks until the post-ACTH cortisol concentration is between 1 and 4 µg/dl. Because the duration of action of trilostane is less than 24 hours, the ACTH response test should be performed within 8 hours of trilostane administration. The trilostane dosage is adjusted based on clinical response and the results of ACTH response tests; the dose is increased if the post ACTH cortisol concentration is more than 4 µg/dl and reduced if it is less than 1 µg/dl. Hypoadrenocorticism can be induced by this drug, and electrolyte abnormalities consistent with mineralocorticoid deficiency can occur. If the dog develops signs of hypoadrenocorticism, trilostane should be discontinued until the signs resolve and the ACTH response test shows an exaggerated response. Some dogs may remain hypoadrenocorticoid for months after discontinuing trilostane. Trilostane is costly and not approved for use in North America.

25. What is the role of Deprenyl (selegiline) in the management of hyperadrenocorticism?

Deprenyl (selegiline) is a monoamine oxidase inhibitor that increases dopamine in the pituitary and inhibits ACTH secretion. Its role in the management of hyperadrenocorticism is limited to PDH, and it appears to be effective in controlling hyperadrenocorticism in about 20% of dogs treated. It does reduce clinical signs or improve the overall condition of a larger percentage of dogs with PDH. Treatment is initiated at 1 mg/kg daily for 2 months. If the response is adequate, this dosage is continued. If clinical signs persist, the dose is increased to 2 mg/kg daily and the effects are evaluated in 1 month. If an inadequate response is seen at that time, alternative treatment should be instituted. Dogs with PDH and concurrent illness should not be treated with selegiline.

26. What is the role of ketoconazole in the management of hyperadrenocorticism?

Ketoconazole is a steroid enzyme inhibitor that is effective for treating ADH and PDH. It is initially administered at 5 mg/kg twice daily for 7 days. If no intolerable effects occur, the dose is increased to 10 mg/kg twice daily, and clinical signs and the results of an ACTH response test are evaluated after 14 days of treatment. The dosage is increased to 15 mg/kg twice daily) if the post-ACTH cortisol concentration is higher than 4 µg/dL, and clinical signs and ACTH response testing are rechecked in 14 days. The maximal dose should not exceed 20 mg/kg twice daily. Side effects include anorexia, vomiting, diarrhea, and hepatic disease. Ketoconazole is effective in about 75% of cases. Daily treatment with ketoconazole is costly.

27. What treatment is recommended for adrenal tumors causing hyperadrenocorticism?

Adrenalectomy is the most effective treatment for adrenal tumors and is curative in 50% of dogs with benign tumors and in many dogs with adrenocortical carcinomas when metastasis has not occurred. Malignant adrenal tumors frequently invade the caudal vena cava, making successful excision difficult. The perioperative mortality for dogs with ADH undergoing adrenalectomy is about 25%. Complications include intraoperative hemorrhage, pancreatitis, sepsis, thromboembolism, poor wound healing, and hypoadrenocorticism.

Medical management of ADH can be accomplished by administration of ketoconazole, trilostane, or mitotane. Only mitotane has an adrenocorticolytic effect, so it may be effective at reducing tumor burden in addition to suppressing cortisol secretion. The dosage and duration of the induction phase of treatment with mitotane are usually higher for dogs with ADH than for those with PDH; for induction treatment, 50 mg/kg daily for 10 to 14 days is recommended. Further treatment is based on the results of ACTH response testing, as was described for PDH. For dogs with ADH, a higher initial maintenance dose (50-75 mg/kg/week) is recommended.

28. What is the prognosis for a dog with hyperadrenocorticism?

The average survival time after diagnosis for a dog with hyperadrenocorticism is about 2 years. Many of these animals die of problems unrelated to hyperadrenocorticism.

28. Hypothyroidism

David L. Panciera

1. What causes hypothyroidism in dogs?

Autoimmune thyroiditis is responsible for destruction of the thyroid gland in approximately 50% of cases. These dogs usually have circulating antithyroglobulin antibodies and occasionally have antibodies against thyroid hormones. Most other cases of hypothyroidism are the result of idiopathic thyroid gland atrophy. The cause is unknown, but long-standing autoimmune thyroiditis has been suspected. Rarely, hypothyroidism results from pituitary disease such as a tumor.

2. What abnormalities are most often evident from the history or physical examination of hypothyroid dogs?

Dermatologic abnormalities, including alopecia, poor hair coat, seborrhea, or pyoderma, are found in about 90% of hypothyroid dogs. Alopecia may initially occur in areas of friction, such as the tail and neck, and eventually spread to involve bilaterally symmetrical areas on the trunk. Obesity and lethargy are common. Lethargy is often reported by owners only in retrospect, when they notice how activity level increases after treatment. Bradycardia or a low-normal heart rate is also common.

3. What neurologic abnormalities are caused by hypothyroidism?

Hypothyroidism can cause localized or generalized peripheral neuropathies as well as abnormalities of the central nervous system. Generalized weakness, hyporeflexia, and decreased conscious proprioception occur with generalized neuropathy, although these signs are typical of peripheral neuropathy due to any cause. Localized neuropathies result in facial nerve and/or vestibular nerve dysfunction. Hypothyroidism-associated neuropathy has also been reported, although rarely, to cause unilateral forelimb lameness. Other clinical signs of hypothyroidism may or may not be present in dogs with neuropathy. Central nervous system abnormalities such as ataxia, hemiparesis, nystagmus, hypermetria, circling, and cranial nerve deficits can also be due to hypothyroidism.

4. Does hypothyroidism have important effects on cardiovascular function?

Myocardial function is impaired by hypothyroidism, but clinical signs are rare. Bradycardia, low-voltage complexes on the electrocardiogram, and decreased myocardial contractility are relatively frequently seen. Rarely, clinical signs of heart failure due to hypothyroidism-induced dilated cardiomyopathy may be seen.

5. Does hypothyroidism cause megaesophagus and laryngeal paralysis?

Megaesophagus and laryngeal paralysis have not been proven to be caused by hypothyroidism. While these problems may occur in hypothyroid dogs, thyroid hormone supplementation rarely if ever resolves the problem.

6. When evaluating a dog for aggression, should hypothyroidism be considered a possible cause?

It appears that a small proportion of dogs with aggression problems have hypothyroidism as an underlying cause. The dogs in which aggression was attributed to hypothyroidism had dominance aggression and few other signs of hypothyroidism. A complete response may not occur with thyroid hormone supplementation alone, and it is recommended that appropriate behavioral modification treatment be instituted concurrently.

7. Is reproductive function affected by hypothyroidism?

Hypothyroidism appears to have little effect on reproduction in the male dog. Little objective information is available regarding the effects of hypothyroidism on female reproduction, although prolonged interestrous intervals, failure to cycle, silent estrous cycles, lack of libido, and prolonged estrual bleeding have been reported to be caused by hypothyroidism.

8. What abnormalities are usually evident on routine laboratory testing of dogs with hypothyroidism?

A mild nonregenerative anemia is found in about one third of hypothyroid dogs, and approximately 75% have an elevated serum cholesterol concentration.

9. How can a diagnosis of hypothyroidism be established in a dog with appropriate clinical signs?

Assuming a dog does not have nonthyroidal illness and does not have a history of recent treatment with a drug that could affect thyroid function, measurement of total T4 is a reasonably accurate test. Serum T4 concentration is below normal in 80% to 90% of dogs with hypothyroidism. About 20% of dogs with normal thyroid function that are tested for hypothyroidism because of compatible clinical signs have a serum T4 concentration below the reference range. Concurrent measurement of TSH is useful in that hypothyroidism is nearly always present in a dog with a decreased serum T4 and elevated TSH concentration. Unfortunately, TSH is normal in 25% to 35% of hypothyroid dogs. Serum free T4 concentration (measured by equilibrium dialysis) is low in 90% to 98% of hypothyroid dogs and is falsely decreased in 6% to 7% of euthyroid dogs, making free T4 the most accurate single test. If T4, free T4, and TSH are all measured, the results will point to an accurate diagnosis in 99% of cases.

10. How important is it to measure free T4 concentrations when testing for hypothyroidism?

Serum free T4 is affected to a lesser degree than serum T4 by nonthyroid illness and by some drugs. It is essential that free T4 be measured by equilibrium dialysis for the results to be valid.

Dogs with moderate to severe nonthyroid illness are almost as likely to have a decreased serum free T4 concentration as total T4 concentration.

11. What is the most likely explanation for finding an elevated serum T4 and/or T3 concentration in a dog suspected of being hypothyroid?

Autoantibodies to T3 and/or T4 can form in dogs with autoimmune thyroiditis. The presence of these antibodies causes false elevation in the measured levels of hormones. This elevation can be mild (bring a low T4 concentration into the normal range) or marked (resulting in marked elevations of T4). This effect is artificial and does not correlate with thyroid hormone concentrations or activity in vivo. If T4 is affected, measurement of free T4 by equilibrium dialysis is necessary to determine if the dog is hypothyroid, because this assay is not affected by the presence of autoantibodies.

12. When hypothyroidism is suspected in a dog with another illness, what is the best method for evaluating thyroid function?

Free T4 is affected to a lesser degree than total T4 in dogs with nonthyroid illnesses, but moderate to severe illness can also lower the concentration of free T4. Resolution of any nonthyroid illness and discontinuation of certain drugs is necessary to accurately assess thyroid function in many cases.

13. What does a positive antithyroglobulin antibody test mean?

Autoimmune thyroiditis is associated with formation of antithyroglobulin antibodies. These autoantibodies are present in 50% to 60% of hypothyroid dogs, and they also may be found in dogs with lymphocytic thyroiditis and normal thyroid function. It is likely that some dogs with antithyroglobulin antibodies and normal thyroid function will develop hypothyroidism, but the frequency of progression to hypothyroidism is unknown.

14. What drugs have significant effects on thyroid function?

Glucocorticoid and sulfonamide drugs have the most substantial effects on thyroid function. Sulfonamide medications in particular can induce hypothyroidism within 1 to 3 weeks of administration. Thyroid hormone concentrations return to normal 1 to 2 weeks after treatment is stopped. Phenobarbital and clomipramine can cause modest decreases in serum T4 and free T4 concentrations.

15. Are there breed differences in the normal ranges for results of thyroid function tests?

In sight hounds, Greyhounds in particular, the normal ranges for serum T4 and free T4 concentrations are lower than the normal ranges for other breeds. Alaskan sled dogs that have undergone extensive training also frequently have serum T3 and T4 concentrations that are lower than standard reference ranges for other breeds. It is likely that other breeds have unique reference ranges for thyroid hormone concentrations.

16. What is the appropriate dosage of levothyroxine supplementation in hypothyroid dogs?

The levothyroxine dosage recommended by this author is 0.022 mg/kg BID. There is controversy regarding the necessity of administering thyroid hormone supplementation in divided doses. However, response to treatment is the final test of the accuracy of the diagnosis of hypothyroidism. Because some investigators have the impression that some dogs respond better to twice daily dosing, the author recommends this dosing regimen for initial treatment. If the clinical response is good, levothyroxine can often then be administered at a reduced dosage of 0.022 mg/kg once daily.

17. Does the formulation of levothyroxine affect response?

There is no evidence that generic levothyroxine preparations are inferior to one of the "brand name" levothyroxine supplements. If switching from one preparation to another, evaluation of the post-pill serum T4 concentration might be indicated, because levothyroxine content and bioavailability might vary from one preparation to another.

18. What is the most appropriate protocol for monitoring treatment of hypothyroidism?

The most important factor to consider in monitoring treatment of hypothyroidism is the clinical response. Improvement in activity and attitude are typically noted within 1 to 2 weeks of instituting treatment. Weight loss also usually begins within a short period after starting levothyroxine. Neurologic signs typically begin to improve within a few days of initiating treatment, but complete resolution of the deficits may require several weeks. Dermatologic manifestations often require months to resolve. Measurement of serum T4 concentration is recommended in all cases and is particularly important if the clinical response is incomplete. The serum T4 concentration typically peaks 4 to 6 hours after levothyroxine administration. The serum T4 concentration should be in the upper end of or slightly above the reference range (40-70 nmol/L if the reference range is 15-50 nmol/L) 4 to 6 hours after a dose is ingested. If the clinical response is poor but the postpill serum T4 concentration is in the desired range, the diagnosis of hypothyroidism may be inaccurate or a concurrent disease may be present.

19. What are the side effects of levothyroxine treatment?

Hyperthyroidism is the only important side effect of levothyroxine treatment. Clinical signs of hyperthyroidism include polydipsia, polyuria, hyperactivity, tachycardia, panting, and weight loss. If these signs are noted, the serum T4 concentration should be determined and no further doses of levothyroxine should be given until the results can be assessed. The levothyroxine should be restarted at 50% of the previous dosage and the dog should be evaluated for renal or hepatic disease, because kidney or liver dysfunction can slow metabolism and excretion of T4.

29. Hyperthyroidism

David L. Panciera

1. What causes hyperthyroidism in the dog?

Hyperthyroidism in dogs is usually due to excessive thyroid hormone secretion by a thyroid tumor. Iatrogenic hyperthyroidism also occurs due to overdosing levothyroxine treatment. Thyroid tumors in dogs are usually malignant carcinomas and adenocarcinomas, and only 10% to 20% of the tumors are functional.

2. What are the clinical signs of canine hyperthyroidism?

Clinical signs of hyperthyroidism in the dog are similar to those of hyperthyroidism in the cat, including weight loss, polyphagia, polyuria/polydipsia (PU/PD), vomiting, diarrhea, behavioral changes, and panting. Many hyperthyroid dogs have a large ventral cervical mass and this is frequently noticed by the owner. Physical examination findings include an enlarged thyroid gland, thin body, muscle wasting, tachycardia, tachypnea, and difficulty swallowing or breathing due to local effects of the thyroid mass.

3. How is hyperthyroidism diagnosed?

A diagnosis of hyperthyroidism is confirmed by finding an elevated serum total T4 concentration in a dog with compatible clinical signs. Some dogs with autoimmune thyroiditis have T4 autoantibodies that cause false elevation of serum T4 concentration on the immunoassays used to measure T4. These dogs may be euthyroid or hypothyroid; hyperthyroidism does not occur as a result of T4 autoantibodies. If there is a question about T4 autoantibodies being the cause of an elevated serum T4 concentration, a test can be performed to detect the autoantibodies or serum free T4 (fT4) can be measured by equilibrium dialysis.

4.   What ancillary testing should be performed in a dog with hyperthyroidism?
Because most thyroid tumors in the dog are malignant and metastasis is found in about 30% of cases, a thorough evaluation for metastasis should be performed. Thoracic radiographs and regional lymph node aspiration or biopsy is indicated. If a ventral cervical mass compatible with an enlarged thyroid gland and elevated total T4 are found in a dog, further evaluation of the cause of the mass is not necessary. Fine needle aspiration is useful, but thyroid tumors are vascular and in some cases bleeding can preclude the acquisition of adequate samples. Incisional biopsy is not recommended.

5.   What is the most appropriate treatment for hyperthyroidism?
When possible, en bloc excision of the tumor is the most effective treatment. Surgery is the best treatment for tumors that are freely moveable and not attached to deep cervical structures, and prolonged survival is likely in such cases, particularly if the tumor is relatively small. Complications of surgery include extensive hemorrhage, damage to surrounding structures (carotid artery, jugular vein, recurrent laryngeal and vagus nerves), and hypoparathyroidism if the tumor is bilateral. External beam irradiation is an effective treatment for nonresectable thyroid carcinomas, with median survival times of 2 years or longer being reported. Radioiodine administration can also be effective, but large doses are required.

6.   What is the prognosis for a dog with hyperthyroidism?
The prognosis for dogs with benign tumors is good if the tumor can be completely excised. Dogs with freely movable malignant tumors that undergo surgery have a median survival time of 36 months. Only 25% of dogs with invasive, nonresectable thyroid tumors are alive 1 year after surgery. External beam irradiation has shown great promise, with 72% of dogs in one study being free of tumor progression 3 years after this treatment.

30. Hypercalcemia

David L. Panciera

1.   What is the significance of an elevated total calcium concentration?
The total serum calcium concentration is routinely measured on serum biochemical analyses. It consists of 3 components. Ionized calcium, the physiologically active form in the circulation, normally accounts for approximately 55% of total calcium. Ionized calcium is important in regulating physiologic functions and in control of parathyroid hormone (PTH) secretion. Approximately 35% of calcium is bound to plasma proteins, and 10% (so-called complexed calcium) is bound to anions, including phosphate, bicarbonate, citrate, sulfate, and lactate. Alterations in plasma protein concentration, blood pH, and anion concentrations can alter total calcium concentration without affecting ionized calcium. Conversely, these factors can affect the concentration of ionized calcium without altering that of total calcium. Therefore an elevated concentration of total calcium does not always reflect an elevated concentration of ionized calcium.

2.   What are the important clinical consequences of hypercalcemia?
Hypercalcemia induces polyuria by inhibiting the action of antidiuretic hormone on the collecting tubules. Hypercalcemia also impairs renal function by reducing glomerular blood flow

through afferent arteriolar vasoconstriction. Hypercalcemia can cause permanent renal dysfunction by inducing renal mineralization, vasoconstriction, and other mechanisms. Calcium-containing uroliths are common in dogs with chronic hypercalcemia. The decreased neuromuscular excitability induced by hypercalcemia can cause weakness, muscle tremors, constipation, and vomiting.

3. What are the common clinical signs of hypercalcemia?

Polyuria and polydipsia are the most common clinical signs of hypercalcemia. Lethargy, inappetence, vomiting, weakness, muscle tremors, and constipation also occur. Signs of lower urinary tract inflammation may be present in dogs with cystic calculi that results from hypercalcemia. Other clinical signs may be present, related either to the primary disease process or to renal failure induced by the hypercalcemia.

4. What are the most common causes of hypercalcemia?

Neoplasia is the most common cause of hypercalcemia, with lymphoma, apocrine gland adenocarcinoma of the anal sac, multiple myeloma, and thyroid carcinoma being the most common. Renal failure is a common cause of elevated total calcium, although the concentration of ionized calcium is usually normal or low. Some dogs with hypoadrenocorticism have mild hypercalcemia. Primary hyperparathyroidism is an uncommon cause of hypercalcemia, and is usually secondary to a solitary parathyroid adenoma or parathyroid gland hyperplasia secreting excessive parathyroid hormone (PTH). Vitamin D intoxication can occur due to ingestion of vitamin D rodenticides, certain plants containing vitamin D compounds, or vitamin D–containing medications. Occasionally, osteolytic lesions can cause a mild increase in serum calcium concentration. Granulomatous diseases, particularly systemic mycoses (blastomycosis), and schistosomiasis can cause hypercalcemia. Laboratory error should always be considered as a cause of a reported elevated serum calcium concentration.

5. What diagnostic testing should be considered when evaluating a dog with hypercalcemia?

The first step is to confirm the hypercalcemia by obtaining another blood sample. Review of a complete history and physical examination, including careful rectal palpation for anal sac or sublumbar lymph node enlargement, usually helps direct further diagnostic testing. Routine complete blood count (CBC), serum chemistry testing, and urinalysis are indicated in every case. The CBC may provide evidence of inflammation associated with granulomatous disease, osteomyelitis, or neoplasia, or of leukemia. Test results may provide some indication of the underlying cause, for example elevated renal values (indicating renal failure), electrolyte abnormalities (indicating hypoadrenocorticism), elevated alkaline phosphatase (ALP) activity (indicating neoplasia or primary hyperparathyroidism), and plasma protein concentration (indicating lymphoid neoplasia or chronic inflammation). Hypophosphatemia or low-normal concentrations of phosphate frequently occur with hypercalcemia due to malignancy and primary hyperparathyroidism, whereas hyperphosphatemia is often found in cases of renal failure and vitamin D toxicosis. Abnormalities identified on the physical examination should be further evaluated by an appropriate method such as fine needle aspiration, biopsy, abdominal radiographs, or ultrasound, as indicated. Thoracic radiographs should be considered early in the diagnostic process, because mediastinal lymphosarcoma is often associated with hypercalcemia. A cause of hypercalcemia is identified in most cases using this approach.

6. What testing should be performed if neoplasia is not identified after a thorough evaluation?

When a thorough evaluation has failed to identify a neoplasm, primary hyperparathyroidism and occult neoplasia are the most likely diagnoses. If an occult neoplasm is suspected, bone marrow aspiration should be considered. A diagnosis of primary hyperparathyroidism is made by documenting an elevated or high normal serum PTH and a concurrent elevation of the concentration of ionized calcium. Measurement of parathyroid hormone-related peptide (PTHrP) can be useful in identifying some cases in which hypercalcemia is due to malignancy. Anal sac adenocarcinoma, some lymphomas, and some other neoplasms will be associated with elevations of PTHrP, although lack of an elevated PTHrP does not rule out malignancy as the cause of hypercalcemia. Cervical ultrasound can sometimes be successful in identifying enlargement of the parathyroid gland, if present, but a high resolution ultrasound transducer and considerable expertise are necessary. If the diagnosis is in question, a therapeutic trial of prednisone, vincristine, or L-asparginase can be attempted, because most cases of lymphoma will respond to this treatment and serum calcium will decrease substantially. This should be a consideration only after exhaustive testing has been performed, because administration of these agents will destroy a lymphoid neoplasm and it will be difficult to make a diagnosis based on examination of a tissue specimen obtained after treatment. Surgical exploration of the ventral cervical area for a parathyroid neoplasm is also a consideration, depending on the degree of suspicion of primary hyperparathyroidism.

7. How is renal function assessed in dogs with hypercalcemia?

Hypercalcemia causes reversible impairment of renal concentrating ability and reduces glomerular filtration rate by causing afferent arteriolar vasoconstriction. As a result, azotemia and isosthenuria can occur without causing permanent renal failure. Alternatively, hypercalcemia can cause irreversible renal damage and result in renal failure. The only practical way to assess renal function in a dog with hypercalcemia is to resolve the hypercalcemia and then reassess renal function.

8. In a dog with hypercalcemia and azotemia, how can one determine if primary renal failure caused the hypercalcemia?

It is important to determine whether primary renal failure caused hypercalcemia or hypercalcemia caused the renal failure. Primary renal failure should be suspected if the elevation in serum calcium concentration is mild to moderate (usually <14 mg/dl), the phosphorus level is elevated, the blood urea nitrogen (BUN) and creatinine concentrations are elevated out of proportion to the degree of hypercalcemia (serum calcium is usually >15-16 mg/dl before permanent renal dysfunction occurs), nonregenerative anemia is present, or there is other evidence of primary renal disease such as small or irregular kidneys. Ionized calcium concentration is typically below or within the reference range in dogs with renal failure, although a mild elevation of ionized calcium concentration is sometimes found. Because serum PTH concentration is often elevated in dogs with renal failure, it can be difficult to differentiate the effects of renal failure from primary hyperparathyroidism.

9. When is emergency treatment of hypercalcemia necessary?

Severe hypercalcemia can induce renal failure, cause mineralization of soft tissues, result in neuromuscular abnormalities, and, rarely, can cause cardiac arrhythmias. Hypercalcemia should be treated aggressively if the serum calcium concentration is more than 16 mg/dl, the calcium concentration multiplied by the phosphorus concentration is more than 70, the dog is dehydrated, the calcium concentration is rapidly increasing, or azotemia is present.

10. What is the most appropriate treatment for severe hypercalcemia?

The goal of treating severe hypercalcemia is to lower the concentration of calcium (and phosphorus, if elevated) to a level that is not dangerous, to correct dehydration, and to resolve any prerenal azotemia that is present. It is unrealistic to expect the serum calcium concentration to normalize in most cases. Intravenous fluid therapy with 0.9% saline is the primary treatment for severe hypercalcemia. Rehydration of dehydrated dogs should be accomplished over a period of 6 to 24 hours, depending on the severity of hypercalcemia, clinical signs, and renal function. The rate of fluid administration should then be adjusted to provide diuresis; this usually results at twice the maintenance rate. If a reasonable decrease in serum calcium is not noted within

24 hours of initiating intravenous fluid therapy, furosemide (2-4 mg/kg) should be administered intravenously (IV). Furosemide should not be given until rehydration is complete. Urine output should be monitored during fluid therapy to ensure that oliguric renal failure has not occurred.

If intravenous administration of fluids and furosemide are not effective in lowering the serum calcium concentration to a safe level, prednisone (2 mg/kg by mouth twice daily) can be administered. Prednisone is most effective in cases of lymphoma, but can induce mild reductions in plasma calcium in most hypercalcemic dogs. Administration of prednisone may make a diagnosis of lymphoma more difficult, so appropriate diagnostic tests should be carried out prior to this treatment. Calcitonin (4-6 IU/kg subcutaneously twice a day) can be also be used. Calcitonin typically results in rapid reduction in plasma calcium concentration and can cause hypocalcemia. If these treatments fail, or if hypercalcemia is likely to continue for a prolonged period, administration of a bisphosphonate should be considered. These drugs inhibit mineral resorption from bone and lower the calcium concentration within 1 to 3 days of administration; the effects last 1 to 4 weeks. Pamidronate (1 mg/kg IV in normal saline administered over 2 hours) has been used successfully in treating hypercalcemia due to malignancy and vitamin D toxicosis in dogs.

11. What is the recommended treatment for primary hyperparathyroidism?
Definitive treatment of primary hyperparathyroidism is usually accomplished by surgical excision of the parathyroid tumor. Alternatively, injection of ethanol into the tumor under ultrasound guidance can be effective. Dogs with serum calcium concentrations above 14 mg/dl are at risk for developing hypocalcemia postoperatively, and administration of a vitamin D compound, with or without oral calcium, is recommended in these cases.

31. Hypocalcemia

David L. Panciera

1. What are the clinical signs of hypocalcemia?
Clinical signs of hypocalcemia are due primarily to increased neuromuscular excitability. The result is tetany, seizures, muscle fasciculations, hyperthermia, stiff gait, weakness, and generalized tremors. Tetany can sometimes be induced by exercise or testing reflexes. Occasionally tetany is localized to specific muscle groups, such as facial muscles, and may be manifest as facial rubbing or pawing due to the pain of cramping. Restlessness and apparent irritability and aggression may occur. Cataracts may occur after prolonged hypocalcemia (usually due to primary hypoparathyroidism); cataracts due to hypocalcemia are located in the anterior and posterior cortical subcapsular area of the lens. Panting or hyperventilation is also sometimes present. In addition to signs of hypocalcemia, clinical signs related to the primary disease may be present.

2. What are the most common causes of hypocalcemia?
Hypocalcemia severe enough to cause clinical signs is usually due to puerperal tetany, iatrogenic hypoparathyroidism, primary hypoparathyroidism, or administration of a phosphate-containing enema. Causes of less severe hypocalcemia include renal failure, pancreatitis, ethylene glycol intoxication, hypoalbuminemia, transfusion of blood with excessive citrate, intestinal malabsorption, and alkalosis.

3. What initial clinical approach should be taken when evaluating a hypocalcemic dog?
A thorough history and physical examination are essential for identifying the cause of

hypocalcemia. History findings that may reveal a cause include recent parturition, exposure to ethylene glycol, administration of a phosphate enema, previous cervical surgery, or symptoms of renal failure or pancreatitis. Physical examination findings that can help determine a specific cause of hypocalcemia include pregnancy or evidence of recent parturition (lactation) and abnormalities related to ethylene glycol ingestion, renal failure, or pancreatitis.

The results of a complete blood count (CBC) and routine serum chemistry tests frequently aid in the diagnosis of a primary disease that could be causing the hypocalcemia, including pancreatitis (leukocytosis, elevated amylase, lipase, liver enzymes), renal failure (azotemia, hyperphosphatemia), hypertonic phosphate enema administration (hyperphosphatemia, hypernatremia), ethylene glycol toxicosis (azotemia, hyperglycemia, metabolic acidosis, increased anion gap), and hypoalbuminemia. In dogs with hypoalbuminemia, the laboratory-reported calcium level can be corrected for the decrease in serum albumin using the following formula:

Corrected calcium = 3.5 − albumin concentration (mg/dl) + serum calcium concentration

4. If a diagnosis is not apparent based on history, physical examination, and routine laboratory testing, what are the possible causes of hypocalcemia and what are the appropriate tests to confirm these possibilities?

If a definitive or presumptive diagnosis is not made based on clinical signs and routine laboratory testing, primary hypoparathyroidism is the most likely cause. It can be confirmed by demonstrating decreased serum levels of ionized calcium in the presence of a serum parathyroid hormone (PTH) concentration below or in the low-normal reference range.

5. When and what emergency treatment is indicated for hypocalcemia?

Emergency treatment for hypocalcemia is indicated when seizures or tetany occur. In these cases, calcium gluconate (10% solution; 1-1.5 ml/kg over 10-20 minutes) should be administered intravenously with close monitoring, including electrocardiographic monitoring for bradycardia, shortened QT interval, and elevated ST segment. If side effects occur, the infusion should be stopped and after the effects resolve, the infusion should be restarted at a lower dose rate. A rapid response to treatment is expected, and the dose can be repeated if signs do not improve or resolve after the initial treatment. The initial intravenous bolus of calcium is followed by a constant infusion of calcium gluconate (6-10 ml/kg over 24 hours), additional boluses of calcium gluconate (1.5-2 ml/kg of a 10% solution every 6-8 hours) or by subcutaneous administration of calcium gluconate (1.5 ml of a 10% solution); the calcium gluconate should be diluted with an equal volume of sterile normal saline solution. Calcium chloride should never be administered subcutaneously because it is irritating.

6. Is there a difference among the calcium preparations for parenteral administration?

Calcium solutions have different concentrations of elemental calcium, so doses must be calculated carefully. Calcium gluconate, supplied as a 10% solution, contains 9.3 mg calcium/ml whereas a 10% solution of calcium chloride has 27.2 mg calcium/ml. Calcium chloride is irritating and may cause severe tissue necrosis if extravasation occurs. Calcium gluconate is preferred because it is less irritating and can be administered subcutaneously with less risk.

7. What are the options for long-term management of primary hypoparathyroidism?

Oral calcium and vitamin D preparations are generally used when long-term management of hypocalcemia is anticipated, as in cases of primary hypoparathyroidism or iatrogenic hypoparathyroidism. Oral calcium is administered initially at a dosage of 25 to 50 mg elemental calcium per day; calcium carbonate is 40% calcium, calcium lactate is 13% calcium, and calcium gluconate is 10% calcium. It is usually not necessary to continue oral calcium supplementation after vitamin D treatment has achieved desired effects.

Vitamin D preparations are used to increase intestinal absorption of calcium. These preparations include dihydrotachysterol and calcitriol. The duration of effect of vitamin D preparations is important, because toxicity due to overdose can cause hypercalcemia and hyperphosphatemia. Dihydrotachysterol (0.02-0.03 mg/kg/day for 2-3 days, then 0.01-0.02 every 24-48 hours) achieves maximal effect in 1 to 7 days; the duration of effect is 1 to 3 weeks. Calcitriol (20-30 ng/kg/day for 3-4 days, then 5-15 ng/kg/day, in 2 divided doses) achieves the maximal effect in 1 to 4 days and has a duration of effect of 2 to 7 days. Initially, the serum calcium level should be measured daily; when the calcium level approaches the low normal range it should be measured weekly until a stable serum calcium concentration is reached, and then every 3 months, with the dose of vitamin D being adjusted to maintain the serum calcium level at or just below the lower limit of the normal range.

8. What are the complications of long-term management of primary hypoparathyroidism?

Hypercalcemia is a common and serious complication of vitamin D supplementation. Prolonged hypercalcemia can cause renal failure and soft tissue mineralization because it is generally accompanied by increased plasma phosphate concentration.

9. After initial emergency treatment of dogs with puerperal tetany, what should be done to prevent recurrence?

Oral calcium should be administered to the bitch for the duration of lactation. If clinical signs of hypocalcemia return, the pups should be weaned.

10. Are treatment recommendations different when managing a dog that has undergone bilateral parathyroidectomy as a consequence of thyroidectomy?

Recommendations for initial treatment with vitamin D and oral calcium are the same. However, the vitamin D dosage can be decreased gradually beginning 2 months after surgery and tapering over the next 6 to 8 weeks. Serum calcium concentration should be measured prior to each dose reduction.

32. Hypoglycemia

David L. Panciera

1. What are the causes of hypoglycemia?

Neonatal hypoglycemia is common, and should be considered in any puppy with nonspecific clinical signs. Hypoglycemia can accompany any neonatal illness that results in anorexia lasting even 24 hours or less. Juvenile hypoglycemia occurs fairly frequently in small-breed dogs younger than 1 year. Hepatic failure and congenital portosystemic shunts can cause hypoglycemia, particularly in young dogs or those with severe hepatocellular dysfunction. Starvation alone is a cause of hypoglycemia by itself only when prolonged (2 weeks or longer), but can contribute to much more rapid development of hypoglycemia in dogs with concurrent illness or preceding cachexia. Sepsis is another relatively common cause of hypoglycemia, and the blood glucose concentration should be measured in any dog that is suspected of having a systemic infection. Exertional hypoglycemia occasionally occurs in dogs after prolonged strenuous exercise; this condition has also been called hunting dog hypoglycemia. Hypoadrenocorticism occasionally causes hypoglycemia to a degree sufficient to cause clinical signs. Hypoglycemia occurs in dogs with hypoadrenocorticism as a result of glucocorticoid deficiency (which may be due to withdrawal of corticosteroids after long-term administration and hypopituitarism), and in these cases, electrolyte abnormalities may be absent. Insulin overdose is a common cause of hypoglycemia in diabetic dogs. Pancreatic islet cell neoplasia (insulinoma) causes severe hypoglycemia due to hypersecretion of insulin. Non–islet cell neoplasia can also cause marked hypoglycemia; hypoglycemia is most likely to be caused by large tumors, such as hepatocellular carcinomas, by splenic neoplasia, or by smooth muscle tumors, particularly of the gastrointestinal tract. Clinicians should avoid diagnosing hypoglycemia based on a single blood glucose measurement in a dog without clinical signs; the diagnosis should always be confirmed by a second fasting blood glucose level.

2.   What clinical signs can be attributed to hypoglycemia?

Physical examination findings typically related directly to hypoglycemia are those related to nervous system dysfunction and include ataxia, weakness, disorientation, collapse, muscle fasciculations, bizarre behavior, seizures, and coma. Hypoglycemia also induces release of cate-cholamines, which causes nervousness and trembling. In many dogs, hypoglycemia is asymptomatic and clinical signs may be related to the primary disease. In these cases the findings are diverse. Peripheral neuropathy has been reported in a few dogs with insulinomas, so weakness, hyporeflexia, proprioceptive deficits, and muscle atrophy will persist in these dogs even in the absence of hypoglycemia.

3.   What is the recommended approach to determining the cause of hypoglycemia?

When hypoglycemia occurs secondary to an obvious systemic disease such as sepsis or overt hepatic failure, no specific evaluation for hypoglycemia is indicated. However, when the cause of hypoglycemia is not obvious from the history and the results of physical examination, and routine tests such as complete blood count (CBC), serum chemistry panel, and urinalysis, the most likely causes are occult hepatic disease, portosystemic shunt, atypical hypoadrenocorticism, insulinoma, and non–islet cell neoplasia. Abdominal radiographs may identify microhepatica due to liver disease or a portosystemic shunt or a mass indicating non–islet cell neoplasia. Abdominal ultrasound can identify hepatic disease, intraabdominal neoplasia, portosystemic shunt, and occasionally a pancreatic mass consistent with insulinoma. Hepatic function tests such as preprandial and postprandial bile acid measurements are indicated when serum chemistry test results indicate hepatic insufficiency, when a portosystemic shunt is suspected, or if no apparent cause is found. An adrenocorticotropic hormone (ACTH) response test should be considered to evaluate for hypoadrenocorticism in young to middle-aged dogs, particularly if lethargy and gastrointestinal disturbances are part of the history, or if no other apparent cause can be found. Measurement of fasting serum insulin concentration to diagnose insulinoma should be performed only after other diseases have been excluded as possible causes of hypoglycemia. The diagnosis is based on finding a serum insulin level in the middle or above the reference range in a hypoglycemic animal (blood glucose concentration of less than about 50 to 60 mg/dl). It may be necessary to fast the animal 4 hours or longer to induce hypoglycemia. If the insulin concentration is in the middle or above the reference range in the presence of hypoglycemia, a diagnosis of insulinoma is likely since minimal insulin secretion is expected with hypoglycemia. It can be confirmed at exploratory laparotomy.

4.   What is the best method of treating hypoglycemia in an emergency situation in the hospital?

If a dog with hypoglycemia is weak, having seizures, in a coma, or showing other signs of severe hypoglycemia, 1 to 2 ml/kg 50% dextrose (diluted to a 25% or less solution if possible) should be administered intravenously (IV) as a bolus. If no improvement is noted after 3 to 5 minutes, another bolus can be administered IV; bolus dosing can be repeated if necessary for an additional 2 to 3 doses. After a response is seen, a continuous infusion of 2.5% to 5% dextrose should be started in most cases to prevent recurrence of hypoglycemia. Some dogs, particularly those administered an overdose of insulin or those with insulinoma, may require administration of a 10% dextrose solution to maintain euglycemia. Hypertonic dextrose solutions may cause phlebitis and should not be administered into a peripheral vein for a prolonged period.

If signs of severe hypoglycemia are still present after this treatment and the blood glucose concentration is normal or elevated, brain injury and cerebral edema may be present secondary to prolonged hypoglycemia. Long-term sequelae of neuroglycopenia include blindness, ataxia, behavioral changes, and coma or obtundation. Treatment with dexamethasone sodium phosphate, 1-2 mg/kg IV, mannitol (0.5-1.0 g/kg IV over 20 minutes), and furosemide (1-2 mg/kg IV) can be administered for cerebral edema, but are unlikely to have much effect. Many dogs with neuroglycopenia recover to some degree.

5. What treatment is recommended if signs of hypoglycemia are not severe?

Frequent feeding of small meals will prevent hypoglycemia in puppies and juvenile small dogs and is useful in dogs with insulinoma. Instructing owners of dogs at risk for hypoglycemia to feed a small meal of the pet's regular food if signs of hypoglycemia are noted is the most effective and safest treatment for mild hypoglycemia. Feeding food rather than a glucose solution is preferable because it will resolve the hypoglycemia for a much longer time. If the dog refuses to eat a meal, a sugar solution such as corn syrup, pancake syrup, honey, or fruit juice can be administered orally. If the dog is unable to swallow, the owner can apply a small amount of sugar solution to the gums and lips, being careful not to allow the dog to aspirate the solution or bite the owner.

6. What treatment alternatives exist if a dog remains hypoglycemic after standard medical treatment?

If the constant infusion of dextrose is not effective in maintaining normoglycemia, glucagon can be given. It is administered initially at a rate of 5 ng/kg/min, which can be increased in increments of 5 ng/kg/min to 20 ng/kg/min or even higher as necessary to maintain the blood glucose concentration above 60 mg/dl.

7. What treatment options are available for management of insulinoma?

The most effective treatment for insulinoma is partial pancreatectomy with removal of the insulinoma and excision of visible metastases. Although this is rarely curative because insulinomas metastasize early, it is often effective at temporarily resolving the hypoglycemia or making medical treatments more effective. Perioperative complications are common and include pancreatitis, hypoglycemia, hyperglycemia, and sepsis. Medical management is indicated if owners decline surgery or if signs persist or recur despite surgery. Feeding 4 to 6 small meals per day of a food that has a low concentration of simple sugars is recommended. Administration of prednisone (starting with a dose of 0.25 mg by mouth twice daily and increasing to as much as 1-2 mg/kg twice daily) is generally recommended at the start of medical treatment to antagonize the effects of insulin. Diazoxide (beginning at 5 mg/kg by mouth twice daily and increasing in 5-mg/kg increments until hypoglycemia is controlled) can be administered to inhibit insulin release in cases where diet and prednisone are ineffective in controlling hypoglycemia. Unfortunately, diazoxide is costly and difficult to procure. Octreotide, a somatostatin analog that inhibits insulin secretion, has been used with limited success in a few cases. The cytotoxic chemotherapeutic agent streptozocin has also been used, although with somewhat discouraging results.

8. What is the prognosis for a dog with insulinoma?

More than 50% of dogs are disease free at 1 year after surgical excision if the tumor was grossly confined to the pancreas. Only about 20% of dogs with evidence of metastasis at the time of surgery are disease free at 1 year.

33. Central Diabetes Insipidus

David L. Panciera

1. What are the causes of central diabetes insipidus?

Central diabetes insipidus is a deficiency of antidiuretic hormone (ADH) secretion by the pars intermedia of the pituitary gland or a deficiency of ADH production by the hypothalamus. The reported causes of deficiency in dogs include neoplasia, trauma, and congenital abnormalities.

2. What clinical signs are caused by diabetes insipidus?

The primary and only clinical signs of diabetes insipidus in most cases are polyuria and polydipsia (PU/PD), which typically are severe. Urinary incontinence is another common complaint and is the result of the marked polyuria induced by diabetes insipidus. Dogs with neoplasia or trauma may have clinical signs related to damage of surrounding structures in the brain. Progression of neurologic abnormalities often occurs in dogs with pituitary neoplasia.

3. How is a diagnosis of diabetes insipidus established?

It is important to thoroughly evaluate a dog with suspected diabetes insipidus for other diseases that could cause PU/PD. Persistent isosthenuria or hyposthenuria confirms the presence of polyuria, while finding a urine specific gravity above 1.030 rules out persistent PU/PD. Hyposthenuria is most frequently found in dogs with central or nephrogenic diabetes insipidus, primary polydipsia, and hyperadrenocorticism. With the possible exception of evidence of dehydration, the complete blood count (CBC) and serum chemistry values of dogs with diabetes insipidus should be normal.

A water deprivation test may be performed for confirmation of the diagnosis.

4. What is the protocol for performing a water deprivation test?

For the results of a water deprivation test to be valid, causes of PU/PD other than central diabetes insipidus, nephrogenic diabetes insipidus, and primary (psychogenic) polydipsia should already have been eliminated. The water deprivation test is contraindicated if the animal is dehydrated, azotemic, or hypercalcemic.

Water can be gradually restricted for 3 days before the water deprivation test to reestablish the renal medullary concentration gradient.

After the dog has fasted for 12 hours, the urinary bladder is emptied by catheterization and urine specific gravity, body weight, and blood urea nitrogen (BUN) are measured. Water continues to be withheld and the above measurements are repeated every 1 to 2 hours until one of the following occurs: urine specific gravity becomes greater than 1.030; weight decreases by 5% or more; azotemia develops; or the dog shows signs of depression, disorientation, or vomiting. The water deprivation test must be terminated if the animal loses more than 5% of its body weight, develops azotemia, or becomes ill; failure to terminate the test when these signs occur may result in life-threatening dehydration and circulatory collapse. Dogs with diabetes insipidus may become dehydrated rapidly.

After completion of the water deprivation test, the dog should be given desmopressin (DDAVP) (5 μg for dogs <15 kg and 10 μg for dogs >15 kg) intravenously (IV) or subcutaneously (SQ). The urine specific gravity should be measured 30, 60, 90, and 120 minutes after DDAVP administration or until the urine specific gravity is above 1.030. At the end of the test, do not allow the dog to drink a large amount of water immediately, because this could result in water intoxication and cerebral edema.

The dog with complete diabetes insipidus will have minimal increase in urine specific gravity (≤1.012) after 5% dehydration. Dogs with partial diabetes insipidus may have a urine specific gravity up to 1.018, but rarely higher. Following administration of DDAVP after 5% dehydration on the water deprivation test, the urine specific gravity typically increases to between 1.018 and 1.030. Renal medullary washout usually prevents further urine concentration.

5. What treatment options exist for diabetes insipidus?

The goal of treatment for central diabetes insipidus is to reduce or eliminate the polyuria. Most cases respond well to administration of DDAVP, 1 to 4 drops of the intranasal preparation (100 μg/ml) once or twice daily. The dose should be adjusted to control the polyuria, although urine concentration may not return to normal. The owner is responsible for monitoring the effects of treatment by observation of water consumption and measurement of urine specific gravity and for adjusting the dose of DDAVP accordingly. Overdosing DDAVP can result in hyponatremia and associated neurologic abnormalities.

SECTION IV BIBLIOGRAPHY

Behrend EN, Kemppainen RJ: Diagnosis of canine hyperadrenocorticism, *Vet Clin N Am Sm Anim Pract* 31:985-1003, 2001.

Briggs CE, Nelson RW, Feldman EC et al: Reliability of history and physical examination findings for assessing control of glycemia in dogs with diabetes mellitus: 53 cases (1995-1998), *J Am Vet Med Assoc* 217:48-53, 2000.

Casella M, Wess G, Hassig M et al: Home monitoring of blood glucose concentration by owners of diabetic dogs, *J Sm Anim Pract* 44:298-305, 2003.

Chew DJ, Nagode LA: Treatment of hypoparathyroidism. In Bonagura JD, editor: *Current veterinary therapy XIII*, Philadelphia, 2000, WB Saunders Co,pp 340-345.

Cohn LA, McCaw DL, Tate DJ et al: Assessment of five portable blood glucose meters, a point-of-care analyzer, and color test strips for measuring blood glucose concentration in dogs, *J Am Vet Med Assoc* 216:198-202, 2000.

Dixon RM, Reid SWJ, Mooney CT. Treatment and therapeutic monitoring of canine hypothyroidism, *J Sm Anim Pract* 43:334-340, 2002.

Drobatz KJ, Casey KK: Eclampsia in dogs: 31 cases (1995-1998), *J Am Vet Med Assoc* 217:216-219, 2000.

Feldman EC, Nelson RW: Diabetes mellitus. In Feldman EC, Nelson RW, editors, *Canine and feline endocrinology and reproduction,* ed 2, Philadelphia, 1996, WB Saunders Co, pp 339-391.

Feldman EC, Nelson RW: Hypercalcemia and primary hyperparathyroidism. In Feldman EC, Nelson RW, editors, *Canine and feline endocrinology and reproduction,* ed 2, Philadelphia, 1996, WB Saunders Co, pp 455-496.

Feldman EC, Nelson RW: Hypocalcemia and primary hypoparathyroidism. In Feldman EC, Nelson RW, editors, *Canine and feline endocrinology and reproduction*, ed 2, Philadelphia, 1996, WB Saunders Co, pp 497-516.

Fineman LS, Hamilton TA, de Gortari A et al: Cisplatin chemotherapy for treatment of thyroid carcinoma in dogs: 13 cases, *J Am Anim Hosp Assoc* 34:109-112, 1998.

Fleeman LM, Rand JS: Management of canine diabetes, *Vet Clin N Am Sm Anim Pract* 31:855-880, 2001.

Gulikers KP, Panciera DL: Influence of various medications on canine thyroid function, *Compend Contin Ed Pract Vet* 24:511-523, 2002.

Hill K, Scott-Moncrieff JC: Tumors of the adrenal cortex causing hyperadrenocorticism, *Vet Med* 96:686-706, 2001.

Kantrowitz LB, Peterson ME, Melian C et al: Serum total thyroxine, total triiodothyronine, free thyroxine, and thyrotropin concentrations in dogs with nonthyroidal disease, *J Am Vet Med Assoc* 219:765-769, 2001.

Kaplan AJ, Peterson ME, Kemppainen RJ: Effects of disease on the results of diagnostic tests for use in detecting hyperadrenocorticism in dogs, *J Am Vet Med Assoc* 207:445-451, 1995.

Kemppainen RJ, Behrend EN: Diagnosis of canine hypothyroidism. Perspectives from a testing laboratory, *Vet Clin N Am Sm Anim Pract* 31:951-962, 2001.

Kerl ME: Diabetic ketoacidosis: pathophysiology and clinical and laboratory presentation, *Compend Cont Ed Pract Vet* 23:220-228, 2001.

Kerl ME. Diabetic ketoacidosis: pathophysiology and clinical and laboratory presentation, *Compend Cont Ed Pract Vet* 23:330-339, 2001.

Kintzer PP, Peterson ME: Treatment and long-term follow-up of 205 dogs with hypoadrenocorticism, *J Vet Intern Med* 11:43-49, 1997.

Klein MK, Powers BE, Withrow SJ et al: Treatment of thyroid carcinoma in dogs by surgical resection alone: 20 cases (1981-1989), *J Am Vet Med Assoc* 206:1007-1009, 1995.

Lifton SJ, King LG, Zerbe CA: Glucocorticoid deficient hypoadrenocorticism in dogs: 18 cases (1986-1995), *J Am Vet Med Assoc* 209:2076-2081, 1996.

Macintire DK: Treatment of diabetic ketoacidosis in dogs by continuous low-dose intravenous infusion of insulin, *J Am Vet Med Assoc* 202:1266-1272, 1993.

Neiger R, Ramsey I, O'Connor J et al: Trilostane treatment of 78 dogs with pituitary-dependent hyperadrenocorticism, *Vet Rec* 150:799-804, 2002.

Pack L, Roberts RE, Dawson SD et al: Definitive radiation therapy for infiltrative thyroid carcinoma in dogs, *Vet Radiol Ultrasound* 42:471-474, 2001.

Panciera DL: Conditions associated with canine hypothyroidism, *Vet Clin N Am Sm Anim Pract* 31:935-950, 2001.

Peterson ME: Medical treatment of canine pituitary-dependent hyperadrenocorticism (Cushing's disease), *Vet Clin N Am Sm Anim Pract* 31:1005-1014, 2001.

Peterson ME, Melian C, Nichols R: Measurement of serum total thyroxine, triiodothyronine, free thyroxine, and thyrotropin concentrations for diagnosis of hypothyroidism in dogs, *J Am Vet Med Assoc* 211:1396-1402, 1997.

Refsal KR, Provencher-Bolliger AL, Graham PA et al: Update on the diagnosis and treatment of disorders of calcium regulation, *Vet Clin N Am Sm Anim Pract* 31:1043-1062, 2001.

Ristic JME, Ramsey IK, Heath FM et al: The use of 17-hydroxyprogesterone in the diagnosis of canine hyperadrenocorticism, *J Vet Intern Med* 16:433-439, 2002.

Roth L, Tyler RD: Evaluation of low sodium:potassium ratios in dogs, *J Vet Diagn Invest* 11:60-64, 1999.

Rumbeiha WK, Fitzgerald SD, Kruger JM et al: Use of pamidronate disodium to reduce cholecalciferol-induced toxicosis in dogs, *Am J Vet Res* 61:9-13, 2000.

Theon AP, Marks SL, Feldman ES et al: Prognostic factors and patterns of treatment failure in dogs with unresectable differentiated thyroid carcinomas treated with megavoltage irradiation, *J Am Vet Med Assoc* 216:1775-1779, 2000.

Van Liew CH Greco DS, Salman MD: Comparison of results of adrenocorticotropic hormone stimulation and low-dose dexamethasone suppression tests with necropsy findings in dogs: 81 cases (1985-1995), *J Am Vet Med Assoc* 211:322-325, 1997.

Vasilopulos RJ, Mackin A: Humoral hypercalcemia of malignancy: diagnosis and treatment, *Compend Cont Ed Pract Vet* 25:129-135, 2003.

34. The Approach to Vomiting and Regurgitation

Anthony P. Carr

1. How can vomiting be differentiated from regurgitation?

Vomiting is an active process whereas regurgitation is the passive expulsion of food from the esophagus. Vomiting will expel the contents of the stomach and also of the proximal small intestine. Typically vomiting is associated with prodromal nausea that is signaled by salivation and restlessness. This is followed by forceful contractions of the abdominal and diaphragmatic muscles. Vomitus will often be yellow tinged if it is mixed with bile. Stomach contents tend to be acidic, whereas regurgitated material may be more alkaline; however, this distinction is often unreliable.

2. What are common causes of regurgitation?

Regurgitation is usually associated with esophageal disease. Regurgitation must be differentiated from dysphagia. Dysphagia can result in ingesta being expelled from the pharynx or oral cavity.

The most common differential diagnoses for regurgitation include esophageal obstruction or megaesophagus. Foreign bodies, of which bones are the most common, can cause obstruction. Obstruction can also occur because of tumors or strictures. The most common causes of strictures are previous foreign bodies, anesthesia-related regurgitation, and medications that become trapped in the esophagus. In very young animals a persistent right aortic arch will also cause regurgitation when solid foods are first taken. Megaesophagus can be acquired or congenital in origin (see Chapter 37).

3. What is the process of vomiting?

Vomiting is a complex process. Vomiting is under control of the vomiting center in the medulla oblongata. The vomiting center receives information from the chemoreceptor trigger zone (CRTZ) in the area postrema (where the blood-brain barrier is weaker), the vestibular apparatus, higher cortical regions, and peripheral receptors (especially in the GI tract). A variety of receptors are involved with vomiting, including dopaminergic receptors in the CRTZ and on afferent nerves in the gut, adrenergic receptors in the vomiting center and CRTZ, cholinergic receptors in the CRTZ and on gut afferents, serotonergic receptors, and histaminergic receptors.

The act of vomiting involves a certain sequence of events. Initially a feeling of nausea is generated. This can be identified in dogs as yawning, salivation, and restlessness. Increased production and swallowing of saliva occurs. The saliva contains bicarbonate, which helps to buffer stomach acid. The lower esophageal sphincter and the cardia then relax. There also is retrograde movement of small intestinal contents into the stomach. The dog then begins to retch, a process in which the diaphragm and other muscles contract while the glottis remains closed. This causes negative intrathoracic pressure, which draws stomach contents into the esophagus.

Active vomiting then occurs when abdominal muscles contract. Contraction of these muscles causes pressure to become positive in the abdomen and when the glottis opens, intrathoracic pressure also become positive, resulting in expulsion of esophageal contents.

4.　What are common causes of vomiting?

Vomiting has many causes (Table 34-1). It helps to divide vomiting between primary GI causes and vomiting secondary to non-GI diseases. Of course, there is the possibility of having overlapping causes. As an example, in dogs with renal failure vomiting can be from the effect of uremic toxins on the CRTZ or because of uremic gastropathy.

5.　What would be the initial approach to a vomiting dog?

The first step would be to differentiate between vomiting caused by self-limiting disorders and vomiting that requires more further diagnostic evaluation and aggressive therapy. This differentiation is made based on the dog's history and the results of the physical examination. A history of chronic vomiting or the presence of abdominal pain, hematemesis, or fever or other signs of a systemic problem is an indication for a more aggressive approach.

A variety of diagnostic tests may be appropriate in a given animal. Radiography is useful in evaluating for GI tract obstruction and for non-GI tract diseases. Abdominal ultrasound can be helpful in evaluating the gut and other abdominal organs. Routine laboratory testing such as complete blood count, serum biochemistry, and urinalysis, can help to rule out systemic problems and any acid-base or electrolyte problems resulting from persistent vomiting. In young dogs that have not been vaccinated or not adequately vaccinated against parvovirus, testing for parvovirus may be considered, especially if the dog is depressed.

Treatment is supportive in most cases of vomiting. Fluids are given parenterally to correct volume deficits, to replace ongoing losses, and to keep the dog hydrated while nothing is given by mouth for a period of time. After vomiting has been controlled, resumption of oral feedings for most dogs starts with small amounts of bland foods.

6.　What antiemetic medications are available and how do they work?

Antiemetic medications are often used in veterinary practice. By reducing nausea they help the animal feel better and by reducing vomiting they halt the loss of fluids and electrolytes caused by persistent emesis. Antiemetic agents can act at various receptors. Some are specific to individual receptors whereas others may influence multiple receptors. Knowledge of each drug's mode of action is important to making appropriate choices in each case.

Table 34-1　*Some Causes of Vomiting in Dogs*

PRIMARY (GI TRACT DISEASE)	SECONDARY (NON-GI TRACT DISEASE)
Acute gastritis	Pancreatitis
GI foreign body	Peritonitis
GI tract ulceration	Uremia
GI tract tumor, especially stomach	Hypoadrenocorticism
Gastric outflow obstruction	Liver failure
Inflammatory bowel disease (IBD)	Lead toxicity
Intussusception	Zinc toxicity
Physaloptera spp.	Drugs (e.g., digitalis, erythromycin, xylazine, aspirin)
Hiatal hernia	Vestibular disease
Parvovirus	Urinary tract obstruction
Dietary indiscretion	Hypercalcemia
Food allergy	

Metoclopramide is a commonly used antiemetic drug. It can be given by intermittent subcutaneous injection (0.2-0.4 mg/kg every 6 hours, subcutaneously [SQ] or intramuscularly [IM]) or as a constant intravenous infusion (1-2 mg/kg/day). The latter mode of administration appears to be more efficacious. This medication predominantly affects the D_2 dopaminergic receptors in the CRTZ and gut. It also affects the 5-HT_3 serotonergic receptors in the CRTZ.

Phenothiazine drugs such as chlorpromazine (0.2–0.5 mg/kg every 8 hours SQ) or prochlorperazine (0.1-0.5 mg/kg every 8 hours SQ or IM) are broad spectrum antiemetics (they have activity at the α_2-adrenergic, D_2-dopaminergic, histaminergic, and cholinergic receptors). However, use can cause hypotension, so blood pressure should be monitored. Sedation is also usually quite pronounced with use of these agents. These medications are a good choice for dogs that fail to respond to metoclopramide. It is possible to use both agents concurrently.

A limited number of medications are specific to the 5-HT_3 serotonergic receptors. Ondansetron (0.5-1.0 mg/kg every 12 to 24 hours, by mouth [PO]) can be helpful in some cases of vomiting associated with stimulation of the CRTZ.

H_1-histaminergic receptor antagonists include diphenhydramine (2-4 mg/kg every 8 hours PO) and dimenhydrinate (4-8 mg/kg every 8 hours PO). These can be used for the treatment of motion sickness or vestibular disease.

Erythromycin at low dosages (0.5-1.0 mg/kg every 8 hours) can also act as an antiemetic by stimulation of the motilin receptors that increase GI motility and promote gastric emptying.

35. The Approach to Diarrhea

Anthony P. Carr

1. How can large-bowel diarrhea be differentiated from small-bowel diarrhea?

Certain criteria help to differentiate the source of diarrhea; they are listed in Table 35-1. Not every case will have every sign. It is also important to remember that mixed forms can occur. This is especially true if small-bowel diarrhea has been present for some time. The dysfunction/malabsorption in the small intestine leads to secondary changes in the large bowel.

2. When considering differentials for diarrhea what are the two primary differential groups?

Diarrhea has many causes. Many times it is due to primary gastrointestinal (GI) tract disease. At times, however, diarrhea can be due to non-GI tract disease such as uremia, liver disease, or hypoadrenocorticism.

3. What pathophysiologic mechanisms lead to diarrhea?

Diarrhea can have various causes such as infections, dietary indiscretions, food allergy and non-GI disease (uremia). The mechanisms by which diarrhea develops can be grouped into secretory mechanisms, osmotic mechanisms, permeability changes, and motility disorders.

Secretory diarrhea usually develops with various infectious agents (*Escherichia coli, Salmonella* spp., etc.) and toxins. This form of diarrhea will not resolve with fasting. The predominant clinical problem with this form of diarrhea is significant fluid and electrolyte loss.

Osmotic diarrhea occurs when increased concentrations of hyperosmolar particles are present in the small and large intestine, overwhelming the ability of the GI tract to resorb water. Common causes include dietary indiscretion and maldigestion. This form of diarrhea is responsive to fasting. The predominant clinical problem is fluid loss.

Table 35-1 *Small Bowel versus Large Bowel Diarrhea*		
CLINICAL SIGN	SMALL BOWEL	LARGE BOWEL
Tenesmus	No	Yes
Frank blood in feces (hematochezia)	No	Yes
Melena	Yes	No
Frequency of defecation	Normal to increased	Markedly increased
Urge	No	Yes
Mucoid feces	No	Yes
Weight loss	Yes	Rarely
Fecal volume	Large	Small

Changes in permeability can result in more severe clinical signs. The increased permeability leads not only to loss of fluids and electrolytes but can also lead to the loss of proteins, blood, and mucus. Generally, changes in permeability are associated with GI tract inflammation.

Although in theory motility disorders can lead to diarrhea, this has been poorly documented in dogs. Hypomotility disorders, which are more common than hypermotility disorders, can be caused by many diseases or other conditions.

4.   What basic laboratory studies are indicated to evaluate diarrhea?

There is no easy answer to this question. A fecal float test is indicated in all cases of diarrhea. This may be the only test needed in uncomplicated cases of acute diarrhea when the dog is not visibly ill. In chronic cases or cases where symptoms are more severe, a complete blood count, serum chemistry profile, urinalysis, and fecal culture are advisable. Imaging studies may be indicated as well. Especially with chronic disease, other diagnostic laboratory studies such as determination of trypsin-like immunoreactivity (TLI), an adrenocorticotropic hormone (ACTH) stimulation test (to rule out hypoadrenocorticism), measurement of serum folate and cobalamin concentrations, and intestinal biopsies may be indicated.

5.   How can biopsies be collected from the GI tract and what are the advantages and disadvantages of each method?

GI tract biopsies are often necessary with chronic disease to establish a more definitive diagnosis. Either full-thickness biopsies or pinch biopsies can be taken. Full-thickness biopsies are usually obtained during exploratory surgery, although they can also be obtained laparoscopically. Pinch biopsies are obtained with endoscopy.

Surgical exploration has certain advantages and disadvantages. Biopsy specimens obtained by this method can be more helpful in diagnosis because they may include all layers of the GI tract. It is also possible to biopsy areas that cannot be reached by endoscopy. Another advantage is that other organs can be examined and biopsied at the same time. The predominant disadvantages of exploratory surgery are that it is more invasive and there is the risk of biopsy site dehiscence. This risk increases considerably when the colon is biopsied or the dog has hypoproteinemia.

Endoscopy often leads to a diagnosis in cases of GI tract disease. The procedure is less invasive than exploratory surgery and there is no risk of wound dehiscence. Endoscopy is preferable for biopsy of the large bowel and in dogs with significant hypoproteinemia. Endoscopy also has the advantage that it allows visualization of the lumen of the GI tract and any abnormal appearing areas. Endoscopy is, however, limited to certain areas of the GI tract (esophagus, stomach, duodenum, proximal jejunum, distal ileum, large intestine) and the biopsy specimens obtained are smaller. Additionally, endoscopy does require the use of special instruments and skill is required to perform a complete endoscopic exam.

ACUTE DIARRHEA

6. What are the clinically significant differences between acute and chronic diarrhea?

Acute diarrhea is a common complaint in small animal practice. Many cases of acute diarrhea are self-limiting, even if mucosal damage is severe, because intestinal epithelial cell turnover is rapid and new, normal epithelial cells will quickly restore normal intestinal function. Treatment need only be supportive and symptomatic, since most animals that die from diarrhea do so not as a result of the underlying cause of diarrhea but from the loss of water and electrolyte imbalance, with subsequent dehydration, acidosis, and shock. In many cases, extensive diagnostic workups are not needed.

In contrast, chronic diarrhea is rarely self-limiting and a diagnosis is needed for optimal treatment. In many cases, biopsy of the GI tract is indicated. Supportive care is less likely to be needed in cases of chronic diarrhea.

7. What are the principles of symptomatic management of acute diarrhea in the dog?

Many dogs with acute diarrhea do not require symptomatic therapy. In those cases, however, when the dog is visibly ill or dehydration is present, it is advisable to initiate more aggressive supportive care.

8. What dietary modification is indicated with acute diarrhea?

Food should be withheld in most cases for 24 to 48 hours; this will be especially effective in dogs with osmotic diarrhea. After this time, a bland diet fed frequently in small quantities is recommended. Then the normal diet is gradually added to the bland diet to allow return to a normal diet.

9. Is fluid therapy indicated with acute diarrhea?

Maintaining fluid balance is vital because diarrhea causes dehydration and the resultant changes in electrolyte and acid-base balance can cause death, especially in puppies. In dogs that are drinking, adequate fluid balance can be maintained by providing them with water. Oral rehydrating solutions can also be used; these combine water with glucose or glycine. The glucose or glycine helps to increase sodium absorption, which in turn increases water absorption.

In dogs that are debilitated, are dehydrated, are vomiting, or have major electrolyte disturbance, intravenous fluid therapy is preferable. In many dogs the subcutaneous route will not provide adequate amounts of fluid. If intravenous fluids are to be used, a minimum laboratory database is indicated to help tailor fluid therapy optimally.

10. When do I use motility modifiers for managing diarrhea? What drugs do I use?

Motility-modifying agents are most appropriate for cases of large-bowel disease, when the dog is not ill and the diarrhea is more of a hygiene problem (e.g., leads to accidents in the house). Narcotic analgesics (loperamide, 0.1 mg/kg every 8-12 hours, diphenoxylate, 0.1-0.2 mg/kg every 8-12 hours) can be effective in treating diarrhea. These medications delay bowel transit time by increasing nonpropulsive contractions and muscular tone of the gut while decreasing propulsive activity. Opiates also influence the transport of water and electrolytes through the intestine and reduce intestinal fluid accumulation, stool frequency, and stool weight (volume). Anticholinergic agents generally are not indicated for the treatment of diarrhea, because they induce ileus.

11. Are locally acting protectants and absorbents indicated for diarrhea therapy?

Bismuth-subsalicylate, kaolin, and activated charcoal are some of the medications that have been recommended for treatment of diarrhea. Salicylate-containing products can be useful in managing secretory diarrhea. Other agents are generally thought not to be efficacious.

12. What should I look for to support the use of antimicrobials in a case of acute diarrhea?

The use of antibiotics with diarrhea is not routinely indicated. However, when extensive damage to intestinal mucosal is suspected, an antibiotic should be used. Mucosal damage is thought to allow penetration of the intestinal wall by bacteria, which are subsequently released into the systemic circulation. Antibiotics are also justified in cases of symptomatic bacterial infection when a known pathogen is diagnosed.

Evidence of extensive mucosal damage includes the following:
- Fever
- Leukocytosis/leukopenia
- Hemorrhagic diarrhea
- Very sick animal
- Positive blood culture

13. What are the clinical signs of hemorrhagic gastroenteritis (HGE)?

The term hemorrhagic gastroenteritis (HGE) refers to a collection of clinical signs. The cause of HGE is variable; often the syndrome is idiopathic. In some cases *Clostridium perfringens* enterotoxin is suspected to be the underlying cause. The dogs show hemorrhagic diarrhea and frequently hematemesis. Marked hemoconcentration may also occur. The onset is acute and dramatic. Hypovolemia is often seen.

14. How is HGE diagnosed?

The appropriate clinical signs, together with a PCV greater than 60%, are consistent with HGE, although this is not an etiologic diagnosis. In most cases when the PCV is elevated, total protein will be normal.

15. How is HGE treated?

Aggressive fluid therapy is vital in these animals; many require initial resuscitation with high dose fluids. After fluid therapy hypoproteinemia may develop, and colloid therapy may be needed. Antibiotics are often used because of the compromised intestinal barrier.

VIRAL DIARRHEA

16. What causes parvovirus infection in dogs?

The inciting virus is canine parvovirus type 2. The virus is highly contagious and resistant to inactivation. The virus is related to feline panleukopenia and mink enteritis virus. The virus attacks host cells that are rapidly dividing.

17. What clinical signs are associated with parvovirus infection?

Clinical signs are variable, and in some cases, none are apparent. In most cases vomiting, profuse diarrhea, pyrexia, anorexia, and depression are noted. This disease can progress to shock and sepsis. The diarrhea is often hemorrhagic, because the intestinal crypts are destroyed, which leads to the villi being denuded of epithelial cells. Marked hypoproteinemia can occur, as can neutropenia due to the virus attacking rapidly dividing cells in the bone marrow. In the past, myocarditis leading to sudden death was seen in puppies after in utero infections, although this phenomenon is no longer seen.

18. How is parvovirus infection diagnosed?

Appropriate clinical signs in a young dog with inadequate vaccination should always raise concern about parvovirus infection. Neutropenia is a highly suggestive sign; not uncommonly, the neutrophil count is less than 1000/μl. In many cases this infection can be definitively diagnosed by an enzyme-linked immunosorbent assay (ELISA) performed in-house on feces.

Usually this assay will demonstrate viral antigen. A weak positive reaction is possible in recently vaccinated dogs. Electron microscopy is an alternative diagnostic tool.

19. How is parvovirus infection treated?

Given the severe fluid losses in these animals, aggressive fluid therapy is required. Hypoglycemia develops frequently and when present, is an indication to add glucose to the intravenous fluids. Antibiotic therapy (ampicillin or cephazolin in uncomplicated cases, ampicillin with an aminoglycoside in cases with sepsis or severe neutropenia) is indicated in all dogs. If vomiting is persistent, use of an antiemetic would be of benefit. Some studies have shown that early enteral alimentation may be a consideration as well. In severely hypoproteinemic dogs, plasma administration can be helpful.

20. What sequelae can occur with parvovirus infection in dogs?

With the marked disruption of the GI barrier, sepsis or endotoxemia can develop. Damage to the intestine can also lead to intussusception.

21. What is the prognosis with parvovirus infection?

If aggressive supportive care is provided, the prognosis is generally good. Concurrent GI tract disease (corona virus infections, GI parasites) leads to a worse prognosis.

22. What clinical signs are seen with corona virus infection in dogs?

The diarrhea with this disease is variable and usually self-limiting.

BACTERIAL DIARRHEA

23. What role do bacteria play in canine diarrhea?

Bacteria are known to be a common cause of diarrhea in all species. There are, however, difficulties determining if a given bacterial species is causing diarrhea in a dog. Many of the pathogenic bacteria are also found in dogs that do not have diarrhea. In some cases there is genetic variability in the bacterial species that can lead to virulence, for instance, the presence of enterotoxigenic *Clostridia*. This genetic variability usually cannot be determined by simple cultures.

24. What role do *Campylobacter* species play in canine diarrhea?

Campylobacter spp. can be pathogens in dogs, predominantly *Campylobacter jejuni, Campylobacter coli, Campylobacter helveticus,* and *Campylobacter upsaliensis*. These species are considered to have zoonotic potential in dogs, even though most human cases of *Campylobacter* infection are contracted from contaminated food, especially poultry. Diarrheic and nondiarrheic dogs can harbor these bacteria, and in many studies isolation rates were similar (up to 50% positive, especially in young kenneled dogs).

25. What are the clinical signs of *Campylobacter* spp. infection?

Signs are variable. Watery to mucoid to hemorrhagic diarrhea can occur, as can an asymptomatic carrier state.

26. How is a *Campylobacter* infection treated?

Either macrolide antibiotics or fluoroquinolones can be used, though most cases would resolve without resorting to antibiotics. Antibiotic therapy is indicated given the zoonotic potential, however. Erythromycin is considered the drug of choice, though it can cause GI upset. Fluoroquinolones can be used, but resistance can develop rapidly.

27. What role do *Salmonella* spp. play in canine diarrhea?

Salmonella is a potential pathogen, although inapparent carrier states commonly occur. This is a potential zoonotic infection. Prevalence rates vary, but in the typical dog population about 1% of dogs will have the bacteria. Higher rates are seen in kennel populations, racing Greyhounds, racing sled dogs, and dogs fed raw-meat diets.

28. What clinical signs are associated with salmonellosis?

Signs are variable, from inapparent carrier state to severe diarrhea/septicemia. Diarrhea can be watery, mucoid, or hemorrhagic. In more severely affected animals, fever, abdominal pain, and sepsis can occur. These animals will often also show changes on CBC such as a neutrophilia with a left shift and evidence of toxic change.

29. How is salmonellosis treated?

For sick animals, supportive care is indicated. Antibiotics should be reserved for more severely affected animals. Antibiotics should probably be given to all dogs that have hemorrhagic diarrhea. Fluoroquinolones are the drugs of choice for this infection.

30. What role does *E. coli* play in canine diarrhea?

It is difficult to ascertain the role that *E. coli* plays in diarrhea, because this organism is often cultured from dogs without diarrhea. Some strains of *E. coli* have virulence factors that can lead to disease developing. Some strains thought to cause diarrhea include enterotoxigenic *E. coli* (ETEC) and enteropathogenic *E. coli* (EPEC).

31. What role does *C. perfringens* play in canine diarrhea?

As with other bacteria, *C. perfringens* is commonly isolated from dogs with or without diarrhea. It is thought that the production of enterotoxin by some strains leads to diarrhea, although nondiarrheic dogs can also have enterotoxin-producing strains of *C. perfringens*. The enterotoxin is released during sporulation of the bacterium.

32. How is *C. perfringens* diarrhea diagnosed?

It is not possible to definitively determine if *C. perfringens* is causing diarrhea. Neither detection of enterotoxin nor large numbers of spores are limited to dogs with diarrhea.

33. What is meant by small-intestine bacterial overgrowth (SIBO)?

Bacteria can be found in the small intestine, and under certain conditions they can begin to proliferate. The abnormal proliferation results in malabsorption and diarrhea. However, there is no universally accepted upper limit for the number of bacteria normally found in the small intestine, and therefore it is impossible to determine the level that represents SIBO.

34. How is SIBO diagnosed?

Quantitative bacterial cultures are necessary to establish a diagnosis, although this is controversial. Elevations in serum folate concentration and decreased serum cobalamin concentration are also suggestive. Response to antibiotic therapy may also allow a presumptive diagnosis, although its diagnostic value is tentative at best.

35. How is SIBO treated?

A variety of antibiotics are used, including amoxicillin, metronidazole, and tylosin.

FUNGAL DISEASE

36. What causes pythiosis?

This disease is caused by infection with *Pythium insidiosum*.

37. Where is pythiosis commonly found?

The geographic distribution of this infection is generally limited to areas near the Gulf of Mexico.

38. What are the clinical signs of this infection and how is it treated?
This infection results in chronic diarrhea. With time, vomiting, anorexia, and progressive weight loss occur. The bowel walls become markedly thickened and obstruction can result.
When possible, surgical excision of affected tissue should be undertaken. Medical management with itraconazole or amphotericin B can be successful, although response rates are low.

39. What is the prognosis with pythiosis?
The prognosis is generally guarded to poor unless affected tissues can be surgically excised with good margins.

40. What GI signs are seen with histoplasmosis?
Histoplasmosis can affect many organs; GI tract involvement is common. The disease results in weight loss, lethargy, and anorexia. Diarrhea is often seen; usually its characteristics indicate large-bowel involvement. Other clinical signs will depend on what other organs are affected.

41. How is GI histoplasmosis diagnosed?
Clinical signs, together with cytologic evidence of *Histoplasma capsulatum* organisms, are diagnostic. A rectal scrape can often be diagnostic in those cases of large-bowel diarrhea. Serologic results are considered unreliable.

PARASITES

42. How are helminth infections diagnosed?
Fecal float tests can be helpful, especially if centrifugation is used. It is, however, important to remember that a negative fecal float test result does not rule out an infection and should never be a reason to not treat with a deworming agent.

43. What roundworms are commonly found in dogs and how are they acquired?
The most commonly found roundworm is *Toxocara canis*. This can be acquired through the fecal-oral or transmammary route or in utero. *Toxascaris leonina* can also be found. It is acquired through the fecal-oral or transmammary route.

44. What clinical signs are seen with roundworms?
Clinical signs are seen almost exclusively in puppies. Severe infestations can result in diarrhea, vomiting, poor nutritional status, and a potbelly. Obstruction can occur.

45. Are roundworms a zoonotic concern?
The ingestion of roundworm eggs by humans can result in visceral larva migrans. This often does not lead to clinical signs, although in some cases blindness can occur.

46. What hookworms are commonly found in dogs and how are they acquired?
The most common hookworm is *Ancylostoma caninum*. Additionally, *Uncinaria stenocephala* can be found. Hookworms are acquired either by the fecal-oral route or the transmammary route.

47. What clinical signs are seen with hookworms?
Diarrhea can occur with this disease. Significant blood and protein loss can also occur, resulting in weight loss, anemia, and hypoproteinemia.

48. Are hookworms a zoonotic concern?
Hookworms can penetrate skin, resulting in dermal larva migrans. There also have been sporadic reports of intestinal disease in humans infected with canine hookworms.

49. What role does *Giardia* play in canine diarrhea?

This parasite can be seen in dogs, though it occurs in dogs with and without diarrhea. Most infections are subclinical. In some cases severe diarrhea can develop.

50. How is *Giardia* diagnosed?

The *Giardia* cysts can be identified on a fecal float test. Motile trophozoites can be seen on fresh fecal smears. There are also highly sensitive fecal ELISA tests available that detect *Giardia* antigen.

51. How is *Giardia* treated?

Metronidazole can be used to treat *Giardia* (25 mg/kg every 12 hours for 5 days). Prolonged use of the drug can result in central nervous system (CNS) disturbances. Fenbendazole is also highly effective in treating this parasite (50 mg/kg every 12 hours for 3 days). Albendazole is also effective; however, bone marrow toxicity has been seen with this drug. Bathing the dog is also recommended to help prevent reinfection.

ADVERSE REACTIONS TO FOOD

52. What is the difference between food allergy and food intolerance?

With food allergy, a true allergic reaction (usually a mix of types I, II, and IV hypersensitivity reactions) occurs. Food intolerance is based on a nonimmunologic reaction.

53. What clinical signs are seen with adverse reactions to food?

The most common sign, especially with food intolerance, is vomiting or diarrhea. Food allergies can result in non-GI-tract signs such as pruritus and urticaria.

54. How is a food allergy diagnosed?

To diagnose a food allergy, an allergic reaction needs to be documented. This is generally clinically not possible.

55. How is an adverse reaction to food diagnosed?

An adverse reaction to food (allergy or intolerance) is diagnosed by means of an elimination diet and challenge. A diet is fed that does not contain elements that the dog has been previously exposed to. This is fed for a period of at least 12 weeks to see if symptoms subside. If the diet is successful, the dog is challenged with the previous diet to see if signs recur. If they do, the elimination diet is started again.

INFLAMMATORY BOWEL DISEASE

56. What is inflammatory bowel disease (IBD)?

IBD refers to variable inflammatory infiltrates in the GI tract and associated clinical signs. The distribution can be focal or generalized. Many diseases can cause GI tract inflammation; however, with IBD, the inflammation is considered idiopathic.

57. What clinical signs are seen with IBD?

Signs will vary with the severity of inflammation. Diarrhea is the most common sign with intestinal IBD. Depending on where there is inflammation, the characteristics may be those of small-bowel, large-bowel, or mixed diarrhea. In severe cases anorexia and weight loss can occur, as well as excessive protein loss.

58. How do you diagnose IBD?

IBD is diagnosed by means of intestinal biopsy.

59. How do you treat IBD?

Treatment will vary somewhat depending on the type of inflammatory cells that predominate and the severity of clinical signs. Dietary modification is commonly used. In some cases food allergy is suspected, and in such cases it is common practice to use antigen limited diets. Alternatively, hydrolyzed diets can be used.

Antibiotics such as metronidazole and tylosin are often used. This can help to treat SIBO (a common condition seen with IBD), which may be partly responsible for the clinical signs. Antibiotics may also change the flora of the GI tract, which might be beneficial if bacterial antigens are responsible for the inflammation.

With IBD it is also common to give antiinflammatory or immune suppressive medications. Corticosteroids are among the most common therapies for IBD. In severe cases azathioprine or cyclosporine can also be considered. In cases of colitis, 5-aminosalicylic acid (5-ASA) can be given. When combined with sulfapyridine, it is called sulfasalazine. In the colon bacteria split the sulfa from the 5-ASA, which can then have a local antiinflammatory effect in the colon.

60. What is meant by eosinophilic enteritis?

This form of IBD is associated with an eosinophilic infiltrate or occasionally with peripheral eosinophilia. This form of IBD is generally more severe and its treatment is more difficult. Given the participation of eosinophils, parasites or allergies could be underlying causes.

61. What is lymphocytic/plasmacytic IBD?

This is the most common form of IBD, with lymphocytes and plasma cells being the predominant intestinal infiltrate. In many cases it can be difficult to determine if a pathologic infiltrate is present because this type of change can be seen in many dogs without clinical signs of IBD. Severity of signs does not have to correlate with how marked the infiltrate is.

62. What is histiocytic ulcerative colitis?

This is a form of IBD in which histiocytes predominate in the intestinal infiltrate. This form of colitis is especially severe and can result in significant weight loss. Ulcers are common, both macroscopically and microscopically.

63. How is histiocytic ulcerative colitis treated?

Previously, immune-suppressive drugs and sulfasalazine were used in treating this disease, although results were not consistently good. Recently treatment with enrofloxacin has resulted in a good response and long-term resolution of clinical signs.

PROTEIN-LOSING ENTEROPATHY

64. What is a protein-losing enteropathy (PLE)?

Protein-losing enteropathies are a diverse group of chronic intestinal disorders characterized by excessive loss of proteins into the GI tract. The most common causes are inflammatory bowel disease and lymphangiectasia, although protein loss can be seen with other GI tract diseases as well, such as neoplasia, parasitism in juvenile animals, and histoplasmosis. Protein loss can also occur acutely with severe exudative enteritis, for instance, with parvovirus infection. The loss of proteins is nonselective; so that both albumin and globulins will be decreased. Other differentials for hypoalbuminemia, such as protein-losing nephropathy or liver disease, usually are not associated with a dramatic decrease in globulins.

65. What is lymphangiectasia?

With lymphangiectasia the lacteals and lymphatic vessels in the mucosa and or submucosa are dilated and can rupture. Proteins and other lymph components are then lost into the GI tract rather than being resorbed. Breeds with predispositions to lymphangiectasia include the Yorkshire

Terrier, Norwegian Lundehund, and Soft-Coated Wheaten Terriers. The cause of this dilation is not always known; rare congenital cases do occur. In most cases the changes are acquired as a result of inflammation, which leads to obstruction of lymph flow. More severe cases will also have dilation of the mesenteric lymph vessels. Lymphangiitis, lymphadenitis, and lipogranulomas are often seen in more advanced cases.

66. What laboratory abnormalities are seen with PLE?

Many changes are nonspecific. Panhypoproteinemia (low globulin and low albumin concentrations) are often present. Decreased serum cholesterol concentrations and lymphopenia are also seen. Fecal concentrations of alpha$_1$-protease can be helpful in documenting PLE.

67. How is a PLE treated?

In those cases where an underlying cause is found, this should be treated. Often if the cause of a PLE is inflammatory bowel disease, the response to glucocorticoids and other immunosuppressive medications is good. If lymphangiectasia is present, treatment centers on dietary intervention. A highly digestible, low-fat, high-calorie diet is optimal. Reducing fat content decreases lymph flow. At one time supplementation with medium-chain triglycerides (MCTs) was recommended because it was thought that MCTs bypassed the lymphatics. Some recent work suggests that this is not the case. In addition, MCT oil generally is poorly palatable.

NEOPLASIA

68. What are common tumors of the canine GI tract?

Unlike cats, lymphoma limited to the GI tract is a relatively rare finding. The most common tumor in dogs is adenocarcinoma. These can occur in the stomach, small intestine, and large intestine. Smooth-muscle tumors (leiomyosarcomas and leiomyomas) are the next most common tumors; they usually are located in the intestine.

69. What is the prognosis for intestinal tumors?

The prognosis for adenocarcinomas is generally poor because surgical resection is rarely curative. On average, survival time is 6 months, though some dogs live longer. With smooth muscle cell tumors, the prognosis is better. Leiomyosarcomas are slow growing, so even if the tumor metastasizes, the survival time may be close to 2 years.

BIBLIOGRAPHY

Hall EJ, German AJ: Diseases of the small intestine. In Ettinger SJ, Feldman EC, editors: *Textbook of veterinary internal medicine,* ed 6, St. Louis, 2005, Elsevier, pp 1332-1378.

Hostutler RA, Luria BJ, Johnson SE et al: Antibiotic-responsive histiocytic ulcerative colitis in 9 dogs, *JVIM* 18;499-504:2004.

Marks SL, Kather EJ: Bacterial-associated diarrhea in the dog: a critical reappraisal, *Vet Clin North Am Small Anim* 33; 1029-1060:2003.

Melzer KJ, Sellon RK: Canine intestinal lymphangiectasia, *Compend Cont Educ Pract Vet* 24; 953-960:2002.

Tams TR: Chronic diseases of the small intestine. In Tams TR, editor: *Handbook of small animal gastroenterology,* ed 2, Philadelphia, 2003, WB Saunders, pp 211-250.

Triolo A, Lappin MR: cute medical diseases of the small intestine. In Tams TR, editor: *Handbook of small animal gastroenterology,* ed 2, Philadelphia, 2003, WB Saunders, pp 195-210.

Washabau RJ, Holt DE: Diseases of the large intestine. In Ettinger SJ, Feldman EC, editors: *Textbook of veterinary internal medicine,* ed 6, St. Louis, 2005, Elsevier, pp 1408-1420.

36. The Approach to Ascites

Anthony P. Carr

1. What clinical signs are associated with ascites?

The clinical signs associated with ascites can be either masked or exacerbated by the signs resulting from the cause of the ascites. As an example, a dog with heart failure and ascites will have exercise intolerance and dyspnea both from the ascites and from the heart disease. In general, significant fluid accumulation in the abdomen will result in cardiovascular (decreased venous return) and respiratory (pressure on the diaphragm limits breathing ability) compromise. Ascites, if significant enough, can result in a fluid wave that can be noted either spontaneously or after ballottement.

2. What are the general pathophysiologic ways in which fluids can accumulate?

Fluid can accumulate because of decreased colloidal pull (generally, hypoalbuminemia), increased resistance to flow (e.g., heart failure or tumor obstruction), increased permeability of the blood vessels, or increased lymphatic leakage.

3. What kinds of fluids can accumulate in the abdomen?

The fluids that can accumulate are blood, chyle, exudates, modified transudates, and pure transudates. Some authors classify hemorrhage as an exudate.

4. What could cause hemorrhage into the abdomen?

Hemorrhage into the abdomen can result either because of a hemostatic disorder or because of a bleeding lesion in the abdomen. Generally only a coagulopathy would result in cavity bleeding; this would not be expected with disorders of primary hemostasis (e.g., thrombocytopenia, von Willebrand's disease). The most common coagulopathy to cause hemoabdomen is vitamin K antagonist rodenticide toxicity. Bleeding into the abdomen with normal hemostasis can occur because of trauma, ruptured blood vessels (e.g., splenic torsion or gastric dilatation-volvulus [GDV]), or bleeding tumors (mainly involving the spleen or liver).

5. What are the characteristics of exudates and what can cause them?

Exudates are rich in protein (>2.5 g/dl) and nucleated cells (>7,000/µl) and have a specific gravity of more than 1.025. They almost always are a result of increased permeability either through inflammation or infection. Nonseptic exudates can result from severe inflammatory conditions such as pancreatitis, bile peritonitis, or uroabdomen (although initially the inflammation would be absent and the fluid would not contain cells or protein). Tumors can also cause nonseptic exudates.

Visible bacteria confirm that a fluid is septic, although neutrophils with signs of degeneration or toxic changes raise the suspicion of an infection even if bacteria are not visible. Septic exudates can result from bile peritonitis (if the bile was infected), gastrointestinal (GI) tract rupture, a penetrating wound, or ruptured pyometra.

6. What is the difference between a transudate and a modified transudate? Name some potential differentials for each.

A transudate is low in specific gravity (<1.015), protein (<2.5 g/dl), and cells (<1500/µl). Modified transudates have specific gravities between 1.015 and 1.025, protein between 2.5 and 6.0 mg/dl, and cell concentrations of less than 7,000 cells/µl. Over time the presence of a pure transudate in the abdomen will lead to peritoneal irritation with resultant increases in protein and cell count. This will change the transudate to a modified transudate.

Pure transudates can be caused by decreased oncotic pressure, such as occurs in dogs with severe hypoalbuminemia (e.g., protein-losing enteropathy, protein-losing nephropathy). In these dogs it is not uncommon to find peripheral edema as well. Low levels of albumin can also be observed with liver disease, although the development of ascites in these dogs is usually exacerbated by the presence of portal hypertension. Portal hypertension can also lead to the formation of a transudate. Portal hypertension can be classified as prehepatic, hepatic, or posthepatic depending on the location of the obstruction to flow. In many dogs with liver disease the lesion can be at multiple sites. Pure prehepatic portal hypertension is associated with restriction of blood flow at the level of the portal vein and results initially in the formation of a transudate.

Modified transudates have higher protein levels and higher cell counts. Hepatic or posthepatic portal hypertension can cause the accumulation of a modified transudate. Posthepatic portal hypertension results when the level of the obstruction to flow is in either the hepatic vein or the caudal vena cava such as by kinking of the vein, right-sided heart failure, or cardiac tamponade. This results in increased hepatic lymph formation in the sinusoids, with subsequent leakage into the abdomen through the capsule of the liver.

7.   What is a chylous effusion?

Chyloabdomen is much more rare than chylothorax. A chylous effusion is milky or it may appear somewhat red if blood is present as well. The fluid often contains many lymphocytes and its triglyceride concentration may be higher than the serum concentration. The fluid accumulates because of leakage in the lymphatic system. The leak can be due to rupture of the thoracic duct, obstruction of lymph flow (e.g., tumor, granuloma, heart failure), or lymphangiectasia.

8.   What would be the initial diagnostic approach in a dog suspected of having ascites?

A thorough history is important in these animals. Duration of signs may be helpful in determining the cause of fluid accumulation. Recent trauma might suggest hemorrhage, diaphragmatic hernia, or bladder rupture as potential causes. Access to toxins such as vitamin K antagonist rodenticides suggests the possibility of hemoabdomen. Because right-sided heart failure is a common cause of ascites, it is important to ascertain if heartworm infestation is present.

Physical examination should generally indicate that fluid is present. If uncertainty exists, radiographs or abdominal ultrasound can be used to confirm the presence of fluid in the abdomen. Physical examination can also be helpful with regard to diagnosing the cause of the fluid accumulation. The jugular vein should be inspected carefully. Distention or a positive hepatojugular reflex (distension of the jugular vein resulting from palpation of the abdomen) suggests increased right atrial filling pressures such as can be seen with right-sided heart failure or cardiac tamponade. A heart murmur might also be suggestive of heart disease. Because dilated cardiomyopathy more commonly causes ascites than other forms of heart failure, it would be expected that the dog would be a large breed. Pathologic arrhythmias such as atrial fibrillation would also tend to point toward heart disease as the cause of ascites. Masses of the spleen or liver may be palpable if smaller amounts of ascites are present. Pain and fever may suggest an infectious/inflammatory cause such as peritonitis. Concurrent jaundice would most likely be consistent with liver disease, whereas pale mucous membranes could suggest hemoabdomen.

Abdominocentesis is warranted in almost all these dogs to determine the type of fluid present. A midline centesis after a surgical preparation near the umbilicus should generally retrieve fluid; if no fluid is obtained, a four-quadrant tap or ultrasound-guided centesis may be needed. The fluid should be analyzed for specific gravity, cell count, and protein content. Bloody fluid should have a packed cell volume (PCV) determined. If PCV of fluid from the abdomen is higher than that of venous blood, hemorrhage into the abdomen has occurred. Blood from a previous hemorrhage should not clot; if it does, the blood originated from inadvertent puncture of an abdominal blood vessel. Cytologic examination of the fluid is indicated to assess for cells present, including tumor cells or infections. Fluid should also be saved for culture, if indicated by cytologic examination.

Imaging studies of the abdomen are indicated, and occasionally imaging of the thorax will be indicated as well. Radiographs may help to detect mass lesions or significant changes in the size of the liver. If a large amount of fluid is present in the abdomen, detail will be lacking and it might not be possible to assess the organs at all. Abdominal ultrasound is valuable in assessing these dogs. This allows assessment of the liver for disease and a general examination of the abdomen to rule out tumors and other disease. Biopsies may also be possible, although a bleeding tendency should be ruled out first.

A complete blood count (CBC), chemistry panel, and urinalysis (to identify proteinuria) are needed to assess these animals. Additional laboratory examinations such as heartworm testing, coagulation profiles, urine protein to urine creatinine ratio, and liver function tests may be needed. If heart disease is a possibility, a cardiac workup with electrocardiography (ECG), thoracic radiography, and echocardiography would be needed.

9. How can ascites be treated?
How best to treat ascites will depend on the kind of fluid present. If it is blood, generally it would not be recommended to remove it because most of it would be resorbed once the bleeding stops. If the bleeding is due to hemorrhage from a ruptured blood vessel or tumor, surgery will be required to stop continued blood loss. Surgery would also be needed in most cases of uroabdomen or septic effusions. Ascites due to heart failure or portal hypertension can usually be managed with diuretics such as furosemide. This can be combined with spironolactone when needed. When ascites is compromising respiratory function or diuretics are not effective in reducing fluid accumulation, drainage is indicated. The goal is to remove as much fluid as necessary to stabilize breathing. Dogs tend to tolerate abdominocentesis well. However, repeated taps can lead to electrolyte shifts and excessive loss of protein.

BIBLIOGRAPHY

King LG, Gelens HCJ: Ascites. *Compend Contin Edu Pract Vet* 14:1063-1073, 1992.
Kruth SA: Abdominal distention, ascites and peritonitis. In Ettinger SJ, Feldman EC, editors: *Textbook of veterinary internal medicine,* ed 6, St. Louis, 2005, Elsevier, pp150-153.

37. Esophageal Disease

Anthony P. Carr

1. What are typical signs of esophageal disease?
Dogs with esophageal disease will often regurgitate. Regurgitation must be distinguished from vomiting. On occasion, dogs will present for respiratory problems caused by aspiration during regurgitation. Dysphagia, salivation, and odynophagia (painful swallowing) are other symptoms that can be present. Esophageal disorders can be secondary to a variety of systemic disorders, so that the clinical signs of these diseases may predominate.

2. What is megaesophagus?
Megaesophagus refers to a generalized hypomotile and dilated esophagus. Megaesophagus can be congenital or acquired, with the latter being most common. This needs to be differentiated from mere dilation (e.g., with aerophagia) and focal involvement. As an example, persistent right aortic arch will cause prolonged esophageal obstruction, which leads to dilation and hypomotility in the area cranial to the obstruction. An insignificant cause of transitory megaesophagus may be observed on thoracic radiographs taken during general anesthesia.

3. What is the most common cause of megaesophagus?

Most cases are idiopathic. The most common cause identified is myasthenia gravis; in most cases, this is a focal form with signs limited to the esophagus. It has been identified commonly in German Shepherds, though any breed can develop this problem.

4. What other causes are there for megaesophagus?

In very young animals, consideration would have to be given to congenital megaesophagus. This is seen with increased frequency in Irish Setters, German Shepherds, Great Danes, Shar-Peis, Miniature Schnauzers, and Fox Terriers.

In adult animals, neuromuscular disease can result in megaesophagus. In addition to myasthenia gravis (generalized or focal form), polymyositis, dysautonomia, and systemic lupus erythematosus can lead to megaesophagus. Hypoadrenocorticism has been linked to this disease as well, both the typical form with mineralocorticoid and glucocorticoid deficiency as well was the atypical form in which only glucocorticoids are lacking. Toxicity from lead and organophosphates are potential causes that need to be ruled out.

5. How is megaesophagus diagnosed?

The diagnosis of megaesophagus is usually straightforward in an animal with appropriate clinical signs. Thoracic radiographs should reveal the dilated and air-filled esophagus. Radiographs should be examined in detail for any evidence of aspiration pneumonia as well. Contrast studies of the esophagus are usually not needed and may not be desirable because of the high risk of aspiration in these dogs. Contrast can help to determine esophageal motility or highlight the organ in those cases in which the esophagus cannot be visualized clearly.

6. What additional tests are indicated once megaesophagus has been diagnosed?

Additional testing will depend on the clinical presentation of the dog. Routine minimum database should include a complete blood cell count, chemistry panel, and urinalysis. An acetylcholine receptor antibody test is indicated in those cases in which a cause is not immediately obvious. Testing for lead or organophosphates may be appropriate. With signs of generalized neuromuscular disease electrodiagnostics (electromyography, nerve conduction studies), muscle/nerve biopsy, and antinuclear antibody testing should be considered. Testing for endocrine disease may also be warranted (hypoadrenocorticism, hypothyroidism).

7. How is megaesophagus managed?

In those cases in which a cause is found, treating the underlying disorder may result in resolution of the megaesophagus. In many cases, however, the esophageal disease may take time to resolve or may remain a permanent problem. Therapy is therefore directed at minimizing complications such as aspiration pneumonia and inadequate nutritional intake.

Feeding several meals daily in an upright position is usually ideal. After feeding, the dog needs to remain in this elevated position for at least 10 to 15 minutes to allow food to move into the stomach. The consistency of the food that is best tolerated varies among dogs. Some will do well with a more gruel-like consistency, whereas others are better managed with meatballs made from canned dog food. Most dogs can be managed conservatively in this manner. If recurrent problems are encountered, placement of a gastric feeding tube should be considered.

Aspiration pneumonia needs to be carefully monitored for. If it develops, antibiotics are indicated. With severe forms, use of intravenous broad-spectrum antibiotic therapy is vital.

8. What is the prognosis with megaesophagus?

Prognosis with megaesophagus is variable. If an etiology can be found that is correctible, then the prognosis may be good. Concurrent pharyngeal dysfunction is of great concern because aspiration pneumonia is more likely if this condition is present.

9. What other common diseases of the esophagus exist?

Esophagitis can occur from irritation from toxic or abrasive materials ingested or from gastric reflux. The latter can occur frequently during anesthesia or deep sedation. Pills and capsules (especially doxycycline) can also lead to esophageal injury if they do not move into the stomach, because of this it is always recommended that food or water be given after oral medications are given. Severe esophagitis can lead to stricture formation.

Foreign bodies can cause mucosal damage leading to esophagitis. Large foreign bodies can lead to obstruction of the esophagus. Bones are frequently involved as are fish hooks (Fig. 37-1).

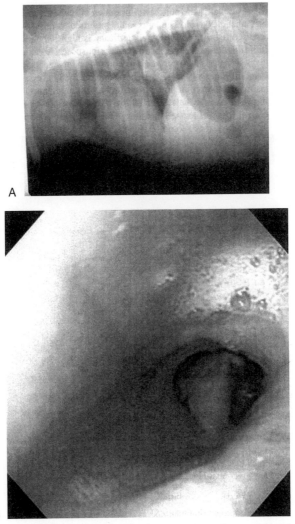

A

B

Figure 37-1. **A,** Lateral radiograph demonstrating a bone in the esophagus caudal to the heart. **B,** Bone foreign body in the esophagus of a dog.

These can penetrate the esophagus leading to mediastinitis and pyothorax. Their removal is generally attempted with endoscopy; surgical intervention with intrathoracic foreign bodies generally does not have a good prognosis. After removal, strictures can develop (Fig. 37-2).

Esophageal strictures are secondary to severe esophageal mucosal injury. A common cause is anesthesia; clinical signs usually begin 1 to 3 weeks afterward. It is assumed that reflux occurs, leading to injury. Foreign bodies, retained medications, and toxic injury have been associated with the development of strictures.

10. How are esophageal strictures managed?

Stricture openings are often small and food cannot be ingested. Bypassing the esophagus with a gastrotomy tube will ensure adequate nutrition. Correction of the stricture is usually either by bougienage or balloon catheter dilation. The latter is the preferred technique. Balloon dilation is associated with a decreased risk of perforation and efficacy is higher than with the bougies. In almost all cases, multiple dilation procedures are necessary for successful management. Initiating therapy for esophagitis is also advisable such as H_2 receptor blocking agents and sucralfate slurry. Omeprazole can be used in place of the H_2 receptor blocking agents because it has a greater ability to suppress gastric acid secretion. Prednisone (0.5 to 1.0 mg/kg/day) has also been used as it may suppress fibrosis; however, the efficacy of this therapy has not been evaluated.

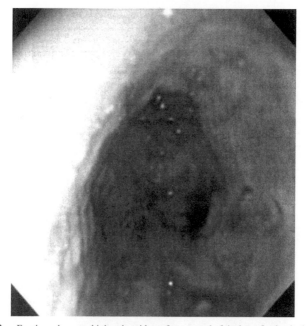

Figure 37-2.   Esophageal mucosal injury is evident after removal of the bone foreign body.

BIBLIOGRAPHY

Jergens AE: Diseases of the esophagus, In Ettinger SJ, Feldman EC, editors: *Textbook of veterinary internal medicine,* ed 6, St. Louis, 2005, Elsevier.

38. Diseases of the Stomach

Anthony P. Carr

GASTRIC DILATION VOLVULUS

1. What is gastric dilation volvulus (GDV)?

GDV must be differentiated from simple dilation in which the stomach is filled with gas, fluid, or ingesta. With a GDV, there is a clockwise rotation of the stomach along its long axis, most commonly 180° though 360° twists can be seen. It is possible that the volvulus results in dilation by trapping gas in the stomach or it may be that dilation of the stomach leads to volvulus. It would seem more likely that volvulus occurs first, because, in most cases, after gastropexy (which prevents volvulus) gastric dilation is rarely seen.

2. Are there any predisposing factors for the development of GDV?

GDVs mainly occur in larger breed dogs, though Basset Hounds, Bulldogs, and Dachshunds can occasionally develop this problem as well. Some of the increased risk may relate to chest conformation in that deep-chested dogs are much more likely to have this problem than are barrel-chested dogs. Ingesting large amounts of food or water at one time might lead to distension of the stomach possibly predisposing to a GDV. Eating rapidly is also thought to contribute to an increased risk of GDV. Exercise after eating has also been considered a potential way that torsion can occur though there are few data to support this contention.

3. What is the pathophysiology of GDV?

After a GDV is established, severe cardiopulmonary compromise occurs. Increased intraabdominal pressure leads to a decreased ability to fully inspire by compromising the function of the diaphragm. Increased pressure also compromises the cardiovascular system. The vena cava is compressed reducing venous return to the heart. The viscera are underperfused and become edematous; if prolonged enough, necrosis can occur, predominantly of the stomach. The short gastric arteries commonly are torn during the volvulus, further compromising blood supply to the stomach. The spleen is also drawn into an abnormal position by the movement of the stomach resulting in splenic congestion and thrombosis. Various substances including endotoxins, myocardial depressant factor, and cytokines are released from the spleen that have a negative effect on systemic cardiovascular function. Shock is a common occurrence as a result. After the stomach is derotated, the tissues are reperfused. This leads to reperfusion injury, mediated mainly by free radicals.

4. What are the clinical signs of GDV?

Dogs usually present with a history of regurgitation, though the owners may interpret this as vomiting. The animals are often anxious and uncomfortable. Abdominal distention may be noted by the owners. On physical examination, the animals often present with signs of shock (tachycardia, weak pulses, delayed capillary refill time, hypotension). Respiratory compromise is evident with shallow, rapid breathing. In most cases the tympanic stomach can easily be found; however, there are some cases of GDV where dilation is minimal.

5. How is a GDV diagnosed?

The clinical signs and signalment are often clue enough to establish a tentative diagnosis of GDV, though this needs to be differentiated from a case of simple dilation. This can be done with radiographs (Fig. 38-1) and the pylorus dorsal to the body of the stomach, though in

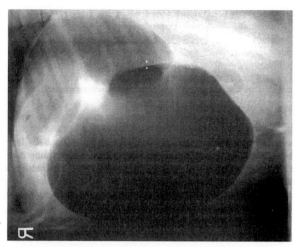

Figure 38-1. Lateral radiograph showing gas distention of the stomach with compartmentalization (double bubble).

compromised animals it may be prudent to stabilize the dog before radiography. Right lateral is the preferred view to use for diagnosis. Check the radiographs carefully for evidence of free air; this could indicate gastric rupture.

6. What emergency interventions are indicated with a GDV?

The goal of treating a GDV is to stabilize cardiovascular function and decompress the dilated stomach. After these goals are achieved the dog is taken to surgery to derotate the stomach and perform a gastropexy to prevent recurrence. Cardiovascular status can be improved by placing large bore intravenous catheters (preferably two). Crystalloids are given at shock doses of 90 ml/kg/hr initially. It is also possible to administer colloids in the resuscitation phase such as 7% hypertonic saline in 6% dextran 70, 5 ml/kg given over 5 minutes. Hetastarch can also be used at 5 to 10 ml/kg over 10 to 15 minutes. If colloids are used, the crystalloid requirement will decrease (20 to 40 ml/kg). Rarely will inotropic support with dopamine or dobutamine be needed.

The next primary goal is to relieve the distension. In animals that are having serious respiratory problems, it may be indicated to do this concurrently with fluid therapy. Opinions vary as to how best to decompress the stomach. Stomach tubing has commonly been recommended. There is the risk of esophageal or stomach rupture if done with too much force, though it can occur with minimal force if the tissue is necrotic. Another alternative is trocarization, which is accomplished with 14- to 16-gauge needles or utilizing an over the needle catheter. The area to be trocarized is percussed, tympany should be evident. The area is clipped and prepped and the needle inserted. This will often relieve enough pressure to significantly improve the dog's cardiovascular status. Decompression in this manner can also make it easier to pass a stomach tube. In my experience, this has been adequate and the dog is stable enough to take to surgery. In rare cases, a temporary gastrostomy can be performed, usually only if there will be significant delay before definitive surgery.

Routine blood work and urinalysis are indicated to rule out concurrent illnesses and to assess for the severity of acid-base and electrolyte abnormalities. Lactate analysis is also helpful. Markedly elevated lactate concentrations are associated with a poorer outcome. Blood pressure should be monitored to assess for efficacy of resuscitation efforts. An electrocardiogram is also recommended. Most arrhythmias develop during anesthesia or postoperatively and do not appear to correlate to outcome. Arrhythmias at presentation do seem, however, to be associated with increased mortality.

7. What surgical options are there for GDV?

Surgery aims to derotate the stomach and perform a gastropexy to prevent recurrence. In addition other procedures may be necessary such as resection of necrotic tissues (especially stomach) or splenectomy. Surgery should be performed as soon as the dog is relatively stable, delay may result in gastric necrosis and other complications.

A midline celiotomy is performed. Often the omentum covers the stomach, a sign of rotation. The stomach is returned to its normal position. If a stomach tube had not been previously passed it is now passed and the stomach lavaged. After this is accomplished, the stomach is assessed for viability. The area along the great curvature is most prone to ischemia. Assessment is subjective and dependent on experience. Areas that are dark gray or black, lack peristalsis, or do not bleed after being incised are probably significantly compromised. Nonviable tissue is either excised via partial gastrectomy or via partial gastric invagination, though the latter is limited to small areas. The spleen should also be assessed for viability. If the spleen is torsed, significant vessel avulsion is present, or the spleen is infarcted, partial or total splenectomy should be performed.

After the stomach has been assessed and any areas of ischemia addressed, a gastropexy is performed. Several methods have been described including belt-loop gastropexy, tube gastropexy, incisional gastropexy, and circumcostal gastropexy. All procedures tend to produce a durable adhesion of the stomach to the body wall. Which technique to use will depend on operator experience and preference.

8. What postoperative monitoring and management are needed?

In the postoperative period, good nursing care is vital. Fluid therapy is needed to maintain perfusion. Any acid-base or electrolyte abnormalities need to be addressed. Potassium will usually have to be added to fluids to prevent hypokalemia. Analgesia is vital as well.

Ventricular arrhythmias occur frequently and the electrocardiogram (ECG) should be monitored continuously. A variety of criteria have been suggested to indicate the need for treatment including absolute number of ventricular premature contractions (VPCs) per minute, number of VPCs in a run of ventricular tachycardia, multifocal VPCs, and R on T phenomenon. The latter especially is considered electrically unstable and may lead to a malignant arrhythmia. However, it is important to know what the goals of antiarrhythmic therapy are in a dog and if the medications being used are able to achieve these goals. If it is thought that the arrhythmia is causing clinical signs (with a ventricular arrhythmia, this would only be the case if the rate was high, so generally higher than 140 or 150 beats/min) treatment is clearly indicated. A good initial choice is lidocaine (bolus of 2-4 mg/kg slow intravenously over 5 minutes followed by a constant rate infusion [CRI] of 50-70 µg/kg/min). Although sudden death can occur, it is unlikely that a medication such as lidocaine or procainamide would prevent this; in fact, studies in humans suggest that they may be proarrhythmic. It has been the author's experience that controlling these arrhythmias may be extremely difficult. It is also important to remember that optimizing the heart's environment will often be helpful in controlling arrhythmias. Maintaining perfusion, correcting acid-base problems, maintaining normal potassium and magnesium concentrations, providing analgesia, and maintaining oxygenation will often be the most important factors in controlling arrhythmias.

Low blood pressure can occur postoperatively. This can compromise organ function and should be treated aggressively. Hypotension can be because of ongoing shock, hemorrhage, or pathologic tachycardias. Gastrointestinal rupture and peritonitis would also lead to hypotensive shock.

Vomiting or recurrent gastric bloating can be noted postoperatively. This can be managed with antiemetics, especially those that are prokinetic such as metoclopramide or low-dose erythromycin. Gastric distension can be addressed with stomach tubing. Some clinicians will place a nasogastric tube for this purpose at the time of surgery. If a tube gastropexy was performed, decompression is easily performed.

If possible coagulation parameters should be assessed. Disseminated intravascular coagulation (DIC) is a common complication of GDV. Treatment with low-dose heparin can be considered, though there are no objective data that show this therapy is of any benefit. Plasma can be given if coagulation values are markedly prolonged or antithrombin III is decreased significantly.

Antibiotics are commonly used in the perioperative period. Broad spectrum antibiotics such as cephalexin (22 mg/kg intravenously every 8 hours) or ampicillin (22 mg/kg intravenously every 8 hours) are adequate in uncomplicated cases. In cases in which peritonitis could develop, a combination of ampicillin with an aminoglycoside (gentamicin 6 mg/kg intravenously every 24 hours) or a fluoroquinolone (enrofloxacin 5-10 mg/kg intravenously every 12 hours) should be administered.

Feeding is started again after 24 to 48 hours. First, small amounts of water are offered; if tolerated, food is given in small amounts frequently. A highly digestible food is preferred. It is important to not overdistend the stomach in these animals.

9.   What is the prognosis for GDV?

Generally if treatment hasn't been delayed and tissues are not necrotic, prognosis is good. Those animals in which stomach necrosis has occurred or a splenectomy has been performed have a guarded prognosis. Arrhythmias at presentation also are associated with a poorer prognosis.

STOMACH TUMORS

10.   What stomach tumors are common in dogs?

Gastric neoplasia is relatively rare, though most tumors that occur have a poor prognosis. Adenocarcinomas are the most frequently diagnosed tumor. Other tumors that can occur include lymphoma, leiomyoma, and leiomyosarcomas. Benign adenomatous polyps can also be seen on occasion. Most cases are seen in older dogs.

11.   What are typical clinical signs of gastric tumors?

Most dogs will present with a chronic history of vomiting, anorexia, and weight loss. Bleeding into the stomach can be present and may be reflected by hematemesis in some animals. In other animals, the blood loss is more chronic leading to a regenerative response, melena, and iron deficiency.

12.   How are stomach tumors diagnosed?

Definitive diagnosis requires biopsy, either surgically or endoscopically (Fig. 38-2). It is recommended that thoracic radiographs be obtained to rule out overt metastatic disease. In addition, abdominal ultrasound is indicated to look for mesenteric lymph node enlargement and evidence of metastasis in the liver.

13.   What therapy is available?

With benign tumors, surgery can be curative. With lymphoma, chemotherapy can result in a good response. With adenocarcinomas, partial gastrectomy can be considered; however, this tumor is rarely resectable.

14.   What is the prognosis with gastric tumors?

With benign lesions prognosis is good if surgery is possible. Prognosis is generally poor with adenocarcinomas; survival times are measured in months.

HELICOBACTER

15.   How common is *Helicobacter* infection and what species of *Helicobacter* infect dogs?

There are various species of *Helicobacter* that have been found in dogs, though the species that infects humans (*Helicobacter pylori*) is not one of them. *Helicobacter heilmannii, Helico-*

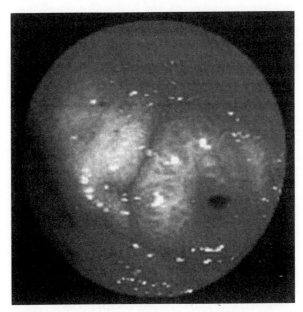

Figure 38-2. Endoscopic image of a gastric adenocarcinoma near the pylorus.

bacter felis, and *Helicobacter bizzozeronii* are some of the canine isolates. Prevalence rates of *Helicobacter* infection vary, but generally are high and can be close to 100% in certain populations.

16. What are the pathologic lesions of *Helicobacter* infections?

In humans, *Helicobacter* infection can result in increased gastric acid secretion, but this does not seem to be the case in dogs. However, infection in the dog does result in an inflammatory response in the stomach. Lymphoid hyperplasia and gastritis are common findings. There may be differences between the various *Helicobacter* sp. and their effect on the stomach. In addition host factors most likely also play a role in determining the severity of lesions. Fibrosis is also associated with infection.

17. What clinical signs are associated with *Helicobacter* infections in dogs?

In most dogs, infection is asymptomatic. Many dogs will have gastritis on biopsy without clinical problems. In some animals, infection is associated with vomiting and other signs consistent with gastritis such as anorexia, hematemesis, and weight loss. Treatment with antibiotics can result in resolution of the clinical signs.

18. How are *Helicobacter* infections diagnosed?

The infection can only be definitively diagnosed with biopsies or brush cytologies of the stomach, with the latter possibly being more sensitive. On light microscopy of cytologic specimens, it is possible to see the spiral organisms using normal stains, including Wright's stain. With biopsy specimens, a hematoxylin and eosin stain is effective; alternatively, a silver stain will highlight spiral bacteria. The biopsy specimens also allow for assessment of inflammation and other abnormalities of the stomach. Detection of urease activity can also point toward infection with *Helicobacter* spp. Generally, a biopsy specimen is placed in agar with a pH indicator. Color change is consistent with the presence of urease-containing bacteria. Culturing, urea breath testing, polymerase chain reaction testing, and serology are other possible diagnostic tests though they are not used extensively in practice.

19. Should *Helicobacter* infections be treated?

This is a controversial topic. There does not seem to be any indication to treat the asymptomatic dog. However, if an animal is diagnosed with gastritis and concurrent *Helicobacter* infection, it may be a consideration to treat for the infection first and see if clinical signs resolve. I have observed this to be the case in my practice. Current information suggests however that cure is not possible so that relapse may well occur.

20. How are *Helicobacter* infections treated?

Antibiotic therapy is helpful in controlling the clinical signs, but, unlike humans, it would appear that cure is unusual and relapses are common. In most cases, a combination of medications is used. Initially amoxicillin (20 mg/kg every 12 hours), metronidazole (15 mg/kg every 12 hours), and bismuth (20 mg/kg every 12 hours) were given in combination for 10 to 14 days. In place of amoxicillin, azithromycin (10 mg/kg every 24 hours) or clarithromycin (7.5 mg/kg every 12 hours) can be used. Famotidine and omeprazole, gastric acid–suppressing drugs, may be prescribed in place of bismuth.

BIBLIOGRAPHY

DeNovo RC: Diseases of the stomach, In Tams TR, editor: *Handbook of small animal gastroenterology*, ed 2, Philadelphia, 2003, WB Saunders.
Leib MS, Duncan RB: Diagnosing gastric *Helicobacter* infections in dogs and cats, *Compend Cont Educ Pract Vet* 27;221-228, 2005.
Simpson K, Neiger R, DeNovo R et al: The relationship of *Helicobacter* spp. infection to gastric disease in dogs and cats, *J Vet Intern Med* 14;223-227, 2005.

GASTRIC MOTILITY DISORDERS

21. What are potential causes of delayed gastric emptying?

Delayed gastric emptying can be mechanical (obstruction) or a functional problem. Mechanical obstructions that are common include foreign bodies, tumors, and antral pyloric hypertrophy. Functional problems are usually caused either by problems with neuronal control of stomach function or smooth muscle function.

22. What clinical signs are associated with delayed gastric emptying?

Vomiting is the most common sign of delayed gastric emptying. Often the vomitus will contain food, even though feeding may have occurred many hours previously. If the problem is chronic or severe, anorexia, weight loss, and abdominal distention can occur.

23. How is the diagnosis of delayed gastric emptying confirmed?

The history should be typical for this disorder with vomiting of food many hours after feeding. Radiography is the most common diagnostic test used to confirm the diagnosis. Barium either as paste or mixed with food can be used. Emptying times are influenced, however, by the food used so that these studies are difficult to standardize. Retention of a barium meal for more than 8 to 10 hours is consistent with delayed gastric emptying. Use of barium-impregnated spheres has been investigated and standardized. These spheres are given with a canned food and serial radiographs are taken to chart the movement of the spheres. This is compared with data from normal dogs. This form of study is more objective than other barium studies.

24. How is antral pyloric hypertrophy treated?

This syndrome is also termed pyloric stenosis or chronic hypertrophic pyloric gastropathy.

Treatment in these animals is with surgery. Pyloroplasty includes removal of excess submucosa to allow the pylorus to become functional again. The Y to U antral advancement flap pyloroplasty is an effective technique.

25. How is primary (functional) delayed gastric emptying treated?

Many treatment options exist. Dietary therapy is often needed. Feeding small meals is preferred. Proteins and fats are less desirable because they slow gastric emptying. Liquid diets can also be of benefit, because liquids will leave the stomach more rapidly than solid foods. A variety of diets may need to be fed to determine which are best tolerated.

In almost all cases, prokinetic medications are required. Metoclopramide (0.2-0.4 mg/kg every 8 hours) can be used. It has central antiemetic effects as well as speeding gastric emptying. A more potent effect with regard to gastric emptying can be achieved with cisapride (0.1 to 1.0 mg/kg every 8-12 hours). Cisapride currently is only available via veterinary compounding pharmacies. Erythromycin at low dosages will also promote gastric emptying by stimulating motilin receptors in the gastrointestinal tract (0.5 to 1.0 mg/kg every 8 hours). Oral ranitidine and nizatidine also have prokinetic effects because they inhibit acetylcholinesterase activity thereby increasing parasympathetic tone.

BIBLIOGRAPHY

DeNovo RC: Diseases of the stomach, In Tams TR, editor: *Handbook of small animal gastroenterology*, ed 2, Philadelphia, 2003, WB Saunders.
Washabau RJ: Gastrointestinal motility disorders and gastrointestinal prokinetic therapy, *Vet Clin North Am Small Anim Pract* 33:1007-1028, 2003.
Washabau RJ, Hall JA: Diagnosis and management of gastrointestinal motility disorders in dogs and cats, *Compend Contin Educ Pract Vet* 19;721-737, 1997.

39. Diseases of the Rectum and Anus

Anthony P. Carr

1. What clinical signs might be associated with diseases of the rectum and anus?

Many clinical signs can be seen with diseases of the anorectum. Table 39-1 lists some of the more common ones.

2. What is the typical signalment for a dog with perineal hernia?

Most dogs with perineal hernias are older and usually male.

3. What clinical signs are seen with perineal hernias?

Clinical signs are varied, though constipation and obstipation are common. Tenesmus and dyschezia are also often noted. Swelling of the perineal region can also be recognized by many owners. In rare cases, the urinary bladder can prolapse into the hernia resulting urinary tract obstruction.

4. How is perineal hernia diagnosed?

Careful rectal palpation, visualization of the hernia, and history are usually adequate to make a diagnosis. During rectal palpation, it is important to note any rectal deviation, sacculation (expansion of the rectal wall on one side), or diverticula (outpouching of mucosa through a rectal wall defect).

Table 39-1 *Clinical Signs of Diseases of the Anorectum*
Dyschezia
Hematochezia
Constipation
Diarrhea
Fecal incontinence
Licking
Scooting
Foul odor
Discharge (purulent, hemorrhagic)
Tenesmus

5. How is a perineal hernia managed?

With mild cases, it may be adequate to use laxatives and stool softeners. Surgical intervention (herniorrhaphy) is indicated in more severe cases. Emergency surgery is indicated if the bladder has prolapsed into the hernia sac.

6. How is a rectal prolapse recognized and managed?

The appearance of a rectal prolapse is classic (Fig. 39-1). An elongated tubular structure protrudes from the anal area. It is important to differentiate it from an intussusception. This can be done by passing a finger or blunt probe between the rectum and the prolapsed tissues. With a prolapse, this would eventually lead to a cul-de-sac.

In most cases, the prolapse is a result of persistent straining (diarrhea, stranguria, anorectal diseases). An important part of therapy is to identify the cause and treat this appropriately. In mild cases, the prolapse can be repositioned, usually under sedation or anesthesia to limit straining. A temporary purse-string suture can be used to limit reprolapse. With extensive prolapse or with nonviable tissue, amputation of the prolapsed tissue is indicated. A colopexy may also be indicated to fix the rectum and colon in place.

7. What tumors occur commonly in the anal region?

Perianal adenomas are the most common tumor of the anal region. Perianal adenocarcinomas and apocrine gland carcinoma of the anal sac represent the malignant tumors of this region.

8. What is the clinical presentation and prognosis with anal sac adenocarcinomas?

Anal sac (apocrine gland) adenocarcinomas are malignant tumors that generally have metastasized before diagnosis. The primary tumor can cause typical signs of anorectal disease. Not uncommonly, however, the main presenting complaints are either because of metastatic disease (obstruction of the pelvis by sublumbar lymph node metastasis) or because of polyuria and polydipsia due to hypercalcemia (50% to 90% of cases).

Prognosis for cure is poor with this tumor. With metastatic disease, survival times are generally shorter than 1 year.

9. What is the clinical presentation and prognosis with perianal adenomas?

Perianal adenomas are benign tumors, though they can become quite large and cause problems such as dyschezia and tenesmus. They can also ulcerate and become infected. They develop under the influence of androgens so that they are most common in older intact males. Cytology of a fine needle aspirate is usually diagnostic.

Prognosis is generally good. Castration will often result in resolution of the tumors. In some cases, surgical removal of the mass may be needed. With large tumors, surgical excision may not

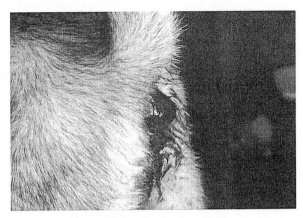

Figure 39–1. Rectal prolapse in a dog.

be feasible. With surgery in this area, there is concern about the development of fecal incontinence.

10. What is meant by a perianal fistula?

Perianal fistulas are sometimes also called anal furunculosis. The disease results in ulcerations and draining tracts of the perianal, anal, and perirectal tissues. This results in typical large bowel signs such as tenesmus, dyschezia, hematochezia, and increased frequency of defecation. The area is quite painful and discharge is often visible (purulent, hemorrhagic). The etiology is undefined, though genetic components may play a role. German Shepherds are clearly overrepresented.

11. How is a perianal fistula managed?

Previous therapies have included surgical excision, laser excision, or cryotherapy, with varying, although often disappointing results. Research indicates, however, that this disease responds to immune suppression. Initially use of high-dose corticosteroids and a high-fiber diet was shown to cause resolution of the problem in 33% of dogs and improvement in 33% of cases. This is an approach therapy worth trying before more invasive or expensive treatments. Further research showed cyclosporine to be a useful therapeutic agent for this disease. Remission of fistulas was achieved after 16 weeks of therapy in 85% of dogs treated. Recurrence is common, however, if treatment is discontinued. Unfortunately, this is an expensive therapy. An effective topical agent is tacrolimus (Protopic 0.1%). It is applied once or twice daily. Approximately 50% of dogs treated in this manner had a complete remission and almost all the rest had a partial remission (greater than 50% reduction in tract area and depth).

BIBLIOGRAPHY

Patterson AP, Campbell KL: Managing anal furunculosis in dogs, *Compend Cont Educ Pract Vet* 27:339-355, 2005.
Sherding RG: Diseases of the large intestine, In Tams TR, editor: *Handbook of small animal gastroenterology,* St. Louis, 2003, Saunders.
Zoran DL: Rectoanal disease, In Ettinger SJ, Feldman EC, editors: *Textbook of veterinary internal medicine,* ed 6, St. Louis, 2005, Elsevier.

40. Pancreas and Pancreatitis

Anthony P. Carr

1.   What function does the pancreas have?
The exocrine pancreas is responsible for the production of inactive zymogens that become active digestive enzymes (e.g., trypsinogen, chymotrypsinogen, proelastases). Some active enzymes are released including lipase and α-amylase. The pancreas secretes products that are necessary for vitamin B_{12} and zinc absorption. In addition, it secretes bicarbonate that helps to buffer the acid entering the duodenum from the stomach. Secretion of pancreatic products is stimulated by cholecystokinin and secretin.

2.   What is autodigestion and what mechanisms are present in the pancreas to prevent this?
Active digestive enzymes would represent a threat to the pancreas. In the active form, they could lead to digestion of the pancreas itself (autodigestion). Because of this, various mechanisms are in place to prevent this catastrophic event from occurring. The majority of pancreatic enzymes are stored and secreted in an inactive form called zymogens. The zymogens are first secreted into the rough endoplasmic reticulum; this segregates the enzymes from substances in the cell that would be capable of activating the enzyme. They are stored for secreting in granules. The activation of zymogens into active enzymes occurs some physical distance from the pancreas, usually in the gut. The pancreatic cells produce a trypsin inhibitor that could inactivate trypsin activity in the cell. The plasma also contains a variety of factors such as α1-antitrypisin and α2-macroglobulin that can inhibit active proteases.

3.   What is the pathogenesis of pancreatitis?
After an insult has occurred that has overwhelmed the ability to prevent autodigestion, inflammation of the pancreas is induced. The enzymes begin to break down the cells and surrounding stroma. Free radicals are generated that cause further damage to the pancreas and surrounding tissues. The inflammation leads to increased permeability, which promotes pancreatic edema. In more severe cases, necrosis of the organ can develop. If the disease is severe enough, multisystemic involvement occurs via the systemic inflammatory response syndrome and by direct effects of circulating active pancreatic enzymes. A generalized increase in permeability results leading to shock, peripheral edema, pulmonary edema, and effusions. Disseminated intravascular coagulation (DIC) can also be a result of the severe injury and inflammation, leading to further organ damage by means of thrombosis.

Depending on many factors, the degree of damage to the pancreas will vary. In general, edematous pancreatitis is differentiated from the hemorrhagic/necrotizing form. The latter has a poor prognosis and is associated with multiple organ involvement, potentially multiorgan failure.

4.   What risk factors are there for developing pancreatitis?
Several risk factors have been identified that predispose to pancreatitis. Small-breed dogs such as Miniature Schnauzers, Poodles, and Yorkshire Terriers appear to be predisposed. In some Miniature Schnauzers the increased risk may be the result of hyperlipidemia, a condition known to occur in this breed. Obesity also appears to be a factor that promotes pancreatitis. Feeding a high-fat meal (dietary indiscretion) may in some cases be an underlying cause.

Certain medications and chemicals are also thought to be associated with pancreatitis. Azathioprine, sulfa drugs, furosemide, and potassium bromide are a few of the drugs that have been implicated as a playing a role. The use of cholinesterase inhibitor insecticides is also suspected of being an initiating event. Corticosteroids have been discussed as a potential cause, though the evidence for this is tenuous. Hypercalcemia (either because of a concurrent illness or from calcium injections) is suspected as well.

Concurrent diseases have been implicated as predisposing factors for pancreatitis. These include hyperadrenocorticism, diabetes, prior gastrointestinal disease, and chronic renal failure, although the association in some cases is uncertain. Any condition that leads to poor perfusion could also lead to pancreatitis. Anesthesia with hypotension would be one such scenario.

5. What clinical signs are associated with pancreatitis?

Clinical signs with pancreatitis can be quite variable. It is possible for the disease to be subclinical. The development of clinical signs is dependent on the severity of the disease. In mild cases, lethargy and anorexia may be noted. In the more severe cases, vomiting, depression, abdominal pain, and fever are commonly seen. Other signs noted on occasion are diarrhea, icterus, dehydration, palpable cranial abdominal mass, arrhythmias, and ascites. The most severe cases will present in shock with hypothermia, prolonged capillary refill time, weakness, or collapse. Tachypnea or dyspnea is often present; this can be from pain, noncardiogenic pulmonary edema, pleural effusion, or pulmonary thromboembolism. Tachycardia can be present because of pain, shock, or arrhythmias.

6. How can imaging help in a dog with pancreatitis?

Imaging can be helpful in establishing a diagnosis and determining if certain complications associated with pancreatitis are present. In addition, imaging is necessary to help rule out some of the major differentials for pancreatitis such as gastrointestinal obstruction, intussusception, bile duct obstruction, and splenic torsion.

Radiography can, on occasion, detect certain changes that suggest pancreatitis, though definitive diagnosis is rarely possible and considerable expertise is needed to appreciate the at-times subtle changes present. This includes loss of detail in the area of the pancreas ("ground-glass appearance"), displacement of the stomach to the left, and widening of the angle between pyloric antrum and proximal duodenum. In more advanced cases, ascites will obscure abdominal detail. Pancreatitis is also a major differential diagnosis for dogs with effusion in the abdomen and thorax. Radiographs can also help to investigate dyspnea or tachypnea in these animals by ruling out pulmonary edema and pleural effusion. Normal thoracic radiographs in a hypoxic animal would also be suggestive of pulmonary thromboembolic disease.

Abdominal ultrasound has proved to be a useful tool with pancreatitis and is one of the more sensitive tests for this disease. Changes suggestive of pancreatitis are an enlarged and hypoechoic pancreas sometimes surrounded by an area of hyperechogenicity that is thought to represent peripancreatic fat saponification and necrosis. Localized effusion in the area of the pancreas can also be seen. The common bile duct may be enlarged due to compression of the duct as it runs through the pancreas. It is also possible to assess for such complications of pancreatitis such as pancreatic pseudocysts or abscesses.

7. What laboratory abnormalities are to be expected with pancreatitis?

The changes noted on laboratory tests will depend on the severity of the pancreatitis. Mild cases may have minimal changes. In more severe cases, multiple abnormalities may be noted. The complete blood cell count will often show changes consistent with inflammation, such as a stress leukogram. With more pronounced inflammation, a left shift will be noted. Neutropenia or a degenerative left shift can be an indication of pancreatic necrosis or sepsis. Low platelet counts may also be seen and this must raise the suspicion that DIC is present.

Multiple changes on serum chemistries can be present. Electrolyte and acid-base changes may be noted depending on the severity and duration of vomiting. Azotemia may be present, either because of dehydration or renal function impairment. Blood glucose can be elevated, potentially mimicking diabetes mellitus. A low blood glucose level would suggest either severe liver dysfunction or sepsis in a dog with pancreatitis. Hepatic enzyme activity may be elevated, as may be bilirubin concentration. This can be from direct injury of the liver close to the pancreas. In addition, blood draining the pancreas is transported to the liver via the portal vein. This blood can contain a variety of inflammatory mediators and activated digestive enzymes. The liver may also be affected by obstruction of bile flow resulting from pancreatic inflammation or fibrosis. On occasion, mild hypocalcemia may be noted; this is thought to be related to peripancreatic fat saponification or hypoalbuminemia.

Coagulation parameters can be altered by pancreatitis. Prolongations of the clotting times (activated partial thromboplastin time [APTT], one-step prothrombin time [OSPT]) are suggestive of DIC, though hepatic function problems can result in this as well. It may be possible to find fibrin degradation products (FDPs) or elevated D-dimer concentrations, together with prolonged clotting times this would be highly suspicious for DIC.

Products from the pancreas may also be found. Amylase and lipase can be variably elevated, though usually only in about 50% to 60% of dogs with pancreatitis. Because these are cleared via the kidney, it is not unusual to see them elevated with renal disease. Lipase can also be dramatically increased in dogs with a pancreatic tumor. Many other diseases have been associated with elevations of amylase or lipase. Canine trypsin-like immunoreactivity has been found to lack the specificity and sensitivity to make it a valuable diagnostic tool. A newer test that has become available is canine serum pancreatic lipase immunoreactivity. This test in preliminary studies appears to be much more sensitive (80%) and possibly also more specific. Further studies will be needed to complete evaluation of this test.

8.   How is pancreatitis diagnosed?

Pancreatitis generally is a clinical diagnosis; definitive diagnosis is only possible through biopsy. An animal with appropriate clinical signs that has laboratory abnormalities or imaging results that are consistent with this disease strongly support the diagnosis of pancreatitis.

9.   What treatment options are available for pancreatitis?

Many treatment modalities for pancreatitis have been investigated, though usually using an experimental model. Most of the treatments have only made a difference if given before inducing pancreatitis. After pancreatitis has been established, there are few treatments that have been proven to be effective in altering outcome.

General supportive care is indicated in addition to appropriate nutritional management (see question 10). The level of supportive care necessary will depend on the severity of signs. Fluid therapy is indicated in almost all cases because the standard therapy for pancreatitis almost always includes nothing per os (NPO) for 24 to 48 hours. In those cases in which shock is present, the goal of fluid therapy is resuscitation and rates of up to 90 ml/kg/hour may be needed short term. Any acid-base and electrolyte disturbances need to be monitored for and addressed if indicated.

Colloidal fluid therapy is indicated in many dogs with pancreatitis. Crystalloids have a short dwell time in the vascular space. Because many dogs with severe pancreatitis have low oncotic pressure or increased vascular permeability, the continued use of high crystalloid fluid rates will exacerbate edema and effusion. Because of this, colloids need to be considered. They also can help maintain blood pressure when crystalloids no longer can. The ideal colloid is plasma that can be given at a rate of 10 to 20 ml/kg. There is a theoretical benefit in that plasma may also contain antiproteases that might help treat pancreatitis. Fresh frozen plasma also contains coagulation proteins and antithrombin III that are of benefit in treating DIC. There are no trials that have shown any benefit of this treatment in human or veterinary patients. Other colloids to consider include dextrans and hetastarch. With severe hypoalbuminemia, human albumin transfusions may also be considered.

Analgesia is a cornerstone of treating pancreatitis. The animal can present with intense discomfort that needs to be addressed aggressively. For mild pain, butorphanol can be given.

Buprenorphine, morphine, oxymorphone, and hydromorphone can be used with more severe pain. A fentanyl patch is another possible way to address analgesia longer term. Dosages are listed in Table 40-1.

Other treatments will depend on the severity of clinical signs. If vomiting or nausea is persistent or severe, use of an antiemetic is indicated (see Chapter 34 for drug dosages). If blood sugar is markedly elevated, the judicious use of insulin can be considered. Many other therapies have been tried, including suctioning gastric contents, stomach acid suppression, peritoneal dialysis, and various pancreatic secretion inhibitors. None has been shown in clinical trials to have any benefit.

10. What is the preferred nutritional management program for dogs with pancreatitis?
Initial management consists of NPO for at least 24 to 48 hours after vomiting has stopped. This should reduce pancreatic secretion and allow the pancreatitis to abate. After the NPO period, water in small quantities is offered. If this is tolerated, small amounts of food can be offered. A low-fat, low-protein diet is preferred to minimize secretory stimulus. If the animal vomits at any time, it is necessary to reinstitute another similar NPO period.

The concern with this approach is that prolonged periods of nonfeeding negatively affect outcome in dogs. If it is necessary to have a second period of NPO, it is important to consider providing nutrition by alternate routes in the near future. One option is partial parenteral nutrition or total parenteral nutrition. Because of the hyperosmolality of the total parenteral nutrition, it is necessary to have a central line to administer it. Another option is to place a jejunostomy tube. This usually is done via surgery, though endoscopic techniques have been described. Enteral nutrition via jejunostomy tube has been shown to be superior to total parenteral nutrition in humans with pancreatitis. This to a large part seems to be the result of a decreased risk of sepsis. Refeeding problems can occur (e.g., hyperlipidemia, electrolyte shifts, hyperglycemia, hypophosphatemia) with either method, and these need to be monitored.

After a dog has had an episode of pancreatitis, it is recommended that a low-fat diet be fed lifelong. In addition it is important to avoid dietary indiscretions and table scraps in these dogs.

11. What complications can occur with pancreatitis?
Pancreatitis in most cases will resolve with no residual effects if properly managed. In severe cases, complications such as DIC or a pulmonary thromboembolism can be seen. Acute respiratory distress syndrome can develop which has a poor prognosis, as does pneumonia. Sepsis is not uncommon and often will be terminal. Multiorgan failure can occur with renal failure being the most readily identified. These more severe cases tend to have pancreatic necrosis and prognosis is guarded.

Some complications develop gradually. Diabetes can be present transient during pancreatitis but may be permanent as well. Severe or protracted pancreatitis could in theory lead to exocrine

Table 40-1 *Analgesics for Pancreatitis*

DRUG	DOSE	ROUTE
Butorphanol	0.2-0.4 mg/kg every 4 to 6 hours	SC, IM (also IV, reduce dose by half)
Buprenorphine	0.005-0.02 mg/kg every 4 to 8 hours	SC, IM, IV
Oxymorphone	0.05-0.1 mg/kg every 4 to 6 hours	SC, IM, IV (up to 0.2 mg/kg if SC or IM)
Fentanyl	3-5 µg/kg every 3 days	Transdermal patch

IM, Intramuscular, *IV*, intravenous, *SC*, subcutaneous.

pancreatic insufficiency. Pancreatic abscesses can develop, and these must be managed surgically. Pancreatic pseudocysts are sterile, fluid-filled cysts in the pancreas that can be seen infrequently in these cases. They often will resolve spontaneously. If not, ultrasound guidance can be used to drain them. The swelling or fibrosis from pancreatitis can compromise the common bile duct sufficiently that surgery may be needed to relieve the obstruction.

12. What neoplasias involve the exocrine pancreas and what is their prognosis?
Tumors of the exocrine pancreas are rare. They are, however, usually quite aggressive and metastasize early. Most are adenocarcinomas either from the duct or acinar cells. Markedly elevated lipase activity can be seen in some of the animals with this tumor. Generally prognosis is poor and few survive 1 year, even with surgical removal.

BIBLIOGRAPHY

Ruaux CG: Pathophysiology of organ failure in severe acute pancreatitis in dogs, *Comp Cont Ed Pract Vet* 22:531-542, 2000.
Simpson KW: Diseases of the pancreas, In *Handbook of small animal gastroenterology*, ed 2, Philadelphia, 2003, WB Saunders.
Williams DA: The pancreas. In Guilford WG, Center SA et al, editors: *Strombeck's small animal gastroenterology*, ed 3, Philadelphia, 1996, WB Saunders.

41. Exocrine Pancreatic Insufficiency

Anthony P. Carr

1. What is exocrine pancreatic insufficiency?
Exocrine pancreatic insufficiency (EPI) is a condition in which the pancreas no longer produces adequate amounts of digestive enzymes. This usually will not occur until more than 90% of the exocrine pancreas has become nonfunctional. Most cases in dogs are caused by pancreatic acinar atrophy, though some may also develop because of chronic pancreatitis. Clinical signs develop because digestion no longer occurs properly, leading to malabsorption with weight loss and diarrhea. Maldigestion and malabsorption does not just result from the enzyme deficiency. The disease also leads to changes in small intestinal digestive processes. Small intestinal bacterial overgrowth (SIBO) is also frequently seen and can contribute to the diarrhea. Low cobalamin levels also occur, which also may play a role with small intestinal disease in these dogs.

2. What is pancreatic acinar atrophy?
Pancreatic acinar atrophy is a condition in which a normal pancreas undergoes atrophy. A familial predisposition in German Shepherds and rough-coated collies has been established. It can, however, occur in any breed, with large-breed dogs being more commonly affected.

3. What is a typical signalment for EPI?
Because pancreatic acinar atrophy is the most common cause of EPI many of the dogs are German Shepherds. They tend to be young animals, usually younger than 2 years.

4. What are the clinical signs of EPI?
Dogs with EPI have profuse diarrhea. The bowel movements are often malodorous. Borborygmus and flatulence are common. These animals will have a ravenous appetite yet continue to lose weight. Poor hair coat is common because of the malnourishment present. On occasion, other signs such as vomiting, coprophagia, pica, and anorexia can be seen.

Routine clinical pathologic tests rarely document abnormalities. Folate levels may be elevated and cobalamin concentration decreased in dogs with EPI. This may be from SIBO; however, the cobalamin deficiency may also occur because the pancreas produces a factor needed for cobalamin absorption that can be lacking in dogs with EPI.

5. How is EPI diagnosed?
EPI is generally diagnosed with pancreatic function tests. Canine trysin-like immunoreactivity (TLI) is the preferred test for EPI. The animal should be fasted 12 hours to collect serum for analysis. Low TLI concentration in dogs with typical clinical signs is considered highly diagnostic. Many other tests have been tried but none is superior to TLI.

6. How is EPI treated?
Treatment of EPI hinges on enzyme replacement and nutritional intervention. Powdered pancreatic enzymes work best and are used at 1 to 2 teaspoons per meal. There is no need to preincubate the food. Alternatively fresh pancreas (50 to 100 g/meal) can be used. Most of the enzymes are destroyed in the stomach, so some dose titration may be needed.

In these animals, it is vital to manage their diet carefully. Initial management can be with a high-quality maintenance diet. If this fails, a fat-restricted, highly digestible diet should be tried. Cobalamin injections can be given (250-500 µg, repeat as indicated by serum levels), especially to those animals that are responding poorly to therapy. Vitamin absorption may generally be inadequate in these dogs, so that use of vitamin supplements is prudent. Antibiotics are indicated if SIBO is suspected to be contributing to poor therapeutic response. Metronidazole, tylosin, and tetracyclines are all good options for this.

BIBLIOGRAPHY

Rutz GM, Steiner JM, Williams DA: Pancreatic acinar atrophy in German shepherds. *Comp Cont Ed Pract Vet* 23;347-356, 2001.
Simpson KW: Diseases of the pancreas, In *Handbook of small animal gastroenterology*, ed 2, Philadelphia, 2003, WB Saunders.
Westermarck EW, Wiberg M: Exocrine pancreatic insufficiency in dogs, *Vet Clin North Am Small Anim Pract* 33:1165-1179, 2003.
Williams, DA: The pancreas, In Guilford WG, Center SA et al, editors: *Strombeck's small animal gastroenterology*, ed 3, Philadelphia, 1996, WB Saunders.

42. Liver
Anthony P. Carr

APPROACH TO THE DOG WITH ICTERUS
1. What is the difference between icterus and hyperbilirubinemia?
Icterus or jaundice are similar expressions and refer to visible hyperbilirubinemia. It is generally possible to see icterus when bilirubin concentrations exceed 2 mg/dl. Areas to inspect for jaundice include the sclera, soft palate, mucous membranes, and the ears. The serum will also be discolored as will urine.

2. Briefly describe bilirubin metabolism.
Bilirubin is a product formed during the degradation of porphyrins, predominantly hemoglo-

bin. Other sources of hemoproteins include myoglobin and cytochromes. In most instances, he-moglobin is the major source of bilirubin in circulation.

Hemoglobin is liberated when senescent red blood cells are phagocytosed by the reticul-oendothelial system, predominantly in the liver and spleen. Iron is removed and reused. The glo-bin is degraded to amino acids that are also reused. Heme is converted to biliverdin. Biliverdin is converted to bilirubin by the enzyme biliverdin reductase. Bilirubin is lipid soluble and enters the circulation where it is bound to albumin (unconjugated bilirubin or indirect bilirubin). The unconjugated bilirubin binds to receptors on hepatocytes is internalized and then conjugated predominantly to glucuronic acid. This water-soluble product is now termed conjugated or direct bilirubin. This is then secreted into the bile canaliculus by means of an active transport process that is the rate-limiting step in bilirubin metabolism. A small percentage of conjugated bilirubin refluxes from the hepatocyte into the circulation. Because conjugated bilirubin is water soluble, it is readily filtered by the kidney and excreted via urine.

Most conjugated bilirubin collects in the gallbladder. On gallbladder contraction, the bilirubin enters the duodenum. The bacteria in the gut then deconjugate it and metabolize it to various other products, including urobilinogens and stercobilin. Some of the urobilinogens are reab-sorbed from the gut. Most are returned to the liver, and a small part is excreted through urine.

3.   Is it useful to differentiate between conjugated and unconjugated bilirubin in clinical cases?

It is tempting to think that this would be useful. Increased unconjugated bilirubin would be expected with hemolytic disease. Conjugated bilirubin would be increased with hepatic or post-hepatic disease. Unfortunately, clinical experience has shown that in dogs these measurements are rarely useful in localizing the cause of icterus.

4.   What is the significance of urobilinogen in the urine?

Urobilinogen is commonly tested for on urine test strips. Its presence has no specific meaning; a negative test could indicate bile duct obstruction (no bile gets to intestine to form urobilinogen). The clinical significance of this is minimal.

5.   How are the common causes of icterus categorized?

Many times, icterus is compartmentalized into prehepatic, hepatic, and posthepatic icterus. Prehepatic icterus would be caused by hemolysis. This would lead to so much hemoglobin being presented to the liver, leading to increased bilirubin production, which eventually overwhelms the capacity of the liver to transport it into bile. Hepatic icterus would be caused by any process that interferes with bile flow. This can be primary liver disease (e.g., cirrhosis, chronic inflammatory liver disease). In rare cases, it can also be seen with inflammatory or infectious diseases outside the liver that inhibit bilirubin transport, such as occurs with sepsis. Posthepatic icterus refers to disease that interferes with bile flow in the larger bile ducts.

6.   What are some potential causes of prehepatic icterus?

Prehepatic icterus is caused by hemolysis. The increased release of hemoglobin overpowers the reserve capacity of the liver to deal with this. In addition, if the anemia is marked enough, the liver will undergo hypoxia, which further reduces the capacity of the liver to deal with hemoglobin. The most common cause is immune-mediated hemolytic anemia. There are many other causes for hemolysis including infections (babesiosis), toxins (lead, zinc), and oxidative injury (onions).

7.   What can cause hepatic icterus?

Almost any form of liver disease can cause icterus if damage is widespread enough.

8.   What can cause posthepatic icterus?

Posthepatic icterus can be caused by a variety of diseases that affect the biliary tract or gallbladder. Common causes include pancreatitis, neoplasia, and gallbladder rupture (trauma or cholecystitis).

9. What would be a reasonable initial diagnostic plan for an icteric dog?

Initially a packed cell volume/total protein (PCV/TP) should be obtained to rule out prehepatic causes of icterus. Generally anemia has to be severe to be the sole cause of icterus. If anemia is not considered the cause, then it is necessary to determine if hepatic or posthepatic disease are present.

Differentiating hepatic from posthepatic icterus can be challenging. History, physical examination, and routine blood work may offer clues that point toward one cause, though it is not possible to establish a definitive answer in this manner. Abdominal ultrasound is an important part of working up icteric dogs. With posthepatic disease, the source of obstruction may become obvious or signs of obstruction (dilation of the biliary tree or common bile duct) may be seen. It is important, however, to remember that it may take 5 or more days to see these changes in acute bile duct obstruction. In addition, gallbladder disease can be visualized at times. With gallbladder perforation, abdominocentesis can be helpful. Ultimately, it may, however, require an abdominal exploratory to obtain liver biopsies and check the integrity of the biliary system.

BIBLIOGRAPHY

Anderson JG, Washabau RJ: Icterus, *Compend Contin Edu Pract Vet* 14:1045–1059, 1992.
Eddlestone SM: Jaundice. In Ettinger SJ, Feldman EC, editors: *Textbook of veterinary internal medicine*, ed 6, St. Louis, 2005, Elsevier.

LIVER DISEASE BASICS

10. What clinical signs are seen with liver disease?

Clinical signs with liver disease can be variable. In some cases, dogs may be severely affected and present in a coma as a result of hepatic encephalopathy. In other cases, the diagnosis may be fortuitous resulting from abnormalities detected on a biochemical profile or finding urate uroliths.

Common clinical findings include lethargy, weight loss, vomiting, anorexia, and diarrhea. With more advanced disease icterus, ascites and symptoms associated with hepatic encephalopathy predominate.

11. What changes on a biochemical profile are expected with liver disease?

Jaundice can be seen with advanced liver disease (see previous section about the dog with icterus). A variety of liver enzyme elevations can be seen with liver disease, though they do not necessarily have to occur. The degree of elevation does not necessarily relate to the severity of the disease. Serum alanine aminotransferase (ALT) is relatively liver specific in dogs. Elevations indicate hepatocellular leakage or necrosis. Marked elevations occur with hepatic necrosis, widespread hepatic neoplasia, and chronic hepatitis. Serum aspartate aminotransferase (AST) is similar to ALT; however, AST is also present in muscle and red blood cells. Alkaline phosphatase (ALP) is an enzyme induced by cholestasis. ALP activity will increase with biliary obstruction as well as with hepatocellular swelling (intrahepatic cholestasis). Isoenzymes occur in bone, liver, intestine, and kidney, though only the bone and liver isoenzymes have half-lives long enough to make them clinically relevant. A corticosteroid induced isoenzyme can also lead to significant ALP activity increases as can certain medications (phenobarbital, phenytoin, primidone). Gamma glutamyltranspeptidase is similar to ALP in its diagnostic importance.

12. Which components of a routine biochemical profile reflect liver function?

Liver enzyme activities do not correlate with hepatic function. Usually liver function tests such as serum bile acids or an ammonia tolerance test are needed to assess liver function properly. There are, however, four values on a biochemical profile that could provide information about liver function. Glucose is partially produced by the liver and with decreased liver function gluco-neogenesis can decrease. In addition, dogs with liver disease are prone to sepsis, which could also decrease glucose concentrations.

Albumin is produced by the liver and represents around 25% of the proteins that the liver synthesizes. Hypoalbuminemia can result as a result of decreased liver function. In addition, albumin is a negative acute-phase reactant. If there is significant inflammation in association with the liver disease, this will reduce albumin synthesis. In many diseases hypoalbuminemia is associated with poorer outcome.

Blood urea nitrogen (BUN) is produced by the liver by conversion of ammonia from the portal circulation. Decreases in BUN occur with extensive liver disease or shunting. BUN concentration is dependent on a number of factors including hydration status (excreted via the kidney), polyuria (will decrease BUN), and nutritional status (increased by protein consumption, decreased by anorexia or consumption of a low-protein diet).

The liver also produces cholesterol. With severe, usually end-stage liver disease hypocholesterolemia can be seen. In many instances of liver disease, however, hypercholesterolemia is seen as a result of cholestasis.

13. How is liver disease confirmed in the dog?

There are a variety of ways to diagnose liver disease in dogs. Cytologic or histopathologic sampling of the liver is required for a definitive diagnosis. Aspirates, needle biopsies, and wedge biopsies are potential ways for obtaining diagnostic specimens. It has been shown that cytology is the least reliable of these techniques. Needle biopsies also often do not concur with results of wedge biopsies. Aspirates and needle biopsies are probably best reserved for cases in which neoplasia is suspected. With inflammatory liver disease, wedge biopsies will have a much higher diagnostic yield.

14. Before biopsy, what additional tests should be considered?

Because liver biopsy can be associated with hemorrhage, it is always advisable to obtain a coagulation panel before biopsy. Dogs with liver disease are prone to coagulopathies, usually because of an inability to produce coagulation proteins. In addition some degree of vitamin K deficiency may also exist. A buccal mucosal bleeding time should also be considered to make sure that primary hemostasis is not impaired.

15. What information can imaging techniques provide in the assessment of liver disease?

Radiography is a good way to assess liver size and to assess for uniform increases or decreases in liver size. On occasion, calcification or gas can be recognized in the liver. Ultrasonography is the most widely used technique to image the liver parenchyma. Ultrasound allows the echotexture of the liver to be assessed. In addition, it is possible to determine if changes are focal or diffuse. With focal lesions, ultrasound-guided biopsies or aspirates may be superior to surgically obtained samples.

CHRONIC INFLAMMATORY LIVER DISEASE

16. What causes chronic liver inflammation in the dog?

In humans, viruses (hepatitis A, B, and C) are the most common cause of inflammatory liver disease. Although there have been studies carried out to identify infectious agents in association with chronic inflammatory liver disease, none have been found that commonly cause disease. On occasion, *Leptospira*, *Bartonella*, and *Histoplasma* can cause significant liver disease, though often the presentation is more acute than chronic. Copper accumulation and drugs can also cause hepatic inflammation. An etiologic diagnosis for most chronic liver disease in dogs is usually not found. In some cases, an immune-mediated phenomenon is suspected. Genetic factors play a role, because certain breeds are more likely to have chronic liver inflammation.

17. What histopathologic changes are seen with chronic hepatitis?

Chronic hepatitis can have many causes, though the histologic changes are often similar. A variable inflammatory infiltrate will be present, with lymphocytes and plasma cells predominating, though neutrophils and macrophages can also be present. There will also be areas of hepatocyte necrosis. Initially, this can be near the limiting plate (piecemeal necrosis). This can extend from the portal vein to the central vein (bridging necrosis). With inflammation and necrosis, fibrosis will develop. This can be extensive enough to connect adjacent portal triads (bridging fibrosis). Biliary hyperplasia is also a common finding as are areas of regeneration (regenerative nodules). After fibrosis progresses sufficiently, cirrhosis develops.

18. Which breeds are predisposed to chronic hepatitis?

Doberman Pinschers, Bedlington Terriers, West Highland White Terriers, and Cocker Spaniels are overrepresented.

19. What treatments are indicated for chronic hepatitis in dogs?

Treatment is best guided by results of a liver biopsy. If an underlying cause is found for the liver disease it should be addressed (e.g., antibiotics for bacterial infections, discontinuation of drugs if toxic hepatopathy). If significant copper is detected, treatments to remove copper or prevent further copper absorption are indicated (see the section on copper storage hepatopathies).

If significant inflammation is observed, antiinflammatory medications are indicated. The most commonly used are glucocorticoids. These medications are effective and inexpensive, though clinical signs of iatrogenic hyperadrenocorticism can develop and their use can result in significant liver enzyme activity elevation. Corticosteroids also reduce fibrosis. Azathioprine is another commonly used antiinflammatory drug. Use of azathioprine reduces the dose of corticosteroids that are required and in can be used as a sole agent for controlling inflammation with hepatitis. Side effects such as bone marrow suppression, pancreatitis, and hepatotoxicity are rare, though they have to be monitored for.

Significant fibrosis would indicate the need for antifibrotic agents. Reduction of inflammation will partially help to reduce fibrosis; however, this may be inadequate. Colchicine (0.03 mg/kg/day) has been used frequently for its antifibrotic activity. It has been shown to be effective in humans; similar information is lacking in dogs. Many dogs treated with this medication will develop gastrointestinal signs such as vomiting and diarrhea. Reducing the dosage and gradually increasing if tolerated can address this. Rarely bone marrow suppression can occur. Zinc is used for minimizing copper absorption from the intestine. It also has some antifibrotic effects.

Several other drugs are used to help protect the hepatocytes from injury, often related to antioxidant effects. Vitamin E is suspected to have some benefits minimizing oxidative injury. S-adenosylmethionine has also been used in dogs. It helps to increase glutathione concentrations in the liver, which helps to reduce oxidative injury. It may be of benefit with toxic liver injury. Milk thistle (silymarin) also has antioxidant effects.

A drug that has multiple effects with liver disease is ursodiol. Ursodiol is a choleretic (increases bile flow) that limits the presence of toxic (hydrophobic) bile acids. Antiinflammatory and immune-modulating effects may also be present.

BIBLIOGRAPHY

Center SA: Chronic liver disease: current concepts of disease mechanisms, *J Small Anim Pract* 40:106-114, 1999.

Cole TL, Center SA, Flood SN et al: Diagnostic comparison of needle and wedge biopsy specimens of the liver in dogs and cats. *JAVMA* 220:1483-1490, 2002.

Mandigers PJJ, van den Ingh TS, Spee B et al: Chronic hepatitis in Doberman Pinschers, *Vet Q* 26:98-106, 2004.

Richter KP: Diseases of the liver and hepatobiliary system. In Tams TR, editor: *Handbook of small animal gastroenterology,* St. Louis, 2003, Saunders.

Roth LR: Comparison of liver cytology and biopsy diagnoses in dogs and cats: 56 cases, *Vet Clin Pathol* 30:35-38, 2001.

Sartor LL, Trepanier LA: Rational pharmacologic therapy of hepatobiliary disease in dogs and cats, *Compend Contin Edu Pract Vet* 25:432-446, 2003.

Wang KY, Panciera DL, Al-Rukibat RK et al: Accuracy of ultrasound-guided fine-needle aspiration of the liver and cytologic findings in dogs and cats: 97 cases (1990-2000), *JAMVA* 224:75-78, 2004.

COPPER STORAGE HEPATOPATHIES

20. What breeds are predisposed to copper storage problems?

Abnormal copper storage can occur in almost any breed. There are, however, clear breed pre-dilections. Bedlington Terriers, West Highland White Terriers, Skye Terriers, Dalmatians, and Turkish Shepherds. Doberman Pinschers will also frequently have elevated copper concentrations in the liver.

In Bedlington Terriers the gene defect of this autosomal recessive trait has been determined. The defect results in decreased biliary excretion of copper. The disease in Bedlingtons does cause liver injury, whereas in other breeds the relationship between copper levels and liver injury is less clear.

21. What diseases are associated with excessive copper storage in the liver?

Copper accumulation is a common occurrence with cholestasis. When too much copper ac-cumulates, it can result in oxidative injury to the liver. Symptoms can vary widely. In many instances the dog may be asymptomatic; elevations in ALT may be present. It is possible to see an acute presentation in Bedlingtons in which acute hepatic failure results. It is also possible to see an acute hemolytic process in association with the liberation of large amounts of copper in this breed. In many cases, a more chronic form develops with progressive liver damage resulting in cirrhosis.

22. How are copper storage problems diagnosed?

It is possible to diagnose the genetic defect that leads to copper storage problems in the Bed-lington Terrier. In other breeds, diagnosis depends on a liver biopsy. It is possible to get a crude idea of the amount of copper in the liver with histopathology. Special stains can enhance the ability to visualize copper in the liver. The most objective is, however, copper quantification from a biopsy. Normal levels should be below 400 mg/kg dry weight liver. In abnormal dogs values greater than 1000 mg/kg are not rare, and at times the values can exceed 10,000 mg/kg dry matter.

23. How are copper storage problems treated?

There are a variety of treatment options for copper storage problems. Diet plays an important role by limiting the amount of copper the dog ingests. Most dog foods contain high levels of cop-per; however, there are some that are low (e.g., Hill's U/D, L/D, Pedigree Hepatic Support).

It is also possible to limit the absorption of copper from the intestinal tract. This can be accomplished by the administration of zinc. Zinc administration leads to the formation of intes-tinal metallothionein, which binds copper in the gut. When these cells die, the copper is excreted with the shed cells. Zinc also helps to remove copper from the liver. Dosage is 5 to 10 mg/kg/day of elemental zinc given approximately 1 hour before feeding. Blood zinc concentration is moni-tored with a goal of between 200 and 400 µg/dl. The major side effect is gastrointestinal upset, with inappropriately elevated zinc concentrations hemolysis could occur.

With severe copper accumulation, aggressive use of chelators is indicated. The two most com-monly used medications are trientine (2,2,2 tetramine, 15 to 30 mg/kg twice daily) or D-peni-cillamine (10 to 15 mg/kg every 12 hours). Penicillamine is not as well tolerated and often will result in vomiting or anorexia.

BIBLIOGRAPHY

Center SA: Chronic hepatitis, cirrhosis, breed-specific hepatopathies, copper storage hepatopathy, suppurative hepatitis, granulomatous hepatitis and idiopathic hepatic fibrosis. In Guilford G, Center SA, Strombeck D et al, editors: *Strombeck's small animal gastroenterology*, ed 3, Philadelphia, 1996, Saunders.

Mandigers PJJ, van den Ingh TS, Bode P et al: Association between liver copper concentration and subclinical hepatitis in Doberman Pinschers. *J Vet Intern Med* 18;647–650, 2005.

TOXIC LIVER DISEASE

24. What drugs are known to cause hepatic disease?

Many drugs can cause toxic injury, usually they are idiosyncratic reactions. Table 42-1 lists selected medications associated with liver disease. In addition, herbal products have the potential for hepatic injury as well.

25. What other toxins can cause liver disease?

Aflatoxins are a classic cause of chronic and often fatal liver disease in dogs. This toxin is usually associated with spoiled food. Amanita mushrooms, heavy metals (lead, zinc, iron), and a variety of other toxins are also implicated as causes of liver disease.

HEPATIC ENCEPHALOPATHY

26. What is hepatic encephalopathy (HE) and what clinical signs are there?

Hepatic encephalopathy represents a syndrome of central nervous signs that develop in dogs with significant hepatic insufficiency. This can be because of chronic liver disease or may be from portocaval shunting. The clinical signs are variable and vary from depression, bizarre behavior, and seizures to coma. The onset of signs can be gradual or acute.

The pathogenesis of HE is somewhat speculative. It does appear that most substances that trigger HE originate from the gastrointestinal tract. Usually the liver would be able to detoxify these substances; however, in the abnormal liver, this no longer occurs adequately.

Ammonia is known to play a role, and administration of ammonia can cause signs of HE to develop in dogs with liver problems. Ammonia is taken up by astrocytes in the brain, which converts it to glutamine. This molecule is osmotically active leading to astrocyte swelling and brain dysfunction. Ammonia is also thought to suppress neuroinhibition, blockade of the GABA receptor complex, and altered membrane transport.

Table 42-1   *Drugs Associated with Liver Disease*

Acetaminophen
Azathioprine
Carprofen
Halothane
Ketoconazole
Mebendazole
Mitotane
Oxibendazole
Phenytoin
Primidone
Phenobarbital
Sulfa drugs, including trimethoprim/sulfa combinations

It has been postulated that other substances from the gut may cause the signs of HE. False neurotransmitters may be produced. Benzodiazepine-like substances are also increased with HE. GABA concentrations rise, which can result in many different central nervous system effects. Short-chain fatty acids, aromatic amino acids, tryptophan, and bile acids may also play a role.

27. What factors predispose to HE?

A variety of risk factors for the exacerbation of HE have been identified. High-protein diets can contribute to signs developing because ammonia is produced during protein digestion. This "meal" can also be blood from gastrointestinal hemorrhage. Constipation can also contribute by allowing more toxins to be absorbed from the colon. Certain types of foods might also contribute by favoring the production of toxins.

The metabolic condition of the animal can also influence the severity of HE signs. Alkalosis will increase brain ammonia uptake. Hypokalemia will also exacerbate the clinical signs, as can hypoglycemia and dehydration. Because of this, diuretics, especially potent ones such as furosemide, need to be used with caution. Medications can also exacerbate HE, especially anesthetic agents.

28. How do you treat HE medically?

The goal of HE therapy is to reduce toxin production/resorption by the gut and to optimize the dog's general metabolic condition to minimize signs of HE. Therapy is instituted as needed to avoid hypoglycemia, hypokalemia, and dehydration. If gastrointestinal bleeding is suspected, appropriate treatment for gastrointestinal ulcers should be initiated with such agents as sucralfate or an H2 blocker (e.g., ranitidine, famotidine).

Toxin production by the gut is managed in several different ways. Enemas are given to reduce colonic contents (5-10 ml/kg). Lactulose is consistently given, either orally or via enema (diluted 1:3 with warm water). Lactulose has several benefits including acidifying the colon (converts ammonia to ammonium, which is not absorbed), acting as a cathartic (reduces dwell time of colonic contents), and positively influencing the bacterial flora of the large intestine (reduce urease containing bacteria and favor lactobacilli). When given orally, the dose is adjusted to produce two to three semiformed stools daily (usually 0.25-0.5 ml/kg two or three times daily).

Antibiotics also play a role in reducing ammonia production by decreasing bacterial counts in the gut. Neomycin is an aminoglycoside that is not absorbed appreciably from the intestine. It is usually given orally but can be added to enemas with or without lactulose. Other antibiotics that can be used include metronidazole (7.5 mg/kg twice daily) and amoxicillin.

29. What role does diet play in controlling HE?

Diet is an important part of managing dogs with chronic HE. Feeding a diet with highly digestible proteins is preferred; however, protein levels should be restricted. Protein restriction should not compromise the nutritional status of the animal. The type of protein also makes a difference, with dairy proteins or soy being preferable over meat proteins. Amino acid profiles may play a role as well with branched chain amino acids being desirable and aromatic amino acids being avoided in dogs with HE.

BIBLIOGRAPHY

Jalan R, Shawcross D, Davies N: The molecular pathogenesis of hepatic encephalopathy, *Intl J Biochem Cell Biol* 35:1175-1181, 2003.
Riordan SM, Williams R: Treatment of hepatic encephalopathy, *New Engl J Med* 337:473-479, 1997.

PORTOSYSTEMIC SHUNTS

30. What is a portosystemic shunt (PSS)?

A PSS is an abnormal connection between the portal vein and the systemic circulation, which can be acquired or congenital. They can be acquired secondary to portal hypertension, a common finding with chronic liver disease and cirrhosis. In this case, multiple shunting vessels are present. PSS can also be a congenital disorder in which usually only a single shunting vessel is present. This vessel most is most commonly located outside the liver or extrahepatic (approximately 75% of cases) rather than intrahepatic. Most cases are associated with a vessel connecting the portal vein with the caudal vena cava. Shunts between the portal vein and azygos vein are also common.

31. Is there a breed predisposition for PSS?

Breeds such as Havanese, Yorkshire Terriers, Miniature Schnauzers, and Maltese appear to be at greater risk for this disease. In these small-breed dogs, extrahepatic shunts are more common. In large-breed dogs, intrahepatic shunts are more common. The exact mode of inheritance for this disorder has not been determined.

32. What are typical clinical signs of a congenital PSS?

Clinical signs with PSS are variable. Most dogs will develop clinical signs early in life; however, some dogs will have few clinical signs. The signs can also be episodic, making the diagnosis difficult.

Most dogs with PSS have a history of doing poorly. Many are small for their age. They often will have waxing and waning neurologic signs, such as depression, seizures, bizarre behavior, head pressing, propulsive activity, and stupor or coma. Polyuria/polydipsia is also commonly observed with PSS. Affected animals can also show poor tolerance of anesthetics and sedatives. In some cases, the animals have a history of lower urinary tract signs secondary to urate urolithiasis. Radiographs may demonstrate a small liver (microhepatica).

33. What are typical laboratory abnormalities observed with a PSS?

A variety of laboratory abnormalities can be seen with PSS. The complete blood cell count can show mild microcytic, normochromic nonregenerative anemia. Morphologically, many target cells and poikilocytes are observed. These abnormalities may be a result of abnormal lipid metabolism, iron sequestration, or iron deficiency.

Liver enzyme elevations (e.g., increased ALP, ALT) are not expected with PSS, though they do occur at times. Most commonly, hypoalbuminemia, hypocholesterolemia, and decreased BUN are observed. Hypoglycemia, especially after fasting, is also frequently noted.

Urinalysis often reveals a low urine specific gravity. Ammonium biurate crystals can be seen and should raise the suspicion of PSS in a non-Dalmatian breed.

Coagulation abnormalities are often observed and it is advisable to screen for these in dogs that are to undergo corrective surgery for PSS.

Liver function tests assays will be markedly abnormal in dogs with PSS. Both serum bile acids (fasting and 2-hour postprandial) and ammonia tolerance tests can be used.

34. Describe the bile acids and ammonia tolerance test.

Serum bile acids and ammonia tolerance are both liver function tests. They will be markedly abnormal with PSS, but may be increased by other causes of hepatic dysfunction.

The dog needs to be fasted for 12 hours before running the bile acid test. Blood is collected at time zero (baseline) and the dog is fed a small meal. Two hours after the meal, a second blood sample is collected. The fast allows the gallbladder to fill with bile. Feeding results in contraction of the gallbladder and emptying of the contents into the small bowel. In the small intestine, the bile acids are resorbed and enter the portal vein. Via the portal vein the bile acids reach the liver, where bile acids are extracted by the hepatocytes. With a shunt, the bile acids bypass the liver and are therefore not efficiently extracted and remain in the systemic circulation.

The animal should also be fasted before running an ammonia tolerance test. Blood is collected to measure the resting ammonia plasma concentration. If elevated, the ammonia challenge is not given. If the resting ammonia concentration is normal, ammonia is administered orally (100 mg/kg of ammonium chloride). A second plasma sample is collected 30 minutes after admini-stration. Because administration of ammonium chloride can often cause vomiting, some clini-cians prefer to administer the ammonia rectally, and plasma is then collected 20 and 40 minutes after administration. The main disadvantage to this test is that ammonia is a labile analyte, so the laboratory analysis needs to be run within a narrow window of collection. There is the additional risk that the exogenously administered ammonia may cause or exacerbate clinical signs of HE.

35. How is a PSS diagnosed?

PSS is suspected based on clinical findings and supportive laboratory results, especially markedly abnormal bile acid or ammonia tolerance test results. Definitive diagnosis, however, requires demonstration of the shunting vessel. This can occur through exploratory laparotomy, contrast radiography (portography), computed tomography, ultrasound, or nuclear scintigraphy. Ultrasonography carried out by a skilled operator is the preferred noninvasive method of making a diagnosis.

Imaging before surgery is ideal to determine if an extrahepatic or intrahepatic shunt is present. The latter is more invasive and technically more challenging. In some cases, a shunt cannot be identified by ultrasound or during exploratory. In this case a portogram is used to try to identify the shunt.

36. How is PSS medically managed?

Medical management for PSS predominantly aims to control signs of HE (see Questions 27-29 in this chapter). Unfortunately, this approach is usually not very successful and most animals are euthanized because of inability to adequately control signs. Most medical management protocols focus on administration of a low-protein diet and the use of agents to reduce the generation and absorption of ammonia within the gastrointestinal tract.

37. How is PSS surgically managed?

Stabilizing the animal's condition before anesthesia is vital. Hepatic encephalopathy should be controlled with appropriate measures. Plasma transfusion should be considered if hypo-albuminemia is present. Fresh-frozen plasma would also be indicated if coagulation abnor-malities are present. Generally, blood transfusions are not needed before surgery; however, blood loss is a possible complication and blood should be readily available for transfusion, if needed.

Many different surgical procedures have been described. Ligation with a suture may be a solution with a single extrahepatic shunt. Complete ligation is often not possible because with complete ligation, portal pressure can increase dramatically leading to ascites, bowel ischemia, and endotoxemia. Partial ligation is more commonly used, and this usually results in dramatic clinical improvement, though a repeat operation to completely reduce the shunt may be required at a later date. Many surgeons prefer the use of implants that gradually reduce the size of the shunt vessel. Both cellophane tape and ameroid constrictors have been used. The ameroid cons-trictor is a circular structure that is placed around the shunt vessel that absorbs water, swelling and thereby progressively constricting around the vessel. Occlusion occurs over a period of 4 to 6 weeks. Cellophane tape elicits an inflammatory response that gradually occludes the shunt ves-sel. This method is slower for shunt occlusion to occur compared with the ameroid constrictor.

With intrahepatic shunts, surgical dissection is needed to identify the shunt. Ligation, ameroid constrictor, or cellophane tape can be used to occlude this vessel as well. Recently, interventional radiology has been used to place thrombogenic coils into these vessels.

A liver biopsy should be collected in all cases. This will help identify any other concurrent liver disease.

38. What are complications of surgery for a dog with PSS?

Complications from surgery can be potentially fatal. Overzealous occlusion of a shunt vessel can result in acute portal hypertension. Clinical signs would include abdominal pain, ascites, vo-miting, and shock.

Seizures sometimes follow surgery. The animals are often not responsive to therapy and more than 50% die or are euthanized. Aggressive anticonvulsant therapy is required if seizures do develop after surgery.

39. What is microvascular dysplasia (MVD)?

Microvascular dysplasia (also termed portal vein hypoplasia without macroscopic shunt) is congenital disease mainly of small-breed dogs [Cairn terriers, Yorkshire terriers]). This disorder results in communication between the systemic and portal vascular system in the liver. Diagnosis is determined through exclusion of multiple or single portosystemic shunts together with biopsy results consistent with MVD.

40. How does PSS differ from microvascular dysplasia?

The clinical presentation of dogs with PSS is somewhat different from dogs with MVD. Dogs with MVD are less likely to have clinical signs and if present they tend to be milder. Elevations of serum bile acids usually are also less dramatic. It is important, however, to note that many dogs with MVD can have PSS concurrently.

DISEASES OF THE GALLBLADDER

41. What clinical signs are seen with gallbladder disease?

Many animals with gallbladder disease will be asymptomatic. Jaundice will develop if there is bile duct obstruction or rupture. Clinical signs can be marked including fever, vomiting, and abdominal pain with bile duct obstruction or infection of the biliary tree.

42. What diagnostic tests are indicated if gallbladder disease is suspected?

General laboratory evaluation of animals with gallbladder disease is indicated. A complete blood cell count may have abnormalities such as neutrophils with toxic changes, neutrophilia, or a left shift that may point toward cholecystitis or biliary rupture. Abdominal radiographs may be of low diagnostic yield, but may reveal a mineralized stone or gas around the gallbladder from emphysematous cholecystitis.

Abdominal ultrasound is a valuable test if gallbladder disease is suspected. Cholecystitis manfests as fluid around the gallbladder. The gallbladder may be thickened, though this is a particularly subjective interpretation. Ultrasound also allows identification of gallstones, bile sludge, and mucoceles. If an infection is considered possible, ultrasound can guide a bile aspirate from the gallbladder for cytology and culture. Bile duct obstruction can be identified with ultrasound, though it takes 5 or 6 days before the intrahepatic bile ducts begin to dilate.

43. What is meant by a mucocele?

A mucocele is also referred to as cystic mucinous hypertrophy of the gallbladder. The gallbladder will be enlarged and filled with echoic material that, unlike sludge, will not move if the dog is moved. Various patterns such as kiwi or stellate have been identified. The gallbladder wall has become markedly thickened and proliferative. At times the gallbladder looks like the omasum of a cow stomach. Mucoceles have been linked to cholecystitis and gallbladder necrosis. This suggests that dogs with mucoceles are at higher risk of gallbladder rupture. The ultrasonographic examination of the gallbladder needs to be focused on detecting any signs of rupture. Generally, a mucocele, if extensive enough, warrants surgical intervention.

44. What is meant by cholecystitis and how is it treated?

Cholecystitis is the inflammation of the gallbladder. It can be sterile; however, is usually infectious in origin. A variety of bacteria may be involved, most of them being of gastrointestinal origin such as *Escherichia coli*, *Enterococcus* sp., *Bacteroides* sp., and *Clostridium* sp. Bacteria (*E. coli*, *Clostridium* sp.) can generate gas, resulting in emphysematous cholecystitis. The disease can be associated with necrosis of the gallbladder wall, leading to rupture.

Treatment is symptomatic. Clinically ill animals may benefit from basic supportive care including fluid therapy. Broad-spectrum antibiotics are indicated. It is preferred to have a gallbladder aspirate for cytology and culture to better guide antibiotic choice. Surgery (cholecystectomy) is warranted in those animals with gallbladder rupture or those animals in which rupture is expected to occur.

45. Do dogs have gallstones and do they cause problems?

Gallstones are an infrequent problem in dogs. They usually are found incidentally on radiographs or abdominal ultrasound. However, most are not mineralized enough to show up on radiographs. The stones can be associated with cholecystitis in which case signs of the infection may predominate. Signs are generally only to be expected if obstruction of the bile duct occurs. In this case jaundice, vomiting, and abdominal pain can be seen. In symptomatic dogs, surgical removal is indicated.

46. What extrahepatic causes of biliary obstruction occur?

The common bile duct transports bile from the gallbladder to the small intestine where it enters it at the major duodenal papilla. Before entering the intestine the bile duct runs in the vicinity of pancreas. It is possible to have disease processes in the bile duct that lead to obstruction such as inflammation, granulomas, gallbladder stones, or tumors. The most common cause, however, is pancreatic inflammation. Infiltrative disease involving the small intestine could also cause obstruction. With complete obstruction of the bile duct, it is important to remember that it may take several days before dilation of the biliary system in the liver becomes apparent sonographically.

47. If the bile duct is obstructed what therapy is possible?

Surgical assessment of the bile duct is required to determine the best therapy. If the bile duct looks healthy and the obstruction can be removed, that may be adequate intervention. In those cases in which this is not possible, cholecystectomy is an option. If the bile duct is damaged, it may be necessary to perform a cholecystojejunostomy.

BIBLIOGRAPHY

Richter KP: Diseases of the liver and hepatobiliary system. In Tams TR, editor: *Handbook of small animal gastroenterology*, 2003, St. Louis, 2003, Saunders.

Section VI
Urinary System
Section Editor: Stanley I. Rubin

43. Acute Renal Failure
Stanley I. Rubin and Mala Erickson

1. What is acute renal failure (ARF)?
- ARF refers to a sudden decline in renal function that occurs over hours to days.
- Disease can involve prerenal, renal, or postrenal elements.
- Hemodynamic, filtration, and excretory failure lead to the accumulation of metabolic toxins as well as fluid, electrolyte, and acid-base imbalances.
- Acute renal failure, as compared with chronic renal failure, is potentially reversible with early diagnosis and supportive treatment.
- ARF must be differentiated from prerenal azotemia, which is usually mild and occurs when there is a decline in glomerular filtration rate (GFR) resulting from decreased renal blood flow, perfusion pressure, or excessive vasoconstriction.
- Damage to the kidney vasculature, tubular epithelium, or interstitium can lead to ARF. Any alterations in renal blood flow can affect GFR and lead to renal damage and disease.
- It is the rate of change in renal lesions and function, not the abruptness with which signs appear, that differentiates acute and chronic renal failure.
- Development of oliguria, declining GFR, increasing serum creatinine, and lack of anemia in a dog known to have normal renal function before onset of the illness is unequivocally ARF.

2. Why are the kidneys prone to injury?
- The kidneys receive about 20% of the cardiac output, with the renal cortex receiving about 90% of that flow.
- Mechanisms that are thought to lead to renal injury include tubular obstruction, increased tubular permeability, and altered renal blood flow.
- Cellular damage from hypoxia can lead to decreased renal blood flow and also affect functioning of the Na+, K+-ATPase pump, leading to cell death.

3. What phases of acute renal failure have been identified?
- Initiation, maintenance, and recovery have been identified as the three phases of acute renal failure.
- Initiation refers to the time of initial insult to the kidneys with parenchymal and tubular epithelium injury. As cell death or necrosis occurs, there is a decline in GFR, loss of urinary concentrating ability, and development of oliguria or polyuria and azotemia. Appropriate therapy during this initial phase may decrease the insult to the kidneys and avoid the development of acute renal failure. This period may last from hours to days, but abnormalities may not be clinically evident.
- Tubular lesions and nephron dysfunction occur during the maintenance phase, which may last for weeks to months. GFR and renal blood flow are decreased, urine production decreases, and uremia may develop.

- During the recovery phase, damaged nephrons may be repaired and there may be compensatory hypertrophy of undamaged nephrons. Tubular injury can be repaired if the basement membranes remain intact and there are viable epithelial cells. Through this phase, which can last weeks to months, there may be improved renal function, but normal function may not be regained. Polyuria often occurs as a response to accumulated water, salt, and osmotically active solutes. Azotemia may resolve during this phase.

4. **What are the major causes of acute renal failure?**
   - Inadequate renal perfusion (e.g, thromboses of renal arteries, severe hypotension from any cause, hyperthermia [heat stroke])
   - Nephrotoxic substances
   - Rapidly progressive forms of specific renal diseases (e.g., glomerulonephritis, infection [pyelonephritis], leptospirosis, urinary tract obstruction)
   - Other miscellaneous conditions (e.g., hypercalcemia)

5. **What drugs have been identified as common causes of acute renal failure?**
   - Aminoglycosides (e.g., neomycin, gentamicin, amikacin) can have a toxic effect on the kidneys by causing tubular necrosis. Interference with phospholipid metabolism in the proximal renal tubule cells leads to release of proteolytic enzymes with resulting cellular damage and cell death. Damage can also occur from increased production of free radicals and altered filtration though the glomerular capillaries. This is a dose- and duration-dependent toxic effect and the damage may be reversible with discontinuation of the drug. High or repeated daily dosing, preexisting renal disease, volume depletion, or exposure to other nephrotoxins can enhance the nephrotoxic effects of aminoglycosides. Concurrent administration of other drugs such as furosemide or misoprostol can worsen the renal damage and their use is contraindicated in treatment of toxicity cases.
   - Nonsteroidal antiinflammatory drugs (NSAIDs) act by reducing prostaglandin and thromboxane production via cyclooxygenase inhibition. Prostaglandins PGE_2 and PGI_2 have vasodilatory actions and help to maintain renal blood flow when systemic blood pressure decreases. NSAIDs can interfere with the kidney's ability to compensate when systemic hypotension occurs. Animals with other risk factors such as dehydration or underlying renal disease have a poorer prognosis. Risk of toxicity can also be higher in animals with congestive heart failure, nephrotic syndrome, diabetes mellitus, renal insufficiency, hypertension, cirrhosis, and those under anesthesia. Renal function should be evaluated before beginning long-term treatment using an NSAID.
   - Angiotensin-converting enzyme inhibitors act by preventing the formation of angiotensin II, a potent vasoconstrictor in the renin-angiotensin-aldosterone system. These substances can preferentially cause dilation of the glomerular efferent arteriole, leading to a decrease in glomerular filtration rate. Animals at greater risk include those with sodium depletion, congestive heart failure, chronic renal insufficiency, or those receiving diuretics.
   - The antifungal drug amphotericin B can have direct toxic effects on renal epithelial cells. It can also cause renal arterial vasoconstriction resulting in a reduction in GFR. Renal function should be evaluated prior to initiating use and during therapy. Maintaining adequate hydration during administration, diluting the drug, and administering the dose slowly over several hours may decrease the risk of acute renal failure. Liposome-encapsulated or lipid-complexed formulations are thought to be less nephrotoxic.
   - The alkylating chemotherapeutic agent cisplatin is concentrated within and mainly excreted by the kidney. It can have dose-dependent, progressive, and irreversible toxic effects by causing renal tubular necrosis. Diuresis with intravenous fluids should be a component of administration to reduce the toxic effects of the drug. Carboplatin, a less nephrotoxic drug, should be considered as an alternative.

6. **What other toxins have been implicated in causing acute renal failure?**
   - Ethylene glycol, which is found in most antifreeze products and in some chemicals used for photographic developing, can cause acute renal failure and gastrointestinal, respiratory, and central nervous system signs. The lethal dose in dogs is 6.6 ml/kg and acute renal failure can occur within 24 to 72 hours of ingestion. Renal tubular injury is caused by the glycolate metabolite of ethylene glycol. The formation of oxalate crystals also causes direct renal tubular damage and can cause obstruction. Other changes with ethylene glycol toxicity include calcium oxalate crystalluria, metabolic acidosis with a high anion gap, azotemia, hyperphosphatemia, hypocalcemia, and hyperkalemia. Diagnosis is based on history of ingestion as well as clinical signs and biochemical abnormalities. Within 12 hours of exposure, serum testing may aid in making the diagnosis. Therapy is aimed at preventing further absorption and to decrease conversion of the ethylene glycol to its toxic metabolites. Use of 4-methylpyrazole or 20% ethanol is considered specific therapy for dogs.
   - Elevated calcium can occur from renal failure or can be a cause of acute renal failure. Presence of hypercalcemia can lead to further renal damage from mineralization of the renal parenchyma. A calcium-phosphorus product greater than 60 is considered a risk factor for tissue mineralization. Further investigation into causes of hypercalcemia should be initiated.
   - There have been published reports of renal toxicity related to ingestion of large quantities of raisins or grapes. A specific toxin or contaminant in products has not been identified. Acute renal failure developed within 24 to 72 hours of ingestion and aggressive management is warranted in cases of known ingestion. Evidence of renal tubular necrosis, metastatic mineralization of tissues, and renal tubular epithelial regeneration has been seen in reported cases.
   - Members of the genus *Lilium,* a plant family that includes the Easter lily and tiger lily, can cause nephrotoxicity when portions of the plant are ingested. Animals may show gastrointestinal signs, neurologic signs, and acute renal failure.
   - Vitamin D toxicosis has historically occurred through exposure to rodenticides containing cholecalciferol (vitamin D_3). The resulting hypercalcemia can lead to acute renal failure. Ingestion of medications containing vitamin D can also be a source of toxin. Management should include saline diuresis, furosemide, and may include the use of bisphosphonates.

7. **What infectious diseases can cause acute renal failure?**
   - Leptospirosis is an infectious, zoonotic disease that can cause acute renal failure as well as hepatic disease. Multiple serovars of *Leptospira interrogans* have been identified as causing acute renal failure including *icterohaemorrhagiae, canicola, pomona, bratislava,* and *grippotyphosa.* Leptospiral organisms can be transmitted through contact with infected urine or exposure to contaminated water or soil. Colonization and replication in the renal tubular epithelium cause direct damage and there can be immune-mediated renal damage through antigenic stimulation. Serologic testing can aid diagnosis by demonstrating rising titers. Supportive care involving fluid support as well as antibiotic therapy are indicated (procaine penicillin, ampicillin, doxycycline).
   - Although it rarely causes acute renal failure, babesiosis (*Babesia canis* and *B. gibsoni*) can cause renal damage via anemic hypoxia, hypovolemia, hemoglobinuric nephropathy, and myoglobinuric nephropathy secondary to rhabdomyolysis. Multiple factors can lead to renal dysfunction in affected dogs.
   - Lyme disease, caused by the spirochete *Borrelia burgdorferi* and transmitted by Ixodes ticks, can cause a severe protein-losing glomerulopathy and acute renal failure although the incidence is unknown. Dogs tend to be younger than those with other glomerulopathies and the disease tends to progress more quickly.

8. **What are some of the risk factors for acute renal failure?**
   - Poor perfusion of renal tissue increases the risk of nephrotoxic and ischemic damage to the kidney. Dehydration and volume depletion are the most significant factors that reduce perfusion.
   - Preexisting renal disease with advanced age.
   - Administration of potentially nephrotoxic drugs or drugs that may enhance nephrotoxicity increases the risk for ARF (e.g., furosemide potentiates gentamicin-induced nephrotoxicity).

9. **What are the typical presenting signs in an animal with ARF?**
   - Acute depression, anorexia, vomiting, and diarrhea are common signs of ARF.
   - Oliguria and less frequently anuria are hallmarks of ARF.
   - Nonoliguric forms of ARF also occur.
   - Acutely uremic dogs are generally depressed, hypovolemic, and hypothermic.
   - Respiratory rate often elevated from metabolic acidosis.

10. **How should I manage an animal suspected to have acute renal failure?**
    - Rule out postrenal causes of azotemia/uremia (e.g., urinary obstruction). Apparent anuria is more likely to be caused by obstruction than by ARF; some urine production usually persists in ARF. Verify that the urethra and bladder neck are not obstructed (pass a urinary catheter, if necessary) and determine that bladder or urethral rupture is not present.
    - Rule out prerenal causes of azotemia. Prerenal azotemia is characterized by being associated with physiologic oliguria. The small volume of urine that is formed has physiologically appropriate characteristics (i.e., highly concentrated [specific gravity >1.035], relatively sodium-poor [urine sodium <10 mEq/L], and creatinine-rich [ratio of urine creatinine to serum creatinine >20]).
    - Always obtain a sample for baseline urinalysis before instituting fluid therapy. Obtaining a urine specimen from an oliguric dog with prerenal adversities (e.g., dehydration) before administering fluid therapy is important for this reason. Animals with prerenal azotemia may have signs that could be produced by uremia (e.g., vomiting), but these signs are usually caused by the condition that led to dehydration (e.g., acute pancreatitis, intestinal obstruction, Addison's disease) more than by uremia per se.
    - When oliguria and azotemia are of prerenal origin, they promptly resolve when the prerenal adversity is treated effectively (e.g., aggressive fluid therapy). Sometimes, differentiation of prerenal and renal oliguria is based ultimately on response to therapy.
    - Seek environmental or medical history of a circumstance or condition that might directly or indirectly produce ARF (e.g., exposure to drug or toxin).

11. **How do I rule in acute renal failure?**
    - The diagnosis of ARF is based on finding compatible clinical and laboratory features.
    - In ARF, the urine that is formed has physiologically inappropriate characteristics (i.e., not highly concentrated [specific gravity 1.007 to 1.017], relatively sodium-rich [urine sodium >25 mmol/L], and creatinine-poor [ratio of urine creatinine to serum creatinine <10]).
    - Renal tubular damage may be indicated by finding casts in the urine.
      Serum biochemical abnormalities typically include the following:
      - Azotemia
      - Hyperkalemia that may be severe and life-threatening.
      - Hyperphosphatemia and metabolic acidosis that tend to be greater in magnitude with comparable degrees of azotemia in ARF than in chronic renal failure.
      - Hypocalcemia, particularly as severity of metabolic derangements, intensifies.
      - Lack of nonregenerative anemia, which is typically observed in chronic renal failure.

12. What are the therapeutic objectives in managing a dog with acute renal failure?
- Minimize further renal injury.
- Correct alterations in extracellular fluid (ECF) volume and repair estimated fluid deficits.
- Manage hyperkalemia.
- Manage acid-base imbalances.
- Use strategies for reduction of nitrogenous waste and the accumulation of uremic toxins.

13. How do I minimize renal injury?
- Discontinue use of potentially nephrotoxic drugs, if possible, or modify dosage appropriately.
- Maintain adequate tissue perfusion; toxic nephropathy is bad enough without superimposing ischemic renal damage.

14. What are the essentials of fluid therapy for ARF?
- Repair estimated fluid deficits. Restore ECF volume to near normal by rapid intravenous administration of an appropriate crystalloid solution.
- Give the calculated volume of fluid needed to repair the estimated deficit in the first 2 to 4 hours, provided the heart can pump it. Lactated Ringer's, normal saline (0.9%), or saline-dextrose combinations are all likely acceptable choices.
- Keep accurate records of animal's weight, volume, and composition of fluids given, and of fluid losses (e.g., urine, vomited fluids, diarrhea, hemorrhage) because meticulous management of fluid balance is required.
- After the animal is rehydrated, match fluid administration to fluid losses, monitor weight carefully, and adjust fluid therapy as conditions may require.
- Determine urine production rate; however, do not catheterize a dog suspected of having ARF unless absolutely essential. Animals with ARF are unusually susceptible to urinary tract infection, and infection is a major cause of morbidity and mortality in animals with renal failure. Urine output can be determined by serial free-catch determinations or with aid of metabolism cage. Crude estimates can be made by palpation, radiographs, or ultrasound. Prevoiding and postvoiding weights of disposable absorbant pads or diapers may give useful measure of urine voided. If catheterization deemed necessary, intermittent catheterization is preferred to an indwelling catheter. When indwelling catheters are used, closed drainage collection systems should be used.

15. What do I do if oliguria persists following correction of fluid deficits?
- If fluid therapy alone fails to convert the dog from oliguria to nonoliguria, consider administration of diuretics (see section on diuretics).
- If oliguria persists for more than a day or two (it usually does, despite efforts to induce diuresis, except in mild cases of ARF), there are two options:
  - Humane euthanasia.
  - Institute dialysis to preserve the animal's life until adequate renal function is restored. This is based on the assumption that the ARF is reversible.

16. When do I use diuretics?
- Diuretics are administered with the goal of converting oliguria to nonoliguria.
- The use of diuretics in the conversion of oliguric to nonoliguric renal failure is controversial. Do not equate an increase in urine flow rates with an improvement in renal function. Diuretic administration is necessary only if the animal is not producing appropriate urine volumes following fluid therapy.
- Furosemide: use 2 mg/kg intravenously; if no response occurs in 2 hours, double dose and repeat.

- Dopamine at a dose of 2 to 5 μg/kg/min in conjunction with furosemide. Dopamine is indicated because it may increase renal blood flow and glomerular filtration rate as a result of renal vasodilatation induced by its beta-adrenergic effect. Dopamine may be diluted in lactated Ringer's solution. A total of 50 mg of dopamine in 500 ml of solution yields a concentration of 100 μg/ml.
- Osmotic agents such as mannitol. The recommended dose of mannitol is 0.5 to 1.0 gm/kg intravenously as a bolus over 15 to 20 minutes. Urine output should improve within 1 hour if treatment is effective. A second bolus may be attempted. Mannitol is effective because it decreases tubular cell swelling, increases tubular flow, and helps to prevent tubular obstruction or collapse. Mannitol also has weak vasodilator properties.

17. How do I manage hyperkalemia?

- The electrocardiogram is a useful tool that provides immediate evidence about the physiologic impact of hyperkalemia on the heart and responses to therapy.
- New technologies have allowed rapid determination of serum potassium concentration in the clinical setting, often in conjunction with blood gas measurements that allow for serial monitoring of critical animals.
- Several therapeutic strategies are used to reduce serum potassium.
- Administration of intravenous fluids will have a dilutional effect.
- Other therapies should be considered immediately if the electrocardiogram indicates severe changes or is worsening despite therapy. An intravenous bolus of sodium bicarbonate (0.5-2 mEq/kg over 5 to 15 minutes) is indicated to treat the hyperkalemia. Intravenous administration of sodium bicarbonate enhances intracellular movement of potassium, thus lowering serum potassium concentration. If there is no response to sodium bicarbonate then calcium gluconate (0.5-1.0 ml 10% calcium gluconate/kg) is administered intravenously over 10 to 15 minutes. Intravenous insulin and glucose may also be used for management of hyperkalemia

18. How do I manage metabolic acidosis?

- Metabolic acidosis associated with ARF is ideally managed by serial assessment of animal's acid-base status.
- An estimate of the base deficit may be based on general severity of azotemia and uremia (i.e., 5, 10, 15, and 20 mEq/L or mmol/L for mild, moderate, severe, and very severe, respectively).
- Administer sodium bicarbonate intravenously. Calculate the initial dosage (i.e., first 2 hours) as 0.3 times body weight (kg) times base deficit (mEq/L or mmol/L). Give half the calculated dosage slowly, over 15 to 30 minutes. Then reassess.
- [0.3 × BW × base deficit] = Calculated dose of sodium bicarbonate
- Use serial assessments of acid-base status, if possible, to adjust therapy according to requirements.

19. How do I manage the uremic gastropathy and vomiting?

- Impaired renal clearance of gastrin leads to hypergastrinemia, excessive stimulation of gastric acid secretion, and gastritis.
- Administer H_2-receptor blocking agents such as cimetidine, ranitidine, or famotidine,
- Use antiemetics that act at the chemoreceptor trigger zone (e.g., metoclopramide [0.2-0.5 mg/kg intravenously, intramuscularly, or by mouth every 6 to 8 hours]) if vomiting cannot be controlled by placing the gastrointestinal tract at rest and giving cimetidine/ranitidine/famotidine.

20. What about nutritional support?

- Nutritional support should also be an element of therapy.

- Malnutrition can lead to impaired immune function, increased susceptibility to infection, delayed wound healing, decreased strength, and poor quality of life. Catabolism can also exacerbate electrolyte and acid-base disturbances.
- Body condition scoring as well as monitoring body weight can help monitor status.
- High-energy diets with moderate protein, potassium, and phosphate would be indicated.
- Oral or enteral feeding may not be possible in a dog with gastrointestinal signs so peripheral parenteral nutrition, total parenteral nutrition, or use of a feeding tube may be necessary.

21. What do I do if the dog suddenly starts producing massive amounts of urine?
- This suggests that the dog is in the diuretic portion of the recovery phase.
- Diuresis may be mild or profound. Match volume of urine produced with fluid therapy or supplementation.
- Hypokalemia may develop if potassium intake is not sufficient, either through diet or intravenous fluids. Supplemental potassium chloride should be added to the intravenous fluids to present severe hypokalemia.

22. What are some indications for renal biopsy in a dog with acute renal failure?
- A renal biopsy should be undertaken under some circumstances to give further definition to the case, which should assist with formulating an accurate prognosis. These circumstances include the following:
  - Lack of a definitive diagnosis
  - Significant and persistent proteinuria
  - Persistence of oliguria beyond 2 to 3 days
  - Persistence of severe uremia or hyperkalemia for 5 to 7 days despite aggressive treatment

23. What is hemodialysis?
Hemodialysis can be considered in dogs with severe oliguria or anuria that cannot be maintained on fluid support, diuretics, and renal vasodilators. Dialyzable toxins and their metabolites can be removed rapidly and completely with dialysis. It is considered particularly effective for treatment of ethylene glycol toxicity. It can also be used for dogs with iatrogenic fluid overload, life-threatening pulmonary edema, or therapies using large fluid volumes. An artificial membrane acts as an exchange surface against which blood and the dialysate are interposed directly across the membrane. Solutes and water move across a semipermeable membrane against concentration gradients. Waste solutes and excessive water loads are removed similarly to what would occur in a normal kidney. There are only a few facilities that offer hemodialysis and the closest institution should be contacted regarding appropriate case selection and referral.

24. What is peritoneal dialysis and how is it performed?
Peritoneal dialysis involves the placement of a crystalloid fluid, the dialysate, into the abdominal cavity to allow equilibration of uremic wastes and excess fluid transfer from plasma with the dialysate, across the barrier of the peritoneal lining. Exchange of solutes depends on the concentration gradient as well as the size of the molecule, peritoneal blood flow, condition of the peritoneal membrane, and time allowed for solute movement. Animals should be well hydrated and normotensive before beginning peritoneal dialysis. A catheter with multiple fenestrations is placed to infuse the dialysate into the peritoneal space. Peritoneal dialysis can be used as an adjunct therapy for treatment of ethylene glycol toxicity as well as in animals with oliguric renal failure from other causes.

25. What is the prognosis for animals with acute renal failure?
- Prognosis depends on the animal's response to initial treatment and intensive therapy. Prolonged monitoring may be needed to predict whether there will be return of renal function.

- Animals with nonoliguric acute renal failure have a better prognosis than those with anuric or oliguric renal failure.
- Those with infectious disease fare better than those with toxic or ischemic acute renal failure.
- Toxin-induced cases do better than ischemia-induced ones because basement membranes are more likely to remain intact.
- Animals have a poor prognosis if preexisting disease is present, there are a high number of complications, several organ systems are involved, there is severe azotemia, or there is a long interval between diagnosis and treatment.
- Older animals tend to have a poorer prognosis.
- The mortality rate has been estimated to be 60% from death or euthanasia in dogs with acute renal failure. Dogs surviving often develop chronic renal failure.

BIBLIOGRAPHY

Cowgill LD, Elliot DA: Acute renal failure. In Ettinger SJ, Feldman EC, editors: *Textbook of veterinary internal medicine, vol 2,* ed 5, Philadelphia, 2000, WB Saunders.
Kraje AC: Helping patients that have acute renal failure, *Vet Med* 97:461-474, 2002.
Lacaze MG, Kirby R, Rudloff E: Peritoneal dialysis: not just for renal failure, *Comp Cont Educ Pract Vet* 24:758-772, 2002.
Thadhani R, Pascual M, Bonventre JV: Acute renal failure, *New Engl J Med* 334:1448-1460, 1996.

44. Chronic Renal Failure

Mala Erickson and Stanley I. Rubin

1. What is the definition of chronic renal failure (CRF)?

Progressive development of polyuria, abnormal but generally stable glomerular filtration rate and elevated serum creatinine, anemia, and small kidneys is unequivocally CRF.

2. What is kidney disease?

- Chronic kidney disease (CKD) is defined as the presence of structural or functional abnormalities in one or both kidneys. Kidney dysfunction usually is irreversible and slowly progressive with function remaining stable or slowly declining over months or years.
- Kidney disease should not be used synonymously with uremia or kidney failure.
- CKD is considered a leading cause of illness and death in dogs with a prevalence reported between 0.5% and 7%.

3. What is the typical signalment of dogs affected by chronic renal failure?

CRF is often considered to occur in older animals, but surveys have shown a mean age of 6.5 to 7 years of age. CRF is considered the most common renal disease in dogs and cats.

4. What are the causes of CRD?

- Congenital and familial causes of CRF reported in Basenji, Bull Terriers, Cairn Terriers, Chow, German Shepherd, Miniature Schnauzer, Standard Poodle, Welsh Corgi, Norwegian Elkhounds, Cocker Spaniels, Samoyeds, Lhasa Apso, Shih Tzu, Beagles, Keeshonden, Golden Retrievers, Blue Merle Collies, Shar-Pei, and Soft-Coated Wheaten Terriers.
- For rational clinical management, the possible causes of CRF that are important to identify are the following:

- Infection, particularly bacterial infection.
- Chronic partial obstruction of the excretory pathway.
- Subacute to chronic nephrotoxins (e.g., hypercalcemia).
- The causes of CRF are numerous, multifactorial, and frequently impossible to determine at the end stage of the disease.

5. What is the clinical course of chronic renal failure?
- In most instances, CRF is the result of a disease that gradually reduces the number of functioning nephrons.
- Surviving nephrons hypertrophy and adaptively change their functional performance in predictable ways that tend to preserve homeostasis.
- Eventually, the consequences of adaptations to maintain homeostasis become noticeable and ordinary measures of renal function become abnormal.
- The earliest change is impaired urine concentrating ability.
- Additional loss of nephrons reduces glomerular filtration rate further and causes azotemia to prevail.
- When the combination of severity and duration of impaired renal function becomes sufficient, signs of an illness (e.g., uremia) develop.
- A rapid or abrupt deterioration in the animal's clinical status may occur.
- Such a "uremic crisis" is characterized by severe azotemia and intensification of uremic signs. Usually, uremic crises are precipitated by changes in extrarenal factors that may be reversible (e.g., dietary indiscretion, water deprivation, vomiting).
- Progressive deterioration of intrinsic functional capacity of the remnant kidneys generally occurs.
- Eventually, residual renal function will be insufficient to sustain life, and a terminal uremic crisis will occur in most cases.

6. What are the sequential stages of renal disease leading to CRF?
1. Kidney disease without insufficiency
2. Kidney insufficiency without failure
3. Kidney failure without uremia
4. Kidney failure with mild to moderate yet stable uremia
5. Uremic crisis of CRF
6. Progression to end stage
7. Death

7. What is azotemia?
- Existence of abnormally high concentration of nonprotein nitrogenous substances (urea, creatinine, and others) in the extracellular fluids, regardless of cause.
- Because nonprotein nitrogenous compounds (including urea and creatinine) are endogenous substances, abnormally elevated concentrations in the serum may be caused by an increased rate of production (by the liver for urea; muscle for creatinine) or by a decreased rate of excretion (primarily by the kidneys).
- Azotemia is a laboratory finding.
- Azotemia may or may not be caused by renal disease; it may be prerenal or postrenal instead of renal in origin.

8. What is uremia?
- Abnormal quantities of urine constituents in the blood caused by the inability to form and excrete urine adequately, and the polysystemic toxic syndrome that occurs as a result of abnormal renal function.
- Uremia is a clinical illness.

- Uremia may or may not be caused by renal disease; it may be postrenal, or occasionally prerenal, instead of renal in origin.
- All uremic animals have azotemia, but some azotemic animals do not have uremia.
- The clinical signs of uremia are nonspecific or gastrointestinal, but a great variety of other clinical signs are observed sometimes.

9.   **What are the typical clinical findings in a dog with chronic renal failure?**
- The onset and range of clinical signs and biochemical events in dogs with CRF may vary depending on cause, severity, duration, rate of progression of uremic state, presence of concurrent disease and the age of the dog.
- Presenting signs may be grouped into a number of organ systems/signs:
  1. Gastrointestinal; anorexia, vomiting, diarrhea
  2. Impaired urine concentrating ability, polydipsia, polyuria, nocturia
  3. Arterial hypertension
  4. Neuromuscular consequences
  5. Ocular consequences
  6. Hemorrhagic consequences

10.   **What are the typical physical examination findings in a dog with CRF?**
- Extreme variability in findings
- Loss of body condition with a historical or detectable loss of body weight
- Hair coat is coarse and lusterless
- Dehydration
- Pale mucous membranes
- Fetid or ammoniacal breath
- On occasion with profound uremia, necrosis of tip of tongue
- Cardiac arrhythmias associated with electrolyte disturbances of advanced uremia
- Tachypnea, associated with metabolic acidosis
- Small, firm kidneys
- Hypothermia

11.   **What are the typical laboratory abnormalities in CRF?**
- Nonregenerative anemia: a progressive hypoproliferative anemia is characteristic of dogs with moderate to advanced CRF
- Stress leukogram
- Hemostatic abnormalities from defective platelet function manifest by prolonged bleeding time
- Azotemia; elevated serum creatinine and blood urea nitrogen
- Hyperphosphatemia
- Metabolic acidosis
- Moderate hyperamylasemia (two to three times normal) and moderate hyperlipasemia (two to four times normal)
- Isosthenuria with inactive urine sediment
- Radiography may reveal small kidneys and osteodystrophy

12.   **What is microalbuminuria?**
- A screening test.
- Microalbuminuria indicates abnormal renal handling of protein
- Results from either reversible or irreversible damage to the glomerular, tubular, or vascular portions of the kidney.
- Persistent microalbuminuria may occur in animals that have stable, subclinical chronic kidney disease, or as an initial sign in animals that will eventually develop progressive chronic kidney disease.

- A urine test is available to detect microalbuminuria; at concentrations that were previously undetectable (E.R.D.–Screen Urine Test, Heska, Ft. Collins, CO).
- A positive test for microalbuminuria does not diagnose a specific underlying condition. Further assessment and follow-up is required.

13. **What should be my clinical approach in a dog with suspected chronic renal failure?**
    - Attempt to rule in CRF by finding evidence of chronic disease
    - History of polyuria and polydipsia prior to the development of signs of uremia
    - Concurrent nonregenerative anemia
    - Osteodystrophy and small, misshapen kidneys
    - Serial assessment of renal function reveals stable or progressive azotemia
    - Rule out potentially treatable causes of continued renal damage
    - Use urinalysis and urine culture to rule out infection; also consider excretory urography and ultrasound to rule out renal infection
    - Use signalment, history, and radiography to rule out partial urinary obstructions (e.g., tumors, calculi)

14. **What do I do if I am uncertain of the diagnosis of chronic renal failure?**
    - Carefully assess dog for presence of prerenal or postrenal factors
    - Consider hypoadrenocorticism as a differential diagnosis
    - Consider nonoliguric acute renal failure
    - Renal biopsy may be required

15. **How can chronic renal failure be differentiated from acute renal failure?**
    - Differentiating chronic from acute renal failure is based on the time course of the disease process.
    - It must be emphasized that it is the rate of change in renal lesions and function, not the abruptness with which signs appear, that differentiates acute from CRF.
    - In CRF, the time course usually exceeds 2 weeks. Animals with CRF often have weight loss, polyuria, polydipsia, poor hair coat, vomiting and diarrhea, and may have small, irregular kidneys noted on palpation or an imaging study.

16. **What gastrointestinal complications can occur with chronic renal failure?**
    - Dogs with chronic renal failure can show anorexia and weight loss as well as nausea, vomiting, and reduced nutrient intake.
    - Vomiting can result from effects of uremic toxins on the chemoreceptor trigger zone within the medulla as well as direct effects on the gastric mucosa.
    - Development of uremic gastropathy has been related to increased levels of gastrin in the stomach which leads to increased gastric acid secretion by parietal cells. Because about 40% of circulating gastrin is metabolized by the kidneys, altered renal function can lead to hypergastrinemia.
    - Uremic stomatitis can also occur with oral ulcerations, necrosis, and sloughing of the anterior portion of the tongue, and uremic breath in affected animals.
    - Uremic enterocolitis may manifest as diarrhea.

17. **How are chronic renal failure and hypertension related?**
    - Arterial hypertension is estimated to occur in between 50% and 93% of dogs with renal failure and also in dogs with glomerular disease.
    - Hypertension can be defined as persistent elevation of either systolic or diastolic blood pressure. For dogs, systolic blood pressure should not normally be greater than 180 mm Hg, whereas diastolic pressures should not normally exceed 100 mm Hg.

- A series of blood pressure measurements should be taken over the course of three hospital visits to determine persistence unless systolic pressures are greater than 200 mm Hg or there is evidence of end-organ injury warranting immediate pharmacologic intervention.

18. What pathologic effects can hypertension cause?

- It is thought that hypertension results from, rather than causes, CRF in small animals.
- Hypertension causes pathology mainly through vascular injury. The eyes, brain, kidneys, and cardiovascular systems are particularly prone to hypertensive injury.
- Animals with uremia may show signs of neurologic disease with altered consciousness, and seizures being the most commonly seen signs—these signs may be cyclic and episodic.
- Hypertension may cause brain ischemia due to local vascular changes or cerebrovascular hemorrhage. With hypertension, ocular changes can also result such as scleral and conjunctival injection and slow pupillary light responses. Ophthalmoscopic examination may show tortuous retinal vessels, papilledema, retinal edema and detachment, and retinal and vitreal hemorrhage. Hyphema and secondary glaucoma may lead to blindness.
- Fundic examination should be performed in all dogs with CRF to look for evidence of ocular disease.
- Hypertension has been shown to speed the progression of CRF.

19. Why are dogs with CRF anemic?

- Dogs with moderate to advanced chronic renal failure usually show a progressive non-regenerative anemia.
- Proposed mechanisms include a shortened red blood cell life span, nutritional abnormalities, erythropoietin inhibitor substances in the plasma of uremic dogs, blood loss, and myelofibrosis.
- Erythropoietin deficiency has been considered the principal cause. Erythropoietin is synthesized by renal peritubular capillary endothelial cells and renal interstitial fibroblasts. Synthesis is stimulated by intrarenal tissue hypoxia resulting from decreased oxygen carrying capacity (anemia) or decreased oxygen content (hypoxia).
- Iron deficiency and chronic gastrointestinal blood loss can also be causes of anemia in animals with CRF.

20. How are phosphorus levels controlled by the kidneys and what changes can result in CRF?

- The kidneys are the main route for phosphorus excretion with net excretion being the net of glomerular filtration minus tubular reabsorption of phosphorus.
- A decline in glomerular filtration rate, with constant dietary intake, will ultimately result in hyperphosphatemia.

21. What is renal secondary hyperparathyroidism?

- A multifactorial disorder characterized by phosphorus retention.
- Hyperphosphatemia, low levels of 1.25-dihydroxycholecalciferol (calcitriol) levels, reduced ionized calcium concentration, and resistance of skeletal system to the effects of parathyroid hormone (PTH).
- Relative to absolute deficiency of calcitriol; the most active form of vitamin D, is formed in renal tubular cells, and its formation is promoted by PTH.
- Early in chronic renal failure, phosphate retention will limit calcitriol production by enzyme inhibition (1α-hydroxylase).
- Impaired calcium absorption related to low serum calcitriol levels plays a role in animals with advanced disease.
- Renal osteodystrophy is seen most often in immature animals and the bones of the skull and mandible may be the most severely affected.

22. **How is calcium balance affected in chronic renal failure?**
   - Hypocalcemia is the most common calcium derangement in animals with CRF.
   - Hypercalcemia can be seen in some cases, although serum total calcium levels may not reflect ionized calcium levels; this may be due to complexation of calcium with organic and inorganic ions such as citrate, phosphate, or sulfate.
   - Hypercalcemia may be a cause or the result of CRF; ionized hypercalcemia can promote renal failure. Animals with ionized hypercalcemia should be evaluated for causes of hypercalcemia such as neoplasia or vitamin D toxicity.
   - Animals with hyperphosphatemia and hypercalcemia are predisposed to metastatic calcification when the Ca X PO_4 product is elevated (higher than 60). Calcification can occur in areas such as the stomach and kidneys as well as the myocardium, lung, and liver.

23. **What aspects of treatment should be considered in animals with chronic renal failure?**
   - Management of animals with CRF should be directed toward correction of fluid, electrolyte, and acid-base abnormalities as well as trying to minimize clinical and pathologic consequences of decreased renal function.
   - Because existing damage cannot be reversed, if possible, therapy should be directed at the primary cause; this is why it is important to screen the renal failure animal for presence of urinary tract infection.
   - Fluid therapy is an important aspect of patient management. Intravenous fluid therapy is indicated for management of uremic crises characterized by severe azotemia and clinical signs of uremia. Therapy for uremic gastropathy should be started because its presence can contribute to malnutrition. Antiemetics (metoclopramide), histamine blockers, as well as tube feeding, may be used.
   - Persistent hypertension should be managed if confirmed through documentation. Angiotensin-converting enzyme inhibitors have renoprotective effects by lowering intraglomerular pressures and reducing proteinuria. Amlodipine besylate, a calcium antagonist, is another option for hypertension management.

24. **How can hyperphosphatemia be treated?**
   - Hyperphosphatemia can be managed through restriction of dietary phosphorus intake, use of intestinal phosphorus binding agents, or a combination of the two.
   - Most prescription diets formulated for management of renal failure are low in phosphorus.
   - Recipes for homemade diets low in phosphorus are available.
   - Dietary restriction alone may not normalize serum PTH levels in dogs with chronic renal failure. Protein-restricted diets are usually lower in phosphorus. If hyperphosphatemia persists despite dietary management, intestinal phosphorus binding agents can be used. These agents interfere with absorption of ingested phosphorus and phosphorus in saliva, bile, and intestinal juices. They should be given with food and be used in combination with dietary restriction. Products may be aluminum based (aluminum hydroxide, aluminum carbonate, aluminum oxide) or calcium based (calcium carbonate, calcium citrate, or calcium acetate). Sucralfate may also aid in binding phosphorus in the intestine.

25. **How can anemia related to chronic renal failure be treated?**
   - Control and treatment of suspected gastrointestinal hemorrhage should be addressed.
   - Iron supplementation may be required for iron deficiency anemia.
   - Transfusions of packed red blood cells or whole blood may be indicated for rapid correction of anemia and repeated transfusions may be necessary for long-term control in some dogs.
   - Recombinant human erythropoietin has also been used.

26. **How can dietary modification be used for managing animals with CRF?**
   - Diet change is recommended at the time of diagnosis based on the evaluation of clinical signs and the presence of azotemia.
   - Diets are formulated to have reduced protein, phosphorus, and sodium content as well as increased B vitamin content and caloric density, with a neutral effect on acid-base balance.
   - Restriction of dietary phosphorus can reduce the severity of hyperphosphatemia secondary to the renal failure.
   - Experimental models of canine chronic renal failure have shown that dietary phosphorus restriction has been linked to prolonged survival and a slower decline in renal function.
   - Dietary fiber increase has also been proposed to enhance gastrointestinal excretion of nitrogenous wastes.
   - Renal function may be preserved through supplementation with omega-3 polyunsaturated fatty acids (fish oils), which can improve renal hemodynamics, minimize proteinuria, and suppress mediators of inflammation and coagulation.
   - Animals may not consume enough fluid to prevent dehydration and flavoring liquids may encourage drinking. Supplemental (subcutaneous) fluids may be a component of home management but there should be close attention to prevent fluid overload.

27. **What about anabolic steroids?**
   - These were used to treat anemia associated with CRF.
   - Controlled studies are lacking.
   - They appear to benefit only a small percentage of animals, have a long delay to onset of action (months), and may be associated with undesirable side effects.

28. **What about giving calcitriol to the animal with CRF?**
   - Administration of active vitamin D or calcitriol in conjunction with proportionate reduction in phosphate intake has been shown to limit renal secondary hyperparathyroidism and its associated skeletal deformities in dogs with experimentally induced CRF.
   - There are reports of favorable impressions after its use in managing dogs with CRF.
   - Calcitriol has the potential to cause hypercalcemia and promote further renal injury.
   - Controlled clinical trials in dogs are lacking.
   - Clinicians should await results of well-designed clinical trials before recommending its use in management of CRF.

29. **Is renal transplantation an option for a dog with CRF?**
   - Renal transplantation is not as well established in dogs as it is in cats.
   - Not an option for dogs at this time because of toxicity and efficacy of immunosuppressive drugs make sufficient immunosuppression more problematic.

30. **What can I tell the owner about prognosis for an animal with CRF?**
   - Start by categorizing the prognosis for the following:
     - Probability of immediate survival (short-term prognosis)
     - Probability of survival over the subsequent months to years (long-term prognosis)
   - Be sure to let the client know that loss of renal function is permanent with CRF; recovery refers to improvement of biochemical deficits and excesses and amelioration of clinical signs rather than recovery of renal function
   - Factors to consider in establishing meaningful prognoses for dogs with CRF include the following:
     - Severity of clinical signs and complications of uremia
     - Probability of improving renal function (e.g., prerenal, postrenal, and newly acquired primary renal conditions)
     - Severity of intrinsic renal functional impairment

- Rate of progression of renal dysfunction with and without therapy
- Age of animal
- Severity of uremic signs is often a relatively good predictor of short-term prognosis
- Severity of renal dysfunction is more useful in establishing a long-term prognosis
- In general, severe renal dysfunction is associated with shorter long-term survival and often a lower quality of life
- The long-term prognosis of dogs with serum creatinine concentrations of 3.0 to 4.0 mg/dl (260 to 350 μmol/L) or less is typically good.

BIBLIOGRAPHY

Brown SA: Evaluation of chronic renal disease: a staged approach, *Comp Cont Educ Pract Vet* 21:752-763, 1999.

Jacob F, Polzin DJ, Osborne CA et al: Clinical evaluation of dietary modification for treatment of spontaneous chronic renal failure in dogs, *J Am Vet Med Assoc* 220:1163-1170, 2002.

Polzin DJ, Osborne CA, Jacob F et al: Chronic renal failure, In Ettinger SJ, Feldman EC, editors: *Textbook of veterinary internal medicine, vol 2*, ed 5, Philadelphia, 2000, WB Saunders.

Vaden S: Microalbuminuria: what is it and how do I interpret it? Proceedings of the twenty-first annual American College of Veterinary Internal Medicine Forum, Charlotte, NC, 2003.

45. Glomerular Disease

Mala Erickson and Stanley I. Rubin

1. **Discuss the basic anatomy of the nephron and glomerulus.**
- The nephron, the functional unit of the kidney, consists of a glomerulus, Bowman's capsule, and a renal tubule.
- Each glomerulus is supplied by an afferent arteriole that connects with an efferent arteriole via the glomerular tuft, a branched capillary system.
- The glomerular capillary lumen is lined by endothelial cells that have pores or fenestrae and the capillaries are surrounded by the glomerular basement membrane (GBM), which serves as the glomerular filter.
- Negatively charged sites on the GBM and the endothelial cells repel anions and prevent passage of high-molecular-weight, noncharged molecules.
- Mesangial cells are phagocytic cells that are thought to remove filtration residues between the GBM and endothelial cells.
- Visceral epithelium lining Bowman's space consists of podocytes with numerous foot processes and is continuous with the proximal tubule. Slit pores between the foot processes serve as another filter.
- Glomeruli prevent passage of molecules with a net negative charge and with a molecular weight greater than 70,000 D.
- One of the major proteins lost in glomerulonephritis is albumin which has a molecular weight of about 65,000 D—it is small enough to pass through the filtration barriers, but its negative charge normally prevents passage.
- Filtrate passes from Bowman's space to the proximal tubule where proteins that escape the glomerular barrier are reabsorbed—a small amount of protein may remain in the urine of dogs.

2.   How does glomerular injury occur?
- Glomerular injury is immune mediated as evidenced by the presence of immunoglobulins and complement factors bound to glomerular structures.
- One proposed mechanism is the deposition or entrapment of preformed circulating antigen-antibody complexes within glomeruli.
- A second proposed mechanism is the entrapment of antigen in the glomerular capillary wall and formation of complexes with circulating antibodies in the glomeruli (in situ).
- With the formation of immune complexes, various events occur causing renal injury including complement activation, neutrophil and macrophage infiltration, platelet aggregation, activation of the coagulation cascade, and fibrin deposition. Oxidants and proteinases are produced by neutrophils, macrophages, and mesangial cells in response to immunoglobulins. Nitric oxide, which can be released by cells during glomerular inflammation, can induce cytotoxicity. Release of platelet-activating factor from platelets, endothelial cells, and mesangial cells can neutralize the negative charges in the glomerular capillary walls and enhance albumin loss in the urine.
- Mediators cause morphologic changes in the glomeruli including mesangial cell and matrix proliferation and GBM thickening. T-lymphocytes are thought to be involved in the resulting glomerular injury with recognition of antigen and subsequent activation.
- Glomerulosclerosis can develop with continued injury.
- Irreversible damage to the glomerulus can lead to a nonfunctional nephron.
- Progressive loss of nephrons can lead to renal failure.

3.   What is glomerulonephritis?
- Glomerulonephritis is a condition that can be idiopathic or secondary to infectious agents, neoplasia, inflammatory disease, endocrine disease, and familial nephropathies.
- It is considered a common cause of proteinuria in small animals.

4.   What is the nephrotic syndrome?
- Coexisting proteinuria, hypoalbuminemia, hypercholesterolemia, and accumulation of transudates interstitially (e.g., edema) or in body cavities (e.g., ascites).
- Massive urinary protein loss that reduces serum albumin to the point (near 10 g/L) that decreased plasma colloid osmotic (oncotic) pressure leads to edema, or ascites produces the nephrotic syndrome.
- The causes of nephrotic syndrome are two types of glomerular diseases: amyloidosis and glomerulonephritis.

5.   How is glomerulonephritis (GN) classified?
- Histopathologic classification of GN may help to differentiate idiopathic from secondary GN.
- It is hoped that histologic classification of a particular case will direct treatment decisions; however, at this point, there is still much to be learned with regard to the biologic behavior of the various forms of GN in the dog.
- Only the kidneys have signs of pathologic involvement in idiopathic GN and no concurrent disease can be found.
- Membranous GN is characterized by a thickened glomerular basement membrane.
- Glomerular hypercellularity with an accumulation of mesangial matrix is seen with proliferative (mesangioproliferative) GN.
- In membranoproliferative GN, there is hypercellularity and increased thickness of the GBM.
- With glomerulosclerosis, there is an increase in matrix and glomerular scarring.

6.   What diseases have been reported to be associated with GN?
- Neoplasia accounts for between 17% and 40% of cases of GN based on various reports.
- Infectious diseases that may be associated with GN include heartworm disease (*Dirofilaria immitis*), ehrlichiosis, and Lyme disease (*Borrelia burgdorferi*).

- GN occurs in dogs with experimentally produced diabetes mellitus, but there has not been evidence of this occurring with natural disease.
- Hyperadrenocorticism (spontaneous and iatrogenic) has been associated with GN.
- Familial glomerulopathies have been reported in Doberman Pinschers, Samoyeds, Rottweilers, Greyhounds, English Cocker Spaniels, and Soft-coated Wheaten Terriers.

7. **Discuss signalment and clinical signs of glomerular disease.**
   - GN is recognized more frequently in dogs, compared with cats, with a reported mean age of 7 years of age.
   - Breeds affected by familial GN may have a younger age of onset.
   - No gender predisposition has been found.
   - The most common reported clinical signs of GN include anorexia, weight loss, and vomiting, with these signs thought to be due to uremia from renal failure.
   - Polyuria and polydipsia resulting from urinary protein loss and loss of functional nephrons.
   - Weight loss.
   - Ascites.
   - Peripheral, dependent or facial edema.
   - Pleural effusion.
   - Signs related to thromboembolism (e.g, acute dyspnea).

8. **How do I work up a dog with suspected nephrotic syndrome?**
   - Determine that the dog has significant urinary protein loss:
     - Abnormal urine protein:creatinine ratio
     - Rule out urinary tract infection. Proteinuria associated with an inflammatory urine sediment (e.g., cystitis, prostatitis) requires resolution of the infection and then rechecking for the presence of the proteinuria. Urine protein:creatinine ratios higher than 10 have been observed in dogs with staphylococcal infection of the lower urinary tract.
   - Investigate the animal as a whole.
   - Glomerulonephropathies are usually secondary to some other disease process in the animal.
   - The primary disease may or may not be identifiable.
   - Faced with the present lack of predictably effective therapy for the glomerular component of disease, the best hope of improving outcome is to discover a potentially treatable underlying disease.
   - A systematic search for disease outside of the urinary system should be conducted.
   - Survey thoracic and abdominal radiographs and abdominal ultrasound are appropriate to look for underlying disease.
   - Rule out chronic infestations, infections, or inflammation, such as the following:
     - Parasites: heartworms, leishmaniasis
     - Bacteria: infectious endocarditis, any chronic infection
     - Fungi: systemic mycoses
     - Viruses: feline leukemia virus, feline immunodeficiency virus
   - Rule out primary immune-mediated disorders (e.g., systemic lupus erythematosus). Check for indications of skin, blood, or joint disease that might have an immunologic mechanism.
   - Rule out disseminated malignancy, especially lymphoreticular neoplasms.

9. **What is the urine protein:creatinine (UP:C) ratio?**
   - To eliminate the effect of urine concentration and to quantify urinary protein loss, a UP:C ratio can be performed.
   - This test should be performed on a urine sample collected by cystocentesis to decrease the likelihood of contamination from the urethra or genitalia.

- A UP:C greater than 1 is considered abnormal and is suggestive of a protein-losing nephropathy, whereas a UP:C of 0.2 to 1 in dogs is considered questionable for protein-losing nephropathy.

10. What are some other causes of proteinuria?

- Physiologic causes of proteinuria can include exercise, seizures, fever, stress, heat or cold, and high activity levels.
- Pathologic nonurinary causes include Bence Jones proteins, hemoglobinuria, myoglobinuria, congestive heart failure, and genital tract inflammation.

11. What is microalbuminuria?

Microalbuminuria indicates abnormal renal handling of protein and usually results from altered glomerular permselectivity, but can also be due to impaired tubular handing of albumin that crosses the glomerular filtration barrier. Persistent microalbuminuria may occur in animals that have stable, subclinical chronic kidney disease or as an initial sign in animals that will eventually develop progressive chronic kidney disease. A urine test is available to detect microalbuminuria (E.R.D.–Screen Urine Test, Heska, Ft. Collins, CO). Persistence of microalbuminuria warrants investigation for evidence of glomerular disease.

12. What is amyloidosis?

- Amyloidosis is characterized by the extracellular deposition of fibrils of polymerized protein subunits, amyloid A protein, which have a characteristic conformation known as a beta-pleated sheet.
- On hematoxylin and eosin staining, amyloid deposits have a characteristic homogenous, eosinophilic appearance.
- With Congo Red staining and viewing under polarized light, amyloid deposits show a green birefringence. Electron microscopy may also be used to evaluate tissues with amyloid deposits.
- Deposits may be systemic or localized with deposits in the brain, lung, or urinary tract reported in dogs. Amyloid A protein has a predilection for kidney, spleen, and liver, with the liver being the most common site for deposits in the dog.
- Most dogs with renal amyloidosis are greater than 5 years of age at diagnosis.
- Familial amyloidosis has been reported in Beagles, Collies, English Foxhounds, and Shar-Peis.

13. When is a renal biopsy indicated?

- To provide a definitive diagnosis of glomerular disease.
- May not be needed if treatment of a potential underlying disease leads to resolution of the proteinuria.
- A biopsy is indicated with severe proteinuria to differentiate between glomerulonephritis and amyloidosis.
- Biopsy information may be useful to make clinical decisions regarding diagnosis, treatment, and prognosis.

14. How are renal biopsies performed?

- Renal biopsies may be collected using one of the following techniques: surgical biopsy, blind or ultrasound-guided percutaneous needle biopsies, or laparoscopy.
- Regardless of which technique is used, biopsies should be taken from the cortex, avoiding the renal hilus and medulla.
- Biopsies should be evaluated using routine light microscopy (hematoxylin and eosin staining for morphology and Congo Red staining to check for the presence of amyloid).

- Samples should always be collected in anticipation of performing routine histopathology, immunofluorescence, and electron microscopy.
- Assessment of coagulation is always performed before biopsy collection.

15. What are potential complications of renal biopsy? What are contraindications to performing a renal biopsy?

- Potential complications of renal biopsy include hemorrhage, hematuria, hydronephrosis, and renal ischemia or infarction. Microscopic hematuria is common for several days after a renal biopsy.
- Perioperative intravenous fluid therapy may decrease the risk of hydronephrosis developing as a result of clot formation in the renal pelvis.
- Contraindications to performing a renal biopsy include bleeding disorders, uncontrollable hypertension, a solitary kidney, renal abscess, pyonephrosis, hydronephrosis, moderate to severe uremia, and small end-stage kidneys.

16. How is glomerulonephritis treated?

- The most logical and possibly most effective form of therapy for GN is *identification and elimination* of the source of antigenic stimulation (e.g., infectious, inflammatory, or neoplastic disease).
- The diagnosis of certain forms of glomerulonephritis (e.g., membranous nephropathy) may indicate specific treatment. The clinician should refer to references for current recommendations. These treatments usually involve regime of immunosuppressive drugs including corticosteroids, other immunosuppressive drugs such as cyclophosphamide, chlorambucil, and cyclosporine.
- Reduction of proteinuria. Angiotensin-converting enzyme (ACE) inhibitors are thought to act by reducing efferent arteriolar pressures, thereby decreasing glomerular capillary hydrostatic pressure and proteinuria. ACE inhibitors can also affect the size of endothelial cell pores, improve lipoprotein metabolism, and have antiinflammatory actions. Use of enalapril in dogs with idiopathic GN has led to a significant reduction in UP:C over 6 months of treatment. Animals should be evaluated for azotemia before and 7 days after beginning treatment with an ACE inhibitor. Development or exacerbation of azotemia during treatment should warrant changing to an alternate ACE inhibitor or to reduce the dosage of enalapril. Benazeprilat, the active metabolite of benazepril, has increased biliary elimination as compared with enalaprilat, the active metabolite of enalapril, which is eliminated mainly by the kidneys.
- Antiplatelet drugs. Aspirin is recommended for dogs with GN because of the role of platelets in glomerular disease.
- Protein restriction is warranted in dogs with GN as is omega-3 fatty acid supplementation. Omega-3 fatty acids may affect thromboxane formation and also decrease proteinuria.
- Sodium-restricted diets are also recommended because of a high frequency of systemic hypertension in affected dogs.

17. What complications can occur with glomerular disease and the nephrotic syndrome?

- Severe protein loss can lead to sodium retention with edema or ascites, hypercholesterolemia, hypertension, hypercoagulability, muscle wasting, and weight loss. Edema or ascites can result due to activation of the renin-angiotensin-aldosterone system and water and salt retention.
- Hyperlipidemia and hypercholesterolemia are thought to occur because of increased hepatic synthesis and decreased protein catabolism. Abnormal lipoprotein lipase function and a decrease in its cofactor, heparan sulfate, can also lead to decreased lipoproteins.
- Hypercoagulability and thromboembolism can result from increased platelet adhesion and aggregation, platelet hyperaggregability with hypercholesterolemia, and loss of antithrom-

bin III in the urine. Altered fibrinolysis can also occur and increased concentrations of large molecular weight coagulation factors (II, V, VII, VIII, and X) can lead to a relative increase in coagulation factors. Thromboembolism may occur in the pulmonary arteries, the most common site, but also in mesenteric, renal, iliac, coronary, or brachial arteries, or the portal vein.

18. What is the prognosis for dogs with GN?
- Dogs with GN have a variable prognosis. Those dogs with azotemia or uremia at initial diagnosis may have shorter survival times. Animals with secondary GN have a better prognosis, assuming the causative disease can be adequately controlled or cured. Median survival times for dogs range from 5 to 1,170 days after initial diagnosis.
- Prognosis for dogs with amyloidosis is poor because of the progressive nature of the disease and resulting chronic renal failure.

BIBLIOGRAPHY

Grant DC, Forrester SD: Glomerulonephritis in dogs and cats: diagnosis and treatment, *Comp Cont Educ Pract Vet* 23:798-804, 2001.
Grant DC, Forrester SD: Glomerulonephritis in dogs and cats: glomerular function, pathophysiology, and clinical signs, *Comp Cont Educ Pract Vet* 23:739-746, 2001.
Grauer GF, DiBartola SP: Glomerular disease. In Ettinger SJ, Feldman EC, editors: *Textbook of veterinary internal medicine, vol 2*, ed 5, Philadelphia, 2000, WB Saunders.
Lees GE, Brown SA, Elliot J et al: Assessment and management of proteinuria in dogs and cats: 2004 ACVIM Forum Consensus Statement (small animal), *J Vet Intern Med* 19:377-385, 2005.

46. Urolithiasis

Mala Erickson and Stanley I. Rubin

1.   What are clinical signs of urolithiasis?
- Clinical signs that may be seen with urolithiasis include hematuria, dysuria, pollakiuria, and inappropriate urination.
- Animals with nephroliths may not show signs or may show lethargy, pyrexia, pain over the lumbar area, anorexia, or a stiff gait.
- Oliguria or anuria may be present with bilateral ureterolithiasis. Small uroliths may pass into the urethra during voiding causing urethral obstruction.

2.   Is crystalluria significant?
- Crystals can be present in urine of dogs and may not be clinically significant.
- Factors that can affect crystalluria include age, diet, urine pH and volume, length of time between voiding, temperature and specific gravity of urine, and concurrent disease.
- Struvite, amorphous phosphates, and oxalate crystals can be found in normal urine samples.
- Bilirubin crystals may be found in concentrated urine samples.
- Urate crystals are commonly seen in urine from Dalmatians and may be seen in animals with liver disease or portosystemic shunts.
- Although crystalluria may indicate a higher risk of developing calculi, it can occur with or without urolithiasis and crystal type does not necessarily indicate urolith type. Crystals can also form in urine when it cools, which should be differentiated from in vivo crystalluria.

3. How do uroliths form?

- Oversaturation of one or more substances eliminated in urine can result in their precipitation and growth. A crystal nidus forms to begin the initiation phase of urolith formation. As urine becomes supersaturated with calculogenic material, nucleation occurs.
- The degree of saturation is affected by the amount of crystalloids excreted by the kidneys, pH of the urine, urine concentration, and presence of substances in the urine that promote or inhibit crystallization. Other substances that can influence formation include the presence of proteinaceous matrix substances with Tamm-Horsfall mucoprotein, red blood cells, white blood cells, epithelial cells, and amorphous material.
- The duration and degree of urine supersaturation, the crystal nidus remaining in the urinary tract lumen, and physical characteristics of the nidus itself are also factors affecting growth of the urolith.
- Once formed, a crystal nidus may be voided or grow within the urinary tract.
- Growth of one crystal type on the surface of another type can also occur giving a urolith of mixed composition.

4. What are the main types of uroliths?

Struvite uroliths are composed mainly of magnesium ammonium phosphate with small amounts of matrix. Most struvite stones in dogs are infection-induced with urea-splitting bacteria such as *Staphylococcus* spp. being most commonly implicated. *Proteus* spp. and *Ureaplasma* are less commonly involved. The enzyme urease hydrolyzes urea in the presence of water to produce a high concentration of ammonia and carbonate ions. Ammonium ions result when ammonia combines with water or hydrogen ions, which leads to an elevated urinary pH, thereby reducing the solubility of magnesium ammonium phosphate and favoring struvite crystal precipitation. Struvite uroliths can form within 2 weeks of induction of a staphylococcal urinary tract infection in dogs. Foreign bodies may also act as a nidus for infection-induced struvite uroliths.

An alkaline urine, diet factors, and genetic predisposition have also been associated with formation of struvite uroliths.

Risk factors for the formation of calcium oxalate uroliths include altered balance between calculogenic minerals such as calcium and oxalate in the urine and inhibitors of crystallization such as citrate, phosphorus, magnesium, potassium, uric acid, Tamm-Horsfall mucoprotein, and nephrocalcin. Most dogs have a urine pH <6.5 at time of diagnosis, and infection does not seem to contribute to oxalate stone formation. Consumption of diets with reduced magnesium that promote formation of acidic urine has also been identified as a risk factor. Excess gastrointestinal calcium absorption as a cause of hypercalciuria and increased levels of oxalic acid from foods such as spinach, rhubarb, peanuts, chocolate, and tea has also been proposed as factors. Phosphorus has a role in minimizing renal production of calcitriol and enhancing excretion of pyrophosphate, an inhibitor of calcium oxalate salts so dietary phosphorus restriction is not desired. Use of urine acidifying medications and hypercalcemia has also been identified as risk factors for calcium oxalate urolith formation.

Ammonium urate uroliths are considered the third most common urolith. Urate calculi are usually small (<1 mm to 1 cm) and are more common in the bladder. These uroliths may contain a mixture of purines including uric acid, sodium urate, or ammonium urate. In dogs, abnormal conversion of uric acid to allantoin will lead to high concentrations of uric acid in serum and urine. Portovascular anomalies and renal tubular reabsorptive deficits have been identified as contributing factors. Urine that is highly acidic with a high urine-specific gravity associated with a diet high in purine precursors are risk factors for urate urolithiasis. Other risk factors include increased concentration of uric acid and increased renal excretion, renal production, urine retention, or production of ammonium by microbial urease.

Cystine uroliths are linked to a hereditary condition affecting renal tubular transport of cystine, a nonessential sulfur-containing amino acid. Cystine is normally freely filtered at the glomerulus and is 99% to 100% actively reabsorbed in the proximal tubule. Solubility of cystine is pH dependent; it is relatively insoluble in acidic urine and becomes more soluble in alkaline urine. Cystinuria and a previous history of cystine urolithiasis are considered predisposing factors. Female Great Danes and Bull Mastiffs have a relatively high occurrence of ammonium urate and cystine stones but a relative lack of struvite uroliths. Other breeds reported with cystine uroliths include Dachshunds, Basset Hounds, English Bulldogs, and Rottweilers with the age at diagnosis ranging from 2 to 7 years.

Calcium phosphate uroliths have been reported in various breeds, including the previously mentioned breeds at risk for calcium oxalate uroliths. They may contain hydroxyapatite and carbonate apatite or as minor components in struvite or calcium oxalate stones. No gender or age trends have been recognized.

Silica uroliths are quite uncommon but have been reported in the German Shepherd and Old English Sheepdog and have been linked to diets high in cereal grains containing silicates (corn gluten, soybean hulls).

Xanthine uroliths are reported after the administration of a xanthine oxidase inhibitor (e.g., allopurinol) for the management of urate uroliths. Xanthinuria has been reported in Cavalier King Charles Spaniels and in Dachshunds and is thought to be due to an inborn error of purine metabolism.

5. What imaging techniques may be used to visualize uroliths?
- Diagnostic imaging should be performed to determine the presence of uroliths in an animal with supportive clinical signs.
- The location, shape, number, and density of any uroliths present can be determined.
- Radiographic and ultrasonographic examinations can be performed to evaluate the animal. Although radiopacity of uroliths can be determined, this will not reliably identify the mineral composition of the stone.
- Contrast techniques can also be used to thoroughly evaluate the urethra for uroliths. Excretory urography involves taking abdominal radiographs after intravenous administration of an iodinated contrast agent. Radiographs are taken at intervals to evaluate renal shape, size, and location to evaluate filling defects in the renal pelvis or ureters. Excretory urography should not be performed in dehydrated animals because of the risk of adverse effects on renal function. Contrast techniques will also allow evaluation of the mucosal surface of the bladder.
- Struvite uroliths are radiopaque and can be visualized on survey radiographs (if they are large enough) as round or disk-shaped structures with a smooth or rough surface.
- Calcium oxalate uroliths are radiopaque although ultrasonography or an intravenous pyelogram may be helpful to visualize renal or urethral calculi.
- Urate and cystine calculi are usually radiolucent, so contrast techniques or ultrasonography may be needed to identify them.
- Retrospective studies have shown that most radiodense stones in dogs are infection-induced struvite uroliths with uroliths >10 mm in diameter being >92% likely to consist of struvite; uroliths >15 mm in any dimension are considered rare.

6. What diagnostics are indicated in an animal with clinical signs of urolithiasis?
- A complete blood cell count and serum chemistry panel should be completed to evaluate the dog for evidence of inflammation or other systemic disease.
- Leukocytosis may be evident in animals with pyelonephritis.
- Azotemia may be present in an animal with urethral obstruction, concurrent renal failure, or prerenal causes.
- Hypercalcemia may be present in some animals with calcium oxalate uroliths.
- A complete urinalysis should be performed and may show signs of inflammation such as hematuria, pyuria, and proteinuria.
- Urine pH can be variable but may be alkaline with a bacterial urinary tract infection.

- Magnesium ammonium phosphate and calcium phosphate uroliths are generally associated with alkaline urine.
- Ammonium urate, calcium oxalate, cystine, and sodium urate uroliths are associated with acidic urine.
- Urine culture should also be performed because urinary tract infections with urease-producing bacteria such as *Staphylococcus* spp. and *Proteus* spp. can cause the formation of struvite uroliths. Altered host defenses from the presence of uroliths can also lead to the development of urinary tract infections with *Escherichia coli* and *Streptococcus* spp.

7. **How common are the various types of uroliths and what breeds are commonly affected?**
   - Various retrospective studies have examined the frequency of the main types of uroliths based on submission for analysis.
   - Struvite uroliths are considered the most commonly analyzed in dogs followed by oxalate with infrequent reports of urate, cystine, and mixed content uroliths. Most struvite stones submitted were from female dogs, with an average age of 5.7 years. Although mixed-breed females were most commonly affected, purebreds with frequent submissions included the Shih Tzu, Bichon Frise, Miniature Schnauzer, Lhasa Apso, and Yorkshire Terrier. Breed associations have also been reported in Pekingese, Cocker Spaniels, Beagles, Pomeranians, and Maltese Terriers. In some dogs, dietary, metabolic, or familial factors rather than urinary tract infections are the cause. Miniature Schnauzers may have an inherited abnormality of local host defenses of the urinary tract leading to an increased susceptibility to urinary tract infections.
   - Calcium oxalate uroliths are considered the second most common type of urolith in dogs. Males are considered to be at an increased risk and the average age of affected individuals is greater (8 years) as compared with dogs with struvite uroliths. Purebred dogs with frequent submissions included the Miniature Schnauzer, Bichon Frise, Lhasa Apso, Shih Tzu, Miniature Poodle, and Yorkshire Terrier. Dalmatians, Labrador Retrievers, English Bulldogs, Cocker Spaniels, and Golden Retrievers have a low prevalence of calculi containing oxalate.
   - Urate uroliths were most commonly from male Dalmatians, although other affected breeds include the Shih Tzu, Miniature Schnauzer, English Bulldog, Yorkshire Terrier, and mixed breeds. The age for a dog with a urate urolith ranges from 3 to 6 years. Consumption of diets high in purines (e.g., liver, beef, sardines) is also considered a predisposing factor. Dalmatians are a high-risk breed with homozygosity for a recessive gene that results in defective urate metabolism. The proximal renal tubules of Dalmatians reabsorb less uric acid than those of other breeds. Despite this difference, only a small number of Dalmatians will develop urate stones and not all stones in Dalmatians are urate. Portovascular (portosystemic shunt) anomalies can predispose to development of urate uroliths.
   - Pure calcium phosphate stones are associated with metabolic disorders such as primary hyperparathyroidism, renal tubular acidosis, and excessive dietary calcium and phosphorus. No gender or age trends have been recognized.

8. **What are the treatment options for uroliths?**
   - Urolithiasis can be treated either medically or surgically depending on the mineral composition.
   - Uroliths within the urethra should be removed by antegrade hydropulsion or retrograde hydropulsion into the bladder. Urethrostomy or urethrotomy may be necessary to remove a urolith that is unable to be dislodged.

9. **How do I medically manage struvite urolithiasis?**
   - Struvite uroliths can be dissolved using a calculolytic diet, which are available from commercial sources.

- Dietary protein is reduced, when feeding a calculolytic diet, which will lead to reduced serum urea and albumin as well as promoting acidic urine. Phosphorus and magnesium are also restricted in dissolution diets.
- Dissolution diets are high in fat, so caution must be used in feeding these diets to dogs prone to obesity, pancreatitis, hyperlipidemia, or heart or kidney disease.
- Medical dissolution of uroliths is considered more difficult in dogs as compared with cats. Contributing factors identified include the high prevalence of infection-induced struvite uroliths, prevalence of fine concentric layers of a urolith with low porosity, and the occasional occurrence of calcium carbonate in struvite uroliths.
- Radiographs should be taken monthly to assess the number, size, and position of the uroliths. Sterile stones may take about 4 weeks to dissolve, whereas stones induced by infection may take more than 3 months to dissolve.
- Antimicrobial treatment should be instituted for dissolution of infection-induced uroliths and continued throughout and for 3 to 4 weeks after dissolution. Selection of antimicrobials should be based on urine culture and sensitivity testing. Urinalyses should be monitored during the dissolution period and serial cultures should be performed to gauge response to therapy.

10. What about management of oxalate stones?

- Calcium oxalate uroliths will not dissolve with medical management, so voiding urohydropulsion or surgery is necessary. Radiographs should be taken to ensure all uroliths have been removed after surgery and follow-up radiographs should be done every 3 to 4 months to detect recurrence, which is common.
- Dietary management through feeding a high-moisture diet with reduced levels of calcium and oxalate should be used to help reduce the risk of recurrence. Alkalinizing agents such as potassium citrate may also be used to promote formation of alkaline urine.

11. How do I manage urate stones?

- For medical management of urate uroliths, the aim is to provide a diet with reduced concentrations of uric acid, ammonium ion, and hydrogen ion. This will lead to a substantial reduction in urinary uric acid and ammonia excretion.
- Allopurinol, a synthetic isomer of hypoxanthine, rapidly binds to and inhibits the action of xanthine oxidase, thereby decreasing the production of uric acid.
- Urine alkalinization can also be achieved through use of sodium bicarbonate or potassium citrate with the goal to maintain a urine pH of about 7.0.

12. How do I manage cystine stones?

- Medical management for cystine uroliths aims to reduce the rate of recurrence through reduction of dietary protein, alkalinization of urine, and use of thiol-containing drugs (e.g., mercaptopurine) to reduce the urine concentration of cystine and increase its solubility.
- Cystine uroliths take between 2 and 4 months to dissolve with medical management.

13. What about other types of uroliths?

- Calcium phosphate stones should be removed surgically because they are not considered responsive to medical dissolution.
- Silica uroliths are not responsive to dissolution, and management involves diet change and enhancing water consumption.

14. What is retrograde urohydropulsion?

- Retrograde urohydropulsion is a technique that can be used to move ureteroliths into the urinary bladder for removal by cystotomy or institution of medical management.
- Radiography should be performed to confirm the presence as well as location, size, and number of uroliths present.

- Animals will usually require sedation or general anesthesia.
- Decompressive cystocentesis before the procedure may be necessary to avoid overdistension of the bladder. A urethral catheter is introduced into the urethra using a flexible catheter; a 1:1 ratio mixture of sterile saline mixed with aqueous lubricant is introduced into the urethral lumen.
- The pelvic urethra is occluded rectally by an assistant and the penile urethra is occluded by digital pressure. This forms a "closed system" from the external urethral orifice to the bony pelvis.
- As the saline solution is injected, there will be an increase in the diameter of the pelvic urethra and the increase in pressure allows ureteroliths to be flushed into the urinary bladder. Digital pressure on the pelvic urethra may aid passage.
- Repeated attempts may be necessary to dislodge uroliths.
- In female dogs, the lumen of the distal end of the urethra is occluded by vaginal palpation to create a closed system. A Foley or Swan-Ganz catheter may be used in females to minimize reflux of saline solution through the external urethral orifice.

15. What is voiding urohydropulsion and how is it performed?

- Voiding urohydropulsion may be another option for removal, depending on the size, shape, and contour of a urocystolith.
- Smooth uroliths tend to pass more easily and stones less than 5 mm in diameter can usually be removed in dogs weighing more than 18 pounds.
- Sedation or anesthesia may be necessary depending on the size of the urethra, larger uroliths can be voided from female dogs than from males of similar size.
- The bladder is distended with sterile saline after passage of a urinary catheter. The catheter is removed and the dog is positioned with the vertebral column approximately vertical. The bladder can be gently agitated to allow gravity to encourage movement of stones into the neck of the bladder. Steady pressure is then applied to the bladder and, after voiding begins, continued pressure is applied.
- The technique uses the dilation of the urethra during the voiding phase of micturition, to help expulsion of urocystoliths through the urethra.

16. What signs might an animal with nephroliths or ureteroliths show? What are treatment options?

- The true incidence of nephroliths is not known because affected animals may be asymptomatic. They are located in the renal pelvis or collecting diverticula.
- Nephroliths may lead to obstruction, pyelonephritis, or injury to the renal parenchyma leading to renal failure.
- Ureteroliths in one or both ureters may cause infection.
- Although animals with nephroliths may be asymptomatic, clinical signs may include hematuria, recurrent urinary tract infections, vomiting, lumbar pain, or uremia.
- Treatment options include surgery, monitoring, and medical dissolution.
- Because nephrotomy can damage tissue and reduce glomerular filtration rate, surgery should only be considered for nephroliths causing clinical signs and complications.
- Nephroliths should be removed if there is evidence of obstruction, recurrent infection, calculi causing clinical signs, progressive nephrolith enlargement, or reduction in renal function.
- Ureteroliths should be surgically removed if there is only one functional kidney or if there is evidence of obstruction such as azotemia, hydronephrosis, or hydroureter.

17. How are uroliths analyzed?

- Uroliths that are voided or removed surgically should be submitted for mineral analysis.
- Physical methods of analysis allow determination of the composition of each layer of the urolith to guide management decisions.

18. **Discuss the relationship between urinary tract infections and development of struvite urolithiasis.**
   - Most struvite uroliths in dogs are induced by infection within the urinary tract.
   - Female dogs are considered to be at greater risk because of the shorter and wider anatomy of the urethra as compared to males. This may allow bacteria to ascend. *Staphylococcus* spp., *Proteus* spp., and *Ureaplasma*, which are urea-splitting bacteria, are often implicated in infections.
   - Urease, in the presence of water, acts to hydrolyze urea to produce ammonia and carbonate. Ammonia then combines with water or a hydrogen ion to form ammonium, which will lead to an elevated (alkaline) urinary pH, thereby reducing the solubility of magnesium ammonium phosphate and favoring the precipitation of struvite crystals.
   - Struvite uroliths can develop in dogs within 2 weeks of experimental induction of a staphylococcal urinary tract infection developing.
   - Uroliths can also cause urinary tract infections by causing trauma to the mucosal lining of the bladder, incomplete urine voiding, and sequestration of microorganisms.
   - Infections with urease-producing bacteria can allow struvite layers to develop over other types of uroliths.

19. **What is lithotripsy and when can it be used?**
   - Lithotripsy involves generation of shock waves that can be transmitted to an animal. The generated waves travel through fluid and soft-tissue structures to reach the surface of a urolith. The energy creates tensile stresses along the surface of the urolith causing cracks and fragmentation with repeated shock waves.
   - Electrohydraulic shock-wave lithotripsy involves transmission of shock waves through a water bath in which the dog is partially submerged.
   - Newer methods are "dry," involving use of a fluid-filled cushion to couple shock waves to the dog. Dry units have a smaller focal zone with a lower peak pressure and may be less effective than the water bath models. The latest models allow movable shock-wave sources to reach uroliths in difficult locations.
   - Extracorporeal shock-wave lithotripsy can be used for treatment of nephroliths or uroliths in some cases. Stones are fragmented by shock waves that are generated outside the body. The dose and frequency of shock waves determine the degree of damage than may be caused through intrarenal hemorrhage.
   - Evaluation of candidates for lithotripsy would include a minimum database, urine culture, coagulation profile, blood pressure measurement, abdominal radiographs and ultrasound, renal scintigraphy, and possibly computed tomography.
   - Procedures are performed under general anesthesia to provide control and analgesia during the procedure. Fluoroscopy and ultrasound are used to localize the stone before treatment. Treatment time takes about 1 hour, depending on the number of sites treated.
   - The strength of shock waves needed and the percentage of cases with nephroliths requiring retreatment vary with the lithotriptor used and the institution.
   - Complications of lithotripsy for nephroliths can include renal swelling, renal or perirenal hemorrhage, vasoconstriction, tubular damage, intrarenal scarring, and renal failure. Damage is dependent on the dose used with the dry lithotriptors requiring higher shock wave doses. Nephrolith fragments may become displaced into the ureters or renal calices on post-treatment imaging.
   - Extrarenal complications can include pain, bowel damage and diarrhea, increased amylase and lipase, and increases in liver enzymes.

20. **What systemic diseases/conditions have an association with urolithiasis?**
   - Hyperadrenocorticism has been identified as a risk factor. Dogs with urolithiasis and hyperadrenocorticism are more likely to have calcium-containing uroliths with a decrease in

renal tubular calcium reabsorption suggested as the mechanism.

- Conditions that predispose to development of urinary tract infections such as anatomic abnormalities, hyperadrenocorticism, and diabetes mellitus may predispose to development of struvite uroliths.

BIBLIOGRAPHY

DiBartola SP: Clinical approach and laboratory evaluation of renal disease. In Ettinger SJ, Feldman EC, editors: *Textbook of veterinary internal medicine, vol 2*, ed 5, Philadelphia, 2000, WB Saunders.

Houston DM, Moore AE, Favrin MG et al: Canine urolithiasis: a look at over 16,000 urolith submissions to the Canadian Veterinary Urolith Centre from February 1998 to April 2003, *Can Vet J* 45:225-230, 2004.

Lane IF: Lithotripsy: an update on urologic applications in small animals, *Vet Clin North Am (Small Animal Pract)* 34:1011-1025, 2004.

Lulich JP, Osborne CA, Bartges JW et al: Canine lower urinary tract disorders. In Ettinger SJ, Feldman EC, editors: *Textbook of veterinary internal medicine, vol 2*, ed 5, Philadelphia, 2000, WB Saunders.

Lulich JP, Osborne CA, Sanderson SL et al: Voiding urohydropulsion—lessons from 5 years of experience, *Vet Clin North Am (Small Animal Pract)* 29:283-291, 1999.

Osborne CA, Lulich JP, Polzin DJ: Canine retrograde urohydropulsion—lessons from 25 years of experience, *Vet Clin North Am (Small Animal Pract)* 29:267-280, 1999.

Seaman R, Bartges JW: Canine struvite urolithiasis, *Compend Contin Educ Pract Vet* 23:407-420, 2001.

47. Urinary Incontinence

Stanley I. Rubin and Mala Erickson

1. **What is urinary incontinence?**
   - Urinary incontinence is defined as involuntary loss of urine from the urinary system. It must be differentiated from inappropriate micturition, which is conscious voiding of urine at inappropriate times or inappropriate locations.
   - **Urge incontinence** results from lower urinary tract irritation, which produces an uncontrollable desire to urinate.
   - **Paradoxical incontinence** is induced by bladder or urethral obstruction (stone or tumor), which allows some urine to leak around the blockage because of pressure within the bladder.
   - **Overflow incontinence** occurs when the bladder cannot contract, but will fill until urine flows passively from the urethra (e.g., lower motor neuron diseases).
   - **Reflex incontinence** is usually caused by an upper motor neuron lesion and results in the bladder filling and emptying normally, but the animal can no longer actively control the process.

2. **What are the major causes of urinary incontinence?**
   - **Congenital.** The most common congenital disorders causing incontinence include ectopic ureter(s), and related anatomic anomalies (patent urachus, pseudohermaphrodites, and urethrorectal fistulae). Congenital malformations of the sacral spinal cord can also cause neurologic dysfunction resulting in a flaccid, overdistended bladder with weak outflow resistance.
   - **Acquired**
     Neurologic. Any disruptions in neurologic pathways from the local neuroreceptors, peripheral nerves, spinal pathways, or higher centers involved in the control of micturition can

disrupt urine storage. Sacral spinal cord lesions including malformation, cauda equine compression, lumbosacral disk disease, or traumatic fractures or dislocation can result in a flaccid, overdistended urinary bladder with weak outflow resistance. Lesions in higher centers including the cerebellum or cerebral micturition center affect inhibition and voluntary control of voiding, usually resulting in urine leakage or frequent, involuntary urination.

Bladder dysfunction. Urinary bladder hypocontractility or poor accommodation of urine during storage may lead to frequent leakage of small volumes of urine. Dysfunction may be caused by urinary tract infection, chronic inflammatory disorders, neoplastic lesions, external compression, and chronic partial outlet obstruction. Congenital urinary bladder hypoplasia may be an adjunct to ectopic ureters or other developmental disorders of the urinary tract.

Urethral disorders. Incompetence of the urethral sphincter mechanism (urethral smooth/ striated muscle, connective tissue) may result from nonneurogenic diseases (bladder, urethra, prostate gland) or neurogenic causes. Urethral incompetence usually results in intermittent urinary incontinence, usually at rest. Urethral disorders may be caused by congenital urethral hypoplasia or incompetence, acquired urethral incompetence (e.g., hormone responsive incontinence), urinary tract infection or inflammation, prostatic disease/surgery, and vestibulovaginal anomaly.

3. What are some of the risk factors for urinary incontinence?

- Spaying/castration increase the risk of development of urethral incompetence. Urethral incompetence may occur months to years after ovariohysterectomy.
- Other characteristics such as bladder neck position, urethral length, and concurrent vaginal anomalies may increase the risk of incontinence in female dogs.
- Disorders causing polyuria may precipitate or exacerbate urinary incontinence.

4. What is a pelvic bladder?

- Dogs whose bladders are located in a more caudal abdominal location in which the bladder neck is caudal to the pectin of the pubic bone can also have urethral sphincter incompetence that results in urinary incontinence.

5. What are the most common clinical signs in dogs with urethral incompetence?

- The most common signs include accumulation of a pool of urine when the animal is recumbent. Involuntary dribbling of urine can occur, but is less commonly observed. Physical examination may reveal accumulation of urine in areas adjacent to the external urethral sphincter (e.g., vestibule). These animals typically void in a normal manner and have a normal postvoiding urine volume in the bladder.

6. What is the most logical approach to evaluation of dogs with urinary incontinence?

- Rule out paradoxical urinary incontinence. Animals with urethral obstruction will sometimes exhibit urinary incontinence because of urine that leaks around the obstruction. Diagnosis would be based on finding urinary retention and direct evidence of the obstruction (e.g., urolith).
- Rule out neurologic disease or dysfunction. A complete neurologic examination should be performed. Animals with spinal cord lesions sufficient to produce upper motor neuron abnormalities of micturition usually have upper motor neuron deficits in their pelvic limbs, too. Animals with sacral cord segment lesions sufficient to cause lower motor neuron (LMN) abnormalities of micturition usually have LMN deficits in the pelvic limbs and perineal area. Animals with peripheral nerve damage sufficient to cause LMN abnormalities of micturition usually have LMN deficits in the perineal area (decreased anal sphincter tone).

- Rule out ectopic ureters or other anatomic abnormalities that allow urine to bypass normal sphincters. Signalment and history are generally strongly suggestive. **Excretory urography** is used to visualize the kidneys and identify the course and termination of the ureters and the urinary bladder. **Retrograde vaginourethrography** will allow visualization of the vaginal vault, urethra, and urinary bladder. Ectopic ureters may fill with contrast media during these retrograde contrast studies. **Double-contrast cystography** may be indicated for full visualization of the urinary bladder and identification of urinary bladder lesions. **Ultrasonographic examination** may be useful in evaluation of the kidneys and urinary bladder to identify masses, hydronepephrosis/hydroureter, and evidence of pyelonephritis or uroliths.
- Urodynamic procedures such as urethral pressure profiles, cystometrography, and electromyography may be considered to assess bladder, urethral, and neurologic function in more depth.
- Urinalysis may reveal evidence of urinary tract infection (bacteriuria, inflammatory urine sediment) or be supportive of a polyuric disorder (low urine-specific gravity).
- Serum biochemistry and hematology may be indicated in dogs with polyuric disorders.
- Assess pharmacologic response to hormones and alpha-adrenergic agonists to rule in a diagnosis of urethral incompetence.

7. **What is the treatment for urinary incontinence?**
- Treat specific disorders directly. Obstructive disorders should be managed as quickly as possible. Primary neurologic disorders may require surgical treatment. Urinary tract infection should be treated with appropriate medical therapy. Ectopic ureters and other congenital anomalies can be surgically corrected; the clinician should be aware that functional abnormalities of urinary bladder storage or urethral competence may accompany this defect. Surgical procedures such as colposuspension, cystourethropexy, and collagen implants have been used in the treatment of incontinence unresponsive to medical therapy.

8. **What drugs are used for the management of urethral incompetence?**
- **Hormones.** Estrogens, usually in the form of diethylstilbestrol, are administered to spayed females. Diethylstilbestrol is usually administered at a dose of 0.1 to 1.0 mg/dog once daily for 5 to 7 days and then once weekly or less as needed to maintain continence. The maximum maintenance dose should not exceed 0.2 mg/kg/wk. Side effects can occur with estrogen administration including increased risk of pyometra and estrogen-sensitive tumors. Bone marrow depression and anemia have occurred with administration of high doses of estrogens to animals; however, these doses are far in excess of what is reported for therapy of incontinence. It is recommended that a complete blood cell count be performed at periodic intervals to monitor for signs of bone marrow toxicity. Testosterone cypionate may be administered at a dosage of 2.2 mg/kg intramuscularly once monthly to male dogs with urethral incompetence. Adverse effects of testosterone administration include prostatic hyperplasia, behavioral changes such as aggression or libido, and may contribute to the development of perineal hernia or perianal adenoma.
- **Alpha-adrenergic agents.** Alpha-adrenergic agonists may be administered for the management of urethral incompetence, alone or in combination with reproductive hormones, where a synergistic effect is sometimes observed. These drugs all have the potential to cause restlessness, tachycardia and hypertension. Ephedrine is administered at a dose of 4 mg/kg every 8 to 12 hours. Many large breed dogs may be started on 25 mg every 8 hours, increasing the dose to 50 mg if there is no clinical response at the lower dose. Phenylpropanolamine has the same potency and pharmacologic properties as ephedrine but seems to cause less central nervous system stimulation. The recommended dose is 1.5 to 2.0 mg/kg twice daily to three times daily. Pseudoephedrine is similar to ephedrine and phenylpropanolamine. The recommended dose is 0.2 to 0.4 mg/kg every 8 to 12 hours or 15 to 60 mg/dog.

- **Other drugs.** Imipramine, a tricyclic antidepressant with anticholinergic and alpha-agonist actions has been used with some success for some dogs with urinary incontinence. The recommended dose is 2 to 4 mg/kg every 12 to 24 hours.

BIBLIOGRAPHY

Adams WM, DiBartola SP: Radiographic and clinical features of pelvic bladder in the dog, *J Am Vet Med Assoc* 182:1212, 1983.

Arnold S, Hubler M, Lott-Stolz G et al: Treatment of urinary incontinence in bitches by endoscopic injection of glutaraldehyde cross-linked collagen, *J Small Anim Pract* 37:163-168, 1996.

Holt PE: Long-term evaluation of colposuspension in the treatment of urinary incontinence due to incompetence of the urethral sphincter mechanism in the bitch, *Vet Rec* 127:537-542, 1990.

Lane IF: Use of anticholinergic agents in lower urinary tract disease, In Bonagura JD, editor: *Kirk's current veterinary therapy*, Philadelphia, 2000, WB Saunders.

Mandigers PJJ, Nell T: Treatment of bitches with acquired urinary incontinence with oestriol, *Vet Rec* 149:765-767, 2001.

Nendick PA, Clark WT: Medical therapy of urinary incontinence in ovariectomised bitches: a comparison of the effectiveness of diethylstilboestrol and pseudoephedrine, *Aust Vet J* 64:117-118, 1987.

Rawlings CA: Colposuspension as a treatment for urinary incontinence in spayed dogs, *J Am Anim Hosp Assoc* 38:107-110, 2002.

Richter KP, Ling GV: Clinical response and urethral pressure profile changes after phenylpropanolamine in dogs with primary sphincter incompetence, *J Am Vet Med Assoc* 187:605-611, 1985.

Scott L, Leddy M, Bernay F: Evaluation of phenylpropanolamine in the treatment of urethral sphincter mechanism incompetence in the bitch, *J Small Anim Pract* 43:493-496, 2002.

White RN: Urethropexy for the management of urethral sphincter mechanism incompetence in the bitch, *J Small Anim Pract* 42:481-486, 2001.

48. Urinary Tract Neoplasia

Stanley I. Rubin and Mala Erickson

1. How common are renal tumors in the dog?
- Primary renal tumors are uncommon and account for less than 2% of all canine cancers.
- Metastatic renal tumors are more common.

2. What are the most common renal tumors in the dog?
- Most renal tumors are malignant
- Carcinoma or adenocarcinoma are most common
- Renal fibrosarcomas, hemangiosarcomas, and undifferentiated sarcomas are also reported
- Bilateral and multiple renal cystadenocarcinomas have been associated with a syndrome of generalized nodular dermatofibrosis described primarily in German Shepherds
- Nephroblastomas may occur in young, middle-age, or older animals
- Metastatic neoplasms

3. What signs are present with renal tumors?
- Usually nonspecific
- Includes weight loss, anorexia, lethargy
- Less commonly abdominal distention, lameness, and pain
- Unilaterally or bilaterally enlarged kidneys
- Hypertrophic osteopathy, a palpable thickening, and warmth in distal long bones may be found

- Pulmonary metastases
- Anemia or polycythemia may be secondary to decreased or increased erythropoietin production
- Neutrophilic leukocytosis may be associated with renal adenocarcinoma

4. **What tests should I perform to make a diagnosis of a renal tumor?**
   - Biopsy will give definitive diagnosis
   - Ultrasound may be useful in identifying renal tumors and guide biopsy

5. **What is the prognosis for renal tumors?**
   - Poor if metastatic disease present
   - Pulmonary metastases detected in 13 of 38 dogs with primary renal tumors

6. **What is the treatment for renal tumors in the dog?**
   - Nephrectomy in dogs with unilateral tumors that have not metastasized

7. **How common are bladder tumors in the dog?**
   - Bladder cancer is uncommon and accounts for less than 2% of all canine malignancies

8. **What is the most common bladder tumor?**
   - Transitional cell carcinoma is the most common primary tumor
   - Other primary tumors include squamous cell carcinoma, leiomyosarcoma, leiomyoma, and rhabdomyosarcoma
   - Bladder may also be invaded by metastatic disease or prostatic neoplasia

9. **What is the cause of bladder tumors?**
   - Likely multifactorial
   - Risk factors include exposure to topical insecticides for flea and tick control, exposure to marshes sprayed for mosquito control, cyclophosphamide administration, female gender, and breed

10. **Are there breeds of dogs reported to be at a higher risk for bladder tumors?**
    - West Highland White and Scottish Terriers
    - Beagles
    - Dachshunds
    - Shetland Sheepdogs

11. **What is the biologic behavior of bladder tumors?**
    - Transitional cell carcinomas are locally invasive, often invading the urethra and other neighboring organs, including prostate, uterus, vagina, and pelvic canal. Metastasis to regional lymph nodes and lung has been described to be present in 16% and 14% of dogs, respectively, at time of diagnosis.

12. **What clinical signs are commonly associated with bladder tumors?**
    - Chronic signs of hematuria, dysuria, pollakiuria
    - Lameness from bone metastasis or hypertrophic osteopathy
    - Signs may have partially or temporarily resolved with antibiotic therapy
    - Physical examination results reported to be normal in 30% of dogs with bladder tumors

13. **How do I make a diagnosis of a bladder tumor?**
    - Neoplastic cells may be found in urine sediment in 30% of dogs
    - Contrast cystography
    - Ultrasound

- Tissue for histopathologic confirmation may be obtained by cystotomy, cystoscopy, or traumatic urethral catheterization

14. What are the treatment options for bladder tumors?
- Surgical excision is usually not possible because of typical trigonal location and urethral involvement of most cases of transitional cell carcinoma
- Medical management is indicated for animals with nonresectable or metastatic tumors

15. What chemotherapeutic options are available for transitional cell carcinoma?
- Cisplatin has been shown to be effective in inducing partial remission or stable disease
- Piroxicam, 0.3 mg/kg/day, has been shown to have antitumor activity in dogs

BIBLIOGRAPHY

Chun R, Knapp DW, Widmer W et al: Cisplatin treatment of transitional cell carcinoma of the urinary bladder in dogs: 18 cases (1983-1993), *J Am Vet Med Assoc* 209:1588, 1996.

Klein MK, Cockerall GL, Withrow SJ et al: Canine primary renal neoplasms: a retrospective review of 54 cases, *J Am Anim Hosp Assoc* 24:443-452, 1988.

Knapp DW: Tumors of the urinary system. In Withrow SJ, MacEwan ED, editors: *Small animal clinical oncology*, Philadelphia, 2001, WB Saunders.

Knapp DW, Richardson RC, Chan TCK et al: Piroxicam therapy in 34 dogs with transitional cell carcinoma of the urinary bladder, *J Vet Intern Med* 8:273, 1994.

Mutsaers AJ, Widmer WR, Knapp DW: Canine transitional cell carcinoma, *J Vet Intern Med* 17:136-144, 2003.

Norris AM, Laing EJ, Valli VEO et al: Canine bladder and urethral tumors: a retrospective study of 115 cases (1980-1985), *J Vet Intern Med* 6:145, 1992.

49. Urinary Tract Infection
Mala Erickson and Stanley I. Rubin

1. How are urinary tract infections (UTIs) localized?
- Upper urinary tract – kidneys and ureters
- Lower urinary tract – bladder, urethra, prostate, vagina

2. What signs will a dog with a UTI show?
- Animals with a UTI may or may not have clinical signs.
- Animals with a lower UTI may show pollakiuria, hematuria, stranguria, dysuria, or inappropriate urination.
- Animals with predisposing conditions such as hyperadrenocorticism or diabetes mellitus may show signs related to the underlying disease.

3. What clinical signs are associated with pyelonephritis?
- May be asymptomatic, depending on whether the condition is acute or chronic, unilateral or bilateral.
- History may reveal signs of polyuria, polydipsia, and renal failure.
- Animals with acute pyelonephritis may exhibit systemic signs of illness including fever, lethargy, and depression.

4. **How common are urinary tract infections?**
   - It has been estimated that 10% to 14% of all dogs will have a bacterial UTI in their lifetime.
   - Fungal UTIs are considered uncommon.
   - Incidence of viral UTIs in small animals is unknown.

5. **What factors can affect urinalysis results?**
   - Urine should be collected and pH should be measured and sediment should be examined within 15 to 60 minutes of collection. Both struvite and oxalate crystals can form in vitro if urine is refrigerated or sits for prolonged periods.
   - In vitro factors such as temperature, time, evaporation, urine pH, and growth of microbial contaminants that produce urease can all influence the formation of crystals in urine samples.
   - Samples should be refrigerated after sample collection if evaluation is delayed. Refrigeration will preserve many of the physical and chemical properties of urine as well as the morphology of urine sediment while minimizing in vitro growth of microbes. Refrigeration may allow increased formation of magnesium ammonium phosphate and calcium oxalate crystals with storage time.
   - Crystals found in stored samples should be confirmed with a fresh urine sample. Storage of urine does not affect pH or specific gravity.

6. **What organisms are typically involved in urinary tract infections?**
   The most common bacterial isolates in UTIs in dogs is *Escherichia coli*, followed by *Staphylococcus* spp., *Proteus* spp., *Klebsiella* spp., *Enterococcus* spp., *Streptococcus* spp., *Pseudomonas* spp., *Mycoplasma*, and *Enterobacter* spp.

7. **What antibiotics are commonly used for treating bacterial infections?**
   - Antibiotic therapy should provide activity at the site of infection and should exceed the amount needed to inhibit the growth of the bacteria involved or kill the bacteria.
   - Antibiotics chosen should reach urinary concentrations that exceed the minimal inhibitory concentration (MIC) of the isolated bacteria by at least fourfold, be easy to administer to ensure client compliance, have few side effects, have a low risk of toxicity, and be relatively inexpensive.
   - Ideally, antibiotic selection should be based on culture and sensitivity testing from urine culture.
   - If sensitivity test results are not available, predictions can be made based on the expected sensitivities of a particular organism. Many urinary tract pathogens have predictable susceptibilities to one or more antibiotics.
   - *Staphylococcus* spp., *Streptococcus* spp., *Enterococcus* spp., and *Proteus mirabilis* are usually susceptible to penicillins (ampicillin, amoxicillin).
   - *E. coli*, *Klebsiella*, and *Enterobacter* are capable of changing their susceptibility patterns within a single bacterial generation, so susceptibility testing should ideally be performed, although a cephalosporin such as cephalexin or a fluoroquinolone is likely to be effective.
   - Antibiotics should be continued for 2 weeks but the length of therapy can be based on follow-up culture results.

8. **What underlying diseases or conditions may predispose to development of UTIs?**
   - Animals with an underlying disease such as diabetes mellitus or hyperadrenocorticism or those receiving corticosteroids or antineoplastic drugs are more susceptible to UTIs.
   - UTIs have been associated with urinary catheterization, which allows introduction of bacteria into the bladder or migration along the catheter surface when remaining indwelling. These bacteria may lead to ascending infection, bacteremia, or sepsis. Incidences between 10.3% and 55% have been reported from hospitalized dogs developing catheter-associated UTIs,

with catheters being in place between 2 and 12 days. The sex of the dog was not a factor, and the bacterial isolates showed minimal antimicrobial resistance. Shorter duration of catheterization may result in a decreased risk of UTI.
- Spinal cord disease leading to paraparesis or tetraparesis may lead to an increased risk.

9. **What laboratory abnormalities can be seen in an animal with a UTI?**
   - Animals with a lower UTI usually do not show changes on a complete blood count and serum biochemistry panel results. Changes may be seen if an underlying disease is also present.
   - A complete urinalysis should be performed on any animal showing signs of lower urinary tract disease. Collection of urine by cystocentesis is preferable to avoid contamination of the sample by the external genitalia. Samples may show altered urine specific gravity, hematuria, and proteinuria. The test pads for white blood cells (WBCs) on commercial urine dipsticks are not considered reliable in small animals. Urine sediment should be examined for WBCs, red blood cells (RBCs), and microbes.
   - Organisms may not be easily identified in dilute urine or there may not be evidence of inflammation if host defenses are compromised by concurrent disease. If there are more than 10,000 rod-shaped bacteria per milliliter of urine, they may be visualized in an unstained urine sediment preparation, whereas there would have to be more than 100,000 cocci bacteria per milliliter to be visualized. Although Gram staining or methylene blue staining may help in diagnosis, urine culture should be performed to confirm a UTI.
   - An animal with pyelonephritis may exhibit leukocytosis and biochemical changes compatible with renal failure if function is compromised.

10. **How is a urine culture performed?**
    - Samples should be obtained before beginning antimicrobial therapy.
    - Therapy should be discontinued for 3 to 5 days before culture being performed if an animal is currently receiving antimicrobials.
    - Urine for culture should ideally be collected by cystocentesis. This will allow differentiation of contaminants from pathogens. If this is not possible, catheterization can be performed with attention to cleaning the external genitalia to prevent contamination.
    - Specimens should be transported in sealed, sterile containers with processing to be completed as soon as possible.
    - Qualitative urine cultures will allow isolation and identification of bacteria.
    - False-positive results may occur if a loop of intestine is inadvertently entered during cystocentesis; this should be suspected if more than one bacterial organism is isolated.
    - Quantification allows the number of bacteria (colony-forming units per unit volume) to be determined and determines their significance. Antimicrobial susceptibility testing to direct treatment decisions should also be done. The agar disk diffusion method or antimicrobial dilution susceptibility test can be used.
    - Urine culture may also be evaluated during the course of antimicrobial treatment to gauge the response to therapy. These may be warranted in dogs with prostatitis, pyelonephritis, immunosuppression, or urinary tract obstruction to verify that the antimicrobial is effective. This may also be considered when using antimicrobials with a high risk of toxicity. Therapeutic cultures may also help to detect early evidence of bacterial resistance. Urine should be sterile if treatment is appropriate.
    - Urine culture may also be obtained 3 to 5 days before discontinuation of therapy and may dictate whether continued treatment is warranted for complicated infections.

11. **What imaging techniques may be warranted in a dog suspected of having a UTI?**
    - Dogs with a UTI may have no abnormal findings when imaging is performed.
    - Abdominal radiographs may be indicated to look for evidence of uroliths, renomegaly, small kidneys, or anatomic defects.

- Pelvic displacement of the urinary bladder ("pelvic bladder") can lead to urinary incontinence and UTI.
- Ultrasonography or contrast studies may also be indicated.
- Endoscopy (cystourethroscopy) may be indicated in some dogs.

12. What are the best imaging techniques to diagnose pyelonephritis?
- Survey abdominal radiographs may reveal uroliths, renomegaly, or small kidneys.
- Excretory urography and ultrasound may reveal dilated renal pelves, dilated pelvic diverticula, dilated ureters, and evidence of outflow obstruction.
- Nuclear imaging studies may be useful but are only available at referral centers.

13. What are some consequences of UTIs?
- UTIs may occur as single episodes or as recurrent or persistent infections.
- Struvite urolithiasis can occur as a consequence of infections with *Staphylococcus intermedius*.
- UTIs can involve the prostate gland in male dogs.
- Pyelonephritis can cause progressive renal injury and renal failure.

14. What are some potential causes for failure of a UTI to respond to antimicrobial therapy?
- Any underlying diseases or defects can interfere with treatment response and should be investigated.
- Therapeutic failure from lack of direct contact between drug and bacteria due to failure of absorption of the drug may be a factor. Bacteria may be walled off within an abscess or within a urolith and thus cannot be reached by the antimicrobial.
- Pyelonephritis with renal scarring, patent urachus, urinary neoplasms, and prostatic involvement may affect response to treatment.
- Concurrent disease, particularly those that result in polyuria, may decrease the antimicrobial concentration in urine.
- If lower urinary tract signs persist despite a negative culture result, further evaluation to assess the urinary tract should be completed to look for nonbacterial causes of a UTI. If the same bacteria are isolated and show in vitro susceptibility to the antimicrobial being used, appropriate administration should be confirmed. Client compliance should be assessed initially to ensure that antimicrobials are being administered correctly. Isolation of a bacterial species that is not susceptible to the current antimicrobial should warrant the suspicion of antimicrobial resistance developing. Acquired resistance of bacteria such as *E. coli*, *Klebsiella* spp., and *Enterobacter* spp. can develop.
- Enrofloxacin use has increased recently and this increased use may select for enrofloxacin-resistant bacteria in urine. Bacteria showing enrofloxacin-resistance may also show resistance to other antibiotics that are commonly used to treat UTIs.
- Culture results showing isolation of a different bacterial species may indicate that treatment of the initial pathogen was effective but predisposed the dog to a superinfection (infection with a resistant pathogen). This may occur if indwelling urinary catheters are used or if there are abnormalities in host defenses.
- After discontinuation of therapy, bacterial relapse or reinfection may occur.
- Relapses refer to recurrences with the same species and strain of bacteria, usually within several weeks of therapy completion. This indicates that the infection was not completely eradicated. Relapses may also indicate poor compliance or poor penetration of drugs to the area. Longer treatment periods should be considered as well as monitoring through reculture of urine.
- Reinfections imply recurrent infections with different pathogens than those initially isolated. Low-dose, chronic antimicrobial therapy may be warranted in cases in which predisposing causes cannot be eliminated, once the pathogen has been eradicated.

BIBLIOGRAPHY

Albasan H, Lulich JP, Osborne CA: Effects of storage time and temperature on pH, specific gravity, and crystal formation in urine samples from dogs and cats, *J Am Vet Med Assoc* 222:176-179, 2003.

Bartges JW: Diagnosis of urinary tract infections, *Vet Clin North Am Small Animal Pract* 34:923-933, 2004.

Blanco LJ, Bartges JW: Understanding and eradicating bacterial urinary tract infections, *Vet Med* 96:776-790, 2001.

Cooke CL, Singer RS, Jang SS et al: Enrofloxacin resistance in *Escherichia coli* isolated from dogs with urinary tract infections, *J Am Vet Med Assoc* 220:190-192, 2002.

Ling GV: Bacterial infections of the urinary tract. In Ettinger SJ, Feldman EC, editors: *Textbook of veterinary internal medicine, vol* 2, ed 5, Philadelphia, 2000, Saunders.

Lulich JP, Osborne CA: Urine culture as a test for cure: why, when, and how? *Vet Clin North Am Small Animal Pract* 34:1027-1041, 2004.

Smarick SD, Haskins SC, Aldrich J et al: Incidence of catheter-associated urinary tract infection among dogs in a small animal intensive care unit, *J Am Vet Med Assoc* 224:1936-1940, 2004.

Section VII
Reproductive Problems
Section Editor: Klaas Post

---

50. Cystic Endometrial Hyperplasia/ Pyometra Complex

Klaas Post

---

1. Define cystic endometrial hyperplasia (CEH).

Cystic endometrial hyperplasia (CEH) is a progressive condition of the uterus that begins with a mucoid discharge during diestrus, through diffuse plasma cell infiltration and cystic hyperplasia, to squamous metaplasia of the endometrium. In the bitch, the 2-to-3-month diestral elevated progesterone plays a major role in producing hyperplasia of the endometrium.

Intact bitches that go through estrous cycles will have repeated exposure of the endometrium to progesterone. The estrogen elevation during proestrus and early estrus will enhance the formation of endometrial hyperplasia.

2. Define pyometra.

Pyometra is defined as an accumulation of purulent exudate in the uterus.

3. What is the role of estrogen and progesterone?

Estrogen priming of the endometrium, followed by progesterone, will increase the risk of developing CEH and pyometra.

4. What is the pathogenesis?

Repeated exposure to estrogen and progesterone will induce either a normal aging process or CEH and secretions of the uterine glands, which are conducive to bacterial growth.

5. Who is susceptible to pyometra?

Pyometra is most often seen in middle-aged, intact bitches 2 to 8 weeks after a heat cycle. Most of these animals have a certain degree of CEH. However, pyometra may also be seen in young bitches that have been treated with estrogen injections for mismating or with progestins for suppression or delay of an estrous cycle.

6. What is the difference between closed and open pyometra?

In open pyometra the cervix is open with a corresponding vaginal discharge. In closed pyometra the cervix is closed and little or no vaginal discharge is noted. In general, the systemic signs are more severe in closed pyometra than in open pyometra.

7. Describe the clinical signs of pyometra.

The clinical signs may differ between open pyometra and closed pyometra. In open pyometra one will observe a varying amount of vaginal discharge, often with a foul odor. The discharge may be mucoid, reddish, purulent, or a combination. The animal may not be very ill.

In closed pyometra, there is little if any discharge, but the bitch may be more systemically ill. Abdominal enlargement is more often noted with closed pyometra.

Signs observed in both open and closed pyometra may be depression, anorexia, vomiting, and diarrhea. Some animals may be polydipsic and polyuric with nocturia. The body temperature can be normal, elevated, or subnormal in the severely toxic animal.

8.   What causes the polydipsia and polyuria?

It is thought that endotoxins produced by *Escherichia coli* may make the renal tubules less sensitive to arginine vasopressin, which causes an inability to concentrate urine (nephrogenic diabetes insipidus). This causes polyuria with a compensatory polydipsia. It is thought that this interference is temporary and corrects itself after appropriate treatment of the pyometra.

9.   What laboratory tests are useful?

A complete blood count (CBC) may reveal changes ranging from mild leukocytosis to a severe degenerative leukocytosis. This is dependent on the chronicity of the pyometra and whether the condition is open or closed. A leukemoid response may be observed in some cases of closed pyometra. A mild nonregenerative anemia may be observed in chronic conditions. Hyperproteinemia due to dehydration and an increase in gammaglobulin concentration may also be detected.

Serum creatinine and blood urea nitrogen (BUN) concentration is usually normal or increased. Specific gravity of urine can be normal, isothenuric, or hyposthenuric. Proteinuria may occur as a result of glomerulonephritis, which occurs in some cases. A urine sample should not be collected by cystocentesis because of the risk of puncture of an enlarged uterus.

Vaginal cytology may reveal numerous degenerative leukocytes and bacteria. This cannot be used as a definitive test because these changes may be observed in other vaginal disorders.

10.   Should a bacterial culture and sensitivity test be done?

It is a good idea to collect vaginal discharge for a bacterial culture and sensitivity. However, before results are back, the dog may have undergone treatment.

11.   Can vaginal discharge from pyometra be confused with the vaginal discharge observed in some brucellosis cases?

This is a possibility. A vaginal slide agglutination test should be done. (See Chapter 52 for diagnosis and pitfalls of test.)

12.   What other tests should be performed to make a diagnosis of pyometra?

The best diagnostic test is ultrasound. Ultrasound will indicate the size of the uterus and its contents and the extent of CEH.

13.   What are the most common bacterial isolates?

In about 75% of pyometras an organism is involved. Approximately 20% of pyometras are sterile. The most common bacteria isolate is *E. coli* with other bacteria such as *Staphylococcus* species or *Streptococcus* species being isolated on a few occasions.

14.   How can pyometra be treated?

The simplest and most satisfactory treatment is ovariohysterectomy. However, medical treatment may be indicated in some cases.

15.   When should medical or surgical treatment be used?

Animals that are younger than 5 years, have breeding potential, and are presenting as open pyometras may be treated medically. For all others, ovariohysterectomy is indicated.

16. How do I treat pyometra medically?

Medical treatment with prostaglandin $F_{2\alpha}$ is used to evacuate the uterine contents. This drug should be administered with great care. $PGF_{2\alpha}$ is contraindicated in cases of closed pyometra because of the possibility of uterine rupture.

Increasing doses of $PGF_{2\alpha}$ (25-250 µg/kg subcutaneously or intramuscularly, 2 to 3 times a day) are administered over a period of 3 to 5 days depending on how much vaginal discharge is observed 45 to 90 minutes after administration. The goal is to note serial reductions in vaginal discharge and to discontinue therapy when there is minimal response to the prostaglandins. Antibiotics are also administered because of the risk of an ascending infection. The most common antibiotics used are trimethoprim-sulfadiazine, ampicillin, and enrofloxacin.

17. Can pyometra be prevented?

All bitches that are not spayed will develop a certain degree of CEH. This may begin at an earlier age in larger breeds than in smaller breeds. Therefore any cycling bitch older than 5 years has the potential to develop pyometra. If medical therapy of pyometra has been successful then it is imperative that the bitch is bred at her next estrous cycle.

18. What is the likelihood of another pyometra developing after medical therapy of pyometra?

After successful medical treatment, a bitch with CEH will most likely develop pyometra again during the diestral period of the next cycle. This is the reason that these bitches should be bred.

19. What is the differential diagnosis for pyometra?

The enlarged uterus could be confused with a gravid uterus if only radiographs were taken before 42 to 45 days of gestation.

Polyuria/polydipsia must be differentiated from other diseases including endocrinopathies and renal failure.

20. What is stump pyometra?

Stump pyometra is a condition in which some of the uterine body is left in situ after an ovariohysterectomy and an abscess develops at that site. It could be a reaction to inappropriate suture material.

In most cases, stump pyometra occurs in conjunction with ovarian remnant syndrome in which estrogen and progesterone are still produced by part of an remnant ovary left after ovariohysterectomy. These have hormonal action on the endometrium of the remnant uterine body.

51. Infertility in the Female Dog

Klaas Post

1. What are the causes of infertility in the female?

If the female is thought to be infertile, make sure that the female is the problem and not the male. It is necessary to obtain a good history about the male and query whether more than one male has been used to get this "infertile" female pregnant or do a semen evaluation. Consider that the female may have been spayed if she was obtained as an adult.

2.　How important is the timing of breeding?

Very important. In 50% to 75% of breedings of so-called infertile females, the optimum time of breeding was not adhered to even though it has been shown that sperm remains viable for up to 8 to 10 days in the normal female reproductive tract. Although the sperm may be viable for 8 to 10 days, it may have a limited period to fertilize the egg.

3.　When is the optimum time for breeding?

The optimum time for breeding is about 4 to 5 days after the luteinizing hormone (LH) peak or 2 to 3 days after ovulation.

4.　What do I look for in the noncycling female?

It is important to note and differentiate between a bitch that has never cycled and the bitch that cycled for a period but now fails to cycle.

5.　What are the causes of infertility in the bitch that never cycled?

It is important to understand that some breeds (larger) may not start cycling until 2 years of age. If a bitch has never cycled, the animal may have a chromosomal abnormality. Karyotyping should be performed if there is a suspicion. Has the animal been spayed? Some bitches may have silent heats in which the external signs of cycling are not present. These animals do ovulate, and when artificial insemination (AI) is performed at the optimum breeding time, the bitch may get pregnant. Could the bitch have an underlying disease such as hypothyroidism or have congenital pituitary abnormalities (e.g., pituitary dwarfism in the German Shepherd)? Other abnormalities such as aplasia of the ovaries may cause a failure to respond to follicle stimulating hormone or LH.

6.　What causes bitches that have previously cycled to stop?

There is always the possibility that age is a factor in cessation of cycles, although it is thought that bitches cycle until they die. In some cases, premature ovarian failure cannot be ruled out. Any long-standing debilitating condition could potentially stop cyclicity in the bitch. Other disorders such as *Brucella canis* infection, hypothyroidism, hyperadrenocorticism, cancer (both ovarian and nonovarian), some viral infections, toxoplasmosis, and immune-mediated disease of the ovaries could stop the estrous cycle.

The medication history, including drugs given both in the past and currently received, must be reviewed. Hormones (progestins and androgens) that were given to postpone or suppress the heat cycle could play a significant role. Other drugs (e.g., anticancer, corticosteroids) may have a serious effect on ovarian function. Drugs that are given for behavior modification may have an effect on cyclicity as well. A bitch that develops an ovarian cyst (progesterone-producing) will stop cycling. These animals will have a consistently elevated serum progesterone concentration.

7.　What are the causes of infertility in the bitch with abnormal cycles/increased interestrous interval?

The first or pubertal cycle may be abnormal and breeding should not be considered during those cycles. With maturity of the bitch, normal cycle patterns will develop. In some animals a normal state does not develop and one can categorize the abnormal cycles as follows:

Prolonged interestrous interval for the breed. Most dogs will cycle between 5 and 10 months with the Basenji being the exception with an interestrous interval of 12 months. The average interestrous cycle is 7 to 8 months. Silent heat or undetected heat cycles are not truly an increased interestrous interval, but an absence of overt signs of cycling. Increased length of the interestrous interval can be associated with hypothyroidism or hyperadrenocorticism. Exogenous administration of glucocorticoids could do the same (e.g., in seasonal allergy where corticosteroid is given during the time the animal is expected to show heat).

Administration of progesterone to delay the onset of heat will increase the interestrous interval, as does a functional luteal cyst of the ovary (ovaries). In some dogs, pregnancy will increase the interestrous interval by 4 to 8 weeks. These dogs will nurse the pups until 6 to 8 weeks of age. It is possible that prolactin may play a protective role and prevent the dog from cycling.

8. What is the cause for shortened interestrous interval?

One of the common causes is a split heat. The bitch will show heat for approximately 1 week; she does not ovulate; the signs regress; and 1 to 8 weeks later she will start heat again, often with ovulation. German Shepherds will show this phenomenon more so than any other breed. Split heat is also observed more frequently in young animals. No treatment is necessary.

In older bitches, this split heat may occur and treatment with gonadotropins may be indicated. Follicular cysts will prolong proestrus/estrus, but because there is no luteal activity, the interestrous interval will be shortened. Those animals with follicular cysts will not ovulate, will go out of heat, and will come in heat sooner than expected. This can also be caused during termination of pregnancy by administration of drugs such as prostaglandins or prolactin inhibitors. The luteal phase is shortened and the animal may come in heat sooner than anticipated.

9. What are the causes of prolonged proestrus/estrus?

Young females during their first few cycles may have external signs of proestrus and estrus for a longer than normal period of time. This condition is usually self-limiting. Animals that have follicular cystic ovaries may have a prolonged proestrus/estrus, but as stated before, the animals do not ovulate, and therefore the luteal phase may be shorter and the interestrous interval will be shorter. Animals that received exogenous estrogen as a mismate may have prolonged proestrus/estrus periods.

Ovarian tumors can cause prolonged estrus. These usually are found in older animals.

10. What if the bitch cycles normally and no offspring are observed?

Timing is important and one must calculate the breeding to take place 2 to 3 days after ovulation. The male must be fertile. The female may have anatomic abnormalities such as strictures in the vestibule/vagina that would prevent the male from penetrating. If penetration is accomplished the cervix has to be patent and stenosis of the cervix could prevent pregnancy. Other abnormalities may involve the uterine horns and or tubes. Strictures preventing semen to enter the tubes or segmental hypoplasia or aplasia of the uterine horns could prevent a pregnancy. Low-grade infection of the uterus and fallopian tubes such as endometritis or salpingitis will make the female infertile. Both bacterial and viral infection such as herpes can play a role in these situations. Hypoluteolism is a condition whereby the progesterone does not remain at a concentration to maintain pregnancy. Progesterone concentration should remain above 2 to 3 ng/ml for maintenance of pregnancy.

52. Brucellosis

Klaas Post

1. What causes brucellosis in the dog?

Brucellosis is caused by *Brucella canis*, a small, intracellular, Gram-negative coccobacillus. *B. canis* primarily causes infections in the dog and wild canids. Human infection caused by *B. canis* occurs.

2.   How is *B. canis* transmitted?

Transmission may occur by the following routes: ingestion or inhalation of infected material, most often in vaginal discharge after an abortion. However, it may occur during coitus. It is believed that the oronasal transmission by aerosols is the most common pathway. Other portals of entry are conjunctival and genital mucous membranes, abrasions in the skin, and maternal placenta.

3.   Will an infected animal shed the bacteria?

Infected animals may secrete the organism in their urine. The bacteria can also be found in secretions from salivary gland, secretions from nasal passages, and vaginal secretions of nonestrous animals and the milk. These are all of minor significance. Organisms in greatest numbers are found in the vaginal discharge of dogs that have aborted a litter.

4.   What role does the uterus play in spreading the organism in nonpregnant bitches?

As a general rule, it is believed that the nonpregnant or diestrous uterus is not a preferred site for multiplication of the organism.

5.   How does it affect the pregnant bitch?

B. canis colonizes epithelial cells of the placenta, which can lead to embryonic or fetal death.

6.   Will all pregnant, infected bitches abort?

No, the bitch may maintain pregnancy and whelp both live and dead pups in the same litter. In most cases, live pups will die shortly after parturition.

7.   What other tissues may become infected in the bitch?

The organism has been identified from kidneys, eyes, meninges, intervertebral discs, and saliva.

8.   What route does the organism follow when it infects the dog?

The organism is phagocytized at portal of entry and carried to lymphatic tissue where they multiply. One to four weeks after infection, a bacteremia develops, which may last from 6 to 64 months. The organism then spreads by the hematogenous route to other organs of the dog.

9.   What are the clinical signs?

Initially, a generalized lymphadenitis, splenitis, abortion, and a vaginal discharge after abortion are seen. Other signs noticed are reproductive failure, fever, fatigue, poor condition, loss of alertness, and failure to perform a task for which the dog is trained.

In the male dog, the organs mostly affected are the testes and epididymides. This causes signs of orchitis and epididymitis, scrotal dermatitis, oligospermia, and infertility. In chronic infections, one may see testicular atrophy associated with teratospermia and eventually spermatogenic arrest.

10.   When is pregnancy terminated as a result of *B. canis* infection?

Pregnancy can be terminated as early as 20 days of gestation, or more typically, between 45 and 59 days of gestation.

11.   How is a definite diagnosis of brucellosis made?

The culture of *B. canis* from infected tissue or blood will yield a definite diagnosis. In the bitch, the gravid or estral uterus, the placenta, and vaginal or uterine (including fetuses) discharge has a high number of organisms. Blood cultures become positive for *B. canis* about 2 to 4 weeks after the infection and this may last for up to 30 months. The organism may also be cultured from bone marrow.

Urine culture for the organism is less likely to be positive in the female than in the male because males tend to have a higher number of organisms in their urine.

12. Is there a screening test available?

Serologic tests such as the rapid slide agglutination test (RSAT) and tube agglutination test (TAT) are readily available. Both tests have the disadvantage that false positives occur because of cross-reactivity with antibodies of other organisms. A second disadvantage is the inability of the tests to detect antibodies until 3 or 4 weeks after the infection occurs.

13. Are there other serologic tests available?

The agar gel immunodiffusion (AGID) and the enzyme-linked immunosorbent assay (ELISA) are available.

14. How do I treat brucellosis?

Treatment of brucellosis is not recommended for most cases. The veterinarian should preface any considerations of treatment with the owner by a conversation that includes informing the client that there is usually a lack of response to treatment, that brucellosis is a zoonotic disease, and that the dog may continue to shed organisms and be a threat to other animals. If a client insists on treating a brucella-positive animal, then spaying or castration should be strongly recommended. Euthanasia is a reasonable recommendation.

15. What therapies have been recommended for brucellosis?

A combination of minocycline at 25 mg/kg orally once per day for a minimum of 2 weeks (12.5 mg/kg twice daily for 2 weeks) and dihydrostreptomycin at 5 mg/kg intramuscularly twice daily for 1 week has been considered the most successful treatment.

A second treatment regimen that has been used is tetracycline hydrochloride at 30 mg/kg twice daily and streptomycin, 20 mg/kg intramuscularly once a day for 14 days. The tetracycline is continued for an additional 14 days.

16. How do I prevent introducing the *B. canis* organism to my kennel?

All new arrivals should be quarantined and test negative for the organism for the initial 8 to 12 weeks after arrival.

17. Is *B. canis* a zoonosis?

Brucellosis poses a threat to both owner and veterinarian. Particularly children, immuno-suppressed people, women of childbearing age, or pregnant women are at risk.

BIBLIOGRAPHY

Austad R, Lunde A, Sjaastad OV: Peripheral plasma levels of oestradiol 17B and progesterone in the bitch during the oestrous cycle, in normal pregnancy and after dexamethazone treatment, *J Reprod Fert* 46:129-136, 1976.

Carmichael LE: Canine brucellosis: an annotated review with selected cautionary comments, *Theriogenology* 6:105-116, 1976.

Carmichael LE, Greene CE: Canine brucellosis. In Green CE, editor: *Infectious diseases of the dog and cat*, Philadelphia, 1990, WB Saunders.

Carmichael LE, Kenney RM: Canine abortion caused by *Brucella canis*. *J Am Vet Med Assoc* 152:605-616, 1968.

Carmichael LE, Soha SJ, Fores-Castro R: Problems with sero-diagnosis of canine brucellosis: dog responses to cell-wall and internal antigens of *Brucella canis, Dev Biol Stand* 56:371-383, 1984.

Christianson LJ. *Reproduction in the dog and cat,* Toronto, 1984, Bailliere Tindall.

Hubbert NL, Bech-Nielsen S, Barta O: Canine brucellosis: comparison of clinical manifestations with serological test results, *J Am Vet Med Assoc* 177:168-171, 1980.

Johnson CA, Walker RD. Clinical signs and diagnosis of *Brucella canis* infection, *Compend Contin Educ Pract Vet* 14:763-773, 1992.

Jones RL: Canine brucellosis in a commercial breeding kennel, *J Am Vet Med Assoc* 18:834-835, 1984.
Nicoletti P: Further studies on the use of antibiotics in canine brucellosis, *Compend Contin Educ Pract Vet* 13:944-947, 1991.
Pollock RV: Canine brucellosis: current status, *Compend Contin Educ Pract Vet* 1:255-267, 1979.
Serikawa T, Iwaki S, Mori M et al: Purification of a *Brucella canis* cell wall antigen rising immunosorbent columns and use of the antigen enzyme-linked immunosorbent assay for specific diagnosis of canine brucellosis, *J Clin Microbiol* 27:837-842, 1989.

53. Prostatic Disease

Stanley I. Rubin and Mala Erickson

1. What are the most common features of prostatic disease in the dog?

- Urethral discharge, hematuria, and rectal tenesmus are the most frequent signs in dogs with prostatic disease.
- Dogs with acute bacterial prostatitis may have depression, anorexia, vomiting, and bloody urethral discharge.
- Straining to urinate, urethral discharge, anorexia, and depression are seen in dogs with prostatic abscesses.
- Recurrent urinary tract infection (UTI) is often a clue to the presence of chronic bacterial prostatitis.
- Dogs with prostatic neoplasia may have decreased appetite, weight loss, urethral discharge, and/or rear limb weakness.
- Dogs are infertile.

2. What are the major categories of prostatic disease?

- Benign prostatic hyperplasia (BPH)
- Acute/chronic prostatitis
- Prostatic abscessation
- Prostatic cyst
- Prostatic neoplasia

3. When should I perform a rectal examination to examine the prostate gland?

- A rectal examination should be routine on any male dog older than 2 years.
- Any male dog of any age with lower urinary tract signs should be examined.

4. How do I perform a rectal examination?

- Simultaneous rectal and caudal abdominal palpation to palpate the prostate per abdomen and to push the prostate toward the pelvic canal
- Best with dog standing

5. Are there any breeds that normally have big prostate glands?

- The Scottish Terrier is reported to have a prostate 4 times larger than that of dogs of similar age and weight.

6. What should be included in the diagnostic workup of a dog with prostatic disease?

- Rectal examination
- Complete blood count

- Serum biochemistry profile
- Radiography
- Culture and cytologic examination of prostatic fluid collected by ejaculate or prostatic wash
- Ultrasound
- Ultrasound-guided fine needle aspiration (possibly)
- Prostatic biopsy

7. Why would I want to evaluate prostatic fluid?
- Cytologically evaluating prostatic fluid and culturing prostatic fluid are useful means of differentiating between BPH, bacterial prostatitis, and prostatic neoplasia.

8. Why is an ejaculate useful?
- Prostatic fluid constitutes the largest volume of an ejaculate and makes up 95% of the volume of an ejaculate. Prostatic fluid is in the third fraction of the ejaculate and is normally clear and acellular.
- Blood may be present in the ejaculates of dogs with bacterial infection, BPH, prostatic cysts and prostatic neoplasia.

9. How do I collect an ejaculate?
1. Some ejaculates may be collected from most intact males by manual stimulation alone. A teaser bitch often aids in collection. The teaser may be in estrus, or an anestrous bitch with pheromone methyl-p-hydroxybenzoate applied to the vulva may be used with the dog.
2. Extrude the penis from the sheath and gently remove any preputial discharge from the penis with gauze sponges and warm water. If any soap or detergent is used, it must be rinsed off with sterile saline and the penis dried. Contamination of the sample with detergent may interfere with the quantitative culture results.
3. A rubber collection funnel (artificial vagina) with attached tube is slipped over the penis with one hand while the other hand holds the sheath retracted. The artificial vagina is placed over the entire penis and bulbis glandis as the male becomes aroused.
4. Pressure is maintained over the bulbis glandis with the hand holding the funnel and the penis is massaged caudal to the bulbis glandis with the other hand.
5. The first two fractions of the ejaculate appear within the first 1 to 2 minutes of collection and are composed of the presperm and sperm-rich fractions. After the first two fractions have passed, a second sterile tube is attached to the collection funnel and the prostatic fraction is collected.
6. Samples of the prostatic fluid are submitted for cytologic evaluation and quantitative bacterial culture.

10. What do I do if I cannot collect an ejaculate?
- Perform a prostatic wash.

11. How do I perform a prostatic wash?
1. The dog is taken out and allowed to void.
2. Light sedation with acepromazine may facilitate the procedure by minimizing physical restraint and decreasing the dog's apprehension.
3. Using aseptic technique, a sterile urinary catheter is passed.
4. The bladder is emptied of urine and flushed several times with sterile saline. The last 5 ml of sterile saline is retained as prostatic massage sample 1.
5. A gloved finger is inserted into the rectum and the catheter is retracted just distal to the prostate. The prostate gland is massaged rectally or abdominally for 1 to 2 minutes. Sterile physiologic saline (5-10 ml) is flushed slowly past the prostatic urethra. The catheter is

then advanced back slowly into the urinary bladder with simultaneous aspiration as the catheter is advanced. This sample is retained as prostatic massage sample 2.

6. Prostatic massage samples 1 and 2 are submitted for cytologic and quantitative microbiologic evaluation.

7. A recently described technique used a microbiological specimen brush in conjunction with prostatic massage to obtain samples for culture and cytologic examination. This technique was found to be useful for the diagnosis of neoplastic, hyperplastic, and bacterial prostatic disease.

12. How do I evaluate the results of a prostatic wash?

- The premassage and postmassage samples are evaluated cytologically and submitted for quantitative culture. Prostatic infection is likely when the postmassage specimen yields a higher bacterial count ($>10^5$ Gram-negative bacterial per milliliter) than the premassage sample. Cytologic evidence of inflammation (increased numbers of neutrophils and macrophages), particularly in the postmassage sample, has correlated well with the presence of infection.

13. When should I collect a prostatic biopsy?

- Biopsy techniques are useful for differentiating neoplastic from inflammatory prostatic disease but are less useful for differentiating infectious from noninfectious, inflammatory prostatic disease.
- A biopsy should be performed when castration does not alleviate prostatomegaly.

14. How are biopsies collected?

- *Direct aspiration of the gland.* It may be guided by ultrasound. Needle aspiration is usually done by the rectal, perirectal, or transabdominal approach, depending on the location of the gland.
- *Core (Tru-cut).* It is performed closed by the perirectal or transabdominal approaches or open after the gland is exposed surgically.

15. Are biopsies ever contraindicated?

- They are contraindicated in the dog with fever or leukocytosis.
- Needle aspiration is potentially dangerous in the dog with acute prostatitis or prostatic abscessation because of the risk of seeding the needle tract with organisms. Aspiration should thus be performed after examination of the prostatic fluid collected by ejaculation or massage.
- Prostatic biopsy has little place in the dog with bacterial prostatitis unless concurrent disease is suspected.

BENIGN PROSTATIC HYPERPLASIA

16. What is benign prostatic hyperplasia (BPH)?

- It is the spontaneous enlargement of the prostate gland in dogs as they age.
- Both hypertrophy and hyperplasia occur with diffuse glandular proliferation and an overall increase in volume and weight of the gland. Small intraparenchymal cysts containing bloody or serosanguinous fluid may form, and as the gland develops increased vascularity, there is an increased tendency for prostatic bleeding.
- It is thought to result from hormonal imbalance (altered estrogen:androgen ratio).
- Prevalence is as high as 50% in all adult dogs by 4 to 5 years of age.
- It is prevented by castration.

17. What are the signs of BPH?

- Tenesmus and constipation (most common)

- Weakness in the hindquarters
- Ribbonlike stool due to partial occlusion of lumen of large bowel
- Bloody urethral discharge, independent of urination
- Hemospermia, infertility
- Decreased libido, reluctance to breed
- Perineal hernia (concurrent condition)
- Symmetrically enlarged prostate that may partially occlude lumen of large bowel
- Prostate that can be palpated abdominally
- No pain

18. How is BPH diagnosed?

- Signalment, history, and physical examination findings indicate prostate enlargement in an otherwise healthy male dog.
- Abdominal radiographs show prostatomegaly.
- Ultrasound examination shows homogenous parenchyma that is normal to slightly hyperechoic with single or multiple, small, fluid-filled parenchymal cysts.
- Prostatic fluid varies in color from clear to red-brown.
- Cytology of ejaculate may reveal changes compatible with hyperplasia, absence of inflammation, and insignificant culture results.
- Signs respond to castration.

19. What is the treatment for BPH?

- *Castration.* Involution of the gland begins within days of surgery. A 50% decrease in size is demonstrable in 3 weeks, and 70% reduction in size is expected by 9 weeks.
- *Medical therapy.* Medical therapy may be used in valuable breeding dogs and for dogs at a high risk for adverse reactions to anesthesia or surgery. Finasteride should be administered at a dose of 0.1 to 0.5 mg/kg/day or as one 5-mg tablet per dog/day for dogs weighing 1 to 50 kg. Finasteride reduces prostatic size but does not adversely affect the libido, semen quality, and fertility.

BACTERIAL PROSTATITIS

20. What are the most commonly isolated organisms causing bacterial prostatitis?

The most common organism is *Escherichia coli,* followed by staphylococci and streptococci.

21. What is the clinical spectrum of a dog with bacterial prostatitis?

- Asymptomatic
- Infertility as a presenting complaint.
- Intermittent episodes of hematuria and dysuria or bacterial UTI
- Mild clinical abnormalities such as pain, fever, and lethargy
- Serious illness with lethargy, anorexia, vomiting, sepsis, shock, and death

22. How is prostatitis diagnosed?

- Pain during rectal palpation
- Asymmetric prostatomegaly if a prostatic abscess is present
- Leukocytosis with left shift
- Serum chemistry result reflecting a reflect systemic illness (e.g., azotemia)
- Urinalysis reveals UTI
- Increased number of red blood cells and white blood cells in prostatic fluid and possibly bacteria within neutrophils
- Large number of single bacterial species revealed by culture of prostatic fluid
- Prostatic enlargement and displacement, indistinct cranial prostatic margins, and prostatic mineralization revealed by radiography

- Diffuse increase in parenchymal echogenicity and abscesses (visible as hypoechoic or anechoic lesions) on ultrasound

ACUTE PROSTATITIS

23. What are the management principles of a dog with acute prostatitis?

- Supportive therapy is indicated for animals that are acutely ill.
- Normally, the blood-prostate barrier is effective in preventing many antibiotics from penetrating into the prostatic parenchyma. In the case of normal acidic prostatic fluid, drugs that are weak bases, such as trimethoprim/sulfa, erythromycin, clindamycin, ciprofloxacin, enrofloxacin, carbenicillin, and chloramphenicol, are able to penetrate into the parenchyma.
- Parenteral enrofloxacin is a good choice for initial therapy while awaiting culture and sensitivity results. Other antimicrobials such as trimethoprim/sulfadiazine and chloramphenicol may also be useful. A combination of ampicillin and gentamicin would also be effective because the blood-prostate barrier is not intact during acute inflammation.
- Prostatic abscesses should be drained surgically by marsupialization, placement of a Penrose drain, partial prostatectomy, or omentalization. Surgery has the potential for high mortality with many complications such as incontinence, chronic draining stomas, peritonitis, septic shock, and death.
- Castration or administration of finasteride is recommended as adjunct therapy.
- Antibiotic therapy should be continued for 2 to 3 weeks.
- Prostatic fluid or urine should be cultured within a few days of discontinuing antibiotics and again 2 to 4 weeks later to be certain that the infection has resolved.

CHRONIC PROSTATITIS

24. What are the features of chronic prostatitis?

- History of acute prostatitis
- Recurrent UTI caused by the same organism
- Recurrent hemorrhagic or purulent urethral discharge, independent of micturition.
- Enlarged, sometimes symmetric, usually nonpainful prostate
- Findings of macrophages in the ejaculate in conjunction with clinical signs of prostatic infection and inflammation
- May be difficult to eradicate

25. What are management principles of chronic prostatitis?

- The blood-prostate barrier is intact, limiting penetration of many antibiotics into the prostatic fluid.
- Choose the antibiotic on the basis of sensitivity of organism.
- Continue antibiotic therapy for at least 4 weeks.
- Evaluate prostatic fluid after discontinuation of antibiotics.
- Castration is an effective adjunct therapy.

26. Why is erythromycin a poor empirical choice for management of bacterial prostatitis?

- The antimicrobial spectrum of erythromycin is against Gram-positive organisms.
- The most common organism isolated is *E. coli,* which is Gram-negative.

PROSTATIC CYSTS

27. What types of cysts are associated with the prostate gland?

- Multiple, small cysts associated with BPH.
- True prostatic cysts. They are thin-walled structures within the prostatic parenchyma containing nonpurulent fluid.

- Paraprostatic cysts. They are thin-walled structures outside the prostatic parenchyma but are attached to the gland by a stalk or adhesions. They develop from remnants of the müllerian duct or as a result of the tremendous enlargement of an existing prostatic cyst.

28. What are the signs of a prostatic cyst?
- Cysts may be asymptomatic.
- Cysts can become extremely large and cause signs by impingement on the bladder or rectum, producing constipation and dysuria, with tenesmus.
- Hematuria, dysuria, and stranguria may develop when cysts become infected or when prostatitis accompanies the disease.
- Local and systemic signs may be present if the cyst is complicated by prostatitis.
- Rarely, a cyst may become infected, rupture, and create a syndrome of acute peritonitis and shock.
- A caudal abdominal mass is detected on physical examination.

29. How do I differentiate a paraprostatic cyst causing a caudal abdominal mass from the urinary bladder?
- Cystography
- Analysis of fluid sample obtained by fine-needle aspiration

30. What is the treatment of a paraprostatic cyst?
- Surgical excision
- Castration

PROSTATIC NEOPLASIA

31. What is the most common prostatic tumor?
- Adenocarcinoma is the most common.
- Other tumors, such as transitional cell carcinoma, rectal and colonic adenocarcinoma, and rectal and colonic squamous cell carcinoma, can locally invade the prostate gland.
- Lymphosarcoma and perianal adenocarcinoma can metastasize to the prostate gland.

32. What signs are associated with prostatic neoplasia?
- It occurs in older male dogs of medium to large breeds.
- The average age at diagnosis is 8 to 10 years
- There may be an insidious history of rear-limb weakness, lumbar pain, dysuria, dyschezia, rectal tenesmus, constipation, hematuria, and weight loss.
- The prostate is enlarged, firm, and irregular. Prostatomegaly in a castrated male dog is highly suspicious of neoplastic disease.
- Urinary obstruction is fairly common in dogs with prostatic neoplasia but rarely occurs in dogs as a result of other prostatic diseases.

33. What is the biologic behavior of prostatic adenocarcinoma?
It is locally invasive and metastasizes to the sublumbar lymph nodes, bony pelvis, and lumbar vertebrae. This causes lumbar pain and pelvic limb lameness or weakness. Lymphatic or venous obstruction may cause pelvic limb swelling.

34. How do I make a definitive diagnosis of prostatic neoplasia?
- Cytologic or histopathologic evidence of neoplasia should be obtained fine-needle aspirate or biopsy.
- Neoplastic cells may be found in samples collected by urethral catheter.
- Neoplasia should be suspected by the finding of a normal-sized or enlarged prostate in a previously castrated male dog.

- Rectal examination may disclose bone pain due to metastases.
- Radiology or sonographic studies may be supportive.

35. What is the prognosis for a dog with prostatic tumors?

- Prognosis is poor. Survival is typically 1 to 2 months after diagnosis.
- Palliative therapy may include surgery, castration, hormonal therapy, chemotherapy, and radiation therapy.
- In one study, therapy with a combination of piroxicam and cisplatin resulted in a complete or partial remission in 71% of dogs.

BIBLIOGRAPHY

Barsanti JA, Shotts EB Jr, Prasse K et al: Evaluation of diagnostic techniques for canine prostatic diseases, *J Am Vet Med Assoc* 177:160, 1980.

Barsanti JA, Prasse KW, Crowell WA et al: Evaluation of various techniques for diagnosis of chronic bacterial prostatitis in the dog, *J Am Vet Med Assoc* 183:219, 1983.

Barsanti JA, Finco DR: Canine bacterial prostatitis, *Vet Clin North Am Small Anim Pract* 9:679, 1979.

Cornell KK, Bostwick DG, Cooley DM et al: Clinical and pathologic aspects of spontaneous canine prostate carcinoma: a retrospective analysis of 76 cases, *Prostate* 45:173, 2000.

Feeney DA Johnston GR, Klausner JS et al: Canine prostatic disease: comparison of radiographic appearance with morphologic and microbiologic findings—30 cases (1981-1985), *J Am Vet Med Assoc* 190:1018, 1987.

Feeney DA, Johnston GR, Klausner JS et al: Canine prostatic disease: comparison of ultrasonographic appearance with morphologic and microbiologic findings—30 cases (1981-1985). *J Am Vet Med Assoc* 190:1027, 1987.

Feeney DA, Johnston GR, Klausner JS: Two-dimensional gray scale ultrasonography: applications in canine prostatic disease, *Vet Clin North Am Small Anim Pract* 15:1159, 1985.

Kay ND, Ling GV, Johnson DL: A urethral brush technique for the diagnosis of canine bacterial prostatitis, *J Am Anim Hosp Assoc* 25:527, 1989.

Ling GV, Branam JE, Ruby AL et al: Canine prostatic fluid: techniques of collection, quantitative bacterial culture and interpretation of results, *J Am Vet Med Assoc* 183:201, 1983.

Ling GV, Nyland TG, Kennedy PC et al: Comparison of two sample collection methods for quantitative bacteriologic culture of canine prostatic fluid, *J Am Vet Med Assoc* 196:1479, 1990.

Olson PN, Wrigley RH, Thrall MA et al: Disorders of the canine prostate gland: pathogenesis, diagnosis and medical therapy, *Comp Cont Ed Pract Vet* 9:613, 1987.

Read RA, Bryden S: Urethral bleeding as a presenting sign of benign prostatic hyperplasia in the dog: a retrospective study (1979-1993), *J Am Anim Hosp Assoc* 31:261, 1995.

Rubin SI: Localizing bacterial infection to the prostate gland. *Vet Medicine* 85:352, 1990.

Rubin SI: Managing dogs with bacterial prostatic disease, *Vet Medicine* 85:387, 1990.

White RA: Prostatic surgery in the dog, *Clin Tech Small Anim Pract* 15:46, 2000.

Section VIII
Polysystemic Problems

Section Editor: Astrid Nielssen

54. Polysystemic Problems: Fever

Astrid Nielssen

1. How is the body's internal temperature determined?

The body's thermoregulatory center is located within the anterior hypothalamus. Central and peripheral thermoreceptors sense changes in the core and peripheral body temperature and relay this information to the central thermoregulatory center. Deviations in temperature above or below the set point of the thermoregulatory center result in the body using mechanisms to either increase heat loss and decrease heat generation or decrease heat loss and increase heat production, respectively.

2. What is the definition of fever?

True fever is defined as an elevated body temperature resulting from an increased thermoregulatory center temperature set point. This is what differentiates fever from hyperthermia, the condition that arises when the body's temperature becomes elevated despite a normal thermoregulatory set point. Hyperthermia arises when the normal heat-dissipating mechanisms of the body are overwhelmed, such as in heat stroke or status epilepticus. Additionally it is not uncommon to see hyperthermia in stressed animals. Body temperature should be rechecked in animals with elevated body temperature to make sure that the elevation is persistent.

3. What are some of the causes of an elevated thermoregulatory set point?

Agents that induce fever (pyrogens) can be either exogenous or endogenous. Examples of exogenous pyrogens include lipopolysaccharides from Gram-negative bacteria, components of Gram-positive bacteria, viral particles, and drugs. Exogenous pyrogens induce fever through their stimulation of the release of endogenous pyrogens; these are products released primarily from host macrophages and lymphocytes. A variety of endogenous pyrogens have been identified including interleukin-1, interleukin-6, and tumor necrosis factor. The endogenous pyrogens bind endothelial cells in the thermoregulatory center and are thought to alter the temperature set point through the production of prostaglandins.

4. What are some of the mechanisms through which the body increases heat production and decreases heat loss?

Muscle contractions, shivering, catecholamine release, and thyroxine production are all mechanisms through which the body increases heat production. Peripheral vasoconstriction, piloerection, postural changes to try and decrease body surface area, and heat-seeking behavior are all mechanisms through which the body decreases heat loss.

5. What is a fever of unknown origin (FUO)?

The current definition of FUO in human medicine is that of fever that has persisted for 2 weeks (or 3 days for immunosuppressed patients) and for which no etiology can be identified despite extensive investigation, including in-hospital evaluation. In veterinary medicine FUO is the term frequently used to describe any febrile state of uncertain etiology that has not responded to a course of empirical antibiotic therapy.

6.   What are some causes of FUO in the dog?

The various causes of FUO in dogs are often organized into categories including:

Infectious:		
	Bacterial:	abscesses, discospondylitis, endocarditis, osteomyelitis, peritonitis, prostatitis, pyelonephritis, pyometra, pyothorax, septic arthritis, brucellosis, leptospirosis, Lyme disease
	Viral:	distemper virus
	Mycotic:	blastomycosis, coccidiomycosis, cryptococcosis, histoplasmosis
	Protozoal:	babesiosis, leishmaniasis, neosporosis, toxoplasmosis, trypanosomiasis
	Rickettsial:	ehrlichiosis, Rocky Mountain spotted fever
Inflammatory:		juvenile cellulitis, pancreatitis
Immune-mediated:		immune-mediated polyarthritis, steroid-responsive meningitis, systemic lupus erythematosus
Neoplastic:		leukemia, lymphoma, multiple myeloma, necrotic tumors
Drug reactions:		ketamine, penicillins, phenobarbital, sulfonamides, tetracyclines
Miscellaneous:		panosteitis, Shar-Pei fever
True FUO:		no known etiology

While the incidence of the various causes of FUO is not well established in canine medicine, immune-mediated and neoplastic diseases are the causes behind a large number of cases.

7.   How should a case of FUO be investigated?

A thorough history and clinical evaluation are essential in these cases. A full history needs to include information on vaccination status, travel, prior trauma or infections, and current medication administration. A careful examination technique with particular attention to oral, dermatologic, fundic, neurologic, and rectal examination; lymph node, joint, and long bone palpation; and thoracic auscultation should be used during the physical examination. Repeated physical examinations throughout the course of the illness may identify a new finding that might help to determine the cause of the fever.

Further workup in these cases should include a complete blood count, serum biochemistry profile, urinalysis, and urine culture. Thoracic and abdominal radiographs can also be helpful in the initial workup. Further diagnostic investigations will depend on initial results but might include cardiac and abdominal ultrasound, blood culture, and potentially more advanced imaging such as computed tomography or magnetic resonance imaging. Serologic testing for infectious or immune-mediated disease may also be indicated. Cytologic assessment of aspirates from any masses, swellings, or body cavity fluids can be performed. Arthrocentesis, lymph node aspiration, and bone marrow aspiration can help to identify occult disease in these body tissues. A cerebrospinal fluid tap and analysis may be indicated if signs of neurologic disease or neck pain are present. Blood and joint cultures can be performed. A skeletal radiographic study can be obtained to rule out occult bone involvement. An exploratory laparotomy can be considered if it is indicated on the basis of earlier diagnostic findings or if all diagnostics have been exhausted and a diagnosis is still not obtained.

8.   How is FUO treated?

If a cause for FUO is identified during the course of the diagnostic workup, then treatment is directed at the cause. In cases where a cause cannot be identified with an initial thorough diagnostic evaluation, a course of treatment with antibiotics may be considered before proceeding with more invasive diagnostics. Without a diagnosis, appropriate antibiotic selection is difficult. However, it may be useful to remember that first- and second-generation cephalosporins, chloramphenicol, and carbapenems are generally effective against Gram-positive bacteria; third-generation cephalosporins, aminoglycosides, fluoroquinolones, and carbapenems are generally effective against Gram-negative bacteria; clindamycin is generally effective against anaerobic bacteria; and tetracyclines are generally highly effective against rickettsial organisms.

If all diagnostic evaluations have been exhausted and a fungal infection is suspected, then an antifungal trial may be considered. Such a trial can be expensive, however, and these drugs are not without potentially serious side effects. Owners need to be informed about these drawbacks before proceeding with such a trial.

If all diagnostic and other therapeutic avenues have been exhausted and no cause for the FUO has been identified, then a corticosteroid trial can be considered. This should only be undertaken with the informed consent of the owner, who must understand that this therapy could result in fatal dissemination of an infectious condition or make an underlying neoplastic condition even more difficult to diagnose. In dogs with steroid-responsive FUO, a positive response is usually seen within 24 to 48 hours of therapy with immunosuppressive doses of corticosteroids.

9.   Should fever be specifically treated?

Fever arises as part of the body's response to infection. It helps to kill or inhibit the growth of microorganisms. It also results in increased leukocyte activity, further helping to eliminate pathogens. Temperatures below 40.3° C in the dog are generally well tolerated and are unlikely to be associated with adverse effects. Because antipyretic medications may impair the defense mechanisms of the host and have well-documented side effects, they are probably best avoided in dogs that are only mildly febrile. Dogs with temperatures above 40.3° C are more likely to have a negative energy balance and inadequate fluid intake. They therefore may benefit from antipyretic therapy.

10.   How can a fever be treated?

Because fever arises from an increased thermoregulatory center set point, mechanical cooling of a truly febrile animal is not appropriate. Such an intervention will only cause the animal discomfort and increase the likelihood that it will have a negative energy balance. Truly febrile dogs do not usually have a temperature above 41.1° C. Dogs with a temperature above 41.1° C likely have hyperthermia, possibly in conjunction with an underlying fever. Temperatures at and above this level can result in serious adverse events and therefore do warrant body cooling and aggressive supportive care.

The most commonly used drugs to lower the thermoregulatory center set point and resolve a fever in dogs are nonsteroidal antiinflammatory drugs (NSAIDs). In addition to lowering the thermoregulatory set point by inhibiting prostaglandin production within the hypothalamus, these drugs can also reduce inflammation and act as analgesics. Corticosteroids are not indicated in the management of fever except in the treatment of specifically diagnosed conditions or as a final-stage therapeutic trial in the management of FUO because their actions can exacerbate underlying infectious diseases.

BIBLIOGRAPHY

Couto CG: Fever of undetermined origin. In Nelson RW, Couto CG, editors: *Essentials of small animal internal medicine*, St. Louis, 1992, Mosby.

Dunn KJ, Dunn JK: Diagnostic investigations in 101 dogs with pyrexia of unknown origin, *J Small Anim Prac* 39:574, 1998.

Feldman BF: Fever of undetermined origin, *Comp Cont Ed* 2:641, 1980.

Guyton AC, Hall JE: Body temperature, temperature regulation, and fever. In Guyton AC, Hall JE, editors: *Textbook of medical physiology*, ed 10, Philadelphia, 2000, Saunders.

Johannes CM, Cohn LA: A clinical approach to patients with fever of unknown origin, *Vet Med* 95:633-642, 2000.

Miller JB: Hyperthermia and hypothermia. In Ettinger SJ, Feldman EC, editors: *Textbook of veterinary internal medicine*, ed 5, Philadelphia, 2000, Saunders.

Ward A: Fever of unknown origin in cats and dogs, *Vet Med* 80:40-52, 1985.

55. Lymphadenopathy

Astrid Nielssen

1. What is meant by the term lymphadenopathy?

The term lymphadenopathy is most commonly used to refer to enlargement of one or more lymph nodes. Lymph node enlargement typically arises secondary to either proliferation of cells arising from within the node or infiltration from cells arising outside of the node. Regional lymphadenopathy is the term used to refer to enlargement of one or more lymph nodes draining a focal anatomic area. Generalized lymphadenopathy is the term used to refer to enlargement of multiple lymph nodes draining multiple anatomic regions.

2. What is meant by the term reactive lymphadenopathy?

When normal lymphoid or mononuclear phagocytic cells within a lymph node proliferate in response to antigenic stimulation, the term reactive lymphadenopathy (or hyperplasia) is used to describe that condition.

3. What are some potential causes of reactive lymphadenopathy?

Any source of chronic antigenic stimulation can result in a reactive lymphadenopathy, including neoplastic disease, infections, and immune-mediated disease.

4. What is meant by the term lymphadenitis?

When inflammatory cells predominate within a lymph node the term lymphadenitis is used to describe that condition. The term suppurative lymphadenitis is used if neutrophils predominate; the term granulomatous lymphadenitis is used if macrophages predominate; and the term eosinophilic lymphadenitis is used if eosinophils predominate.

5. What are some potential causes of lymphadenitis in the dog?

Suppurative lymphadenitis can result from bacterial or fungal infections, enlarging tumors, infarction, or immune-mediated disease. Granulomatous lymphadenitis can result from certain bacterial and fungal infections, chronic immune-mediated diseases, foreign bodies, protozoal infection, or algal infection. Eosinophilic lymphadenitis can result from chronic allergic skin disease, parasitism, mast cell tumors, and phycomycosis.

6. What is meant by the term infiltrative lymphadenopathy?

When neoplastic or inflammatory cells infiltrate and displace the normal population of cells within a lymph node, this condition is referred to as an infiltrative lymphadenopathy.

7. Which lymph nodes are palpable during physical examination of the dog?

Mandibular, prescapular, superficial inguinal, and popliteal lymph nodes are routinely palpable in healthy dogs. Axillary lymph nodes are also sometimes palpable in healthy dogs. Lymph nodes that may become palpable when sufficiently enlarged include the facial, retropharyngeal, mesenteric, and sublumbar nodes.

Enlarged lymph nodes are typically firm, euthermic, and nonpainful on palpation, unless lymphadenitis is present, in which case the nodes may be soft and warm, and palpation may be associated with discomfort. Dogs with lymphadenitis or neoplastic disease may have extracapsular adhesions, resulting in reduced mobility of the node.

8. How should a dog with lymphadenopathy be investigated?

A thorough history and physical examination can help to identify possible causes for the lymphadenopathy, as well as the extent of the disease. Regional lymphadenopathy should prompt especially close investigation for local disease. Marked lymphadenopathy (lymph nodes greater than 5 times normal size) occurs most commonly with lymphosarcoma and lymphadenitis, although it can also occasionally be seen in dogs with salmon poisoning. Mild lymph node enlargement is typically seen more often with other diseases.

A minimum database (complete blood count, serum biochemistry profile, and urinalysis) is indicated for the workup in most of these dogs, particularly those with generalized lymphadenopathy. Cytologic assessment of lymph node aspirates can often provide conclusive diagnoses in many cases, although histopathologic analysis of a biopsy specimen may be required in others. Additional investigations that may be indicated in individual cases include diagnostic imaging (radiographs and ultrasound), serologic testing, immunologic testing, bone marrow aspiration, and culture of tissue sample.

9. How should a dog with lymphadenopathy be treated?

Treatment and prognosis are dependent on the underlying cause of the lymph node changes. Surgical excision of abscessed lymph nodes may be of benefit in some cases.

BIBLIOGRAPHY

Couto CGL: Lymphadenopathy and splenomegaly. In Nelson RW, Couto CG, editors: *Essentials of small animal internal medicine*, St. Louis, 1992, Mosby.

Couto CG, Hammer AS: Diseases of the lymph nodes and the spleen. In Ettinger SJ, Feldman EC, editors: *Textbook of veterinary internal medicine*, ed 4, Philadelphia, 1995, Saunders.

Fox PR, Petrie JP, Suter PF: Peripheral vascular disease. In Ettinger SJ, Feldman EC, editors: *Textbook of veterinary internal medicine*, ed 5, Philadelphia, 2000, Saunders.

Thomas JS: Disease of lymph nodes and lymphatics. In Morgan RV, Bright RM, Swartout MS, editors: *Handbook of small animal practice*, Philadelphia, 2003, Saunders.

56. Joint Disease

Astrid Nielssen

1. What categories of disease can affect joints?

Diseases of the muscles, tendons, or ligaments associated with a joint; articular fractures; developmental and congenital disorders (e.g., osteochondrosis desiccans, hip dysplasia); metabolic, dietary, and endocrine abnormalities; neoplasia (e.g., synovial cell sarcoma); and various arthritides can all be associated with joint dysfunction and disease.

2. What are the definitions of arthropathy and arthritis?

An arthropathy is any disease affecting a joint. An arthropathy can affect a single joint (monoarticular arthropathy or monoarthropathy) or many joints (polyarticular arthropathy or polyarthropathy). Arthritis is defined as any condition causing inflammation within a joint. Arthritis can also be described as affecting one (mono) or multiple (poly) joints.

3. How can arthritis be classified?

Arthritis can generally be classified as either primarily inflammatory or noninflammatory in nature. Systemic signs of illness can be seen in association with inflammatory joint diseases and can include fever and lethargy. Inflammatory joint diseases can be either infectious or immune-mediated and are characterized by inflammatory changes within the synovium and synovial fluid. Immune-mediated joint diseases are typically further categorized, based on radiographic findings, as either erosive or nonerosive. Although commonly referred to as arthritis, degenerative joint disease is noninflammatory. It is associated with degenerative changes in the joint cartilage, absence of inflammation in the synovium or synovial fluid, and absence of systemic signs of illness.

4.   What are some of the possible causes of infectious polyarthritis?

Numerous agents have been identified as causing arthritis in the dog, including fungi, bacteria (including *Borrelia burgdorferi* and bacteremic conditions such as those associated with endocarditis and discospondylitis), bacterial L-forms, rickettsial infections (*Ehrlichia* spp., *Rickettsia rickettsii*), mycoplasma, protozoal agents, and viruses. Although a polyarthropathy is most commonly identified in association with these infections, a septic monoarthropathy in the dog may be seen in association with direct organism inoculation into the joint, resulting from trauma or other such insult. Identification of these various agents depends on obtaining a complete clinical and medical history, thorough physical examination, and appropriate diagnostic imaging and laboratory investigations (including cytologic assessments, serologic testing, and cultures).

5.   What is erosive polyarthritis?

The most common form of erosive polyarthritis in the dog is canine rheumatoid arthritis (RA). It is a rare condition seen most commonly in young to middle-aged small-breed dogs. Like all of the immune-mediated arthropathies, the most distal joints are typically affected first and most severely. Lameness, joint swelling, and systemic symptoms such as fever, lethargy, and inappetance can be seen. With time, significant joint deformity can arise in affected dogs. The cause of RA is unknown, although autoimmune and immune-mediated processes are known to be involved. Antiglobulin antibodies (referred to as rheumatoid factor) are involved. The role of immune system changes associated with a response to chronic antigenic stimulation, such as with canine distemper virus infection, is still speculative at this time.

Other forms of erosive polyarthritis that do not fit into the definition of RA have also been identified in the dog. An erosive polyarthropathy in Greyhounds has been identified. It is associated with typical symptoms of RA but also with low to negative rheumatoid factor and antinuclear antibody titer levels.

6.   How is rheumatoid arthritis diagnosed?

Typical historical and clinical findings, appropriate synovial fluid analysis results ($>5 \times 10^9$/L white blood cells, predominantly neutrophils, poor mucin quality, negative culture), and typical radiographic changes help to heighten the suspicion for a diagnosis of RA. A positive rheumatoid factor test result is present in 25% to 75% of dogs with RA. It can also be positive in dogs that do not have RA, so a positive result alone is not diagnostic for this disease. Radiographic changes that can be seen with rheumatoid arthritis include periarticular joint swelling; joint effusion; collapse of the joint space; destruction of subchondral bone; and, in advanced cases, hypertrophic exostoses, fibrous ankylosis, and angular limb deformities. Synovial membrane biopsy specimens may reveal villous hypertrophy, synovial hyperplasia, and mononuclear cell infiltration.

7.   What is nonerosive immune-mediated polyarthritis (IMPA)?

IMPA appears to be a type III immune reaction, resulting from the deposition of antigen-antibody complexes within the synovial membrane and causing activation of the inflammatory cascade. Nonerosive IMPA can be associated with systemic lupus erythematosus, chronic infections, lymphocytic-plasmacytic synovitis, neoplasia, and other chronic inflammatory disease. It can also be idiopathic in nature.

8. How is nonerosive IMPA diagnosed?

Dogs with nonerosive IMPA may have signs associated with the underlying disease process. Signs associated with joint disease are similar to those seen in dogs with erosive IMPA and can include fever, inappetance, lethargy, and lameness. The most distal joints are most frequently affected. Neck pain may be noted, either because of the intervertebral joints being affected or because of the concurrent presence of meningitis. Lymphadenopathy and muscle wasting may also be noted.

A minimum database (a complete blood count, serum biochemistry profile, and urinalysis) is recommended in all cases of suspected IMPA. Further diagnostic tests may be indicated on the basis of associated symptoms and suspected underlying diseases. Arthrocentesis of multiple joints is recommended to assess joint fluid. Normal joints should contain less than 3×10^9 white blood cells per liter. Joint radiographs can help to differentiate erosive from nonerosive disease. Serologic testing may be indicated depending on the dog's geographic location and concurrent signs. Further immunologic testing may also be indicated based on the presence of other clinical signs. Only when all other causes of IMPA have been ruled out can a diagnosis of idiopathic IMPA reasonably be made.

9. How is IMPA treated?

Any underlying causes of IMPA that are identified during diagnostic investigations are treated as indicated. Except in certain geographical locations, many infectious causes of IMPA are responsive to doxycycline. Therefore trial therapy may be a consideration, especially if extensive titer testing is not pursued. If an infectious cause of IMPA has been ruled out, then immunosuppressive therapy is indicated in the management of these immune-mediated conditions. Because of the list of differential diagnoses, it is not possible to completely rule out an infectious cause. Owners should be informed that immunosuppressive therapy could result in an infectious disease being unmasked with potentially severe adverse effects. Prednisone at immunosuppressive dosages (2 to 4 mg/kg/day) is usually the cornerstone of therapy. Should a complete remission not be obtained after 2 to 3 weeks of this therapy, as demonstrated by persistently abnormal joint fluid obtained by follow-up arthrocentesis, then additional cytotoxic drug therapy (azathioprine, cyclophosphamide, and chlorambucil) can be considered. Gold salts are reserved for refractory cases and should not be used in combination with cytotoxic drugs. RA typically requires combination therapy and is often refractory to treatment.

10. What is degenerative joint disease?

Degenerative joint disease is a consequence of damage that arises from normal stresses placed on abnormal cartilage or from abnormal stresses placed on normal cartilage (such as occurs with hip dysplasia). It can also occasionally result from trauma, hemophilia, or joint denervation. It is a disease that typically manifests clinically as slowly progressive joint pain, joint stiffness, and decreased range of motion in affected joints. It can result in the thinning of joint cartilage and joint effusion, and the production of periarticular osteophytes.

11. How can degenerative joint disease be treated?

Lifestyle changes (weight reduction, low-impact activities), palliative treatment with nonsteroidal antiinflammatory drugs, administration of chondroprotective agents, and potentially even surgical interventions may all be used in the management of degenerative joint disease.

BIBLIOGRAPHY

Bennett D: Immune-based non-erosive inflammatory joint disease of the dog. 1. Canine systemic lupus erythematosus, *J Small Anim Pract* 28:871, 1987.
Bennett D: Immune-based non-erosive inflammatory joint disease of the dog. 3. Canine idiopathic polyarthritis, *J Small Anim Pract* 28:909, 1987.

Bennett D, Kelly DF: Immune-based non-erosive inflammatory joint disease of the dog. 2. Polyarthritis/polymyositis syndrome, *J Small Anim Pract* 28: 891, 1987.

Bennett D, May C: Joint diseases of dogs and cats. In Ettinger SJ, Feldman EC, editors: *Textbook of veterinary internal medicine*, ed 4, Philadelphia, 1995, Saunders.

Carr AP, Michels G: Identifying noninfectious erosive arthritis in dogs and cats, *Vet Med* 92:804, 1997.

Carr AP, Michels G: Treating immune-mediated arthritis in dogs and cats, *Vet Med* 92:811, 1997.

Hulse DA, Johnson AL: General principles, techniques, and nonsurgical joint disease. In Fossum TW, editor: *Small animal surgery*, St. Louis, 1997, Mosby.

Magne ML. Swollen joints and lameness. In Ettinger SJ, Feldman EC, editors: *Textbook of veterinary internal medicine*, ed 4, Philadelphia, 1995, Saunders.

Rouse JK: Diseases of joints and ligaments. In Morgan RV, Bright RM, Swartout MS, editors: *Handbook of small animal practice*, Philadelphia, 2003, Saunders.

57. Edema

Astrid Nielssen

1. What is edema?

Edema refers to the excess accumulation of fluid within the tissues of the body. Edema can arise as a result of intracellular fluid accumulation. Most frequently, however, it arises as a result of fluid accumulation within the interstitial space.

2. What can cause edema resulting from intracellular fluid accumulation?

Intracellular fluid accumulation can arise when the normal transmembrane sodium gradient is not maintained. This is due to ionic pump dysfunction, a condition that can result from compromised blood flow to a tissue, or inflammation, a condition that can increase membrane permeability. The increased sodium concentration that arises in the cell draws water into the cell via osmosis and can result in marked cellular swelling.

The edema caused by intracellular swelling is typically nonpitting edema.

3. What can cause edema resulting from extracellular fluid accumulation?

There are two general causes of edema that result from extracellular fluid accumulation: increased capillary filtration and a failure of adequate lymphatic drainage. The most common causes fall into the increased capillary filtration category.

Increases in capillary permeability, hydrostatic pressure, or decreased osmotic pressure can all result in an increased capillary filtration rate. Causes of increased capillary permeability include immune reactions (e.g., histamine release), toxins, bacterial infections, ischemia, and burns. Causes of increased capillary hydrostatic pressure include high venous pressure (e.g., heart failure, venous blockage) or excessive fluid and sodium retention (e.g, acute renal failure). Decreased plasma colloid osmotic pressure results from a decreased plasma protein level, predominantly if albumin is decreased. This can be due to a failure of production (e.g., with hepatic failure) or an increased loss (e.g., with nephrotic syndrome, protein-losing enteropathy, vasculitis) of these proteins.

Edema associated with diminished lymphatic drainage (also called lymphedema) can be either primary or secondary in nature (see question 4). Edema associated with lymphatic obstruction can be especially severe because the proteins that are leaked into the extracellular space have no other means by which to be removed and provide an increased osmotic pull within the interstitium.

The edema caused by interstitial fluid accumulation is typically a pitting edema.

4. What is meant by the terms primary and secondary lymphedema?

Primary lymphedema refers to the interstitial fluid accumulation that arises from congenital abnormalities in the lymphatics or lymph nodes. This condition is rare and is most commonly associated with aplasia or dysplasia of the proximal lymph nodes or popliteal lymph nodes in the hindlimbs of young dogs. The edema may be transient or permanent and affect only the hind-limbs, or be more generalized.

Secondary lymphedema refers to the interstitial fluid accumulation that arises from acquired abnormalities of the lymphatics or lymph nodes. Some of the more common causes of acquired lymphatic obstruction include extralymphatic obstruction by tumors, surgical or other trauma, lymphangitis, and lymphadenitis.

5. How should cases of lymphedema be investigated?

A careful history and physical examination can yield many clues as to the potential underlying cause of lymphedema. A history of polydipsia and polyuria may be reported in the hypercalcemic dog with mediastinal lymphoma and pitting edema of the head, neck, and forelimbs resulting from tumor-associated obstruction of the cranial vena cava, a form of secondary edema referred to as precaval syndrome. Sublumbar lymphadenopathy may be identified in a dog with bilateral hindlimb edema. A minimum database (complete blood cell count, serum biochemistry profile, and urinalysis), a heartworm antigen test, local radiographs and ultrasound imaging, fine needle aspirates or biopsy of involved lymph nodes, affected tissues, or masses can also be valuable in the workup of the dog with lymphedema. Lymphangiography may also be indicated in the diagnostic investigation in some cases.

7. How should lymphedema be treated clinically?

Cases of secondary lymphedema are best addressed by management of the underlying condition. Animals with primary lymphedema or secondary lymphedema that cannot be resolved with treatment of the underlying disorder can be managed with pressure bandages and meticulous skin care to prevent secondary infections and complications. Additional medications that can be considered include benzopyrones (e.g., rutin), corticosteroids, and fibrinolysin inhibitors. Surgical treatment options include lymphangioplasty, lymphaticovenous shunts, and superficial to deep lymphatic anastomosis.

8. What mechanisms help to prevent the formation of edema?

Three primary factors help to prevent edema from forming. These include a low compliance of the interstitium, a remarkable ability for the lymphatics to increase flow thereby improving drainage, and the increased interstitial protein absorption resulting from increased lymphatic flow which thereby decreases the interstitial colloid osmotic pressure.

BIBLIOGRAPHY

Couto CG: Lymphadenopathy and splenomegaly, In Nelson RW, Couto CG, editors: *Essentials of small animal internal medicine*, St. Louis, 1992, Mosby.

Couto CG, Hammer AS: Diseases of the lymph nodes and the spleen, In Ettinger SJ, Feldman EC, editors: *Textbook of veterinary internal medicine*, ed 4, Philadelphia, 1995, WB Saunders Company.

Fossum TW, Miller MW: Lymphedema. Etiopathogenesis, *J Vet Intern Med* 6:283, 1992.

Fossum TW, King LA, Miller MW et al: Lymphedema. Clinical signs, diagnosis, and treatment, *J Vet Intern Med* 6:312, 1992.

Fox PR, Petrie JP, Suter PF: Peripheral vascular disease, In Ettinger SJ, Feldman EC, editors: *Textbook of veterinary internal medicine*, ed 5, Philadelphia, 2000, WB Saunders.

Guyton AC, Hall JE: The body fluid compartments: extracellular and intracellular fluids; interstitial fluid and edema, In Guyton AC, Hall JE, editors: *Textbook of medical physiology*, ed 10, Philadelphia, 2000, WB Saunders.

Thomas JS: Disease of lymph nodes and lymphatics, In Morgan RV, Bright RM, Swartout MS, editors: *Handbook of small animal practice*, Philadelphia, 2003, WB Saunders.

58. Paraneoplastic Syndromes

Astrid Nielssen

1. What is a paraneoplastic syndrome?

Paraneoplastic syndromes are various regional and systemic physiologic, metabolic, and anatomic alterations that arise as a consequence of an underlying neoplastic disease. Examples of some abnormalities that can arise from a malignancy include hypercalcemia, hyperviscosity, hyperhistaminemia, hypoglycemia, inappropriate secretion of antidiuretic hormone, hypertrophic osteopathy, fever, and cachexia. Signs of the paraneoplastic syndrome may be what actually prompt veterinary evaluation in the first place, and not signs directly associated with the tumor itself. Persistence or recurrence of the signs associated with a paraneoplastic syndrome may also be indicative of treatment failure and tumor regrowth.

2. Why is hypercalcemia sometimes identified in the canine cancer patient?

Cancer is the most common cause of hypercalcemia in the dog, and can be seen as a consequence of a wide variety of neoplasms, including most commonly lymphosarcoma. The mechanisms by which tumors produce hypercalcemia are incompletely understood and can vary, but can include increased bone resorption or increased gut and renal calcium absorption caused by production of parathyroid hormone or a parathyroid hormone-like protein (PTHrp), prostaglandins, calcitriol, and osteoclast-activating factor or osteoclast activating factor–like agents. Clinical signs are often associated with the renal effects of hypercalcemia and can include polyuria and polydipsia. Other clinical signs can include inappetence, vomiting, constipation, bradycardia, hypertension, muscle weakness, and neurologic signs including coma and seizures resulting from the effects of the high calcium levels on the gastrointestinal, cardiovascular, and neurologic systems. Treatment is directed at the underlying malignancy and, depending on the severity of the hypercalcemia, supportive treatments aimed at lowering serum calcium levels including saline diuresis, furosemide treatment, and prednisone administration; calcitonin and pamidronate may be indicated.

3. What is hyperviscosity syndrome?

Hyperviscosity syndrome is seen as a result of poor circulation due to increased protein levels or cell concentrations in the blood. Increased protein levels can be seen with neoplasms such as a multiple myeloma. Increased cell concentrations can be seen in such clonal disorders as leukemias and polycythemia vera. Hyperviscosity syndrome can result in an increased cardiac workload and compromised renal function as a result of poor perfusion. Central nervous system (bizarre behavior, seizures), and ophthalmic symptoms (tortuous retinal vessels, retinal hemorrhage, retinal detachment) can also be seen as a result of hypoxia. Hyperglobulinemias can also result in bleeding disorders as a result of the excessive protein levels inhibiting platelet function or functioning as coagulation factor inhibitors. Definitive treatment is directed at the underlying neoplasm. Supportive therapy to decrease viscosity such as parenteral fluid therapy, plasmapheresis and phlebotomy (in cases of polycythemia vera) may also be indicated.

4. Why is hyperhistaminemia sometimes identified in canine cancer patients?

Increased levels of histamine can be seen in association with mast cell tumors that degranulate as a result of cellular injury. This can be caused by trauma, chemotherapy, or temperature changes. Symptoms are associated with the action of histamine at both the H_1 and H_2 receptors and can include cutaneous erythema, pruritus, hypotension, bronchoconstriction, anaphylaxis, and gastrointestinal hemorrhage. Treatment to stabilize the mast cells with H_1 (e.g., diphenhydramine) and H_2 (e.g., cimetidine, ranitidine) blockers as well as prednisone may be of benefit in these animals. Definitive therapies include surgical excision of the tumor.

5. Why is fasting hypoglycemia sometimes identified in canine cancer patients?

Although an insulinoma is the most common neoplasm associated with marked hypoglycemia in the dog, other tumors including hepatic tumors, hemangiosarcoma, lymphoma, and leiomyosarcoma, can also be associated with this finding. Although insulinomas cause hypoglycemia as a result of excessive secretion of insulin, other neoplasms may cause this syndrome through secretion of an insulin-like substance, increased glucose use by the tumor, and impairment of normal hepatic gluconeogenesis or glycogenolysis. Signs of neurologic disease are the most commonly identified signs associated with hypoglycemia. Treatment is directed at elimination of the underlying neoplasm (usually with surgical excision) and supportive care to palliate the hypoglycemia.

6. What is the syndrome of inappropriate secretion of antidiuretic hormone (SIADH)?

SIADH arises when a neoplasm ectopically secretes an ADH-like molecule or when the hypothalamus itself inappropriately secretes excessive ADH (can sometimes be seen in response to certain chemotherapy drugs such as vincristine), resulting in the retention of excessive free water. It is an uncommon syndrome in canine cancer patients. Clinical pathologic findings include serum hypoosmolality and hyponatremia not accompanied by hyposthenuria, sustained natriesis, normal renal and adrenal gland function, and the absence of dehydration. Signs associated with this disorder can include inappetence, vomiting, and weakness, and can progress to seizures and coma. Treatment is directed at elimination of the underlying neoplasm or drug and water restriction in mild cases. More aggressive therapies may be necessary in severe cases and include hypertonic saline, furosemide, and demeclocycline administration.

7. What is hypertrophic osteopathy?

Hypertrophic osteopathy (also referred to as hypertrophic pulmonary osteopathy) is a condition that arises when periosteal new bone is formed, localized to the terminal epiphyses of the long bones and the phalanges, affecting all four limbs. This condition is most commonly associated with a primary or metastatic intrathoracic neoplasm, although it is also occasionally noted in association with other lung disease and extrathoracic neoplasms. Dogs affected with this syndrome may demonstrate lameness and warm, painful swelling of the affected bones. The cause of this syndrome is unknown but suspected to be neurovascularly mediated. Elimination of the pulmonary tumor may resolve the syndrome, whereas glucocorticoids may temporarily palliate it. Intrathoracic vagotomy has also been reported to be helpful.

8. Why are fevers seen in association with neoplastic diseases?

A persistent or recurrent fever may be noted in the canine cancer patient, potentially in association with necrotic tumors or secondary infections. However, it can also be noted in animals in which such complications are not present, either as a result of pyrogens produced by the tumor itself or through lymphokines that are produced in response to tumor-associated immune system activation. The persistence of significant fever can be associated with increased morbidity. Diagnostic investigations should rule out other potential causes of pyrexia, and any identified conditions managed appropriately. Effective therapy of the underlying malignancy should resolve the fever. If necessary, symptomatic therapy of the fever with nonsteroidal antiinflammatory drugs may help to alleviate clinical symptoms associated with this paraneoplastic condition.

9. What is cancer cachexia?

Cancer cachexia is likely the most common paraneoplastic syndrome in veterinary medicine. It arises from derangements in fat, protein, and carbohydrate metabolism and results in weight loss, muscle wasting, and immune system dysfunction. It is most commonly associated with inappetent or anorectic dogs. The exact pathophysiologic changes associated with this syndrome are unknown, but it is believed that tumor-associated hormonal or cytokine-mediated changes may play important roles. It is unquestionably associated with high morbidity. Ensuring adequate and appropriate nutritional intake may help to minimize complications associated with this syndrome.

BIBLIOGRAPHY

Bergman PJ: Paraneoplastic syndromes, In Morgan RV, Bright RM, Swartout MS, editors: *Handbook of small animal practice*, Philadelphia, 2003, WB Saunders.

Fox LE: The paraneoplastic disorders, In Bonagura JD, Kirk RW, editors: *Kirk's current veterinary therapy XII*, Philadelphia, 1995, WB Saunders.

Morrison WB: Paraneoplastic syndromes and the tumors that cause them, In Morrison WB, editor: *Cancer in dogs and cats*, Philadelphia, 1998, Lippincott Williams & Wilkins.

Ogilvie GK: Paraneoplastic syndromes, In Ettinger SJ, Feldman EC, editors: *Textbook of veterinary internal medicine*, ed 5, Philadelphia, 2000, WB Saunders.

Vail DM, Ogilvie GK, Wheeler SL: Metabolic alterations in patients with cancer cachexia, *Compend Contin Educ Pract Vet* 12:381, 1990.

Section IX
Hemolymphatic Disorders
Section Editor: Astrid Nielssen

59. Canine Lymphoma
Astrid Nielssen

1. What is lymphoma?

Lymphoma (also referred to as malignant lymphoma or lymphosarcoma) is defined as the malignant proliferation of lymphoid cells, originating from outside of the bone marrow, in solid organs such as lymph nodes, liver, or spleen. It is the origin of this malignancy from outside of the bone marrow that differentiates lymphoma from lymphoid leukemias. Lymphoma is the most common hematopoietic malignancy in dogs.

2. What are the predisposing factors for, and causes of, the development of canine lymphoma?

Most dogs with lymphoma are middle-age or older (6 years or older). An increased incidence of this disease in certain breeds such as Boxers, Scottish Terriers, Basset Hounds, Airedale Terriers, Chow Chows, German Shepherds, Poodles, Saint Bernards, English Bulldogs, Beagles, and Golden Retrievers has been reported. No sex predilection has been reported.

The cause of lymphoma in dogs is unknown and suspected to be multifactorial in nature. Although some studies have shown an association between pesticide use and magnetic field exposure, and an increased incidence of this disease in middle-age, related purebred dogs, the significance of these associations is controversial.

3. How is canine lymphoma classified and staged?

Canine lymphoma can be classified by anatomic site, histologic or cytologic phenotype, and immunophenotype. Clinical stage can be established based on the World Health Organization (WHO) clinical staging guidelines for domestic animals with lymphoma.

The four anatomic classification sites include the following:

1. Multicentric: generalized lymph node, hepatic, splenic, or bone marrow involvement.
2. Alimentary: solitary, diffuse, or multifocal gastrointestinal tract infiltration, hepatic, splenic, or mesenteric lymph node involvement.
3. Extranodal: renal, central nervous system, cutaneous, any organ or tissue.
4. Mediastinal (thymic): mediastinal lymphadenopathy or bone marrow involvement.

More than 80% of canine lymphoma cases will be multicentric in nature. Mediastinal lymphoma is the least commonly seen form of canine lymphoma.

There are many histologic and cytologic grading schemes that can be used (e.g., Kiel, National Cancer Institute Working Foundation) to grade canine lymphomas based on tumor architecture, mitotic index, and cellular features. Regardless of which scheme is used, most canine lymphomas correlate to medium and high-grade non-Hodgkin's lymphomas in human beings.

Immunophenotyping of canine lymphomas is used to determine whether the tumor is of B- or T-cell origin. Approximately 70% to 80% of canine lymphomas are of B-cell origin. Approximately 20% to 30% are of T-cell origin, and rarely are non-B, non-T cell tumors identified.

The WHO clinical staging for domestic animals with lymphoma guidelines are as follows:

Stage I: Single lymph node involvement

Stage II: Multiple lymph node involvement in a regional area

Stage III: Generalized lymphadenopathy

Stage IV: Hepatic or splenic involvement (with or without stage III)

Stage V: Bone marrow or blood involvement or any nonlymphoid organ (with or without stage I to IV)

All stages are further substaged depending on whether clinical signs of disease are absent (substage a) or present (substage b).

4. What are the most common historical complaints made by owners of dogs with lymphoma?

Most dogs (more than 80%) with lymphoma are not clinically ill at the time of diagnosis (WHO substage a). Of the minority of dogs that are WHO substage b at presentation, the most common clinical complaints include nonspecific signs such as inappetence, weight loss, and lethargy. Other more specific clinical signs may reflect the particular anatomic location of the tumor burden in each individual case. Those dogs with paraneoplastic hypercalcemia (10%-20% of dogs with the multicentric form of lymphoma, up to 40% of the dogs with mediastinal lymphoma) may show polydipsia, polyuria, and other less specific clinical signs associated with their elevated serum calcium levels. Dogs with severe bone marrow involvement may have significant peripheral cytopenias and have clinical signs associated with that complication (e.g., infection resulting from neutropenia, hemorrhage resulting from thrombocytopenia, anemia).

5. Which aspects of the physical examination are of particular importance for the dog suspected to have lymphoma?

All accessible lymph nodes should be carefully palpated for enlargement; this includes performing a digital rectal examination. Thorough abdominal palpation can help to identify hepatomegaly, splenomegaly, renomegaly, or abnormalities in the gastrointestinal tract, and potential abdominal lymph node enlargement. Conscientious thoracic auscultation may help to identify pulmonary involvement or the presence of a pleural effusion. Mucous membrane evaluation may identify pallor, icterus, or petechiae. An ocular examination, including fundic evaluation, is also essential because as many as 50% of dogs with lymphoma can have ocular changes associated with their disease.

6. How is a diagnosis of canine lymphoma obtained?

The cornerstone of lymphoma diagnosis in the dog is microscopic confirmation of the disease. The cytologic evaluation of fine-needle aspirates from enlarged lymph nodes by a clinical pathologist may be adequate to make the diagnosis in most cases. It is important to avoid aspirating lymph nodes draining reactive areas (e.g., the submandibular lymph nodes) to prevent confusion between reactive hyperplasia and lymphoma on cytologic assessment. Cytologic analysis of aspirates from affected organs (e.g., liver, spleen, kidneys) or of fluids (pleural, abdominal, cerebrospinal fluid) may also provide the diagnosis. A tissue biopsy for conclusive histologic confirmation of lymphoma will be necessary in some cases of lymphoma.

7. What diagnostic investigations are indicated in the workup of the canine lymphoma patient?

A complete blood cell count, serum biochemistry panel, urinalysis, thoracic and abdominal radiographs, abdominal (or thoracic) ultrasound, and bone marrow aspirate and core biopsy are indicated to thoroughly stage a canine lymphoma patient. Additional investigations (e.g., cerebrospinal fluid tap) may be appropriate depending on the particulars of a given case. The minimum database collected for a dog whose owners are contemplating chemotherapy should include a complete blood cell count, serum biochemistry profile, and urinalysis.

8. What therapy is indicated for the management of canine lymphoma?
Canine lymphoma is a systemic disease and therefore is best managed with chemotherapy. In the rare cases of focal disease, surgery or radiation therapy may be considered. In these cases, systemic disease usually does develop months to years later. Adjunctive chemotherapy may be initiated at the time of local treatment or delayed until the development of systemic disease in these cases.

9. What are the expected survival times of canine lymphoma patients?
The average survival time of untreated dogs after the diagnosis of lymphoma is 4 to 6 weeks. The large number of chemotherapy protocols available for the treatment of canine lymphoma is associated with different remission rates and median survival times. The most complex chemotherapy protocols combine cyclophosphamide (C), doxorubicin (H for hydroxydaunorubicin), vincristine (O for Oncovin), and prednisone (P). Remission rates are around 80% with the various CHOP protocols and median survival time is 12 months. Approximately 20% to 25% of dogs will be alive 2 years after the initiation of therapy with these protocols. Single-agent chemotherapy with doxorubicin alone results in remission rates in approximately 75% of cases and a median survival time of 7 months. Prednisone administered alone at immunosuppressive doses (2 mg/kg/day by mouth) can result in short-lived remissions of 1 to 2 months. It is important to warn clients that the administration of prednisone before the administration of a more aggressive course of chemotherapy may result in shorter remission and survival times.

10. What factors influence response to chemotherapy in canine lymphoma?
The presence of signs of clinical illness (WHO substage b) and having a T-cell lymphoma are two well-established negative prognostic indicators for canine lymphoma patients. Other factors that have been reported to convey a poorer prognosis include cranial mediastinal lymphadenopathy, hypercalcemia (although this may be associated with the increased incidence of T-cell tumors in hypercalcemic dogs), prior prolonged glucocorticoid therapy, male sex, low proliferation rate, and P-glycoprotein expression. WHO stage, with the exception of advanced stage V disease, does not likely significantly affect clinical prognosis. Histologic grade is of uncertain prognostic significance.

BIBLIOGRAPHY

Dhaliwal RS, Kitchell BE, Messick JB: Canine lymphosarcoma: clinical features, *Compend Contin Educ Pract Vet* 25:572, 2003.
Dhaliwal RS, Kitchell BE, Messick JB: Canine lymphosarcoma: diagnosis and treatment, *Compend Contin Educ Pract Vet* 25:584, 2003.
Thomas JS: Diseases of lymph nodes and lymphatics, In Morgan RV, Bright RM, Swartout, MS, editors: *Handbook of small animal practice*, ed 4, Philadelphia, 2003, WB Saunders.
Vail DM: Hematopoietic tumors, In Ettinger SJ, Feldman EC, editors: *Textbook of veterinary internal medicine*, ed 5, Philadelphia, 2000, WB Saunders.
Vail DM: Lymphoma, In Feldman BF, Zinkl JG, Jain NC, editors: *Schalm's veterinary hematology*, ed 5, Philadelphia, 2000, Lippincott Williams and Wilkins.
Vail DM: Treatment and prognosis of canine malignant lymphoma, In Bonagura JD, editor: *Kirk's current veterinary therapy XII*, Philadelphia, 1995, WB Saunders.
Vonderhaar MA, Morrison WB: Lymphoma, In Morrison WB, editor: *Cancer in dogs and cats*, Philadelphia, 1998, Lippincott Williams & Wilkins.

60. Hemangiosarcoma

Astrid Nielssen

1. What is hemangiosarcoma (HSA)?

HSA (also referred to as hemangioendothelioma or angiosarcoma) is a highly aggressive malignant neoplasm of the blood vessel endothelial cells. It is a cancer that can be found in almost any organ, but in dogs is found most often in the spleen. Other common primary anatomic locations include the right atrium, cutaneous, and subcutaneous tissues. Some forms of cutaneous/subcutaneous HSA appear to have a lower metastatic potential and less aggressive biologic behavior.

2. What are the predisposing factors for the development of canine HSA?

Older dogs (8 years or older) and large breed dogs (German Shepherds, Pointers, Boxers, and Labrador and Golden Retrievers) are overrepresented for the visceral forms of the disease. Some investigators have also reported an increased incidence in male dogs.

Middle-age or older dogs (4 years and older) and Whippets, Basset Hounds, and Dalmatians are overrepresented for the dermal forms of the disease. Sun exposure may contribute to the development of this form of the disease.

3. How is canine HSA staged?

Splenic HSA can be categorized by a three-stage classification scheme. The stages are as follows:

Stage I: Tumor confined to the spleen.
Stage II: Ruptured splenic tumor with or without regional lymph node involvement.
Stage III: Distant lymph node or other tissue metastases.
Hemoperitoneum or splenic rupture is associated with a worse prognosis.

A three-stage classification scheme for canine cutaneous/subcutaneous HSA has also been proposed, with the different stages associated with differing prognoses. The stages are as follows:

Stage I: Primary tumor confined to the dermis.
Stage II: Primary tumor involving the hypodermis with or without dermal involvement.
Stage III: Primary tumor with underlying muscular involvement.

Stage I tumors have been associated with a greater than 2-year median survival time with surgery alone, whereas stage II and III tumors have been associated with median survival times between approximately 6 and 10 months, respectively, when treated with surgery alone.

4. What are the most common complaints made by owners of dogs with HSA?

Owners may report the sudden onset of collapse or weakness associated with splenic tumor rupture. Cardiac HSA may result in signs of right-sided heart failure associated with pericardial effusion and tamponade. Other signs of visceral HSA depend on the anatomic location of the primary tumor or its metastases. Metastases arise most commonly in the liver, omentum, mesentery, and lungs, but can also arise in the kidney, brain, muscle, peritoneum, lymph nodes, adrenal glands, and diaphragm. The common concurrent presence of extensive coagulation abnormalities may also result in signs associated with a hemorrhagic diathesis.

With cutaneous disease, owners may report noticing a dark red to purple superficial plaquelike to raised lesion. These lesions are most commonly identified in hairless regions such as the ventral abdomen. Subcutaneous lesions can occur anywhere and can range from soft fluctuant to firm masses. Discoloration and ulceration are common with these lesions.

5. How is a diagnosis of canine HSA made?

The diagnosis of canine HSA is often strongly suspected based on classic clinical history and presentation, results of a complete blood count and coagulation profile, radiographic and ultrasonographic findings. Cytologic analysis of fine-needle aspirates or impression smears can occasionally be helpful in making the diagnosis, although analysis of effusions is a low-yield diagnostic. Ultimately, a diagnosis of HSA needs to be confirmed with histopathologic testing.

6. What diagnostics should be performed in the dog suspected to have HSA?

Recommended diagnostic tests include a minimum database (complete blood cell count, serum biochemistry profile, and urinalysis), coagulation profile, thoracic and abdominal radiographs, abdominal and cardiac ultrasound, and an electrocardiogram. Common abnormalities noted on the complete blood count include regeneration with or without concurrent anemia, red blood cell fragmentation and acanthocytosis, thrombocytopenia, and neutrophilia. Approximately 50% of dogs with visceral HSA may have sufficiently extensive coagulation abnormalities to suggest the presence of disseminated intravascular coagulation or a localized tumor associated consumptive coagulopathy (localized consumptive coagulopathy or Kasabach-Merritt syndrome); therefore all dogs with suspected HSA should have a coagulation panel assessed. Three radiographic views of the thorax should be obtained to assess for the presence of thoracic metastases. Abdominal radiographs and ultrasound are useful imaging techniques to further stage this disorder. Because one quarter of dogs with splenic HSA have right atrial HSA, an echocardiogram is also a helpful diagnostic tool. Arrhythmias are common with splenic involvement, and may be seen with cardiac HSA, therefore making an electrocardiogram also part of the database in these animals.

It is important that even dogs with suspected cutaneous or subcutaneous HSA have a full staging workup done before the decision to proceed with surgical intervention because those primary tumors can metastasize to the viscera and conversely visceral forms of HSA can metastasize to the skin or subcutis.

7. How should canine HSA be treated?

Surgery for cutaneous and subcutaneous canine HSA is recommended. Adjunctive doxorubicin-based chemotherapy should be administered to those animals with stage II or III disease. Radiation therapy for localized stage II and III disease might also be a reasonable consideration.

With respect to visceral HSA, splenectomy alone in cases in which this organ is involved results in median survival times between 19 to 65 days. Excision of right atrial tumors results in a median survival time of 4 months. The addition of doxorubicin-based chemotherapy to surgery improves median survival times to roughly 6 months, provided there is no evidence of gross metastasis at the time of surgery. If gross metastasis is present at the time of surgery, median survival time is prolonged to only 2 months with adjunctive doxorubicin-based chemotherapy.

The most effective chemotherapy protocol for HSA has not yet been established. Traditional protocols combined vincristine or cyclophosphamide and doxorubicin. The addition of cyclophosphamide or vincristine has not been shown to result in longer median survival times than doxorubicin alone.

BIBLIOGRAPHY

Chun R: Evidence based medicine for canine hemangiosarcoma, ACVIM 18th annual meeting, Seattle, WA, 2000.

Clifford CA, Mackin AJ, Henry CJ: Treatment of canine hemangiosarcoma: 2000 and beyond, *J Vet Intern Med* 14:479, 2000.

Morrison WB: Blood vascular, lymphatic, and splenic cancer, In Morrison WB, editor: *Cancer in dogs and cats*, Philadelphia, 1998, Lippincott Williams & Wilkins.

Ogilvie GK, Powers BE, Mallinckrodt CH et al: Surgery and doxorubicin in dogs with hemangiosarcoma, *J Vet Intern Med* 10:379, 1996.

Page RL, Thrall DE: Soft tissue sarcomas and hemangiosarcomas, In Ettinger SJ, Feldman EC, editors: *Textbook of veterinary internal medicine*, ed 5, Philadelphia, 2000, WB Saunders.

Rishniw M, Lewis DC: Localized consumptive coagulopathy associated with cutaneous hemangiosarcoma in a dog, *J Am Anim Hosp Assoc* 30:261, 1994.

Ward H, Fox LE, Calderwood-Mays MB et al: Cutaneous hemangiosarcoma in 25 dogs: a retrospective study, *J Vet Intern Med* 8:345, 1994.

61. Approach to the Bleeding Dog

Astrid Nielssen

1. How should the bleeding animal initially be assessed?

It is essential that all hemorrhaging dogs be carefully examined at presentation to ensure that they are clinically stable. Intravenous crystalloids, colloids, or blood products, as well as other supportive care measures, may be needed to stabilize animals demonstrating signs of cardiovascular shock. Dogs with hemorrhage that can be decreased through therapeutic measures, such as the application of focal pressure or tourniquets, should have such measures applied. If possible, efforts should be made to try and collect any necessary laboratory samples before the initiation of supportive or other therapies that might alter their results (e.g., collect any samples for coagulation testing before the administration of blood products). Care must be taken to avoid iatrogenic injuries to the dog (intramuscular injections, cystocentesis, using the jugular vein for blood draws). After the animal is clinically stable, it is then essential, based on clinical history and examination findings, to attempt to determine whether the hemorrhage is the expected consequence of a traumatic injury, or whether or not further investigation into a possible underlying hemostatic disorder is indicated.

2. How can a dog's history be of value in determining the cause of a coagulopathy?

A thorough history is absolutely essential in assessing the dog suspected of having a coagulopathy. Puppies with a prior history of bleeding episodes, a family history of bleeding, and puppies of certain breeds may be likely to have an inherited coagulopathy. Farm dogs may have been exposed to an anticoagulant rodenticide. Aspirin or other nonsteroidal antiinflammatory medication administered by an owner may cause sufficient platelet dysfunction to result in a bleeding problem.

3. What findings on general physical examination might help indicate the nature of an animal's bleeding disorder?

Detection of petechiae, ecchymoses, or mucosal hemorrhage (e.g., gingival hemorrhage) indicates disorders of primary hemostasis, such as a thrombocytopenia or thrombocytopathia (abnormal platelet function). Large-volume hemorrhages into body cavities such as those resulting in hemothorax, hemoabdomen, and hemarthrosis are typical of disorders of secondary hemostasis, such as clotting factor deficiencies.

4. What in-clinic diagnostics can be useful in assessing the animal suspected of having a bleeding problem?

1. Packed cell volume/total protein determination: Used to assess the degree of blood loss suffered by a dog, although it is important to be aware that the values of the dog with acute hemorrhage are not likely to yet reflect the true extent of the blood loss.
2. Assessment of a blood smear: Used to estimate if adequate numbers of platelets are present.

3. Activated clotting time: Used to assess the intrinsic coagulation system. It is similar to, but less sensitive than an activated partial thromboplastin time. It can be reasonably run in almost any practice. Normal dog values are in the range of 60 to 90 seconds.
4. Buccal mucosal bleeding time: Used to evaluate the time it takes for a surface buccal mucosal incision to stop bleeding. It is a test of primary hemostasis. A double blade device is most commonly used to make the incisions in dogs. Normal buccal mucosal bleeding time is between 2 and 4.5 minutes in the dog.

5. How can additional coagulation tests be run if rapid access to the necessary laboratory is not available?
With a little preparation and attention to detail, most clinics can manage to send out samples for coagulation testing. Advance consultation with the appropriate laboratory to receive specific instructions regarding appropriate sample collection and shipping is recommended. Be careful to avoid hemolysis during collection of any samples for coagulation testing and be sure to be exact with respect to the ratio of blood to anticoagulant. Take care to ensure hemostasis occurs at all venipuncture sites. Most samples will likely need to be immediately centrifuged after collection and the plasma collected and frozen before shipping. Plastic tubes and pipets should be used for this process.

BIBLIOGRAPHY

Boudreaux MK: Platelet and coagulation disorders, In Morgan RV, Bright RM, Swartout MS, editors: *Handbook of small animal practice*, Philadelphia, 2003, WB Saunders.
Brooks M: Coagulopathies and thrombosis, In Ettinger SJ, Feldman EC, editors: *Textbook of veterinary internal medicine*, ed 5, Philadelphia, 2000, WB Saunders.
Couto CG: Disorders of hemostasis, In Nelson RW, Couto CG editors: *Essentials of small animal internal medicine*, St. Louis, 1992, Mosby.
Couto CG: Spontaneous bleeding disorders, In Bonagura JD, editor: *Kirk's current veterinary therapy XII*, Philadelphia, 1995, WB Saunders.
Hohenhaus AE: Bleeding disorders in dogs and cats, Proceedings of the ACVIM 17th annual meeting, Chicago, IL, 1999.

62. Anemia

Astrid Nielssen

1. What is anemia?
Anemia is defined as a decreased hemoglobin concentration, hematocrit, or total red blood cell count. It results in a decrease in the oxygen carrying capacity of the blood and compromised tissue oxygen delivery. In dogs, anemia can be categorized as mild, moderate, severe, or very severe. A mild anemia corresponds to a hematocrit of 30% to 37%, a moderate anemia to a hematocrit of 20% to 29%, a severe anemia to a hematocrit of 13% to 19%, and a very severe anemia to a hematocrit of less than 13%.

2. What causes anemia?
The causes of anemia can be thought of as occurring in one of the following three main categories:
1. Decreased production of red blood cells
2. Increased loss of red blood cells
3. Increased destruction of red blood cells

3. **What are some causes of the decreased production of red blood cells in the dog?**

There are a large number of causes of decreased red blood cell production. These can be divided into causes associated with conditions within the bone marrow itself (primary causes) or causes outside of the bone marrow (secondary causes). Primary bone marrow disorders resulting in decreased red blood cell production include toxicities arising from chemotherapeutics, immunosuppressants, estrogens, various other drugs, infectious diseases (e.g., chronic ehrlichiosis), marrow fibrosis, myelophthisis, ineffective erythropoiesis, and stem cell disorders including immune-mediated destruction of red blood cell precursors. Secondary causes of decreased red blood cell production include endocrine disease (e.g., hypothyroidism, hypoadrenocorticism), metabolic disease (e.g., renal disease, portosystemic shunt), nutritional deficiencies (e.g., iron or cobalamin deficiency), and chronic inflammatory disease.

4. **What are some causes of increased red blood cell loss in the dog?**

Traumatic injuries, gastrointestinal disease resulting in ulceration, excessive parasitism, ruptured tumors, and coagulopathies can all result in significant red blood cell loss.

5. **What are some causes of increased red blood cell destruction in the dog?**

Red blood cell destruction can arise as a result of various toxins (e.g., onions, zinc), certain infectious agents (*Babesia* spp.), metabolic defects, and cellular fragmentation (e.g., fibrin strand injury), or it can result from immune-mediated hemolysis.

6. **How are anemias classified morphologically?**

Mean cell volume (MCV) and mean cell hemoglobin concentration (MCHC) can be used to classify anemias based on red blood cell morphology. Macrocytic hypochromic, normocytic normochromic, and microcytic hypochromic are the three patterns of anemia identified most commonly in the dog and can typically be associated with regenerative anemias, nonregenerative anemias, and iron-deficiency anemias, respectively.

7. **What is meant by a regenerative anemia?**

The term *regenerative* indicates that the bone marrow is responding appropriately to the decreased total red blood cell mass by increasing red blood cell production. This is evidenced in the complete blood count by the presence of reticulocytes. Reticulocytes can be seen within 2 to 4 days after the onset of an anemia. Regenerative anemias can be seen with anemias caused by either red blood cell loss or increased red blood cell destruction. The absolute reticulocyte count is the best way to determine if an anemia is regenerative. The percentage reticulocytes is multiplied by the red blood cell number (per microliter) and then this is divided by 100 to determine the reticulocytes per microliter. A value greater than 60,000 is considered consistent with regeneration.

8. **How should the anemic animal be assessed?**

A thorough history, physical examination, and complete blood cell count, including a reticulocyte count and careful blood smear evaluation, are essential. Additional tests that might be indicated can be determined based on these initial results, but could include a serum biochemistry profile, a urinalysis, specific endocrine testing, a fecal flotation and occult blood test, bone marrow evaluation, a coagulation profile, and serum iron assays.

9. **How does the body compensate for anemia?**

The body has many compensatory mechanisms in place to help improve oxygen delivery to tissues in the presence of an anemia. Animals that have had enough time for these mechanisms to be fully activated are able to better compensate for their disease and are therefore commonly far less symptomatic at the same hematocrit level than are animals that have very acute disease. This is why animals with anemias resulting from decreased red blood cell production are less likely to display profound signs of anemia than are those with anemias resulting from acute increased red blood cell loss or destruction. Compensatory mechanisms include decreased red blood cell oxygen affinity through the increased production of 2,3-diphosphoglycerate, decreased tissue perfusion to nonvital organs, increased cardiac output primarily through an increase in heart rate, and increased erythropoietin secretion.

BIBLIOGRAPHY

Ahn AH, Cotter SM: Approach to the anemic patient, In Bonagura JD, editor: *Kirk's current veterinary therapy XII*, Philadelphia, 1995, WB Saunders.

Aird B: Clinical and hematological manifestations of anemia, In Feldman BF, Zinkl JG, Jain NC, editors: *Schalm's veterinary hematology*, ed 5, Philadelphia, 2000, Lippincott Williams & Wilkins.

Fisher DJ: Disorders of red blood cells, In Morgan RV, Bright RM, Swartout MS, editors: *Handbook of small animal practice*, Philadelphia, 2003, WB Saunders.

Rogers KS: Anemia, In Ettinger SJ, Feldman EC, editors: *Textbook of veterinary internal medicine*, ed 5, Philadelphia, 2000, WB Saunders.

Tvedten H, Weiss DJ: Classification and laboratory evaluation of anemia, In Feldman BF, Zinkl JG, Jain NC, editors: *Schalm's veterinary hematology*, ed 5, Philadelphia, 2000, Lippincott Williams & Wilkins.

63. Polycythemia

Astrid Nielssen

1. What is polycythemia?

Polycythemia (erythrocytosis) is defined as an increase in the number of red blood cells per liter above the normal range.

2. What is the difference between relative and absolute polycythemia?

Relative polycythemia is characterized by the presence of an increased hematocrit with a normal total red blood cell number. It can be the result of abnormal fluid balance resulting in decreased plasma volume as might be seen in dehydration, or it might arise secondary to splenic contraction.

Absolute polycythemia is characterized by the presence of an increased hematocrit with an increased total red blood cell number.

3. What can cause absolute polycythemia?

Absolute polycythemia can be further characterized as being primary (polycythemia vera, polycythemia rubra vera) or secondary in nature. Secondary polycythemia results from excessive production of erythropoietin. The excessive erythropoietin might arise in response to systemic hypoxia resulting from cardiac disease, pulmonary disease, or a hemoglobinopathy. This is an appropriate physiologic response to tissue hypoxia. In other cases of polycythemia, there is increased erythropoietin secretion without systemic hypoxia. This might occur as a result of diseases in the kidney such as a renal carcinoma. In human beings, this form of secondary polycythemia has also been identified with other types of tumors and nonneoplastic renal disease.

4. What is polycythemia vera?

Primary polycythemia is considered to be a myeloproliferative disorder, resulting from the clonal expansion of erythroid precursors, which do not require, or require little, erythropoietin for development. This is a rare condition in the dog; relative and secondary causes of polycythemia are diagnosed far more frequently. Historical signs reported for dogs diagnosed with polycythemia vera include red mucous membranes, congested scleral vessels, weakness, hemorrhage, and various neurologic signs. The latter three signs most commonly arise as a result of hyperviscosity syndrome.

5. How should a dog with polycythemia be investigated?

The possibility of a relative polycythemia is ruled out on the basis of historic and clinical findings. Diagnostics often indicated for the workup of a dog with secondary polycythemia include a complete blood cell count, serum biochemistry profile, urinalysis, arterial blood gas, thoracic and abdominal radiographs, cardiac and abdominal ultrasound, bone marrow aspirate, and serum erythropoietin level to rule in or out the various differential diagnoses (e.g., cardiopulmonary disease, renal tumors, other neoplasms) that can result in a secondary polycythemia. The exclusion of any causes of secondary polycythemia and typically a low to normal serum erythropoietin level are findings consistent with a diagnosis of primary polycythemia vera.

6. How should polycythemia be treated?

Relative polycythemia from dehydration can be treated with the correction of fluid deficits and management of the underlying disorder. Polycythemia resulting from splenic contraction is not of clinical consequence.

In cases of appropriate secondary polycythemia (e.g., secondary to cardiopulmonary disease), reduction of the hematocrit may not be indicated, and therapy directed at the primary clinical disease may be all that is warranted. If clinical signs are associated with the polycythemia, however, small volume phlebotomy (5 ml/kg at a time) coinciding with replacement of the blood volume by intravenous crystalloids may be performed. In cases of inappropriate secondary polycythemia, treatment of the underlying disease should be instituted if possible, the dog stabilized by phlebotomy (10-20 ml/kg), and the blood replaced by an equivalent volume of crystalloids.

Primary polycythemia vera can be treated with long-term therapeutic phlebotomy and iron supplementation. The goal of therapy is to maintain the hematocrit in the high to normal range and alleviate signs associated with the polycythemia. Another treatment option is oral hydroxyurea therapy with or without occasional therapeutic phlebotomy. At some institutions, radioactive ^{32}P may be available, with long-term control of this disease possible with a single treatment.

BIBLIOGRAPHY

Campbell KL: Diagnosis and management of polycythemia in dogs, *Compend Contin Educ Pract Vet* 12:543, 1990.
Couto CG: Erythrocytosis, In Nelson RW, Couto CG, editors: *Essentials of small animal internal medicine*, St. Louis, 1992, Mosby.
Meyer HP, Slappendel RJ, Greydanus-van der Putten SWM: Polycythemia vera in a dog treated by repeated phlebotomies, *Vet Q* 14:108, 1993.
Peterson ME, Randolph JF: Diagnosis of canine primary polycythemia and management with hydroxyurea, *J Am Vet Med Assoc* 180:415, 1982.
Smith M, Turrel JM: Radiophosphorus (^{32}P) in the treatment of bone marrow disorders in dogs, *J Am Vet Med Assoc* 194:98, 1989.
Vail DM: Hematopoietic tumors, In Ettinger SJ, Feldman EC, editors: *Textbook of veterinary internal medicine*, ed 5, Philadelphia, 2000, WB Saunders.
Watson ADJ: Erythrocytosis and polycythemia, In Feldman BF, Zinkl JG, Jain NC, editors: *Schalm's veterinary hematology*, ed 5, Philadelphia, 2000, Lippincott Williams & Wilkins.

64. Neutropenia

Astrid Nielssen

1. What is neutropenia?

Neutropenia in the dog is defined as less than 2.9×10^9 neutrophils per liter.

2. What can cause neutropenia?

The following are the three main categories of causes for neutropenia:
1. Decreased production
2. Increased use due to excessive tissue demand or accelerated destruction
3. A shift in neutrophils from the circulating pool to the marginal pool (pseudoneutropenia)

3. What are some common causes of decreased neutrophil production?

Chemotherapeutic, immunosuppressant, or other drugs, irradiation, toxins, infections such as canine parvovirus or ehrlichiosis, stem cell disorders, marrow fibrosis, or myelophthisis are all potential causes of decreased neutrophil production in the dog.

A cyclic neutropenia, typically accompanied by cyclic decreases in the products of other cell lines, is a documented congenital abnormality seen in some Gray Collies or Gray Collie crosses. It is suspected that this disorder is the consequence of a defect in granulocyte colony-stimulating factor postreceptor signal transduction.

4. What diseases are associated with the neutropenia caused by overwhelming tissue demand or accelerated neutrophil destruction?

Acute severe inflammatory conditions, often caused by Gram-negative bacteria can result in neutropenia from an increase in the efflux of neutrophils from the circulating pool into the tissues.

Immune-mediated neutrophil destruction is possible and may be idiopathic (primary) in nature, or secondary to drug administration, infection, neoplasia, or other concurrent immune-mediated disease. Immune-mediated neutrophil destruction has not been well documented in the dog.

5. What can cause pseudoneutropenia in the dog?

In addition to the increased efflux of neutrophils into tissues caused by Gram-negative infections, endotoxins can also reduce the neutrophil count by causing neutrophils to shift from the circulating to the marginal pool. Anaphylaxis is another, although uncommon, cause of this phenomenon.

6. How should the neutropenic animal be managed clinically?

A thorough clinical history, physical examination, and various diagnostic investigations (complete blood cell count, serum biochemistry profile, urinalysis, serologic testing, diagnostic imaging, and bone marrow evaluation) may be necessary to establish the cause of the animal's neutropenia. After a diagnosis has been established, aggressive appropriate therapy directed at the primary disorder is the best way of correcting the neutropenia. Although human recombinant granulocyte-colony stimulating factor is available and can be used in dogs to stimulate neutrophil production, it is a foreign protein and eventually elicits the production of a neutralizing antibody, which may then cross-react with the dog's endogenous granulocyte-colony stimulating factor. Therefore it is not appropriate for the long-term management of the neutropenic canine patient.

Animals with a neutrophil count lower than 1.0×10^9/L are at high risk for opportunistic infections and may benefit from aggressive broad-spectrum antibiotic prophylaxis.

BIBLIOGRAPHY

Allen WM, Pocock PI, Dalton PM, et al: Cyclic neutropenia in collie, *Vet Rec* 138:371, 1996.
Avalos BR, Brody VC, Ceselski SK, et al: Abnormal response to granulocyte colony-stimulating factor (G-CSF) in canine cyclic hematopoiesis is not caused by altered G-CSF receptor expression, *Blood* 84:789, 1994.
Boone LI: Disorders of white blood cells, In Morgan RV, Bright RM, Swartout MS, editors: *Handbook of small animal practice*, Philadelphia, 2003, WB Saunders.
Farris GM, Benjamin SA: Inhibition of myelopoiesis by serum from dogs exposed to estrogen, *Am J Vet Res* 54:1374, 1993.
Jacobs G, Calvert C, Kaufman A: Neutropenia and thrombocytopenia in three dogs treated with anticonvulsants, *J Am Vet Med Assoc* 212:681, 1998.
Meyer DJ, Harvey JW: Evaluation of leukocyte disorders, In Meyer DJ, Harvey JW, editors: *Veterinary laboratory medicine*, ed 2, Philadelphia, 1998, WB Saunders.
Moore FM, Bender HS: Neutropenia, In Feldman BF, Zinkl JG, Jain NC, editors: *Schalm's veterinary hematology*, ed 5, Philadelphia, 2000, Lippincott Williams and Wilkins.
Weiss DJ: Leukocyte disorders and their treatment, In Bonagura JD, editor: *Kirk's current veterinary therapy XII*, Philadelphia, 1995, WB Saunders.

65. Thrombocytopenia

Astrid Nielssen

1.   What is thrombocytopenia?

Thrombocytopenia in the dog is defined as a platelet count of less than 200×10^{12}/L.

2.   What can cause thrombocytopenia?

The causes of thrombocytopenia can be divided into the following three major categories:
1. Decreased production
2. Increased consumption or destruction
3. Abnormal platelet distribution

In addition there are dog breeds that can have low platelet counts as a variation of normal, one example being the Cavalier King Charles Spaniel. Approximately one third of the Cavalier King Charles Spaniel breed may have platelet counts that are lower than 100×10^{12}/L but greater than 50×10^{12}/L. The platelets are typically macrocytic in these dogs. There is no recognized increase in bleeding tendency in affected dogs. Greyhound and Shiba Inu dogs may also have lower platelet counts than those usually seen with other dog breeds.

3.   What are some causes of decreased platelet production?

Platelet production defects are an uncommon cause of thrombocytopenia in the dog and when present are typically present in association with other cytopenias. Potential causes of marrow production defects in the dog include infectious agents (canine parvovirus, distemper virus, ehrlichia), vaccination (typically a mild transient response arising 3-5 days after vaccination and not associated with any bleeding tendencies), drug therapy (chemotherapeutics, immunosuppressants, estrogens, sulfa antibiotics), irradiation, toxins, dysthrombopoiesis associated with myelodysplasia, and immune-mediated destruction of megakaryocytes.

4. What are some causes of increased platelet consumption or destruction?

Thrombocytopenia due to increased platelet consumption can be seen in cases of severe trauma or hemorrhage. The thrombocytopenia is usually mild and transient. Clinical conditions that cause generalized activation of the coagulation cascade or extensive damage of the endothelium, potentially even resulting in disseminated intravascular coagulation, can also cause a thrombocytopenia. These mechanisms for platelet consumption likely play a role in the thrombocytopenias identified in dogs with many systemic inflammatory diseases and infections including babesiosis, ehrlichiosis, Rocky Mountain spotted fever, and adenovirus type I infection.

Increased platelet destruction can arise from direct injury by certain infectious agents (distemper virus) or drugs or may be due to immune-mediated mechanisms.

5. What is immune-mediated thrombocytopenia?

Immune-mediated thrombocytopenia (IMT) typically results from antibody mediated platelet destruction by the mononuclear-phagocyte system. Primary (idiopathic, autoimmune) IMT does not have an apparent etiology, is not associated with any underlying conditions, and arises when antibodies develop against platelet autoantigens. Although dogs of many breeds and ages have been diagnosed with IMT, the mean age of dogs with this disorder is approximately 6 to 7 years, and females and Cocker Spaniels appear to be overrepresented. Secondary IMT arises when an underlying associated condition or therapy triggers the immune-mediated platelet destruction.

6. What are some potential causes of secondary IMT?

Secondary IMT may arise as a result of an antibody response directed toward non-self antigens that are nonspecifically adsorbed to the surface of circulating platelets. Infectious agents, drugs, novel antigens associated with malignancies, and circulating immune complexes have the capacity to become adsorbed onto the platelet surface and trigger this response. High levels of circulating immune complexes can be seen as a result of some infectious diseases, vaccination, drug therapies, neoplasia, or in association with other autoimmune disorders.

Alloimmune thrombocytopenia is another form of immune-mediated platelet destruction that can result in significant thrombocytopenia. The only form described in the dog is posttransfusion alloimmune thrombocytopenia (posttransfusion purpura). The thrombocytopenia may arise shortly after the transfusion, possibly as the result of passively transfused donor antiplatelet alloantibodies, or it may occur approximately 1 week after the transfusion, possibly as the result of the triggering of the production of an antidonor platelet antibody that shares reactivity against the recipient platelets.

7. What is the cause of thrombocytopenia associated with abnormal platelet distribution?

Splenic sequestration of platelets can result in a circulating thrombocytopenia. In a normal state of health approximately 30% to 40% of the total platelet mass may be stored within the spleen. In pathologic conditions associated with marked splenic enlargement (e.g., hypersplenism), the percentage of splenically stored platelets can rise to as high as 90%. Hypothermia, hypotension, and endotoxemia may all also cause transient splenic platelet pooling.

8. What signs are likely to be reported in dogs that are demonstrating signs associated with their thrombocytopenia?

Clinical signs associated with thrombocytopenia are usually not noted until the platelet count falls below 30×10^{12}/L unless there is a concurrent disorder contributing to platelet dysfunction or coagulation abnormalities. Clinical signs associated with severe thrombocytopenia can include epistaxis, petechiae, ecchymoses, melena, hematochezia, hematemesis, mucosal bleeding, hematuria, and nonspecific signs of anemia such as weakness, lethargy, and inappetence.

9. How should the thrombocytopenic dog be worked up?

Because the diagnosis of primary IMT is one of exclusion, a thorough history, physical examination, and diagnostic workup are essential. A thorough history should include obtaining a full drug, vaccination, travel, and medical history. During the physical examination, extra care should be paid to identifying any conditions that may suggest an underlying disorder such as fever, organomegaly, lymphadenopathy, or joint effusions.

Initial diagnostic investigations include a complete blood cell count along with a careful blood smear evaluation, and possibly a manual platelet count to, among other things, rule out spurious causes of thrombocytopenia (e.g., platelet clumping). Dogs with IMT frequently have less than 10 $\times 10^{12}$ platelets per liter. Mean platelet volume may be increased, normal, or decreased in dogs with IMT. Dogs may be noted to be anemic, either from hemorrhage or from the concurrent disorder of immune-mediated hemolytic anemia. Complete blood cell count abnormalities suggestive of underlying disease include other concurrent cytopenias, an inflammatory leukogram, intracellular or extracellular parasites, and aberrant red blood cell morphology. A serum biochemistry profile, urinalysis, coagulation profile, serologic and immunologic screening tests, and advanced imaging may all be useful in investigating these animals. Bone marrow evaluation can also be essential in ruling out disorders causing production failure. Thrombocytopenia is not a contraindication to bone marrow aspiration. Platelet antibody assays are not widely available and not widely used because of difficulties associated with the transport and stability of samples. The identification of antiplatelet antibody simply indicates the process of immune-mediated platelet destruction, it does not rule out all the various causes of secondary IMT.

10. How should the thrombocytopenic dog be treated?

All dogs with thrombocytopenia should be treated with appropriate supportive care as their conditions dictate. Care should be taken to avoid any medications that might further compromise platelet function (e.g., nonsteroidal antiinflammatory drugs) and trauma should be minimized.

Dogs with underlying identifiable conditions associated with their thrombocytopenia should receive specific therapy for that disorder along with appropriate supportive care. The cornerstone of therapy for dogs with idiopathic IMT is immunosuppressive doses of corticosteroids (2 mg/kg prednisone by mouth twice daily). Various other medications have also been used in the management of idiopathic IMT including azathioprine, cyclophosphamide, vincristine, and danazol. Cyclosporine, splenectomy, and human immunoglobulin G have been used in dogs not responding to traditional therapy.

11. What is the prognosis for dogs with thrombocytopenia and how should they be monitored?

The prognosis for dogs with thrombocytopenia associated with an underlying condition depends on the nature of their underlying disease and their response to therapy. They are monitored with follow-up platelet counts until their level normalizes. As many or more than 50% of dogs with idiopathic IMT will respond fully to therapy and have a complete recovery. Others may respond, but then relapse and require ongoing maintenance therapy. A reasonably low percentage (<20%) are poor responders, and either they may die of hemorrhage or other complications from their disease, or they may be euthanized as a result of the prolonged clinical course of their disease. Dogs with idiopathic IMT are typically kept in hospital and monitored with platelet counts every 24 to 48 hours until their platelet number is equal to or greater than 75 $\times 10^{12}$/L. They can then be followed as outpatients. After a dog with idiopathic IMT has responded fully to therapy (platelet count equal to or greater than 200×10^{12}/L), its medications can slowly be tapered down over the following months provided follow-up platelet counts continue to be within the normal range.

BIBLIOGRAPHY

Grindem CB: Infectious and immune-mediated thrombocytopenia, In Bonagura JD, editor: *Kirk's current veterinary therapy XIII*, Philadelphia, 2000, WB Saunders.

Grindem CB, Breitschwerdt EB, Corbett WT et al: Epidemiologic survey of thrombocytopenia in dogs: a report on 987 cases, *Vet Clin Pathol* 2:38, 1991.

Lewis DC, Meyers KM: Canine idiopathic thrombocytopenic purpura, *J Vet Intern Med* 10:207, 1996.

Mackin A: Canine immune-mediated thrombocytopenia-part I, *Compend Cont Educ Pract Vet* 17:515, 1995.

Mackin A: Canine immune-mediated thrombocytopenia-part II, *Compend Cont Educ Pract Vet* 17:353, 1995.

Scott MA: Immune-mediated thrombocytopenia, In Feldman BF, Zinkl JG, Jain NC, editors: *Schalm's veterinary hematology*, ed 5, Philadelphia, 2000, Lippincott Williams & Wilkins.

Weiss DJ: Platelet production defects, In Feldman BF, Zinkl JG, Jain NC, editors: *Schalm's veterinary hematology*, ed 5, Philadelphia, 2000, Lippincott Williams & Wilkins.

Zimmerman KL: Drug-induced thrombocytopenias, In Feldman BF, Zinkl JG, Jain NC, editors: *Schalm's veterinary hematology*, ed 5, Philadelphia, 2000, Lippincott Williams & Wilkins.

66. Immune-Mediated Hemolytic Anemia

Astrid Nielssen

1. What is immune-mediated hemolytic anemia (IMHA)?

IMHA is an antibody-mediated disease that results in the premature destruction of red blood cells. In most cases, the red blood cell destruction occurs primarily in the mononuclear phagocytic system within the spleen and liver, a process referred to as extravascular hemolysis. In some cases, when the antibody is capable of directly fixing complement, intravascular hemolysis can also occur.

2. What is the difference between primary and secondary IMHA?

As with immune-mediated thrombocytopenia, IMHA can be categorized as being either primary or secondary. Primary, or idiopathic, IMHA (to be referred to as autoimmune hemolytic anemia, AIHA, in the rest of this section) does not have an apparent etiology, is not associated with any underlying conditions, and arises when antibodies develop against red blood cell autoantigens. At its most basic level, AIHA is the result of the loss or dysfunction of mechanisms of normal immunologic tolerance. Secondary IMHA arises when an underlying associated condition or therapy triggers the immune-mediated red blood cell destruction. This can occur as a result of antigenic agents adsorbed to the red blood cell membrane (drugs, infectious agents, immune complexes). It can also arise when a condition or disease process alters the red blood cell membrane, either exposing new antigens or altering existing ones, so as to result in an immune response directed against those epitopes. Infection with agents that carry epitopes similar to those on the red blood cell membrane may also result in the production of an antibody that reacts with self-antigen (antigenic mimicry).

3. What are some of the causes of secondary IMHA?

Secondary IMHA can be seen as a reaction to certain drugs (penicillins, cephalosporins, trimethoprim-sulfadiazine, procainamide), toxins, infectious agents (ehrlichia, other bacterial infections), parasites (heartworm), neoplasia, and systemic autoimmune disease.

Neonatal isoerythrolysis, another form of IMHA, is rarely recognized in the dog, likely as the result of the absence of significant naturally occurring pathogenic red blood cell antigen antibodies. Neonatal isoerythrolysis results from the presence of passively transfused maternal antibodies with specificity for paternally determined red blood cell membrane epitopes. For this complication to arise in pups, the bitch would have to have been previously sensitized by a mismatched blood transfusion or antigen exposure during an earlier pregnancy or labor. It is because of the possible presence of red blood cell alloantibodies that bitches that have had litters, or dogs that have received prior blood transfusions, should not be used as blood donors.

4.   Are certain dogs predisposed to AIHA?

A genetic influence predisposing to the development of this disease is strongly suspected. An increased incidence is reported in several breeds including Cocker Spaniels, English Springer Spaniels, Lhasa Apsos, Old English Sheepdogs, Poodles, and Shih Tzus. The Cocker Spaniel has been most consistently overrepresented in the literature. There is suspected to be an increased incidence in female dogs, and although the disease can happen in dogs of any age, the mean age at presentation is approximately 6 years.

5.   What are the most common clinical signs of IMHA?

Clinical signs of IMHA can include weakness, lethargy, anorexia, pale or icteric mucous membranes, tachycardia, tachypnea, splenomegaly, and possibly fever. Owners may report having noticed discolored urine (from either bilirubinuria or hemoglobinuria) or stool (as a result of increased bilirubin excretion).

6.   What abnormalities are typically noted on the minimum database (complete blood count serum, biochemistry profile, and urinalysis) from an animal with IMHA?

Typical hematologic findings include a regenerative anemia with reticulocytosis, spherocytosis, anisocytosis, polychromasia, and a reactive leukocytosis with a neutrophilia and a left shift. Thrombocytopenia is also commonly seen and can be due to concurrent immune-mediated thrombocytopenia or to increased platelet consumption due to thrombosis or disseminated intravascular coagulation. Abnormalities commonly noted on the serum biochemistry profile include elevations in the total bilirubin and liver enzyme levels. The urinalysis typically reveals bilirubinuria. Other abnormalities associated with either underlying disease conditions or clinical conditions may also be noted.

7.   What are the best ways of determining if a dog has IMHA?

Diagnosis is based on characteristic hematologic findings and commonly either a positive saline slide-agglutination test result or a positive direct antiglobulin test result (DAT test, Coombs' test).

A saline slide-agglutination test, consisting of mixing one drop of the animal's anticoagulated blood with two or three drops of saline on a slide, and observing for the presence of persistent autoagglutination, can be performed while initially assessing the animal. If obvious agglutination is not evident, the slide should be checked under the microscope for microagglutination. A positive result is consistent with a diagnosis of IMHA.

The DAT test is the definitive way of identifying erythrocyte bound antibodies or complement, although it is positive in only approximately 60% to 80% of cases of AIHA. It is performed on EDTA anticoagulated blood and either with polyvalent species-specific sera (specific from immunoglobulin G, immunoglobulin M, and C3) or with reagents specific for each of these agents alone. It is performed at 37°C and often also at 4°C to assess for the presence of cold-reacting agglutinins. The most common DAT result pattern for AIHA is high levels of immunoglobulin G, with or without the other immunoreactants, at both 37°C and 4°C. A negative result can arise for a number of reasons, including insufficient bound antibody or complement, technical mistakes, improper testing temperature, prior corticosteroid therapy, and drug associated IMHA.

No other diagnostic tests used to detect antibodies or complement on the surface of canine red blood cells (e.g., flow cytometry, a direct enzyme linked antiglobulin test) are in widespread clinical use. Because AIHA and secondary IMHA are both antibody- and complement-mediated processes, no diagnostic test that simply identifies the presence of these immunoreactants is going to differentiate between these disorders.

8.   What ancillary diagnostic tests should be considered in the animal with IMHA?

Because there is no definitive diagnostic test for the diagnosis of AIHA, a thorough history, physical examination, and diagnostic workup are essential. A full drug, vaccination, travel, and medical history should be obtained. During the physical examination, extra care should be paid to identifying any conditions that may suggest an underlying disorder. A serum biochemistry profile, urinalysis, serologic and immunologic screening tests, and advanced imaging (thoracic and abdominal radiographs, abdominal ultrasound) are useful in investigating these animals and identifying possible underlying conditions. A bone marrow evaluation may be useful in cases of a nonregenerative anemia (that has had adequate time to regenerate) or in other cases in which a marrow disease is suspected. A coagulation profile is also suggested in cases of IMHA because a large number of dogs with AIHA have significant coagulation abnormalities, and many fulfill criteria for disseminated intravascular coagulation.

9.   How is IMHA treated?

All dogs with IMHA should be treated with appropriate supportive care as their conditions dictate, including blood transfusions as needed to ensure that they maintain adequate tissue oxygen delivery and to decrease the physiologic stress associated with compensation for a severe anemia. There has been no substantive evidence to support the old adage that transfusing animals with IMHA adds "fuel to the fire" and worsens their hemolytic crisis or contributes to the development of thromboembolic complications. Ultimately, the decision to transfuse should be based on the animal's clinical condition and the laboratory values. A posttransfusion hematocrit goal of 20% to 25% is reasonable to maintain the drive for red blood cell regeneration and minimize iatrogenic complications.

Dogs with underlying identifiable conditions associated with their IMHA should receive specific therapy for that disorder along with appropriate supportive care. Treatment of AIHA involves immunosuppressive or immunomodulating drugs aimed at halting the immune-mediated hemolysis. The first line of therapy for dogs with AIHA is immunosuppressive doses of corticosteroids (2 mg/kg prednisone by mouth twice daily). Several other medications have also been used in the treatment of AIHA, particularly in the more severe clinical cases, including cyclophosphamide, azathioprine, danazol, and cyclosporine. Plasmapheresis, human immunoglobulin G, and splenectomy have also been used in the treatment of this condition. No studies have revealed any clear benefit to the use of any of these adjunctive therapies in the treatment of canine AIHA, although some have indicated an increased risk of death associated with the use of cyclophosphamide. Given the high incidence of thromboembolic complications in dogs with AIHA, heparin prophylaxis had been suggested to potentially be of benefit in preventing this frequently devastating complication. Clinical evidence identifying a benefit of this therapy, or providing information with respect to an appropriate dosage in these cases, is lacking.

10.   How should dogs with IMHA be monitored?

Monitoring recommendations for animals with secondary IMHA are determined by the nature and gravity of their underlying disease. AIHA is a heterogeneous condition, with animals having a wide gradation in the severity of their illness. Obviously, the degree of monitoring and supervision in AIHA cases will therefore be dictated by the clinical condition of the individual dog. Care needs to be taken with each animal, however, to carefully monitor hematocrits and complete blood cell counts for evidence of gradual improvement and eventual remission of disease. After the hemogram has normalized, then attempts can be made to gradually (over months) taper down and potentially discontinue the animal's medications. It is essential that close monitoring be continued during the tapering process so that any evidence of disease recurrence can be identified promptly and therapy modified appropriately. Follow-up monitoring of serum biochemistry profiles and urinalyses may also be necessary in some cases to monitor for the potential side effects of certain medications. Even after all therapies have been discontinued, ongoing lifelong monitoring of survivors is likely indicated.

11. What is the long-term prognosis for dogs with IMHA?

The prognoses for dogs with secondary IMHA will again depend on the nature and severity of their underlying disease process and their response to treatment. Mortality rates for AIHA vary widely from study to study, ranging from 18% to 70%, but the lower mortality rates were often seen in studies that did not follow animals past the time of initial hospital discharge, therefore resulting in an underestimation of the true mortality associated with this disease. One of the most common causes of death or euthanasia in these animals is thromboembolic disease (most commonly, pulmonary thromboembolic disease). A relatively high recurrence rate of AIHA is suspected in dogs surviving their initial episode, although information in the literature is lacking on this subject.

BIBLIOGRAPHY

Barker RN: Anemia associated with immune responses, In Feldman BF, Zinkl JG, Jain NC, editors: *Schalm's veterinary hematology*, ed 5, Philadelphia, 2000, Lippincott Williams & Wilkins.
Day MJ: Immune-mediated hemolytic anemia, In Feldman BF, Zinkl JG, Jain NC, editors: *Schalm's veterinary hematology*, ed 5, Philadelphia, 2000, Lippincott Williams & Wilkins.
Day MJ: Serial monitoring of clinical, haematological and immunological parameters in canine autoimmune haemolytic anemia, *J Small Anim Prac* 37:523, 1996.
Klag AR, Giger U, Shofer FS: Idiopathic immune-mediated hemolytic anemia in dogs: 42 cases (1986-1990), *J Am Vet Med Assoc* 202:783, 1993.
Klein MK, Dow SW, Rosychuk RAW: Pulmonary thromboembolism associated with immune-mediated hemolytic anemia in dogs: 10 cases (1982-1987), *J Am Vet Med Assoc* 1295:246, 1989.
Miller E: CVT update. Diagnosis and treatment of immune-mediated hemolytic anemia. In Bonagura JD, editor: *Kirk's current veterinary therapy XIII*, Philadelphia, 2000, WB Saunders.
Scott-Moncrieff JCR, Reagan WJ, Snyder PW et al: Intravenous administration of human immune-globulin in dogs with immune-mediated hemolytic anemia, *J Am Vet Med Assoc* 210:1623, 1997.
Stewart AF, Feldman BF: Immune-mediated hemolytic anemia. Part II. Clinical entity, diagnosis and treatment theory, *Compend Contin Educ Pract Vet* 15:1479, 1993.

67. Coagulopathies

Astrid Nielssen

ACQUIRED

Anticoagulant Rodenticide Intoxication

1. Which activated coagulation factors become deficient with warfarin and other vitamin K antagonists and why?

Factors II, VII, IX, and X all require posttranslational carboxylation for activation. The carboxylation of these proteins requires the presence of active vitamin K and results in the conversion of active, reduced vitamin K, by vitamin K epoxidase, to its inactive epoxide form. Vitamin K epoxide reductase then converts the inactive oxidized form back to the active form. Anticoagulant rodenticides competitively inhibit vitamin K epoxide reductase, preventing the regeneration of active vitamin K, and therefore inhibiting the production of functional vitamin K–dependent coagulation factors. Anticoagulant factors C and S also rely on vitamin K for posttranslational modification and activation.

2. How long after exposure to an anticoagulant rodenticide do clinical signs of a coagulopathy arise?

Typically, the onset of clinical symptoms occurs a few days after exposure, when all of the four affected coagulation factors have become profoundly deficient. The half-lives of the factors vary (41, 6.2, 13.9, and 16.5 hours for factors II, VII, IX, and X, respectively) and so it is possible for signs to arise earlier, in association with the depletion of factor VII. Clinical signs do not often arise this early, however, perhaps because the concurrent inhibition of anticoagulant protein C activity (half-life 8-10 hours) balances the loss of the procoagulant factor VII.

Clinical signs are those of disorders of secondary hemostasis: large volume hemorrhage, body cavity bleeds, and the absence of petechiae, ecchymoses, or mucosal bleeding.

3. What diagnostic findings may be noted in a case of anticoagulant rodenticide intoxication?

Typically with anticoagulant rodenticide intoxication, both the prothrombin time and activated partial thromboplastin time are prolonged at the time of clinical presentation, although because of the short half-life of factor VII, early in the course of the intoxication, only the prothrombin time may be prolonged. The animal's complete blood cell count may reveal a nonregenerative anemia secondary to acute hemorrhage, but typically there is no significant aberrant red blood cell morphology. The platelet count is typically within normal limits but can be mildly to severely decreased in some cases. Antithrombin III and fibrinogen levels and the thrombin time are typically normal. A mild increase in the level of fibrin degradation products (FDPs) may be present. An alternative test to one-stage prothrombin time (OSPT) is PIVKA (proteins induced by vitamin K absence or antagonism). This test represents a diluted OSPT with greater sensitivity to decreased factor levels. The test is not specific to anticoagulant rodenticides; it will be elevated with many other coagulopathies that affect the vitamin K–dependent factors.

4. Are there any other conditions that can result in vitamin K–dependent factor deficiencies?

Diseases of the liver, pancreas, or alimentary tract that result in decreased vitamin K absorption, or severe dietary vitamin K deficiency can result in a coagulopathy.

5. How are cases of vitamin K antagonism or deficiency treated?

Initial stabilization therapy (fluids, blood products) is required for many of these animals. Care must be taken to minimize physical trauma. Thoracocentesis is not performed in those animals with hemothorax unless it is resulting in respiratory compromise. Vitamin K supplementation is implemented, often subcutaneously initially (never intravenously because it can cause anaphylaxis when administered via this route), and then as an oral maintenance therapy. Dogs with vitamin K deficiency as a result of diminished absorption require ongoing parenteral therapy. The recommended dose of vitamin K varies, but the newer generation of anticoagulant rodenticides requires higher doses and more prolonged treatment. Higher doses of vitamin K have been associated with a Heinz body anemia in some dogs. A prothrombin time can be used to assess the efficacy of therapy and should be determined 2 days after the discontinuation of therapy to ensure that the duration of treatment was adequate.

Disseminated Intravascular Coagulation

6. What is disseminated intravascular coagulation (DIC)?

DIC results from the generalized activation of the coagulation system, resulting in widespread microthrombosis. The resulting capillary injury further shifts the coagulation system into a procoagulant state and results in further consumption of procoagulant and anticoagulant factors. The older term used for DIC, consumptive coagulopathy, appropriately described a central feature of this disorder.

A mixed bleeding pattern (symptoms of abnormalities in both primary and secondary hemostasis) can be seen in dogs with DIC because of the decrease in both platelets and coagulation factors in combination with circulating inhibitors of hemostasis (e.g., FDPs). Dogs with DIC may occasionally present with the primary clinical signs of thrombosis.

7.   What can cause DIC?
There are a large number of conditions that can cause DIC. Some more frequently identified causes in the dog include neoplasia, hepatosplenic disease, systemic infections, heartworm infection, extensive tissue trauma, cardiovascular shock, heat stroke, and envenomation.

8.   How is DIC diagnosed?
A diagnosis of DIC is made on the basis of appropriate historic and clinical findings and typically a minimum of a total of three of the following laboratory abnormalities: thrombocytopenia, prolonged activated partial thromboplastin time and prothrombin time, elevated FDPs (or D-dimers, an FDP seen only with fibrinolysis of polymerized fibrin), decreased fibrinogen levels, and decreased antithrombin III activity.

9.   How is DIC treated?
DIC should be initially treated with aggressive efforts to restore effective tissue oxygenation and promote adequate capillary blood flow. Crystalloids, colloids, inotropes, and vasodilators can all be used to try and accomplish this. Therapy can then be directed at addressing the underlying disorder, if this is possible. Additional supportive therapies can include enteral nutrition to try and maintain the integrity of the gut wall and prevent bacterial translocation, and oxygen supplementation if respiratory compromise is present. Blood product therapy can be used to address anemia, an insufficiency of coagulation factors, and antithrombin III deficiency. Heparin therapy to increase the activity of what antithrombin III is present can also be implemented.

Liver Disease

10.   Why do diseases affecting the liver often result in abnormalities of the coagulation system?
The liver is the site of synthesis of all the coagulation factors except for factor VIII (factor VIII is synthesized in the hepatic sinusoidal endothelial cells and elsewhere) and is also crucial in the synthesis of the various anticoagulant and fibrinolytic proteins. It is also the organ in which these products are often activated, degraded, and cleared. Given these facts, it is not surprising that most dogs with significant hepatopathies have abnormalities in their coagulation profiles.

INHERITED

Hemophilia

11.   What are hemophilias A and B?
Hemophilias A and B are inherited coagulopathies resulting from deficiencies in functional factors VIII and IX (Christmas factor), respectively. They are both X-linked disorders, with clinical signs of disease identified in males and the rare homozygous female. The carrier heterozygous female does not demonstrate signs of the disorder.

12.   What are the clinical signs of hemophilia A and B?
Both disorders result in signs associated with disorders of secondary hemostasis. With hemophilia A, mildly affected animals with factor activity higher than 5% do not tend to have notable bleeding tendencies. Those with factor activity between 2% and 5% can demonstrate

prolonged hemorrhage resulting from minor trauma. Those with factor activity less than 2% can have severe, spontaneous hemorrhage. With hemophilia B, severity of disease is associated with the size and activity of the animal, with larger and more active dogs tending to demonstrate the most severe clinical signs.

13. How are hemophilia A and B diagnosed?

The prothrombin time is within normal limits and the activated partial thromboplastin time is prolonged for both hemophilia A and B. The addition of normal fresh serum (which contains factor IX, but not factor VIII) to the animal sample can correct the activated partial thromboplastin time of the animal with hemophilia B but not A. However, definitive diagnosis of hemophilia A or B requires specific factor assays.

14. How is hemophilia A treated?

Basic supportive care and avoidance of trauma is essential for these dogs. Cryoprecipitate or fresh frozen plasma can be used to increase factor VIII levels and minimize bleeding. Cryoprecipitate contains 10 times more factor VIII per unit volume than plasma and is therefore a more effective way to deliver this factor to the dog without having to be concerned about volume overload. Red blood cell transfusion, either with fresh whole blood or packed cells, may also be indicated in the markedly anemic dog. Clinical benefits with the use of deamino-D-arginine vasopressin (DDAVP) or fibrinolytic inhibitors in animals with hemophilia A have not yet been convincingly identified. Use of the human factor VIII concentrate in these animals cannot be recommended, given that as a foreign protein from another species, it is almost certain to elicit a profound neutralizing antibody response that could diminish the efficacy of any future therapies.

15. How is hemophilia B treated?

Appropriate therapy for dogs with hemophilia B is similar to that for dogs with hemophilia A, with the exception that cryoprecipitate should not be used in these dogs because it does not contain significant concentrations of factor IX.

16. How can these diseases be prevented?

Unfortunately, coagulation studies cannot be used to try and identify females that are carriers for hemophilia A. With hemophilia B, however, most heterozygotes have factor IX activity levels in a range that falls above that of the affected animals and below that of unaffected individuals, thereby making this a reasonable screening test to identify most carriers. DNA analysis is now also available to screen for carriers of these disorders in selected breeds.

von Willebrand's Disease

17. What is von Willebrand's disease (vWD)?

Von Willebrand's factor (vWF) is a multimeric protein of varying size that supports platelet adhesion at areas of endothelial injury. In dogs, this protein is primarily produced in endothelial cells. Deficiency of this protein, or a deficiency in the larger multimers, can result in a disorder of primary hemostasis called vWD. vWD is inherited in an autosomal manner.

18. How is vWD classified?

vWD is typically classified into three categories as follows:

Type I: All multimers decreased; severity varies from mild to severe.

Type II: Disproportionate decrease in high molecular weight multimers; generally severe.

Type III: Undetectable levels of multimers; severe.

Type I occurs most commonly and is the type typically identified in Doberman Pinschers, Welsh Corgis, and German Shepherds.

19. How is vWD diagnosed?

vWD should be considered as a differential diagnosis for any animal suspected of having a bleeding tendency. Clinical signs consistent with a disorder of primary hemostasis despite a normal platelet count, a prolonged buccal mucosal bleeding time, and the absence of evidence of other concurrent disorders, should prompt the performance of a specific assay for plasma vWF to confirm the presence of this disorder. Genetic testing is available in some breeds.

20. How is vWD treated?

Basic supportive care and avoidance of trauma is essential for these animals. Cryoprecipitate or fresh frozen plasma can be used to increase vWF levels and minimize bleeding. Cryoprecipitate contains between 5 and 10 times more vWF per unit volume than plasma, and is therefore the safest and most effective product to use to rapidly increase vWF levels. Red blood cell products may also be indicated in the markedly anemic dog. DDAVP can be administered to try and increase endothelial release of stored vWF, an action thought to be mediated through V_2 vasopressin receptors. The hemostatic improvements last only in the range of hours, and repeated DDAVP administrations lose their effectiveness. DDAVP may be used in affected animals before surgery or during a bleeding crisis to try and minimize hemorrhage. Measuring a dog's buccal mucosal bleeding time before and 1 hour after DDAVP administration can help to determine whether it may be of clinical benefit in that animal. Dogs with vWD types II and III do not tend to respond as significantly to this therapy. Administration of DDAVP to blood donor dogs 1 hour before blood collection has been suggested as a method to increase vWF levels in the donated blood.

21. How can these diseases be prevented?

Quantitative vWF assays have proved useful in identifying carrier dogs in many cases. DNA analysis is now also available to screen for carriers of this disorder in selected breeds.

BIBLIOGRAPHY

Boudreaux MK: Platelet and coagulation disorders, In Morgan RV, Bright RM, Swartout MS, editors: *Handbook of small animal practice*, Philadelphia, 2003, WB Saunders.

Brooks M: Coagulopathies and thrombosis, In Ettinger SJ, Feldman EC, editors: *Textbook of veterinary internal medicine*, ed 5, Philadelphia, 2000, WB Saunders.

Carr AP, Panciera DL: Von Willebrand's disease and other hereditary coagulopathies, In Bonagura JD, editor: *Kirk's current veterinary therapy XIII*, Philadelphia, 2000, WB Saunders.

Kirby R, Rudloff E: Acquired coagulopathy VI: disseminated intravascular coagulation, In Feldman BF, Zinkl JG, Jain NC, editors: *Schalm's veterinary hematology*, ed 5, Philadelphia, 2000, Lippincott Williams & Wilkins.

Mansell P: Hemophilia A and B, In Feldman BF, Zinkl JG, Jain NC, editors: *Schalm's veterinary hematology*, ed 5, Philadelphia, 2000, Lippincott Williams & Wilkins.

Prater MR: Acquired coagulopathy I: avitaminosis K, In Feldman BF, Zinkl JG, Jain NC, editors: *Schalm's veterinary hematology*, ed 5, Philadelphia, 2000, Lippincott Williams & Wilkins.

Prater MR: Acquired coagulopathy II: liver disease, In Feldman BF, Zinkl JG, Jain NC, editors: *Schalm's veterinary hematology*, ed 5, Philadelphia, 2000, Lippincott Williams & Wilkins.

Section X
Infectious Diseases

Section Editor: Gregory C. Troy

---

68. Antifungal Therapy

Gregory C. Troy and David Clark Grant

---

1. What groups of compounds are commonly used in the treatment of fungal infections in the dog?

The major groups of compounds include natural agents such as griseofulvin, amphotericin B and its lipid formulations, and synthetic agents including iodides, pyrimidine inhibitor (flucytosine), azoles (ketoconazole, itraconazole, fluconazole, voriconazole), allylamine derivative (terbinafine), mannoprotein complexing agents, ergosterol synthesis blockers, and chitin/glucan synthetase inhibitors (lufenuron and caspofungin) (Table 68-1).

2. What is the mechanism of action of amphotericin B on fungal cells?

Amphotericin B is a fungistatic agent. It works by binding to ergosterol in the fungal cell wall. This action results in an increased permeability of the cell wall. This drug also binds to cholesterol in mammalian cell membranes to a lesser degree and is responsible for some of the toxicities associated with amphotericin B.

3. What is the major toxicity of amphotericin B?

Nephrotoxicity occurs in most dogs treated with this agent. The nephrotoxicity is characterized by vasoconstriction, reducing glomerular filtration rate (GFR), and by effects on the distal tubular area of the nephron. Distal tubular dysfunction results in metabolic acidosis because of a failure to excrete hydrogen ions. Dogs have metabolic acidosis and are unable to acidify the urine maximally. Polyuria and compensatory polydipsia develops. Serum urea nitrogen and creatinine concentrations may become elevated, and when greater than 50 mg/dl, therapy with the drug should be discontinued until these abnormalities resolve. In most instances, renal function returns to normal after therapy cessation unless high levels of amphotericin B are administered.

4. What can be done clinically to lessen the nephrotoxicity of amphotericin B?

The animal should be well hydrated before administration of this drug. Saline loading of dogs can be used before administration of the drug. The drug should be administered over 2 to 4 hours.

5. What is the mechanism of action of the triazole agents?

The triazole compounds are fungistatic drugs that inhibit ergosterol synthesis, altering cell membrane functions and leading to cell death and failure of replication.

6. What are the major differences in the triazole compounds for treatment of mycotic infections?

The major differences in these compounds are related to their bioavailability, solubility, and spectrum of action. This group of drugs is weak dibasic agents that are insoluble in water, with the exception of fluconazole.

Text continued on p. 394

Table 68-1 Summary of Antifungal Compounds Used to Treat Certain Mycotic Diseases in Dogs

CLASS OF DRUG	MECHANISM OF ACTION	GENERIC NAME	BRAND NAME	FORMULATION	TOXICITY	SYNERGY WITH OTHER ANTIFUNGAL AGENT	DOSE(S)	FUNGAL DISEASE(S)
Polyene Antibiotic	Inhibition of ergosterol synthesis disrupting cell membrane functions	Amphotericin B	Fungizone	Intravenous, oral	Nephrotoxic, phlebitis	Triazoles	0.25 to 0.50 mg/kg every 48 hour intravenously Total dose 3 to 10 mg/kg	B, H, Cox, Cr, Asp
		Amphotericin B Lipid Complex	Abelcet	Intravenous	Same as above		2 to 3 mg/kg every 24 hours	B, H, Cox, Cr, Asp
		Amphotericin B cholesteryl sulfate	Amphotec Amphocil	Intravenous	Same as above			B, H, Cox, Cr, Asp
		Amphotericin B liposomal	AmBisome	Intravenous	Same as above		1 mg/kg 3× week Total dose 12 mg/kg	B, H, Cox, Cr, Asp
Pyrimidine Analogue	Inhibition of synthesis of DNA and RNA proteins	Flucytosine	Ancobon	Oral tablets and suspension	Bone marrow suppression vomiting, diarrhea erythremic dermatitis, alopecia	Amphotericin	25 to 50 mg/kg by mouth every 8 hours Dose must be adjusted in renal disease	Can, Cr, Asp

Azoles Triazoles	Inhibits ergosterol biosynthesis by inhibiting lanosterol 14 alpha demethylase, altering cell membrane and function	Ketoconazole	Nizoral	Oral	GI signs, vomiting, diarrhea, hepatic enzyme elevations, cutaneous vasculitis	10 to 20 mg/kg every 12 hours	B,H,Cr,Cox, Spor, Asp
		Clotrimazole	Lotrimin	1% topical	Cellulitis	1.5 g/trx	Nasal Aspergillosis
		Enilconazole	Imaverol*	10% topical solution		10 mg/kg every 12 hours for 7 to 10 days	Nasal Aspergillosis
		Fluconazole	Diflucan	Tablet, oral suspension, intravenous prep		5 to 10 mg/kg every day by mouth	Cr, Cox

*Imaverol is not currently licensed in the United States.

B, Blastomycosis; Cr, cryptococcosis; H, histoplasmosis; Cox, coccidioidmycosis; Sp, sporotrichosis; Can, candidiasis; Asp, aspergillosis; Pyth, pythiosis; M, mucormycosis; trx, treatment.

Continued

Table 68-1 *Summary of Antifungal Compounds Used to Treat Certain Mycotic Diseases in Dogs—cont'd*

CLASS OF DRUG	MECHANISM OF ACTION	GENERIC NAME	BRAND NAME	FORMULATION	TOXICITY	SYNERGY WITH OTHER ANTIFUNGAL AGENT	DOSE(S)	FUNGAL DISEASE(S)
		Itraconazole	Sporanox	Tablet and solution, intravenous	Photo-sensitization, hepatitis, vomiting, diarrhea, cutaneous vasculitis		2.5 mg/kg every 12 hours or 5 mg/kg every 24 hours for 60 to 90 days	B, H, Cox, Cr, Spor Pyth
		Voriconazole	Vfend	Oral, intravenous		Amphotericin, Caspofungin	10 mg/kg every 24 hours for 6 to 9 months	Asp, Cr, Can, H, Cox
		Posaconazole	Noxafil	Capsule, tablet, liquid				Asp, Can, Cr
Iodide	Mechanism is unknown	Sodium or potassium iodide	Sodium iodide	Oral 20% solution	Iodism – anxiety Panting Tachycardia Vomiting		40 mg/kg every 8 hours	B, H, Cox, M Spor

Class	Mechanism	Generic name	Trade name	Route	Side effects	Drug	Dose	Treatment
Allylamine	Blocks ergosterol biosynthesis by inhibiting squalene epoxidase	Terbinafine	Lamisil	Oral	Gastrointestinal toxicity Hepatitis	Amphotericin	5 to 10 mg/kg every 24 hours	Pyth, Cr
Competitive inhibitor chitin synthase	Inhibition of chitin synthesis	Lufenuron	Program	Oral	Vomiting Lethargy Pruritus	Azole	5 to 10 mg/kg every 24 hours	Cox, B
		Nikkomycin	Nikkomycin Z	Oral		Fluconazole Itraconazole		H, B, Cox
Echinocandin	Inhibition of B-glucan synthase in fungal cell wall	Caspofungin acetate	Cancidas	Intravenous		Amphotericin	70 mg intravenously Day 1 50 mg for 13 days	Can, Asp, H, C

*Imaverol is not currently licensed in the United States.

B, Blastomycosis; *Cr*, cryptococcosis; *H*, histoplasmosis; *Cox*, coccidioidomycosis; *Sp*, sporotrichosis; *Can*, candidiasis; *Asp*, aspergillosis; *Pyth*, pythiosis; *M*, mucormycosis; *trx*, treatment.

7. How are the triazoles administered?

Most drugs are in a tablet formulation, but parenteral itraconazole is available as a cyclo-dextrin solution that has better absorption. Ketoconazole and itraconazole are better absorbed in an acidic environment and are best given with meals. H2 blockers should not be administered with these two drugs.

8. What are the major side effects of the azoles?

The major side effects are gastrointestinal in nature and are characterized by inappetence, vomiting and elevated liver enzymes (predominantly alanine aminotransferase [ALT]). Because these drugs have effects on endogenous steroid synthesis, hair coat changes and suppression of cortisol and sex hormones may also occur. These drugs are teratogenic and mutagenic and should not be administered to pregnant bitches.

Itraconazole can result in a cutaneous vasculitis in dogs that is characterized by an erythremic, ulcerative dermatitis. Skin lesions usually regress after the drug is discontinued.

9. What can be done clinically to lessen the hepatotoxicity of the azoles?

There are no effective ways to prevent this complication of therapy. Sequential monitoring of the animal and of biochemical markers (liver enzymes—alanine aminotransferase [ALT], alkaline phosphatase [ALP], and total bilirubin) may allow the veterinarian to detect elevations that could suggest impeding problems associated with these compounds.

10. How effective are the chitin inhibitors in treatment of dogs with mycotic infections?

There are a few reports in the veterinary literature on use of lufenuron in the treatment of dermatophytes, blastomycosis, and coccidioidomycosis. Some effectiveness has been shown in a reduction of the duration of therapy.

BIBLIOGRAPHY

Groll AH, Gae-Banacloche JC, Glasmacher A et al: Clinical pharmacology of antifungal compounds, *Infect Dis Clin N Am* 17:159-191, 2003.
Grooters AM, Taboada J: Update on antifungal therapy, *Vet Clin N Am (Sm Anim Pract)* 33:749-758, 2003.
Kerl ME: Update on canine and feline fungal diseases, *Vet Clin N Am (Sm Anim Pract)* 22:721-747, 2003.

69. Canine Infectious Diseases

David Clark Grant and Gregory C. Troy

SUMMARY OF DIAGNOSTIC TECHNIQUES

A multitude of infectious diseases are encountered in small animal veterinary practice and, as such, numerous diagnostic tests and techniques are used in their diagnosis. Some of the commonly used techniques and tests available in small animal infectious disease diagnosis are discussed in this chapter. Specific tests for the diseases discussed in this chapter are summarized in Table 69-1.

1. How are antigens and antibodies detected?

Serologic testing refers to the detection of endogenous antibodies directed against a particular infectious agent or detection of actual infectious antigens. Numerous techniques are used in this process. Serologic antigen detection is considered more diagnostic of infection than antibody detection because antibodies can be present in animals that were previously infected. Additionally, serologic antibody tests are more likely to have cross-reactivity with antibodies directed at other, closely related agents. Therefore high single antibody titers, or demonstration of a four-fold increase in serum antibody titers, are generally required to support active infection.

The enzyme linked immunosorbent assay (ELISA) is a commonly used rapid method of detection of antibodies or antigens. This methodology is used in commercial test kits intended for "in-house" use. *Dirofilaria* (antigen), *Ehrlichia* (antibody), and *Borrelia* (recombinant product that detects antibody) infections can be detected in practice settings with these kits. Individual test characteristics are important for the practitioner to understand, because false-positive and false-negative tests results are not uncommon when there is a lack of quality control in their performance.

Fluorescent antibodies (FAs) can also be used to detect antibodies or antigen. These are not performed as an in-house test. A fluorescing molecule is first bound to antibodies specific to an organism or antibody being evaluated. These are then applied to serologic, histologic, or cytologic specimens. If the organism or antibody of interest is present in the sample, fluorescence will be seen when evaluated. Fluorescent techniques have some subjectivity to their interpretation and the practitioner should be confident of individual laboratories performing these interpretations. Diseases diagnosed with this methodology include distemper, rabies, pseudorabies, Lyme disease, Rocky Mountain spotted fever (RMSF), ehrlichiosis, plague, and tularemia.

The ability of antigen or antibody to cause agglutination of red cells or other materials is used for detection of some infectious diseases. Latex agglutination is used in a kit for cryptococcal antigen detection. Agar gel immunodiffusion (AGID) and complement fixation (CF) are used to detect antibodies against some of the pathogenic fungi. In general, these two tests lack sensitivity and specificity and therefore identification of the organism is important.

The availability of polymerase chain reaction (PCR) as a method of detection is gradually increasing in veterinary medicine. Minute amounts of DNA or RNA can be detected with nucleic acid primers specific to the organism and then multiplied via rounds of replication to produce enough material for electrophoretic analysis. As a result, PCR tests can detect infections in tissues with low concentrations of antigen and detect differences in species within a genus. Along with the incredible sensitivity of these tests comes a greater effect on results if contamination occurs. Whole blood can be collected from dogs and tested via PCR for *Bartonella* and *Ehrlichia* species. Blood or joint fluid can be tested for *Borrelia*. Urine or renal tissue can be tested for *Leptospira*. Other PCR tests for canine infectious diseases are likely to become commercially available in the near future.

2. How do you collect cytologic samples?

Lymph node and tissue aspiration are simple, inexpensive, and frequently rewarding techniques used to diagnose cases of fungal infection. A 22-gauge needle is applied to a 12-cc syringe. The needle is then inserted into the affected tissue, and either it is redirected through the tissue numerous times ("woodpecker" technique), or a light amount of suction is applied by drawing back to the 2- or 3-cc mark on the syringe. Suction is released and the needle withdrawn. The needle is removed from the syringe, air drawn into the syringe, the needle reattached, and the fluid forced out of the syringe onto a slide, culture swab, or into a glass tube depending on the intended purpose of the sample. In the case of cytology, a simple smear is made. Cytologic samples can be used for direct visualization of *Histoplasma*, *Blastomyces*, *Coccidioides*, *Cryptococcus*, *Neorickettsia helminthoeca*, *Ehrlichia*, and *Clostridium*. With application of FA techniques, cytologic samples can be used to verify *Yersinia* and *Tularemia* infections.

Conjunctival scrapings can be used for cytologic diagnosis of distemper. Scrapings are collected by first removing mucus and tears from the inferior conjunctiva with a cotton tip applicator. A heat-sterilized blunt metal spatula or dull scalpel blade is then used to repeatedly scrape the superficial layer of conjunctiva until a small amount of tissue can be lifted off, applied to a glass slide, and smeared. This usually causes erythema of the conjunctiva and a slight amount of

Table 69-1 Summary of Laboratory and Diagnostic Tests Used for Infectious Diseases

DISEASE	ORGANISM	DIAGNOSTIC TECHNIQUES	SAMPLE
Bacterial Diseases			
Plague	*Yersinia pestis*	1. Anaerobic culture 2. Immunofluorescent cytology 3. Hemagglutination titers	1. Fluid or tissue 2. Immunofluorescent 3. Serum
Leptospirosis	*Leptospira interrogans* (serovars *canicola, bratislava, icterohaemorrhagiae, pomona, grippotyphosa*)	1. Microscopic agglutination titers 2. Histology (FA) 3. PCR 4. Aerobic culture	1. Serum 2. Affected tissue (kidney, liver) 3. Blood, urine 4. Blood, urine, renal, or hepatic tissue
Tetanus	*Clostridium tetani*	1. Anaerobic culture 2. Cytology	1. Affected tissue 2. Affected tissue
Lyme disease/ borreliosis	*Borrelia burgdorferi*	1. Antibody titers (ELISA, FA)	1. Serum
Rickettsial Diseases			
Salmon poisoning	*Neorickettsia helminthoeca*	1. Cytologic identification 2. Fecal smear, flotation, sedimentation	1. Lymph node aspirate 2. Feces
Ehrlichiosis	*Ehrlichia canis*	1. Cytologic identification 2. Antibody titers (FA, ELISA) 3. PCR	1. Blood, buffy coat preps, lymph node aspirates, bone marrow aspirates, joint, and CSF aspirates 2. Serum 3. Blood, serum, and tissues
Rocky Mountain spotted fever	*Rickettsia rickettsii*	1. Antibody titers (FA)	1. Serum

Fungal Diseases

Disease	Organism	Diagnostic Method	Sample
Histoplasmosis	*Histoplasma capsulatum*	1. Cytologic identification	1. Aspirate (lymph node, lung), bronchial fluid, rectal scraping
		2. Histologic identification	2. Affected tissues
		3. Antibody titers (AGID, CF)	3. Serum
Blastomycosis	*Blastomyces dermatitidis*	1. Cytologic identification	1. Aspirate (lymph node, lung), bronchial fluid, tissue imprint (skin lesions)
		2. Histologic identification	2. Affected tissues
		3. Antibody titers (AGID)	3. Serum
Cryptococcosis	*Cryptococcus neoformans*	1. Cytologic identification	1. Exudate or tissue imprint (nasal, cutaneous), CSF
		2. Antigen titers (LA)	2. Serum, urine, CSF
		3. Histologic identification	3. Affected tissues
Coccidioidomycosis	*Coccidioides immitis*	1. Antibody titers (AGID, ELISA, CF)	1. Serum
		2. Cytologic identification	2. Bronchial fluid, aspirates (lung, bone, lymph node)
		3. Histologic identification	3. Affected tissues

Viral Diseases

Disease	Organism	Diagnostic Method	Sample
Distemper	Canine distemper virus	1. Antibody titers (ELISA), PCR	1. Serum, CSF
		2. Cytology (FA)	2. Conjunctival scraping
		3. Histologic identification	3. Affected tissues
Rabies	Rabies virus	1. Histopathology (FA)	1. Brain
Infectious canine hepatitis	Canine adenovirus 2	1. Cytology/histopathology	1. Liver, Kidney
Pseudorabies	Pseudorabies virus	1. Cytology (FA)	1. Brain, tonsil
		2. Virus isolation	2. Brain, tonsil

FA, Fluorescent antibodies; *PCR*, polymerase chain reaction; *CSF*, cerebrospinal fluid; *ELISA*, enzyme-linked immunosorbent assay; *AGID*, Agar gel immunodiffusion; *LA*, latex agglutination; *CF*, complement fixation.

bleeding. Slides are sent for distemper fluorescent antibody staining. Using routine in house stains, the slides can be evaluated for characteristic intracytoplasmic distemper virus inclusions.

Rectal scrapings can be useful for detection of histoplasmosis (Fig. 69-1). This is performed by passing a gloved finger or cotton-tipped applicator into the rectum and scraping the mucosa repeatedly. The finger or applicator is removed and the tip lightly rolled on a slide for staining with routine in house stains.

Tracheal washes can be used for diagnosis of fungal and bacterial infections. A 16- to 18-gauge, 12-inch through-the-needle catheter is needed. The needle is either inserted between tracheal rings either in the distal third of the cervical trachea large dogs or in the cricothyroid ligament (space just cranial to the firm ventral ridge of the cricoid cartilage) in medium-size dogs. The area of puncture is prepared aseptically and sterile gloves are worn. Dogs that weigh less than 20 pounds are best sampled by passing a sterile red rubber catheter through a sterile endotracheal tube. After the needle is inserted and the catheter advance through it, the needle is withdrawn a short distance out of the skin. One to 10 ml of sterile saline is infused. When the animal coughs, aspirate to collect wash material. This can be repeated several times if needed. The catheter is removed and typically no bandaging is needed. Subcutaneous emphysema can occur. The fluid is used for cytologic analysis and culture as indicated.

3.   How do you collect and evaluate cerebrospinal fluid (CSF)?

CSF is collected in a much more refined manner and must be handled with care. Cytologic preparations are best interpreted by an experienced cytologist and made after cytocentrifugation to concentrate the low quantity of cells into a small area. The fluid must be analyzed within a short period before cellular degradation. Therefore a laboratory capable of handling CSF should be identified before collection and be reachable within 30 minutes. The atlantooccipital cistern is the most useful site of collection for most central nervous system (CNS) infections. After anesthesia has been induced and the site aseptically prepared, the dog is placed in lateral recumbency (right lateral for a right dominant person) with the neck flexed to open the atlantooccipital cistern. The space is identified as a subtle depression in the center of a triangle made by placing the left thumb on the right wing of the atlas, the left middle finger on the left wing, and the index finger on the occipital protuberance. This correlates to the cranial aspect of the

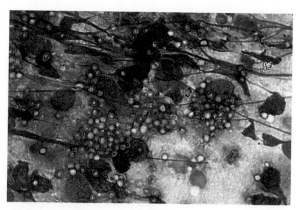

Figure 69-1.   Rectal scraping from a dog presented with clinical signs of chronic large bowel diarrhea and weight loss. Cytologic examination reveals large numbers of intracellular and free *Histoplasma capsulatum* organisms.

atlas. A 22-gauge, 1.5- to 2.5-inch spinal needle is then slowly inserted into this space with the needle nearly 90° to the spine and directly on midline with the bevel directed cranially. It is uncommon to completely insert a 1.5-inch needle into a dog of any size. The stylet is removed intermittently to evaluate for flow so that the needle is not advanced into the cord or brain stem. If frank blood appears, the needle has been placed off midline and the needle should be removed. After CSF flows from the needle, it should be aseptically collected by allowing it to drip into an empty glass tube. Approximately 1 to 2 ml is required for most diagnostic tests. The needle is then removed. Cell counts, cytologic evaluation, and fluorescent antibody techniques can be applied to CSF for detection of canine distemper virus antigens. Titers for distemper, *Ehrlichia canis*, RMSF, *Cryptococcus*, and other infections can be determined and compared with serum concentrations for diagnosis. Fluid can be submitted for cultures.

VIRAL DISEASES
Canine Distemper
4. What is the etiologic agent of canine distemper?
Canine distemper is caused by a single stranded RNA containing *Paramyxovirus* virus.

5. How do animals acquire the infection?
Canine distemper virus (CDV) is acquired from infective aerosol respiratory secretions.

6. What is the pathogenesis of the disease?
The virus attaches to the upper respiratory epithelium. Local replication occurs in mononuclear cells and spreads to local lymph nodes and tonsils, and then to other lymphoid containing organs and epithelial tissues. Hematogenous dissemination results in infection of other epithelial organs and the CNS. Animals that mount an adequate humoral and cell-mediated response clear the virus. If immunity of the dog is inadequate, then spread of the virus to other tissues, skin, glandular tissue, epithelium of the gastrointestinal tract, and respiratory and urinary system occurs and clinical signs become evident. Shedding of virus from infected dogs may be of short or long duration, depending on the dog's immunologic status and response.

7. What are the major clinical manifestations of canine distemper?
Major clinical signs develop in young animals usually younger than 16 weeks. The most common systems affected by canine distemper include respiratory, gastrointestinal, skin and nervous systems.

Ocular and nasal discharges are present in early stages of the disease, and are usually associated with concomitant constitutional signs such as fever, lethargy, and anorexia. If the dog's immunity is inadequate, secondary bacterial infections result in purulent ocular and nasal discharges and cough. Respiratory distress may be observed in severely infected animals.

Gastrointestinal signs such as vomiting and diarrhea may be observed because of the local replication of virus in these tissues. Enamel hypoplasia can be noted in young animals that were previously infected with canine distemper and subsequently develop neurologic signs.

Dermatologic signs such as impetiginous dermatitis in young dogs, or nasal and footpad hyperkeratosis may be noted. Pustular dermatitis is reported to be a good prognostic indicator but is not a consistent observation.

Neurologic signs in dogs are due to acute or chronic encephalitis. Manifestations include seizures, cerebellar and vestibular signs, paraparesis, tetraparesis, and myoclonus. Myoclonus and the classical "chewing gum fits" are features that are almost pathognomonic for this disease, but other CNS disease can produce similar clinical manifestations. However, if these signs are observed in a susceptible, unvaccinated young dog, it would lend more credence to canine distemper infection. Ocular manifestations associated with canine distemper infection include conjunctivitis, keratitis, optic neuritis, and keratoconjunctivitis sicca.

8. What are the major laboratory abnormalities associated with canine distemper?

Leukopenia may be observed early in the disease and may persist in dogs with progressive disease and early neurologic manifestations. A mild anemia and thrombocytopenia have also been reported in the early stages of infection. Leukocytosis and neutrophilia result when secondary opportunistic infections are present.

Viral inclusions can be observed in erythrocytes, lymphocytes, and other mononuclear cells. These appear as round to oval gray/blue intracytoplasmic bodies. No major biochemical abnormalities are consistently noted.

9. What are major means of diagnosis of CDV infection?

A compatible history and clinical signs are usually supportive of a diagnosis of acute canine distemper. Lack of proper vaccination in a young animal should also increase the clinical suspicion. Chronic neurologic disease from canine distemper infection is difficult to differentiate from other causes of acquired seizures and paresis, based solely on historical and physical findings.

CSF analysis in dogs with acute encephalitis usually shows increases in protein concentration and increased mononuclear cells, predominately lymphocytes. Detection of anti-CDV antibody in the CSF is the most definitive evidence of distemper encephalitis, provided that blood contamination is minimal during collection. If blood contamination is present in CSF, serum, and CSF antibody titers for CDV and canine parvovirus can be measured and their corresponding CSF to serum ratios computed. If the ratio for CDV antibodies exceeds that of parvovirus, then a diagnosis of CDV infection is plausible (see Chapter 4). Immunocytology and immunohistochemistry can be used to detect viral antigen in tissue samples. Conjunctival, tonsillar, and respiratory samples may reveal a positive fluorescence test early in the course of disease before antibody titers increase. This technique may also be applied to tissue samples obtained at the time of biopsy or necropsy.

Serum titers can be detected by ELISA methodology. Immunoglobulin (Ig)M antibodies can be detected in both acute and chronic encephalopathies from canine distemper and is more definitive than IgG antibodies. IgG antibodies only denote that the animal has been exposed to the virus, either naturally or through vaccination.

A seminested reverse transcriptase PCR has also been used to detect viral antigen in fresh and formalin fixed tissues to aid in the detection of canine distemper.

10. What therapies are used to treat canine distemper?

There is no known effective antiviral therapy that moderates the disease. Supportive therapies consist of control of opportunistic infections and include, antibacterial therapy, and antiprotozoal therapy. Opportunistic infections reported include *Bordetella* spp., *Salmonella* spp., *Toxoplasma gondii*, and *Neospora caninum*.

Attention to general hygiene, fluid balance, and nutrition is also important. Cleaning of ocular and nasal discharges, application of ophthalmic preparations to prevent exposure keratitis, and a good high protein and caloric diet are all beneficial.

11. What is the best method of prevention of canine distemper?

Vaccination is typically started at approximately 6 weeks to avoid lapse in protection in puppies with maternal antibody titers that are waning. Boosters are administered every 2 to 3 weeks until the dog is 16 weeks of age. The decline of maternal antibodies is predictable based on the maternal antibody titers by use of nomogram that shows the rate of antibody decline and the expected time for optimal vaccination. At least two vaccines should be administered to all dogs in the initial preventative program.

12. What type of vaccines should be used for vaccination?

Several different vaccines are available that provide active immunization of animals. These include modified live, inactivated whole virus, subunit products, and recombinant vector–based vaccine. Use of heterologous vaccination with measles virus can provide temporary immunity in animals younger than 6 weeks.

13. What is the duration of immunity in dogs that recover from canine distemper infection?
Postinfection immunity from canine distemper infection is reported to last at least 7 years.

14. What type of disinfectants should be used in households where infected dogs have resided?
This virus is susceptible to most common disinfectants including sodium hypochlorite and the quandary ammonium compounds.

Canine Adenovirus Infections

15. What clinical syndromes do canine adenovirus (CAV-1 and CAV-2) agents cause in dogs?
There are two different and distinct adenoviruses that infect dogs. CAV-1 causes infectious hepatitis and upper respiratory disease, whereas CAV-2 predominately results in an acute upper respiratory disease. CAV-2 is one viral agent incriminated in the canine "kennel cough" complex.

16. How are adenoviruses transmitted to dogs?
These viruses are shed in most body secretions from acutely infected dogs. Contact of susceptible dogs with contaminated fomites results in oronasal exposure. The virus replicates in tonsils and lymphoid tissues of the oral cavity and then disseminates hematogenously to other tissues and organs.

17. What are the major clinical manifestations of adenovirus infections in dogs?
CAV-1 infections can be commonly asymptomatic infections, based on serologic surveys, or cause acute or chronic disease syndromes. These syndromes are related to organ injuries of the liver, kidneys, eyes, and respiratory tract. The predominant organ injury with CAV-1 is the liver, where it causes hepatic necrosis. Clinical signs related to hepatic injury include fever, vomiting, diarrhea, hepatic enlargement, and abdominal pain. If the dog mounts an effective immune response early in the disease, hepatic injury may be limited. In dogs with severe hepatic necrosis, disseminated intravascular coagulation (DIC) may result and cause a hemorrhagic diathesis. Partial immune responses in infected CAV-1–infected dogs can result in a chronic hepatopathy, characterized by persistent hepatic inflammation.

Renal injury also occurs in CAV-1 infection but is subclinical. The virus localizes in the glomerular vasculature and later leads to immune complex deposition and proteinuria. Virus persists in the renal tubular epithelium and a mild interstitial nephritis can develop. Clinical signs of renal involvement are not usually significant.

Ophthalmologic signs occur in some naturally infected dogs. Keratitis and uveitis develop from virus replication and antibody production within this tissue. Mild to severe corneal edema can develop. CAV-1 can eventually result in secondary glaucoma from obstruction of the ocular drainage angle from inflammatory debris. Ocular changes may be the only clinical sign noted in mild cases of CAV-1 infection. These ocular lesions are not always reversible in the dog on its recovery.

Respiratory involvement with CAV-1 and CAV-2 infections result in mild to moderate respiratory signs and produce a dry hacking cough and abnormal lung sounds. Interstitial pneumonia may be complicated with secondary bacterial infection in severely infected, susceptible dogs.

Severe CAV-1 infection can produce neurologic signs from hemorrhage and activation of the clotting system associated with vasculitis and from hepatic failure (hepatoencephalopathy).

18. What laboratory findings are common with adenovirus infections in dogs?
Laboratory abnormalities depend on the severity of injury to the liver, kidneys, eye, and vascular endothelium. Hemogram changes include leukopenia and thrombocytopenia. In severe

infections, DIC and associated coagulation abnormalities can be observed with increases in activated partial thromboplastin time, one-stage prothrombin time, fibrin degradation products, and D-dimer concentrations.

Hepatic enzyme elevations depend on the severity of infection and the host immune response to infection. Increases in alanine aminotransferase (ALT) and alkaline phosphatase (ALP) are usually present, with ALT concentrations being greater than ALP concentrations. Hyperbilirubinemia is not a feature of the acute hepatic syndrome because most dogs that recover do so rapidly. In animals with viral persistence causing chronic hepatic inflammation, this finding may be present along with other biochemical abnormalities associated with a chronic hepatopathy (decreased serum urea nitrogen, albumin and glucose, increased ALT, ALP, and total bilirubin).

Dogs infected with CAV-2 infections do not have any consistent laboratory abnormalities, except in cases of secondary respiratory bacterial infection in which an inflammatory leukogram may be present.

19. How are adenovirus infections diagnosed?

A clinical diagnosis of CAV-1 infection is difficult, but should be suspected when young, unvaccinated dogs are presented with an acute onset of gastrointestinal signs and elevated liver enzymes. Dogs presenting with this compatible history are often suspected of having toxicosis. Evidence of a hemorrhagic diathesis in dogs with the aforementioned signs and laboratory abnormalities consistent of DIC lend additional support for an acute hepatopathy with activation of the clotting pathways. CAV-1 can be isolated by viral isolation from oropharyngeal swabs, but this is not a viable diagnostic test for most clinical cases.

Histologic examination of the liver reveals an acute centrilobular to panlobular necrosis. Evidence of hemorrhage may be widespread in dogs that exhibit signs compatible with DIC. Intranuclear, acidophilic inclusion bodies can be identified in dogs that die from CAV-1 infection.

20. How can adenovirus infections be prevented in dogs?

Vaccination with CAV-1 and CAV-2 modified live vaccines are highly effective in preventing disease. CAV-1 modified live virus (MLV) may result in ocular and renal lesions; therefore, a CAV-2 MLV is used to provide a heterotypic antibody response that is protective. Administration of two doses of MLV vaccine beginning at 8 to 9 weeks of age is recommended. Because of the duration of immunity with MLV, booster vaccination is not always required.

Pseudorabies

21. What is the etiologic agent causing pseudorabies?

Pseudorabies, also known as Aujeszky's disease or mad itch, is caused by an α-herpesvirus.

22. How do dogs and cats contract pseudorabies?

Infection is acquired when the dog ingests infected tissues. Whereas other mammals can be transient reservoirs of the virus, pigs are the predominant reservoirs of the disease and can have subclinical infections. Dogs can also contract pseudorabies by biting infected pigs or eating raw infected meat. Dogs are not a source of infection for other dogs. After ingestion, the virus ascends nerve fibers in the area of inoculation in a retrograde fashion, ultimately infecting the brain stem and cranial nerve nuclei.

23. Is there a geographic distribution of this disease?

Pseudorabies is found worldwide but is more common in areas with a high population of pigs.

24. What are the most common clinical manifestations of pseudorabies?

Ptyalism was the most common clinical sign of pseudorabies in dogs and was reported in 100% of cases in one retrospective study. In the same report, all dogs had exposure to pigs. Restlessness, anorexia, ataxia, wandering aimlessly, tachypnea, dyspnea, vocalizing, and pruritus were associated with the disease in more than 50% of dogs with pseudorabies. Muscle spasms, vomiting, aggressiveness, trismus, dysphagia, and abnormal papillary light responses can also be seen. Death routinely occurs within a short period after the first clinical signs become apparent.

25. What are the most common laboratory abnormalities observed?

Hematologic or biochemical abnormalities are not consistently identified in dogs with pseudorabies infection.

26. What are the best methods to diagnose this disease?

Clinical signs and a history of exposure to pigs should raise a degree of suspicion of the disease. Antemortem diagnosis is uncommon as the disease is rapidly fatal. Postmortem diagnosis is accomplished with fluorescent antibody testing or virus isolation from affected tissues.

27. What is the most effective therapy?

There is no effective treatment for pseudorabies.

28. How can pseudorabies be prevented in dogs?

Animals should not be allowed exposure to pigs or access to uncooked pork tissues. There are no available vaccines for dogs or cats in the United States.

Rabies

29. What is the etiologic agent of rabies?

This is a viral disease of mammals. The virus belongs to the genus *Lyssavirus* in the family Rhabdoviridae.

30. How do dogs contract the disease?

The disease is transmitted from the bite of an infected animal through its saliva to a susceptible animal. Domestic dogs are considered to have moderate susceptibility to this viral infection.

After the virus is injected into tissue, the virus replicates within tissues myocytes and then enters surrounding nervous tissue. The virus spreads in motor and sensory neurons by axonal spread to the central nervous system. After the central nervous system is infected, the virus disseminates to other body tissues via peripheral, sensory, and motor neurons. Salivary glands eventually become infected; from there, the viral disease can then be transmitted to other susceptible animals. Not all animals infected with rabies are efficient in the transmittal of this disease through their saliva.

31. What wildlife species are the important reservoirs for maintaining rabies in the United States?

Depending on the region of the country, skunks, foxes (gray, Arctic, and red), raccoons, and bats account for most of the wildlife species reported with rabies. The number of cases reported in 2001 increased among bats, cats, skunks, rodents/lagomorphs, and swine and decreased among dogs, cattle, foxes, horses/mules, raccoons, and sheep/goats. The relative contributions of the major groups of animals were as follows: raccoons (37.2%; 2767 cases), skunks (30.7%; 2282), bats (17.2%; 1281), foxes (5.9%; 437), cats (3.6%; 270), dogs (1.2%; 89), and cattle (1.1%; 82).

32. What are the major clinical manifestations of rabies infection in the dog?

Clinical signs vary and are mainly neurologic in nature. Ptyalism, dysphagia, and an inability to swallow may suggest pharyngeal, esophageal, or a gastrointestinal disorder, but these are the result of neurologic dysfunction. In the early states of rabies, behavioral changes are present. These changes are subtle and are not always noticed by the owner or veterinarian.

Furious and paralytic forms of the disease are described in dogs. These clinical manifestations are arbitrary and are used to describe changes in the dog's behavior during progression of the disease. The furious form of the disease in dogs is characterized by aggression to people, animals, or inanimate objects. Dogs may appear excitable, bark, or attack imaginary objects. Ataxia or incoordination precedes the more dramatic clinical neurologic signs. Seizures, coma, and paralysis are evident before the animal succumbs of the disease.

33. What is the best method of diagnosis of rabies in dogs?

On the basis of current methods, the most rapid and sensitive test for detecting rabies is the direct fluorescent test on brain tissue. The head from the suspected dog should be cooled and maintained on ice and not frozen. Specimens of the medulla, cerebellum, and hippocampus are used for the direct FA test.

Conventional histopathologic examination of brain tissue does not always provide confirmation of the disease because changes are mild. Acute polioencephalitis is observed early in the course of the disease, with a necrotizing encephalitis in progressive infections. Presence of intracytoplasmic inclusions, or Negri bodies, may be observed in the hippocampus and Purkinje cells of affected dogs. Special stains may be required to demonstrate these structures more readily.

34. How can you prevent rabies infection in dogs?

The first step is to prevent contact of dogs with wildlife reservoirs such as skunks, foxes, and raccoons. Vaccination of dogs is highly effective and should be performed based on current recommendations by the National Association of State Public Health Veterinarians.

Vaccination is recommended with a vaccination approved by the Food and Drug Administration at 3 months of age and 1 year later. Booster vaccinations after the initial two vaccinations should be performed in accordance with local public health laws with an approved product, either annually or every 3 years.

35. What should be done if a vaccinated dog is bitten by an animal that is definitively diagnosed with rabies?

Procedures vary slightly and depend on local public health laws. Contact with local health officials should be established before any action of suspected animals.

RICKETTSIAL DISEASES

Ehrlichiosis

36. What species of *Ehrlichia* infect dogs?

The taxonomy of the *Ehrlichia* species has recently changed and is based on an objective classification scheme of the sequences of 16S ribosomal genes. The genus *Ehrlichia* belongs in the family Anaplasmataceae, which contains three other genera: *Anaplasma, Neorickettsia,* and *Wolbachia.* The *Ehrlichia* genus contains *Ehrlichia canis, Ehrlichia chaffeensis,* and *Ehrlichia ewingii. Ehrlichia phagocytophila, Ehrlichia equi,* and *Ehrlichia platys* are now classified in the genus *Anaplasma,* along with the agent of human granulocytic ehrlichiosis. These latter three *Ehrlichia* species have similar nucleotides and are considered by some to be the same organism.

The genus *Neorickettsia* now contains the organisms formally named *Ehrlichia sennetsu* and *Ehrlichia risticii,* along with the agent of that causes salmon poisoning in dogs, *N. helminthoeca.*

37. What is the geographic distribution of ehrlichiosis?

These agents have a worldwide distribution that is related to the distribution of vectors for the specific infective agent.

38. How are the *Ehrlichia* species transmitted to dogs?

The most common means of transmission for the *Ehrlichia* species infecting dogs is through salivary secretions of infected ticks. *Neorickettsia risticii* (old taxonomy name: *E. risticii*) is infective to the horse by the ingestion of *N. risticii*–infected trematode stages, either free in water, or in an intermediate host, such as aquatic animals. The true means of transmission in the dog is not definitively known.

39. What are the common vectors for the disease in dogs?

E. canis: *Rhipicephalus sanguineus*
E. chaffeensis: *Amblyomma americanum, Dermacentor variabilis*
E. ewingii: *A. americanum, R. sanguineus*
Anaplasma equi + HGE: *Ixodes pacificus, Ixodes scapularis*
Anaplasma phagocytophila: *Ixodes ricinus*
Anaplasma platys: *R. sanguineus*
N. risticii: Infected metacercaria of snails, aquatic insects

40. What are the most common clinical manifestations of disease?

Clinical manifestations of ehrlichiosis vary from asymptomatic cases to severe and life-threatening infections. Asymptomatic infection is common in endemic areas and has been demonstrated by a high level of seropositivity in dogs. Clinical signs of ehrlichiosis depend on the stage of the disease present (acute, subacute, and chronic phases), the infecting agent, host response and presence of coinfections with other vector-borne or related diseases (*Babesia* infection, RMSF, and *Bartonellosis* infection).

Constitutional signs such as fever, weight loss, lethargy, lymphadenopathy, and depression are common in the acute stages of the disease. Bleeding diathesis is observed in approximately 50% of dogs and may consist of epistaxis, melena, hematuria, petechial, and ecchymotic hemorrhage from associated thrombocytopenia, and platelet dysfunction associated with hypergammaglobulinemia. Additional clinical signs include polyarthritis, uveitis, and CNS signs (ataxia, vestibular signs, and seizures). Lameness from polyarthritis is observed in some dogs infected with certain species of *Ehrlichia* (*E. ewingii*). Renal disease and failure may also result from glomerulonephropathy induced by chronic antigenic stimulation.

41. What laboratory abnormalities are commonly observed with ehrlichiosis?

A nonregenerative anemia and thrombocytopenia are commonly observed abnormalities present on the hemogram. Biochemical changes include hyperproteinemia characterized by hypergammaglobulinemia and hypoalbuminemia. Monoclonal or polyclonal gammopathies can be identified and can be confused with neoplastic processes. Renal involvement may cause azotemia and proteinuria due to immune complex glomerulonephropathy.

Lymph node cytologic examination commonly reveals a reactive plasma cell hyperplasia. Bone marrow aspirates may reveal hypercellularity and hypocellularity of certain cell lines and increased number of plasma cells.

42. What laboratory tests are useful in the diagnosis of ehrlichiosis?

Evaluation of peripheral blood smears, buffy coat smears, lymph node cytologic examination, and bone marrow may be of diagnostic help in the acute stage of disease. Morula can be observed and are noted in buffy coat smears and lymph node cytology. Joint fluid analysis may reveal the presence of morula depending on the infective species.

Detection of antibodies against ehrlichiosis is the most commonly used laboratory method for detection of infection. Indirect fluorescent antibody titers (IgG) increase early in the disease (7-28 days). Acutely infected animals may not seroconvert. Repeating the indirect fluorescent antibody (IFA) test in 2 to 3 weeks is indicated when clinical signs are compatible with ehrlichiosis.

Serologic cross reactivity does occur among the various species but certain *Ehrlichia* species may not be detected by routine IFA testing with *E. canis* antigen. A positive serologic cross reactivity can be noted with infections with *E. canis, E. ewingii,* and *E. chaffeensis. A. platys, A. equi,* and *N. risticii* are unlikely to be detected with the IFA test for *E. canis*. A specific IFA titer cutoff point is not universally accepted as defining infection. A significant IFA titer may range from less than 1:20 to 1:80 depending on the specific laboratory. A commercially available in-house ELISA test for *E. canis* uses a value of less than 1:100.

Western blot analysis and PCR testing can be performed to identify specific infecting species. These methods may be useful when a positive IFA test is present and there is a strong clinical suspicion of disease. Coinfections occur in dogs with reports of *Rickettsia rickettsi* and *Babesiosis* and *Bartonellosis* species being detected.

Antibodies detected against the *Ehrlichia* species does not equate with active disease. Antibodies persist for extended periods in infected and treated dogs. Persistence of clinical signs and hypergammaglobulinemia may indicate ineffective treatment protocols. Antibodies are not protective against reinfection.

43. What is the treatment for ehrlichiosis?

Several drugs are used for therapy and include tetracycline, chloramphenicol, imidocarb dipropionate, and amicarbalide. Tetracycline, oxytetracycline, doxycycline, and minocycline are the most commonly used agents. A course of doxycycline (10 mg/kg every 24 hours) for 28 days is recommended for dogs. Imidocarb dipropionate is as effective as doxycycline and can be administered at 5 mg/kg intramuscularly, two doses 2 weeks apart.

There is some controversy regarding how animals should be monitored after treatment. PCR testing is the only clinically available means of determining whether an animal was effectively cured, but a positive PCR test result does not equate with viable organisms. If there is doubt whether the dog is cured after treatment, PCR testing should be performed after antibiotic therapy has been discontinued for 2 weeks. If a positive PCR test result is still evident, additional therapy should be administered or another anti-ehrlichia agent should be used (imidocarb).

Rocky Mountain Spotted Fever

44. What is the etiologic agent of RMSF?

R. rickettsii is the only spotted fever rickettsial species known to be pathogenic in the United States in dogs.

45. How is RMSF transmitted to dogs?

This disease is a vector-borne disease. The organism is transmitted to dogs during the feeding period of the tick. *Dermacentor andersoni* and *D. variabilis* are the most common natural hosts, reservoirs, and vectors for this disease. Other tick vectors reported to transmit RMSF include *A. americanum*, *R. sanguineus*, and *Haemaphysalis leporispalustris*.

46. What are the major clinical manifestations of RMSF in the dog?

Most cases are presented during the spring to early fall seasons (March to October). Clinical signs are usually acute in nature. Young and purebred dogs are overrepresented in several reports. Fever, anorexia, lymphadenopathy, and petechial and ecchymotic hemorrhages may be present. Hemorrhage may be present on the skin and other mucous membranes. Retinal hemorrhage is commonly noted on ophthalmologic examination. Peripheral edema can result from the associated vasculitis. Polyarthralgia and myalgia are common. Neurologic signs include altered mental states, vestibular signs, paresis, and seizures.

47. What are the common laboratory abnormalities associated with RMSF?

Hemogram changes include a mild anemia, leukocytosis with a left shift, and thrombocytopenia. Thrombocytopenia is reported to be the most commonly observed laboratory abnormality in infected dogs. In some instances, prolongation of the activated partial thromboplastin time, increased fibrin degradation products and D-dimers may be observed and are consistent with DIC.

Biochemical changes include increased ALT, ALP, aspartate aminotransferase (AST), and hypercholesterolemia. Creatine kinase levels may be increased because of muscle involvement. Hypoalbuminemia is common and is associated with the vasculitis and subsequent leakage of serum proteins. Azotemia may be present and indicate prerenal and renal involvement. Urine sediment examination usually reveals proteinuria, hematuria, and pyuria because of associated glomerular and tubular injuries.

If CSF is analyzed, increases in protein are mild with increases in polymononuclear cells. Joint fluid analysis may reveal an increase in mononuclear cells and protein concentration.

48. How is RMSF diagnosed?

Compatible clinical signs, laboratory findings, and serologic tests are used in most cases to arrive at a diagnosis. Serologic testing is the mainstay of diagnosis of this disease. Direct fluorescent staining of infected tissue obtained by biopsy can detect infection early in the disease, before serum antibody titers become positive. PCR on blood and tissue specimens can also be used to detect antigen, but is not commercially available at this time.

Several serologic tests are available and include the microimmunofluorescent antibody and ELISA. The MicroFA test can detect IgM and IgG antibodies. IgG titers are usually less than 1:64. A fourfold IgG titer increase is required to document active infection and this generally becomes positive at 2 to 3 weeks after infection. IgG antibodies may persist for months after infection. IgM antibodies can be detected approximately 1 week after infection and decrease after 4 to 8 weeks. IgM antibody titers higher than 1:8 on a single titer may be compatible with active infection.

49. What is the current treatment for RMSF?

Therapy is considered to be rickettsiostatic. Tetracycline, oxytetracycline, doxycycline, minocycline, chloramphenicol, and fluoroquinolones have been used as effective therapy. Tetracyclines and fluoroquinolones should not be used in animals younger than 6 months. Antibiotic therapy should be given for approximately 10 to 14 days. Antibiotic therapy early in the course of the disease may blunt the serologic response to infection and may lead to erroneous interpretation of test results.

Supportive care with intravenous fluids and plasma are indicated in dogs presented with shock and associated coagulation disorders. Judicious use of these agents is indicated because the associated vasculitis may result in fluid extravasation. Neurologic manifestations may require use of anticonvulsant therapy.

50. Are dogs immune to reinfection with *R. rickettsii*?

Most animals that recover from infection are suspected to be immune to reinfection for some period.

51. How can RMSF be prevented?

Vector control is important and is best accomplished with topical or systemic tick control treatments of permethrin, fipronil, or seasonal dips with limited access to tick-infested areas. Impregnated dog collars have also some to be beneficial in the control of the vectors.

Salmon Poisoning Disease

52. What is the etiologic agent causing salmon poisoning disease?

The etiologic agent is *N. helminthoeca*, a Gram-negative coccoid to coccobacillary member of the family Rickettsiaceae. The organism infects the fluke *Nanophyetus salmincola*. This fluke requires three hosts to complete its life cycle. First, it infects the snail, *Oxytrema silicula*. Eventually, the cercaria leaves the snail and penetrates the skin of fish in the Salmonidae family. Other fish and the Pacific giant salamander are also susceptible to this organism. Replication in the salmon occurs predominantly in the kidneys. Metacercaria within the kidneys then are ingested when dogs eat the salmon. A similar yet less severe disease called Elokomin fluke fever is caused by a similar, but yet to be named organism that is carried by the same fluke.

53. How do dogs acquire infection with *N. helminthoeca*?

Transmission occurs when dogs eat infected salmon or other susceptible fish, but only about half of the time is fish ingestion known to have occurred. Dogs can have infections of both *N. helminthoeca* and *N. salmincola* or only the latter. Rickettsemia occurs soon after intestinal infestation by *N. salmincola* and the organisms disseminate to lymphoid tissues and most organs.

54. Is there a geographic distribution of this disease?

Yes. Salmon poisoning disease is limited to the geographic range of *O. silicula* and extends from California north to Vancouver Island.

55. What are the most common clinical manifestations of disease?

Dogs typically show clinical signs approximately 1 week after ingestion of infected fish. Clinical signs include fever, depression, anorexia, generalized lymphadenopathy, acute vomiting and diarrhea, dehydration, and severe weight loss. Temperature gradually decreases to normal or subnormal over 4 to 8 days. Without treatment, dogs typically die within 10 days.

56. What are the most common laboratory abnormalities observed?

Although no consistent hematologic or biochemical patterns are reported, thrombocytopenia, lymphopenia, increased alkaline phosphatase, and decreased albumin occur in more than 50% of dogs.

57. What methods are used to diagnose this disease?

Suspicion of the disease is based on appropriate history and clinical signs. Because of the rapid progression of the disease, treatment may be required before a full diagnostic workup can be completed. Diagnosis is accomplished by fine-needle aspiration cytology of affected lymph nodes and is effective in 86% of cases in one series of reports. *N. helminthoeca* organisms are obligate intracellular cocci or coccobacilli with a purple color within mononuclear cells using Giemsa stain or commonly used Diff-Quik techniques. Detection of the eggs of *N. salmincola* by direct fecal smear, sedimentation, or flotation techniques is indirect evidence of infection with *N. helminthoeca*.

Fecal flotation procedures are reported to be sensitive but are performed differently than for common intestinal parasite analysis (sodium nitrate or zinc sulfate); thus commercial laboratories may be useful if the direct smear fails to elucidate the eggs. The light brown eggs have a single, poorly apparent operculum, a small knob at the opposing end, are approximately 90 μm long, and are shed beginning 5 to 8 days after ingestion.

58. What is the most effective therapy?

Hospitalization for supportive treatment with intravenous fluids and antiemetics is usually required. Because anorexia and vomiting are common parenteral sulfonamides, penicillin, doxycycline, or oxytetracycline (7 mg/kg intravenously, three times daily) can be used. Oral drugs, typically doxycycline (10 mg/kg, twice daily) or tetracycline (22 mg/kg, three times daily), can be given after vomiting has remitted. The cure rate with tetracycline was reported to be 91%. Antimicrobials are given for approximately 1 week. *N. salmincola* is cleared with oral praziquantel administered once subcutaneously at the labeled dose.

59. How can salmon poisoning be prevented?

Preventing animals from eating raw or undercooked fish is the best preventative. No vaccine is available.

BACTERIAL DISEASES

Leptospirosis

60. What are the etiologic agents that cause clinical disease?

Multiple serovars are responsible for disease in dogs and include *Leptospirosa interrogans* sensu stricto, *Leptospirosa icterohaemorrhagiae, Leptospirosa canicola, Leptospirosa pomona, Leptospirosa bratislava, Leptospirosa autumnalis, Leptospirosa hardjo,* and *Leptospira kirschneri grippotyphosa.*

61. What are the naturally occurring reservoirs of the disease?

Each agent has a different primary wildlife or domestic animal reservoir species and includes the rat, mouse, cow, swine, skunk, and opossum.

62. How is leptospirosis transmitted?

Dogs normally become infected by contact with infected urine. The organism can also penetrate intact mucosal membranes.

63. What are the most common clinical presentations of leptospirosis in dogs?

Clinical manifestations of the disease in the dog are dependent on the serovar causing infection and host immunity. Infections may be associated with peracute death, or an acute disease process characterized by vomiting, diarrhea, icterus, and bilirubinuria. Hemorrhagic tendencies may be present and result in hematemesis, melena, hematochezia, epistaxis, and petechiation. Urine output is usually reduced in animals that experience acute renal failure. Certain serovars have been temporally associated with chronic diseases, most notably chronic active hepatitis and chronic renal disease.

64. What are the most common laboratory abnormalities?

The major laboratory abnormalities are usually the result of the associated vasculitis. Leukocytosis, thrombocytopenia, increased one-stage prothrombin time, activated partial thromboplastin time, elevated fibrin degradation products or D-dimers, elevated liver enzymes (ALT > ALP), bilirubinemia, bilirubinuria, renal azotemia, and inflammatory urine sediment can be seen. Urine output may be reduced to oliguria or anuria.

65. How is leptospirosis diagnosed?

Diagnosis of leptospirosis is based on clinical manifestations and serologic testing. The microscopic agglutination test or ELISA test methodology are the most commonly used methods used. Whole cell preparations are usually used as the antigen. A single microscopic agglutination test titer of 1:800 or greater or a fourfold increase in microscopic agglutination test (MAT) titers that are specific to a serovar is compatible with active infection. Vaccination with bacterins may also result in measurable titers but are not usually of the magnitude of the infecting serovar. IgM and IgG titers parallel increases with the MAT. IgM titers are usually present early in the disease and are more specific than IgG titers. Titers are usually the highest to the infecting serovar but cross-reactivity can cause numerous serovar titers to be increased. Early antibiotic therapy may blunt the serologic response.

Isolation of the organism from blood or urine can be attempted, but because of the fastidious nature of the organism, it requires considerable attention to sterility of sample procurement and transport to a laboratory. Organisms can be isolated from healthy dogs and is therefore not in itself indicative of leptospirosis.

PCR techniques are being used in a research setting and have been recently patented for use. Validation of this method and use in clinical patients is lacking but shows promise for future.

66. What is the treatment for leptospirosis?

Antibiotic therapy should be initiated early in the disease. Ampicillin or penicillin should be used and reduces leptospiremia within a short period. These antibiotics do not eliminate carrier states. Tetracycline, doxycycline, and macrolides have been shown to eliminate the carrier state. Fluoroquinolones are effective in vitro and in vivo, but clinical studies with these agents have not been conducted.

Supportive care for dehydration should include intravenous fluids and antiemetics. Ancillary treatments to increase urine output in cases of oliguric or anuric acute renal failure may include osmotic and loop diuretics, though whether they influence outcome is uncertain. If DIC is present, plasma transfusions and low-dose heparin may be considered.

67. How can leptospirosis be prevented?

Reduce contact with primary hosts and with infected urine. This should include control of contact with rats, mice, swine, cattle, and wildlife species. Vaccines with *Leptospira* bacterins are available, but do not always prevent infections with other serovars. Bacterins have recently been shown to reduce the incidence of the carrier state in challenge studies and to produce immunity for 6 to 12 months after two vaccinations.

68. Is leptospirosis a zoonotic disease?

Yes, leptospirosis is a zoonotic disease and type Bio2 containment procedures will effectively reduce the risk of contracting the disease. Hand-washing procedures were effective in one study. Gloves and eye protection should be used because these organisms can penetrate intact mucous membranes. Treatment of contaminated areas should include use of detergent agents and treatment with iodophor disinfectants.

Canine Lyme Disease or Borreliosis

69. What is the etiologic agent of Lyme disease?

Borrelia burgdorferi, a spirochete that infects a wide range of mammals and birds including humans, dogs, cats, cows, horses, and blackbirds.

70. How is *B. burgdorferi* transmitted?

The organism is transmitted by the bite of infected ticks into the skin of animals. The organism then disseminates to other organ tissues. The major genus of ticks reported to transmit the disease is the *Ixodes* species. *I. scapularis* and *I. pacificus* are the most commonly reported vectors.

71. What are the major clinical manifestations of the disease in dogs?

Clinically, dogs have an acute onset of fever, depression, and lameness. Lameness is usually monoarticular and is attributable to an acute suppurative arthritis. Experimentally, this arthritis is usually in the leg closest to the tick bite. Transient lameness occurs, but multiple joints can be affected over time. Reports of cardiac arrhythmia (bradyarrhythmia) and a rapidly progressive renal disease are described but are poorly documented in the veterinary literature. The renal manifestations include a membranoproliferative glomerulonephritis that is characterized by azotemia, hypoalbuminemia, and proteinuria.

72. Is there a geographic distribution of the disease?

The disease is mainly found in the northeastern, mid-Atlantic, and upper north-central regions, and in several counties in northwestern California. This geographic distribution is similar to states that have a high incidence of borreliosis in human beings.

73. What methods are used in the diagnosis of the disease?

Culture of skin tissue and joint fluid can be performed, but is not a highly productive method and requires special media and specialized laboratory techniques.

Serologic methods used in the diagnosis of Lyme disease include IFA, ELISA, kinetic ELISA (KELA), Western blot analysis, and PCR. IgM and IgG antibodies can be detected by use of a whole-cell extract of *B. burgdorferi* as the antigen. Serologic prevalence of infection is high in dogs within endemic areas and cross-reactivity of antibodies occur in dogs infected with other spirochetes and disease processes.

Antibody detection to a conserved immunodominant region of VlsE (antigenic variation lipoprotein of *B. burgdorferi*) has been found to be sensitive and specific for the diagnosis of Lyme disease in man and dogs. This antibody is not affected by vaccination with Osp A and whole-cell vaccines and serologic titers decrease with effective treatment.

74. Can dogs transmit the disease to human beings?

B. burgdorferi cannot be directly transmitted to humans. The agent requires a vector (tick) that may be carried on animals resulting in people having a greater exposure to the tick and thereby the infective agent.

75. What are the major laboratory abnormalities noted in dogs that are infected?

Mild to moderate leukocytosis can be noted on the hemogram. Specific biochemical abnormalities are not present unless infection causes renal disease. In cases with renal involvement azotemia, hypoalbuminemia, and proteinuria are observed. Cytologic evaluation of joint fluid usually reveals a mild to moderate suppurative inflammatory reaction.

76. What is the treatment for Lyme disease?

Amoxicillin, doxycycline, azithromycin, and the third-generation ceftriaxone are recommended for 14 to 21 days. There is no clinical benefit of prolonged antibiotic therapy in human beings and whether this applies to treatment of infected dogs is unknown at present.

Plague

77. What is the etiologic agent of plague?

Plague is caused by *Yersinia pestis*, a Gram-negative, coccobacillus, anaerobic bacterium.

78. How do dogs become infected with this agent?

Transmission to dogs is through ingestion of infected reservoir animals. Reservoirs for the disease are rabbits and rodents, such as prairie dogs and squirrels. Fleas are the primary vector among rodents and may transmit *Y. pestis* to dogs and cats. Inhalation of respiratory droplets from infected animals can also transmit the plague. Therefore dogs and cats can transmit the *Y. pestis* to humans either directly through secretions or indirectly by carrying rodent fleas.

79. Is there a geographic distribution of this disease?

Plague occurs in many countries. Semiarid climates near deserts are common habitats. Within the United States, plague is limited to the western part of the country (e.g., Arizona, New Mexico, Nevada, Oregon, Washington, Utah, California, Hawaii). Diagnosis of the disease is more common during the summer months.

80. What are the most common clinical manifestations of disease?

Plague occurs in three forms and includes local (buboes), septicemic, and pneumonic forms. Clinical signs of bubonic plague are lethargy, anorexia, fever, and lymphodenomegaly (known as bubo) especially when involving the submandibular nodes. Signs of shock and DIC may occur in septicemic forms that can progress to other forms of the disease. Pneumonic plague occurs as a sequel to bubonic or septicemic forms, or after inhalation of infected respiratory droplets. Clinical signs of pneumonic forms consists fever, tachypnea, dyspnea, cough, and depression. Pneumonic plague carries the worst prognosis in man.

81. What are the most common laboratory abnormalities observed?

Marked leukocytosis is observed in dogs with the septicemic form. Other laboratory abnormalities may be observed if DIC or vital organ involvement results from infection.

82. What are the best methods to diagnose this disease?

Visualization of the organism and a positive culture are the most definitive method of diagnosis. Fine-needle aspiration of affected lymph nodes or tissues can be used to identify the bipolar, coccobacillus organism with the use of Gram-staining technique. These samples can also be used to inoculate transport media, or stored in blood tubes to be used for culture. Acquisition of infected tissue can be used in a similar manner through touch preparation cytology and with submission for culture. Cytologic preparation can be submitted for fluorescent antibody testing. Passive hemagglutination titers can be used if the disease is suspected, but the organism cannot be detected. Care should be used when handling samples as plague can be transmitted through cuts, mucous membrane exposure, and inhalation.

83. What is the most effective therapy?

Worker safety should be kept in mind when treating an animal suspect, or having been exposed to organism. Handlers should wear gloves, masks, and protective clothing. Fleas should be eliminated from the dog as part of the treatment protocol. Infected dogs should be isolated and the cage should be disinfected regularly. Public health officials should be contacted if a diagnosis of plague is made.

In vivo tests of antibiotic efficacy in animals have not been undertaken in dogs; thus, drugs used to treat human beings are recommended. Tetracyclines are given most commonly for the bubonic form and appear to have the highest cure rate at doses ranging from 50 to 500 mg per day. Therefore in dogs, a standard dose of 25 mg/kg every 8 hours is recommended. Gentamicin and chloramphenicol are considered the most effective antibiotic therapy in man. These antibiotics as well as trimethoprim-sulfadiazine, trimethoprim-sulfamethoxazole, and lincomycin have been used for treatment in cats. Antibiotics are recommended for a minimum of 21 days. Penicillin and its derivates may not be efficacious. Treatment recovery takes from 1 to 10 days.

84. How can the plague be prevented?

Pets should not be allowed access to carcasses and rodent populations should be controlled. Flea preventative should be used to minimize exposure of humans and pets to rodent fleas. Vaccination failed to prevent bacteremia and death in cats, but it is unknown whether this prevention method is useful in dogs.

Tetanus

85. What is the etiologic agent?

The etiologic agent is *Clostridium tetani*, an anaerobic, spore-forming, Gram-positive bacillus. This organism produces a neurotoxin during its vegetative growth phase in animals that results in the production of clinical manifestations.

86. How do dogs become infected with this agent?

This agent can be isolated from the feces of many animals and numerous environmental sources. The organism enters sites in the animal usually through traumatic injury. The organism replicates, when anaerobic conditions are present, and the exotoxin is absorbed in the circulation producing clinical signs.

87. What toxin produces clinical manifestations?

Two neurotoxins are produced by the organism but only tetanospasmin is known to bind to nervous tissues and produce clinical signs. This neurotoxin inhibits release of glycine and gamma-aminobutyric acids, the neurotransmitters of inhibitory neurons of the CNS.

88. What clinical manifestations are common in the dog?

Dogs are relatively resistant to the effects of the toxin compared with other domestic species. Clinical manifestations are the result of the toxin producing a local or systemic blockade of motor neurotransmission. Muscle contractures (risus sardonicus [smile]) or a rigid contraction of the masticatory muscles (trismus) may be observed when local tetanus involves the muscles of the head. Stilted gait, muscle contractures, and lameness may be present when systemic signs predominate.

89. How is tetanus diagnosed in dogs?

Compatible history of trauma and a physical examination that reveals a local injury coupled with clinical suspicion. Compartmentalized gas in a region of injury may be supportive of a diagnosis. Anaerobic culture can be confirmatory if required.

90. What treatments are most effective for tetanus?

Prolonged therapy is required in dogs and the level of financial commitment can be significant. Antitoxin (antitetanus equine serum) can be used in an attempt to neutralize the neurotoxin. Intravenous administration of antitoxin provides a more rapid response, but may produce anaphylactoid reactions. Debridement of wounds, coupled with antibiotic therapy and supportive care, are most commonly used. Antibiotic therapy should consist of a penicillin or synthetic derivative (amoxicillin, ampicillin, or amoxicillin-clavulanic acid).

Sedatives or muscle relaxants can help control reflex muscle spasms. Chlorpromazine and acetylpromazine are effective. Barbiturates (pentobarbital, phenobarbital) can be used to control spasms and seizures. Methocarbamol, diazepam, baclofen, and dantrolene have been used clinically to provide relief of muscle rigidity until recovery become apparent.

Maintenance of fluid balance and nutrition is important until clinical recovery is apparent. Esophagotomy and gastrotomy tubes to provide adequate fluid and nutritional support have improved recovery in dogs.

91. What is the prognosis for dogs with tetanus?

In dogs with local disease, the prognosis is guarded to good. In dogs in which there are systemic signs of disease, the prognosis is guarded to poor for recovery.

Tularemia

92. What is the etiologic agent of tularemia?

Francisella tularensis, a Gram-negative, non–spore-forming bacillus. There are two different strains: Type A and Type B.

93. What is the difference between the strains Types A and B?

The difference in the Type A and Type B strains is related to the transmission cycle of the disease. Type A strains are found in North America and involve the tick-rabbit cycle, whereas Type B strains involve involves rodents, ticks, mosquitoes, and environmental factors.

94. How is tularemia transmitted to dogs?

Dogs are infected by consumption of infected animals, most notably rabbits.

95. What are the major clinical manifestations of tularemia?

Few reports of tularemia are in the veterinary literature. Dogs can exhibit fever, lymphadenopathy, lethargy, and acute death. Ocular signs are also reported and include uveitis, keratitis, and conjunctivitis.

96. How is tularemia diagnosed?

Isolation of the organism is the most definitive method for diagnosis and is performed on exudates and in tissue samples. Direct fluorescent antibody technique can be used on these samples as well. Serologic testing by use of agglutinating antibodies and ELISA techniques are other alternatives.

97. What is the treatment for tularemia in dogs?

Efficacy of antibiotic therapy in dogs is unknown. The aminoglycosides (gentamicin and streptomycin) are considered the treatment of choice in man. Additionally, tetracycline, chloramphenicol, and the fluoroquinolones may be effective, but controlled studies are lacking in dogs.

98. Is tularemia a zoonotic disease?

Yes, there are reports of dogs and cats transmitting the disease to human beings. Most instances involve cat bites and scratches. Dogs' saliva and aerolization of the organism were possible modes of transmission in some reports in man.

FUNGAL DISEASES

Blastomycosis

99. What is the etiologic agent of blastomycosis in dogs?

Blastomyces dermatitidis is a dimorphic fungus found in the soil. Sandy, acidic soils are more likely to contain *Blastomyces* species, and infections are more common in areas close to water and in excavated land.

100. What is the geographic distribution of the disease?

The major distribution of this disease is along the Mississippi, Missouri, and Ohio River valleys. Endemic areas are also located in the south central and southeastern United States.

101. How do dogs become infected with this agent?

Dogs inhale infective conidiophores. These conidia are phagocytized by macrophages where they transform from the mycelial to yeast form. Replication occurs mainly in terminal bronchioles of the lung. If host response is adequate, the infection may be primarily confined to the pulmonary parenchyma and tracheobronchial lymph nodes. Failure of an adequate cellular immune response in susceptible animals results in dissemination of the infection to extrapulmonary sites.

There are reports of direct inoculation of this agent into the skin of dogs and through the bite of infected animals.

102. Are there any predispositions reported to this disease?

Large-breed male dogs of the hound and sporting breeds are overrepresented, which is attributed to their outdoor activity as a risk factor.

103. What are the most common clinical findings in dogs and cats?

Infection with blastomycosis can remain confined to the respiratory tract or disseminate to other extrapulmonary systems. Fever, inappetence, tachypnea, dyspnea, and cough are frequently observed systemic and respiratory signs. Clinical signs associated with disseminated disease include generalized lymphadenopathy, skin lesions (nodular and draining tracts), ocular signs (uveitis, panophthalmitis, retinal detachments), and lameness (bone pain, draining tracts). Less frequently systems involved with blastomycosis include urinary tract signs (dysuria, prostatomegaly, testicular enlargement) and the central nervous system (depression and seizures).

104. What are the most common laboratory abnormalities observed with blastomycosis?

In cases in which respiratory signs predominate, a mild anemia and leukocytosis may be observed. Hyperproteinemia and hypergammaglobulinemia are common findings and are the result of increases in acute and chronic inflammatory proteins. Hypercalcemia is reported with this fungal infection and may be the result of osteolysis or granulomatous disease that produce an activated vitamin D.

105. How is blastomycosis diagnosed in dogs?

Demonstration of the organism is the most common method of definitive diagnosis (Fig. 69-2). Imprints of draining skin lesions or tracts and fine-needle aspirates of lymph nodes, eyes, lung and bone lead to diagnosis in approximately 50% of cases. Even normal-size, peripheral lymph nodes can contain organisms demonstrable on aspiration cytology. In some cases, tissue biopsy of affected lymph nodes, skin, ocular tissue, bone, and CSF fluid may yield a diagnosis.

Radiographs of the thorax commonly reveal a diffuse nodular bronchointerstitial pattern and hilar lymphadenopathy (Fig. 69-3). Bone lesions are characterized by osteoproliferation and osteolysis of metaphyseal regions and are difficult to differentiate from primary or metastatic bone tumors.

Serologic testing for antibodies can be performed. A combination of a compatible history, clinical signs, radiographic findings, and serology can be used as criteria for a diagnosis when demonstration of organisms has failed. The agar gel immunodiffusion test for detection of an antigen of *Blastomyces dermatitidis* is one test with a reported sensitivity and specificity of more than 90%. Anti–WI-1 antibodies can be detected by radioimmunoassay (RIA) in dogs with blastomycosis and were found to be highly specific for infection.

106. What is the treatment for blastomycosis in dogs?

Amphotericin B and itraconazole are considered the drugs of choice for treatment. Because of the route of administration and associated nephrotoxicity, amphotericin B is not used frequently but is indicated when a rapid response is required because of the severity of clinical signs (see Chapter 38). Itraconazole is as effective as amphotericin B with reduced toxicity and can be administered orally. Itraconazole should be administered for at least 60 days or for 1 month after resolution of all clinical signs. Recurrence of clinical signs may occur in approximately 20% of cases treated with either amphotericin B or itraconazole.

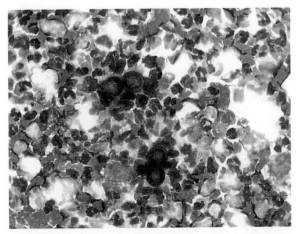

Figure 69-2. Urine sediment from a dog with acute respiratory signs, multiple draining skin lesions, panophthalmitis, prostatic enlargement, and urinary incontinence revealing *Blastomyces dermatitidis* organisms on examination.

107. What is the prognosis for a dog with blastomycosis?

Approximately 70% of dogs are cured with antifungal treatment. Brain and diffuse lung involvement are negative prognostic indicators. Worsening of respiratory signs, if present, is expected during the early phase of treatment and only 50% of dogs with severe pulmonary involvement will survive. Approximately 20% of treated dogs will relapse.

Coccidioidomycosis

108. What is the etiologic agent?

Coccidioides immitis, a saprophytic soil fungus.

109. Does this disease have a particular geographic distribution?

The organism is found in Sonoran life zones, areas with sandy and alkaline soils, high temperature, and low rainfall. In the United States, the disease is more prevalent in the southwestern portions of the country.

110. Are there any clinical predispositions of this disease?

Dogs of larger breeds and male dogs housed outdoors are overrepresented.

111. How do dogs become infected with this agent?

Dogs become infected by inhalation of infective arthroconidia into the respiratory tract. Arthroconidia enlarge into spherules producing endospores that are released into pulmonary tissues and bronchial lymph nodes. If the dog is unable to mount an appropriate cellular immune response, dissemination of the organism occurs to extrapulmonary tissues. A few cases are reported in which the organism was injected into the subcutaneous tissues to produce local infection.

112. What are the clinical manifestations of this disease?

The infection in dogs may be asymptomatic, characterized only by lethargy and fever. In dogs with an inappropriate immune response, a mild to severe respiratory syndrome occurs. This syndrome is characterized by fever, weight loss, and cough. In approximately 20% to 40% of

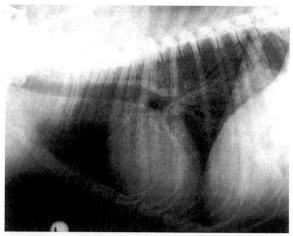

Figure 69-3.   Lateral (**A**) and ventrodorsal (**B**) thoracic radiographs of a dog presented for acute respiratory signs from blastomycosis revealing a diffuse, miliary, interstitial pattern.

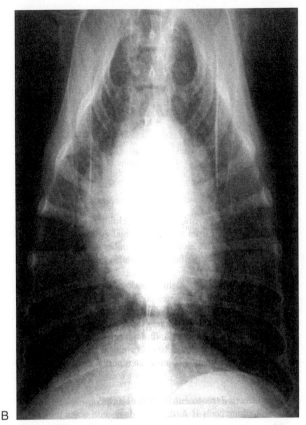

B

Figure 69-3, cont'd For legend see opposite page.

cases, the disease becomes disseminated to extrapulmonary tissues. Major sites of dissemination include regional lymph nodes, bone, central nervous system, or parenchymal organs.

If the infection spreads to bone, osteomyelitis occurs and can be clinically apparent as lameness and swelling over the infected site. Draining fistula may develop over sites of osteomyelitis.

Ocular lesions are not uncommon in disseminated disease. The disease is most frequently associated with signs referable to the anterior segment of the eye, such as iritis and granulomatous uveitis. Posterior segment involvement can result in blindness. Subsequent evidence of glaucoma may be present from the inflammatory response.

113. What are the radiographic findings in dogs with coccidioidomycosis?

In most cases, a diffuse interstitial pattern is present with a mixed interstitial-alveolar or interstitial-bronchovascular pattern. Hilar lymphadenopathy may be marked. In cases of dissemination of this infection to bone, osteomyelitis of the appendicular skeleton is seen. Most boney lesions are located in the distal diaphysis, metaphysis, and epiphysial region and are productive in nature (Fig. 69-4).

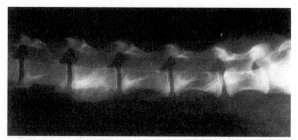

Figure 69-4.   Lateral spinal radiograph of a dog presented for paraparesis infected with *Coccidioides immitis*, revealing an osteoproductive lesion of the fourth lumbar vertebral body.

114. What are the best methods for diagnosis of coccidioidomycosis?

Demonstration of the organism from tracheobronchial aspirates, draining skin lesions, or in biopsy samples is the most definitive method. The number of organisms is low in tissues and exudates, and special stains such as periodic acid-Schiff allow for better demonstration of the organism. Spherules are the form of the organisms noted and are seen as variably sized, round, 10 to 80 μm, double-walled structures containing endospores (Fig. 69-5).

Serologic tests are useful in the diagnosis of this disease especially in cases in which there is fever of unknown origin, suspicion of fungal infection, and failure to demonstrate the organism. Agar gel immunodiffusion or ELISA techniques for detection of IgM and IgG antibodies are most common. IgM antibodies rise initially and may persist for some time. IgG antibodies increase later in the disease process and have been correlated with dissemination of disease and prognosis. Rising CF titers higher than 1:32 has been reported to indicate active and progressive disease and a poor prognosis.

115. What is the most effective treatment for this disease?

Treatment of coccidioidomycosis is difficult. In dogs with acute respiratory signs, amphotericin B may provide a more rapid response than the triazole compounds (see Chapter 68). Ketoconazole and itraconazole are the most useful of the triazole antifungal agents for use in the dog. These drugs should be given past the point of resolution of all clinical and radiographic signs. In some dogs with disseminated disease, long-term therapy and daily maintenance therapy may be required. It is not uncommon to have relapses and a need for ongoing maintenance antifungal treatment.

Chitin synthesis inhibitors (lufenuron, Nikkomycin Z) and echinocandins (caspofungin) have been used to treat this fungal infection in dogs, experimental animal models, and in man, as adjuvant therapy with amphotericin B and the triazoles with promising results.

116. What is the prognosis for coccidioidomycosis?

The prognosis for a cure with disseminated infection is guarded as relapses are common. Without treatment disseminated infection is commonly fatal. The prognosis for localized respiratory infection is good with treatment.

Cryptococcosis

117. What is the etiologic agent?

Cryptococcus neoformans var. *neoformans* and var *gattii* and *grubii*, antigenic variants of the dimorphic fungus. *Cryptococcus bacillispora* is also reported to cause disease in dogs.

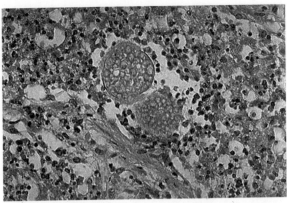

Figure 69-5.   Cytologic preparation of a fine-needle aspirate from the lung of a dog with diffuse respiratory lesions on radiographic examination showing a spherule of *C. immitis.*

118. How do dogs acquire infection with this agent?

These organisms can be isolated from the nasal cavity of healthy dogs and cats but are usually from inhalation of basiphores found in the environment. The organism replicates within the nasal or pulmonary cavities. Dissemination of the infection can occur through lymphatic or hematogenous routes to extrarespiratory tissues. Direct extension can occur to the CNS by direct extension through the cribriform plate.

119. Is there a geographic distribution of this disease?

Warm and arid climates. In the United States, the organism is ubiquitous, with foci within the southern and southwestern United States.

120. What are the most common clinical manifestations of disease?

Cryptococcosis is 10 times more prevalent in the cat. In the dog, cryptococcosis is reported in young dogs of the larger breeds. Pulmonary, ocular, and CNS involvement are more frequently observed in the dog. Respiratory signs include tachypnea, dyspnea, and coughing. CNS signs include altered behavior, ataxia, paresis, cranial nerve deficits (nystagmus, vestibular, optic neuritis), and seizures. Anterior and posterior uveitis may also be observed in dogs with CNS involvement. Lymphadenopathy can be present and commonly involve the submandibular lymph nodes when the nasal cavity is affected.

121. What are the most common laboratory abnormalities observed?

Because this disease is often localized to the nasal cavity or CNS, there are few consistent abnormalities. In dogs, CSF fluid may reveal an increase in protein content with demonstration of the organism. Inflammatory cells may be increased in CSF, but this response is usually mild to moderate. Ocular paracentesis may show inflammatory cells and the organism.

122. What are the best methods to diagnose this disease?

Demonstration of the organism is the preferred method of diagnosis. The organism can be noted in imprints made from skin lesions, imprints, or biopsy of nasal lesions, aspirates of enlarged lymph nodes, and CSF and bronchoalveolar lavage fluids (Fig. 69-6).

Radiographs or alternate imaging studies of animals with nasal involvement commonly reveal a soft-tissue density in the nasal cavity. Pulmonary lesions may be observed with fine miliary densities present.

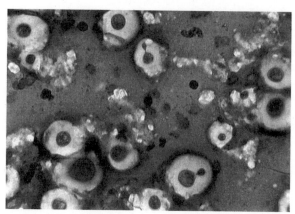

Figure 69-6.   An India ink cerebrospinal fluid preparation from a dog presented with multifocal central nervous system disease. The capsule of this organism is clear and does not stain with this preparation.

Serology is also useful when clinical signs are suggestive of the disease. Antibody levels are usually elevated when the animal is presented with clinical signs, but detection of serum antigen has a higher sensitivity and specificity for the disease. The latex cryptococcal antigen agglutination test is usually higher than 2 in cases of cryptococcus and ranged from a median of 2048 to 4096 in one study of 58 animals with cryptococcosis. Antigen titers decrease with therapy but are slower to decrease than clinical response. Recommendation is to continue therapy until the titer is lower than 2 or has decreased at least by 32 times or 32-fold.

123. What is the most effective therapy for cryptococcosis?

Effective therapy depends on the primary lesions in the animal. Central nervous system involvement is best treated with fluconazole, a water soluble imidazole (see Chapter 68). This agent penetrates the blood brain barrier more effectively than other triazole agents. In theory, the inflammatory responses within the CNS may allow penetration of other antifungal agents. Ketoconazole, flucytosine, and amphotericin B are other antifungal agents used to treat CNS and disseminated disease.

124. What is the prognosis for *Cryptococcus* infection in dogs?

If the disease is localized to the nasal cavity or pulmonary tissue the prognosis is guarded. In dogs with CNS infections, the prognosis is guarded to poor.

Histoplasmosis

125. What is the etiologic agent of histoplasmosis in dogs?

Histoplasma capsulatum, a dimorphic soil-borne fungi.

126. What is the major geographic distribution of histoplasmosis?

Most cases are reported from the central United States in the Ohio, Missouri, and Mississippi River valley basins.

127. How do dogs become infected with this agent?

Inhalation of microconidia that eventually lodge in the lower respiratory airways. The yeast is phagocytosed by mononuclear cells and undergoes intracellular replication. Dissemination of the infection occurs through the lymphatic and hematogenous routes.

128. Are there age, breed, and sex predilections for this disease in dogs?

This disease is common in young dogs; there is no noted sex predilection, but there are reports of a higher incidence in the hunting or sporting breeds.

129. What are the most common clinical manifestations of histoplasmosis in dogs?

General signs of infection include fever, anorexia, and weight loss. Respiratory and gastrointestinal signs predominate. Respiratory signs include tachypnea, dyspnea, and cough. Gastrointestinal signs include weight loss, predominately large bowel diarrhea (tenesmus, mucus, and hematochezia). Additional signs include hepatomegaly, icterus, and lymphadenopathy.

130. What are the most common methods used for diagnosis of this disease in dogs?

Demonstration of the organism is the preferred method because of a lack of reliable serologic tests. The organism is most commonly noted in tracheobronchial secretions or samples, fine-needle lymph node aspirates, rectal scrapings or gastrointestinal biopsy samples, fine-needle hepatic aspirates or biopsies, and bone marrow aspirates (see Fig. 69-1).

Laboratory findings commonly include nonregenerative anemia, elevated liver enzymes (ALT, total bilirubin), and hypoalbuminemia. These signs are nonspecific and usually relate to the chronicity of the disease process.

Thoracic radiographs may demonstrate a diffuse, interstitial pattern with miliary and nodular densities. Hilar lymphadenopathy may be noted as well.

131. What is the most effective treatment for histoplasmosis?

Depending on the clinical condition of the animal amphotericin B, itraconazole and fluconazole may be indicated. In cases in which clinical signs are severe, initial therapy may consist of amphotericin B (see Chapter 68).

BIBLIOGRAPHY

Arceneaux KA, Taboada J, Hosgood G: Blastomycosis in dogs: 115 cases (1980-1995), *J Am Vet Med Assoc* 213:658-64, 1998.
Bradsher RW, Chapman SW, Pappas PG: Blastomycosis, *Infect Dis Clin N Am* 17:21-40, 2003.
Centers for Disease Control and Prevention (CDC): Lyme disease—United States, 1999, *MMWR Morb Mortal Wkly Rep* 50:181-185, 1999.
Chiller TM, Galgiani, JN, Stevens DA: Coccidioidomycosis. *Inf Dis Clin N Am* 17:41-57, 2003.
Cohn L: Ehrlichia and related infections, *Vet Clin N Am (Sm An Pract)* 33:863-884, 2003.
Dumler JS, Barbet AF, Bekker CPJ et al: Reorganization of genera in the families Rickettsiaceae and Anaplasmataceae in the order Rickettsiales: unification of some species of Ehrlichia with Anaplasma, Cowdria with Ehrlichia and Ehrlichia with Neorickettsia, descriptions of six new species combinations and designation of Ehrlichia equie and "HGE agent" as subjective synonyms of Ehrlichia phagocytophila, *Int J Syst Evol Microbiol* 51: 2145-2165, 2001.
Jenkins SR, Auslander M, Conti L et al: Compendium of animal rabies prevention and control, *J Am Vet Med Assoc* 222:156-161, 2003.
Johnson LR, Herrgesell EJ, Davidson AP et al: Clinical, clinicopathologic, and radiographic findings in dogs with coccidioidomycosis: 24 cases (1995-2000), *J Am Vet Med Assoc* 222:461-466, 2003.
Kerl ME: Update on canine and feline fungal diseases, *Vet Clin N Am (Sm Anim Pract)* 22:721-7474, 2003.
Klasasen HLBM, Molkenboer MJCH, Vrijenhoek MP et al: Duration of immunity in dogs vaccinated against leptospirosis with a bivalent inactivated vaccine, *Vet Microbiol* 195:121-135, 2003.
Klein BS, Squires RA, Lloyd JK et al: Canine antibody response to Blastomyces dermatitidis WI-1 antigen, *Am J Vet Res* 61:554-558, 2000.
Kordick S, Breitschwerdt EB, Hegarty BC et al: Coinfection with multiple tick-borne pathogens in a Walker Hound kennel in North Carolina. *J Clin Microbiol* 37:2631-2638, 1999.
Krebs JW, Noll HR, Rupprecht CE et al: Rabies surveillance in the United States during 2001, *J Am Vet Med Assoc* 221:1690-701, 2002.
Langston CE, Heuter KJ: Leptospirosis: a re-emerging zoonotic disease, *Vet Clin N Am (Sm Anim Pract)* 33:791-807, 2003.

Legendre AM, Rohrbach BW, Toal RL et al: Treatment of blastomycosis with itraconazole in 112 dogs, *J Vet Intern Med* 10:365-371, 1996.

Mack RE, Becovitch MG, Ling CV et al: Salmon diseases complex in dogs—a review of 45 cases, *Calif Vet* 44:42-45, 1990.

Macy DW: Plague. In Greene CE, editor: *Infectious diseases of the dog and cat*, ed 2, Philadelphia, 1998, WB Saunders.

Malik R, McPetrie R, Wigney DI et al: A latex cryptococcal antigen agglutination test for diagnosis and monitoring of therapy for cryptococcosis, *Austral Vet J* 74:358-364, 1996.

Malik R Wigney DI, Muir DB et al: Cryptococcus in dogs: a retrospective study of 20 consecutive case, *J Med Vet Mycol* 33:291-297, 1995.

Monroe WE: Clinical signs associated with pseudorabies in dogs, *J Am Vet Med Assoc* 195, 599-602, 1989.

Neer TM, Breitschwerdt EB, Greene RT et al: Consensus statement on ehrlichial disease of small animals from the infectious disease study group of the ACVIM, *J Vet Int Med* 16:309-315, 2002.

Willis AM: Canine viral infections, *Vet Clin N Am (Sm Anim Pract)* 30:1119-1133, 2001.

Warner RD, Marsh WW: Rocky Mountain spotted fever, *J Am Vet Med Assoc* 221:1413-1417, 2002.

Worsmser CP, Ramanathan R, Nowakowski J et al: Duration of antibiotic therapy for early Lyme disease, *Ann Intern Med* 138:697-704, 2003.

Index

A

A-a gradient, 210
AAI (atlantoaxial instability), 32-33
Abdominal ultrasound
  of gallbladder, 303
  in pancreatitis, 289
Abdominocentesis, 274
Abducens nerve, 5
Absolute polycythemia, 375
Accessory nerve, 6
ACE inhibitor. *See* Angiotensin-converting enzyme
    inhibitor
Acepromazine, 172
Achalasia, cricopharyngeal, 156
Acid, bile, 301
Acidosis
  in acute renal failure, 310
  ketoacidosis, 234-237
ACTH test
  in hyperadrenocorticism, 242
  in hypoadrenocorticism, 238
  in hypoglycemia, 256
Actinomyces, 213
Activated charcoal for diarrhea, 265
Activated clotting time, 373
Acute heart failure
  chronic versus, 88
  findings in, 82
Acute prostatitis, 352
Adenoma, perianal, 286
Adenocarcinoma, anal sac, 286
Adenovirus infection, 401-402
Adrenal disorder
  hyperadrenocorticism, 241-246
  hypoadrenocorticism, 232
Adrenocorticotropic hormone
  in hyperadrenocorticism, 242-244
  in hypoadrenocorticism, 238
  in hypoglycemia, 256
Adulticide, heartworm, 133
Adverse reaction, to food, 270
Afterload in heart failure, 85
Agar gel immunodiffusion, 395
Age, heartworm treatment and, 134
Aggression in hypothyroidism, 247
Airway disorder
  bacterial colonization and, 196-197
  bronchial, 184-189
  large, 177-184
  nodular, 157
  tracheal, 177-184

Airway disorder—*Continued*
  collapse as, 177-179, 180f, 180t
  hypoplastic, 180-182, 181t, 182f
  laceration as, 182-183
  upper, 167-173
    brachycephalic airway syndrome as, 168-171
    foreign body causing, 167-168
    laryngeal paralysis as, 171-173
    laryngeal tumor as, 173-175
    tracheal tumor as, 175-176
Alanine aminotransferase
  in adenovirus infection, 402
  in hyperadrenocorticism, 241
  in liver disease, 295
  in Rocky Mountain spotted fever, 407
Albendazole, 207t
Albumin
  in liver disease, 296
  renal failure and, 314-315
Albuterol
  for bronchitis, 186t
  for tracheal collapse, 180t
Alimentary lymphoma, 367
Alkaline phosphatase
  in adenovirus infection, 402
  in heartworm disease, 132
  in hyperadrenocorticism, 241
  in hypercalcemia, 251
  in liver disease, 295
  in Rocky Mountain spotted fever, 407
Alkylating chemotherapy, 306
Allergic rhinitis, 151-152
Allergy, food, 270
Alopecia in hypothyroidism, 246
Alpha-adrenergic antagonist, 333
Alveolus, heartworm and, 132
Amikacin, 306
Aminoglycoside
  in gastric dilation volvulus, 282
  for infective endocarditis, 123
  renal failure caused by, 306
5-Aminosalicylic acid for irritable bowel disease, 271
Amlodipine in mitral valve disease, 67
Ammonia tolerance test, 301
Ammonium urate urolith, 325
Amoxicillin
  in *Helicobacter pylori* infection, 284
  for rhinitis, 145
Amoxicillin-clavulanic acid
  for pyothorax, 215
  for respiratory infection, 196

Page numbers followed by f indicate figures; t, tables.

Amphotericin B, 390t
  for blastomycosis, 415
  in coccidioidomycosis, 418
  in cryptococcosis, 22
  for histoplasmosis, 421
  renal failure caused by, 306
  toxicity of, 389
Ampicillin for endocarditis, 123
Amrinone, 86
Amylase, 290
Amyloidosis, 322
Anabolic steroid in chronic renal failure, 318
Anal disorder, 285-287
Anal sac adenocarcinoma, 286
Analgesia in pancreatitis, 290-291, 291t
Ancylostoma caninum, 206
Anemia, 373-375
  assessment of, 374
  causes of, 373-374
  in chronic renal failure, 316, 317
  classification of, 374
  compensation for, 374-375
  definition of, 373
  in ehrlichiosis, 405
  immune-mediated hemolytic, 381-384
Anesthesia
  for foreign body, 167
  for laryngeal paralysis, 172
Angiography, 209
Angiostrongylus vasorum, 204-205
Angiotensin-converting enzyme inhibitor
  for dilated cardiomyopathy, 112
  in dilated cardiomyopathy, 113
  in glomerulonephritis, 323
  in heart failure, 85, 89
  in mitral valve disease, 67, 68
  renal failure caused by, 306
Antibiotic
  for diarrhea, 266
  for discospondylitis, 48
  in ehrlichiosis, 406
  in gastric dilation volvulus, 282
  in *Helicobacter pylori* infection, 284
  in hepatic encephalopathy, 300
  for infective endocarditis, 123-124
  for irritable bowel disease, 271
  for leptospirosis, 410
  nasal tumor and, 163
  in plague, 412
  for pneumonia, 202
  for pyothorax, 215
  for respiratory infection, 196
  for rhinitis, 145
  for urinary tract infection, 337, 339
  in urolithiasis, 328
Antibody
  antithyroglobulin, 238
  detection of, 394-395
  in ehrlichiosis, 405
  in glomerular injury, 320
  in Rocky Mountain spotted fever, 407

Antibody coefficient in toxoplasmosis, 27
Anticoagulant rodenticide intoxication, 386-387
Anticonvulsant drug, 9-14
Antidiuretic hormone, 365
Antiemetic
  in acute renal failure, 310
  for gastrointestinal disorder, 261-262
Antifibrotic agent, 297
Antifungal therapy
  for aspergillosis, 149-150
  drugs for, 389, 390t-393t, 394
  renal failure caused by, 306
Antigen
  detection of, 394-395
  in ehrlichiosis, 405-406
  in glomerular injury, 320
Antigen testing
  in canine distemper viral encephalitis, 28
  for heartworm, 128, 140
Antigenemia, heartworm, 129-130, 135
Antihistamine, 152
Antiinflammatory drug
  for bronchitis, 186t
  for nasal tumor, 165-166
  renal failure caused by, 306
Antimicrobial
  for diarrhea, 266
  in urolithiasis, 328
Antiplatelet drug
  in glomerulonephritis, 323
  in thromboembolism, 210
Antithyroglobulin antibody test, 238
Antitussive
  for bronchitis, 186t
  for respiratory infection, 196
  for tracheal collapse, 180t
Antral pyloric hypertrophy, 284-285
Anuria, obstruction causing, 308
Anxiety in heart failure, 87
Aortic stenosis, subvalvular, 94, 99-100,
        100f
  hypertrophic cardiomyopathy versus, 115-116
Aortic valve, 118
AR (allergic rhinitis), 151-152
ARF (acute renal failure), 305-312. *See also* Renal
        failure, acute
Arginine vasopressin, 91
Arrhythmia
  in gastric dilation volvulus, 280-281
  respiratory sinus
    heart failure and, 82
    in mitral valve disease, 62
Arterial blood gas
  in parenchymal disease, 192
  in thromboembolism, 209
Arterial hypoxemia, 209
Arteritis, steroid responsive, 49-50
Arthritis
  classification of, 359-360
  definition of, 359
  infectious, 360

Arthritis—*Continued*
   nonerosive immune-mediated polyarthritis,
      360-361
   rheumatoid, 360
Arthropathy, 359
Artificial vagina, 349
Ascites, 273-275
   in mitral regurgitation, 70
ASD (atrial septal defect), 105
Aspergillosis, 145-150
Aspiration
   of lung, 202
   lymph node, 395
   transtracheal, 199
Aspiration biopsy of lung tumor, 220
Aspirin
   in glomerulonephritis, 323
   in heartworm disease, 133-134, 136
   for infective endocarditis, 125
   in thromboembolism, 210
Assay, enzyme-linked immunosorbent, 395
Atlantoaxial instability, 32-33
Atrial enlargement, 68
Atrial fibrillation, 113
Atrial natriuretic peptide, 91
Atrial septal defect, 105
Atrial wall in cardiac tamponade, 75f
Atrophy in spinal cord disease, 31t
Aujeszky's disease, 402-403
Auscultation
   in dilated cardiomyopathy, 110
   in patent ductus arteriosus, 94-95
   of tracheal tumor, 176
   in ventricular septal defect, 103
Autodigestion, pancreatic, 288-289
Avulsion, branchial plexus, 15
Azathioprine
   for immune-mediated hemolytic anemia, 383
   in thrombocytopenia, 380
Azithromycin, 284
Azole, 391t-392t, 394
Azotemia
   definition of, 313
   in ehrlichiosis, 405
   hypercalcemia and, 252
   renal failure versus, 305, 308

B
Babesiosis, 307
Bacterial infection
   diarrhea in, 267-268
   leptospirosis as, 409-410
   Lyme disease as, 410-411
   meningoencephalitis, 19-20
   overgrowth, 268
   plague as, 411-412
   prostatic, 351-352
   respiratory, 196-204
   tetanus as, 412-413
   tularemia as, 413-414
Bacterial meningoencephalitis, 19-20

Bacterial rhinitis, 145-146
Bacteroides
   cholecystitis and, 303
   in pyothorax, 213
Balloon cardiac catheterization, 93
Bartonella, 296
Basset Hound, urolithiasis in, 326
Beagle
   bladder tumor in, 335
   heart disease in, 93
   urolithiasis in, 327
Bedlington Terrier
   copper storage disease in, 298
   hepatitis in, 297
Belgian Shepherd, 44
Benazepril
   for dilated cardiomyopathy, 112
   in mitral valve disease, 67
Benign pericardial effusion, 79
Benign prostatic hyperplasia, 350-351
Benzodiazepine, 13-14
Benzopyrene, 217
Beta-adrenergic antagonist
   in dilated cardiomyopathy, 112, 113
   in heart failure, 89
   in hypertrophic cardiomyopathy, 116
Biceps reflex, 3
Bichon Frise
   conformational disorder in, 155
   patent ductus arteriosus in, 94
   primary ciliary dyskinesia in, 189
   urolithiasis in, 327
Bile acid in portosystemic shunt,
      301
Biliary obstruction, 304
Bilirubin
   icterus and, 293-294
   metabolism of, 294-295
Biochemical profile in liver disease, 295-296
Biopsy
   in diarrhea, 264
   in *Helicobacter pylori* infection, 283
   of laryngeal tumor, 174
   liver, 297
   of lung tumor, 220, 221
   of nasal tumor, 163
   for neosporosis, 26f
   prostatic, 350
   renal, 322-323
   in rhinitis, 144-145
Bismuth in *Helicobacter pylori* infection,
      284
Bismuth-subsalicylate for diarrhea, 265
Bladder
   pelvic, 332
   tumor of, 335-336
   urinary incontinence and, 332
Blastomycosis, 397t
   radiography of, 416f, 417f
Bleb, 158
Bleeding, approach to, 372-373

Bleeding diathesis in ehrlichiosis, 405
Bleeding disorder
    acquired, 384-386
    hereditary, 386-388
Bloating, 281
Blood
    in discospondylitis, 48
    heartworm in, 126-127
    in pericardial fluid, 78
    in pleural effusion, 217
Blood-borne disease, 125-141. *See also*
        Heartworm
Blood count
    in diabetes, 229
    in hemangiosarcoma, 371
    in hypercalcemia, 251
    in hypocalcemia, 254
    in pancreatitis, 289
    in pyometra, 342
    in thrombocytopenia, 380
Blood culture
    in brucellosis, 346
    in infective endocarditis, 120-121
Blood gas
    in parenchymal disease, 192
    in thromboembolism, 209
Blood pressure
    chronic renal failure and, 315-316
    in gastric dilation volvulus, 281
Blood urea nitrogen
    in liver disease, 296
    in pyometra, 342
Border Collie
    conformational disorder in, 155
    primary ciliary dyskinesia in, 189
Bordetella bronchiseptica, 196
Borrelia burgdorferi, 410-411
    diagnostic tests for, 396t
    polyarthritis in, 360
    renal failure caused by, 307
Boston Terrier
    brachycephalic airway syndrome in, 169
    conformational disorder in, 155
Botulism, 16-17
Bouvier des Flandres, laryngeal paralysis in, 171
Boxer
    cardiomyopathy in, 108
    conformational disorder in, 155
    dermoid sinus in, 34
    infective endocarditis in, 118
    subvalvular aortic stenosis in, 99
Brace for atlantoaxial instability, 33
Brachycephalic airway syndrome, 168-171
    age and, 169
    cause of, 169
    definition of, 168
    diagnosis of, 169
    predisposition to, 169
    progression of, 169-170
    signs of, 169
    surgery for, 170

Brachycephalic breed, conformational disorder
        in, 155
Brain
    head deviation caused and, 5
    seizure and, 8-9, 8t
Brain natriuretic peptide, 91
Branchial cyst, 157
Branchial plexus, avulsion of, 15
Breeding, infertility and, 343-345
Bronchial compression in mitral valve disease, 61,
        68
Bronchial mineralization, 190
Bronchiectasis, 187-189, 188f
Bronchitis, 184-187
Bronchoalveolar lavage, 201
Bronchodilator
    for bronchitis, 186t
    for tracheal collapse, 180t
Bronchoesophageal fistula, 190
Bronchoscopy
    in bronchitis, 185
    complications of, 201
    indications for, 201
Brucellosis, 345-348
    discospondylitis and, 48-49
Buccal mucosal bleeding time, 373
Bull Terrier, laryngeal paralysis in,
        171
Bulldog
    conformational disorder in, 155
    pulmonic stenosis in, 101
Bull Mastiff
    conformational disorder in, 155
    primary ciliary dyskinesia in, 189
    urolithiasis in, 326
Buprenorphine, 291t
Butorphanol
    for bronchitis, 186t
    in pancreatitis, 291t
    for tracheal collapse, 180t
Bypass, cardiopulmonary, 100

C
Cachexia, 365-366
Calcitonin, 253
Calcitriol
    in chronic renal failure, 318
    for hypocalcemia, 255
Calcium
    in chronic renal failure, 317
    hypercalcemia and, 250-253
        cancer and, 364
    hypocalcemia and, 253-255
    renal failure caused by, 307
Calcium channel blocker in mitral valve disease,
        67
Calcium gluconate, 254
Calcium oxalate urolith, 325, 327, 328
Calcium phosphate urolith, 328
Calculus, urinary. *See* Urolithiasis
Campylobacter, 267

Cancer. *See also* Tumor
  cachexia in, 365-366
  hypercalcemia in, 364
Canine adenovirus infection, 401-402
Canine distemper virus, 194-195, 399-401
Canine herpesvirus, 194, 195
Canine infectious tracheobronchitis, 194
Canine influenza, 194
Canine viral distemper encephalitis, 27-29
Capillaria aerophila, 204, 205-206
Capillary, glomerular, 319
Captopril
  for dilated cardiomyopathy, 112
  in mitral valve disease, 67
Cardiac catheterization, for congenital heart
    disease, 93
Cardiac disease. *See also* Heart; Heart failure
  congenital, 94-107
  of mitral valve, 59-70. *See also* Mitral valve
  pericardial, 71-81. *See also* Pericardial disease
Cardiac hemangiosarcoma, 370
Cardiac output, 73
Cardiac tamponade
  consequences of, 73
  drugs for, 76-77
  manifestations of, 73-74
  pericardiocentesis for, 77-79
Cardiogenic versus parenchymal disease,
    193
Cardiomyopathy
  ascites and, 274
  dilated, 107-114
    auscultation of, 110
    in Boxers, 108
    in Cocker Spaniels, 109
    definition of, 107
    in Doberman Pinchers, 108
    echocardiography of, 111, 111f
    electrocardiography in, 111
    heart failure in, 82-83
    occult, 108-109
    pathogenesis of, 107-108
    radiography of, 110-111, 110f
    taurine and, 109-110
    treatment of, 112-114
  hypertrophic, 114-117
Cardiopulmonary bypass, 100
Cardiovascular system
  in gastric dilation volvulus, 280
  in hypothyroidism, 247
L-Carnitine, 112
Caspofungin acetate, 393t
Castration for benign prostatic hyperplasia,
    351
Catecholamine derivative, 86
Catheter brush analysis, 202
CAV-2, 194, 195
CAV-1 infection, 401-402
Cavalier King Charles Spaniel
  mitral valve disease in, 60, 67-68
  urolithiasis in, 326

Cavitary lesion, pulmonary, 158
CDV (canine distemper virus), 194-195, 399-401
Celiotomy, 281
Central diabetes insipidus, 258-260
Central nervous system. *See also* Neurological
    disorder
  aspergillosis and, 149
Central venous pressure in pericardial disease, 76,
    80
Cephalexin, 282
Cephalosporin, 123
Cerebellum
  in globoid cell leukodystrophy, 35
  postural reaction deficits and, 7
Cerebral lesion, 7
Cerebral phaeohyphomycosis, 22-23
Cerebrospinal fluid
  in bacterial meningoencephalitis, 19-20
  collection of, 398-399
  in cryptococcosis, 22
  in distemper viral encephalitis, 28
  in globoid cell leukodystrophy, 35
  in granulomatous meningoencephalitis, 23
  in phaeohyphomycosis, 22
  in Rocky Mountain spotted fever, 407
  in steroid responsive meningitis-arteritis, 49
  in syringohydromyelia, 36
  in toxoplasmosis, 26
Cervical spondylomyelopathy, 41-43
Cervical tracheal collapse, 177
Chelator in copper storage disease, 298
Chemodectoma, 79
Chemoreceptor trigger zone, 261
Chemotherapy
  for granulomatous meningoencephalitis, 24
  for hemangiosarcoma, 371
  for lung tumor, 222
  for lymphoma, 369
  for nasal tumor, 165
  for pulmonary metastasis, 225
  renal failure caused by, 306
Chest tube
  for pyothorax, 215
  removal of, 216
Chiari-type malformation, 36
Chihuahua
  conformational disorder in, 155
  primary ciliary dyskinesia in, 189
  tracheal collapse in, 177
Chinese Shar-Pei
  conformational disorder in, 155
  primary ciliary dyskinesia in, 189
Chloramphenicol
  in ehrlichiosis, 21
  in Rocky Mountain spotted fever, 407
Cholecystitis, 303-304
Cholesterol
  in glomerulonephritis, 323-324
  in liver disease, 296
CHOP protocol in lymphoma, 369
Chorda tendineae rupture, 69

Chow Chow
  conformational disorder in, 155
  primary ciliary dyskinesia in, 189
Chronic bronchitis, 186-187
Chronic diarrhea, 265
Chronic hepatitis, 296-297
Chronic inflammatory liver disease, 296-297
Chronic paraparesis, 52f
Chronic prostatitis, 352
Chronic versus acute heart failure, 88
Chyloabdomen, 274
Chylothorax, 213-214, 214f, 217
Chylous effusion, 274
Ciliary dyskinesia, 155, 189-190
Cleft palate, 155, 157
Click, midsystolic, 61-62
Clindamycin
  for infective endocarditis, 123
  for protozoal meningoencephalitis, 27
  for rhinitis, 145
Closed pneumothorax, 216-217
Closed pyometra, 341-342
Clostridium, cholecystitis and, 303
Clostridium botulinum, 16-17
Clostridium perfringens, 268
Clostridium tetanus, 412-413
Clotrimazole, 391t
  in aspergillosis, 149-150
Clotting factor deficiency
  in disseminated intravascular coagulation, 385-386
  in liver disease, 386
Clotting time, 373
Cluster seizure, 9
Coagulation
  in hemangiosarcoma, 371
  in pancreatitis, 290
  in portosystemic shunt, 301
  in thromboembolism, 209
Coagulopathy, 384-388
  acquired, 384-386
  in adenovirus infection, 402
  bleeding in, 372-373
  disseminated intravascular, 385-386
    in gastric dilation volvulus, 282
  hereditary, 386-388
  in liver disease, 386
Cobalamin, 293
Coccidioidomycosis, 397t, 416-418, 418f, 419f
Cocker Spaniel
  dermoid sinus in, 34
  dilated cardiomyopathy in, 109
  immune-mediated hemolytic anemia in, 382
  pimobendan in, 90
  primary ciliary dyskinesia in, 189
  urolithiasis in, 327
Codeine for bronchitis, 186t
Collapse, tracheal, 177-179, 180f, 180t
Collie
  exocrine pancreatic insufficiency in, 292
  lymphoplasmacytic rhinitis in, 153

Colloidal fluid therapy in pancreatitis, 290
Colonization, airway, 196-197
Complement fixation, 395
Complete blood count
  in diabetes, 229
  in hemangiosarcoma, 371
  in hypercalcemia, 251
  in hypocalcemia, 254
  in pancreatitis, 289
  in pyometra, 342
  in thrombocytopenia, 380
Complications
  of brachycephalic airway surgery, 170
  of bronchoscopy, 201
  of intervertebral disc surgery, 38
  of laryngeal paralysis surgery, 173
  of pancreatitis, 291
  of pericardiocentesis, 78
  of portosystemic shunt, 302
  of renal biopsy, 323
  of tracheal collapse, 178
  of transtracheal washing, 200-201
Compression in mitral valve disease, 61, 68
Computed tomography
  in aspergillosis, 147
  in cervical spondylomyelopathy, 43
  in cryptococcosis, 22-23
  in discospondylitis, 48
  of foreign body, 168
  in intervertebral disc disease, 39
  in lumbosacral spondylomyelopathy, 45, 46f
  for lung tumor, 219-220
  of nasal tumor, 164
  in phaeohyphomycosis, 22-23
  in rhinitis, 144
  of tumor, 50
Conformational disorder, 154-159
  branchia cyst as, 157
  classification of, 155
  cleft palate as, 157
  cricopharyngeal achalasia as, 156
  differential diagnosis of, 157
  flail chest as, 157-158
  history of, 155-156
  Kartagener's syndrome as, 157
  nasal dermoid sinus cyst as, 156
  pectus excavatum as, 157-158
  predisposition for, 155
  pulmonary cavitary lesion as, 158
  swimmer pup and, 155-156
Congenital disorder
  of heart, 93-106. *See also* Heart disease
  of spinal cord, 32-36
  urinary incontinence with, 331
Congenital laryngeal paralysis, 155
Congestive heart failure
  in heartworm disease, 137
  infective endocarditis and, 124
  in mitral valve disease, 68-69
Conjunctival scraping, 395
Conjugated bilirubin, 294

Conscious proprioception, 1-2
Constrictive pericardial disease, 79-80
Contamination of blood sample, 120
Contraction, ventricular premature, 281
Coonhound paralysis, 16
Copper storage hepatopathy, 297-299
Core biopsy of lung tumor, 221. *See also* Biopsy
Corticosteroid
    for allergic rhinitis, 151
    for atlantoaxial instability, 33
    for immune-mediated hemolytic anemia,
      383
    for irritable bowel disease, 271
    for liver disease, 297
    for lymphoplasmacytic rhinitis, 154
    for perianal fistula, 287
    in spinal trauma, 53
    in thrombocytopenia, 380
    for tracheal collapse, 179
Cortisol:creatinine ratio, 242
Corynebacterium, 213
Cough
    in bronchitis, 184
    in mitral valve disease, 61
COX-2 inhibitor for nasal tumor, 165-166
Cranial nerve
    evaluation of, 6
    function of, 5-6
Creatinine
    cortisol:creatinine ratio and, 242
    protein:creatinine ratio and, 321-322
    in pyometra, 342
Crenosome vulpis, 204
CRF (chronic renal failure), 312-319. *See also*
    Renal failure, chronic
Cricopharyngeal achalasia, 156
Cromolyn sodium for allergic rhinitis, 152
Cryptococcosis, 397t, 418-420
    intracranial, 21-22
Crystalloid for gastric dilation volvulus, 280
Crystalluria, 324
CT. *See* Computed tomography
Culture
    in brucellosis, 346-347
    in discospondylitis, 48
    in infective endocarditis
      of blood, 120-121
      of urine, 121
    in Lyme disease, 410
    nasal tumor and, 163
    in rhinitis, 145
    urine, 338
Curve, glucose, 231-233
Cutaneous hemangiosarcoma, 370
Cyanotic heart disease, 105-106
Cycle, estrous, 344-345
Cyclooxygenase-2 for lung tumor, 222
Cyclophosphamide
    for immune-mediated hemolytic anemia,
      383
    in thrombocytopenia, 380

Cyclosporine
    for immune-mediated hemolytic anemia, 383
    for perianal fistula, 287
    for rhinitis, 152
Cyst
    branchial, 157
    nasal dermoid sinus, 155
    pericardial, 71
    prostatic, 352-353
    pulmonary, 158
Cystic endometrial hyperplasia/pyometra complex,
    341-343
Cystine urolith, 325-326, 328
Cystography, double-contrast, 333
Cytology
    in aspergillosis, 147, 148f
    in bronchitis, 185
    of lung tumor, 221
    in lymphoma, 368
    of pericardial fluid, 78
    sample collection for, 395, 398
    transtracheal, 199-200, 200f

D

D-dimer in thromboembolism, 209
Dachshund
    bladder tumor in, 335
    conformational disorder in, 155
    primary ciliary dyskinesia in, 189
    urolithiasis in, 326
Dalmatian
    conformational disorder in, 155
    copper storage disease in, 298
    laryngeal paralysis in, 171
    primary ciliary dyskinesia in, 189
    urolithiasis in, 327
Danazol
    for immune-mediated hemolytic anemia, 383
    in thrombocytopenia, 380
DAT test, 382
DCM (dilated cardiomyopathy), 107-114
DDAVP, 259
Death
    hypertrophic cardiomyopathy causing, 116
    Interceptor treatment and, 138
Decompensated heart failure, 82, 88
Decompression
    in gastric dilation volvulus, 280
    for intervertebral disc disease, 38
Deep pain perception, 32
    in intervertebral disc disease, 41
Degenerative disease
    joint, 361
    of mitral valve, 59-70. *See also* Mitral valve
    myelopathy as, 43-44
    myxomatous valvular, 59
    spinal, 36-46
Dehydration in ketoacidosis, 235
Delayed gastric emptying, 284-285
Demographics of heartworm disease, 126
Depigmentation in aspergillosis, 148, 148f

Deprenyl, 245
Dermacentor tick, 16
Dermatologic disorder
  in distemper, 399
  in hypothyroidism, 246
Dermoid sinus, 33-34
Dermoid sinus cyst, nasal, 155
Desmopressin, 258
Desoxycorticosterone pivalate, 239
Dexamethasone for hypoglycemia, 257
Dextrose, 256-257
Diabetes insipidus, 258-260
Diabetes mellitus, 229-237
  cause of, 229
  clinical findings in, 229
  diagnosis of, 229
  diet in, 230
  exercise and, 230
  glucose control in, 230-233
  hypoglycemia in, 234
  insulin for, 230-231
  insulin resistance in, 234
  ketoacidosis in, 234-237
  oral hypoglycemic drugs for, 230
Dialysis, 311
Diaphragm, conformational disorder of, 155
Diaphragmatic hernia, pericardioperitoneal,
    71-72
Diarrhea, 263-272
  acute, 265-266
  bacterial, 267-268
  diagnosis of, 264
  in exocrine pancreatic insufficiency, 292
  food intolerance causing, 270
  fungal, 268-269
  irritable bowel disease, 270-271
  large-bowel versus small-bowel, 263, 264t
  malignancy causing, 272
  parasites causing, 269-270
  pathophysiology of, 263-264
  protein-losing enteropathy causing, 271-272
  viral, 266-267
Diazepam
  in heartworm disease, 137
  for status epilepticus, 14
DIC (disseminated intravascular coagulation), 282,
    385-386
Diet
  in acute renal failure, 310-311
  in chronic renal failure, 318
  in copper storage disease, 298
  in diabetes mellitus, 230
  in diarrhea, 265
  in exocrine pancreatic insufficiency, 293
  in gastric dilation volvulus, 282
  in glomerulonephritis, 323
  for heart failure, 90
  in hepatic encephalopathy, 300
  in hypoglycemia, 257
  in megaesophagus, 276
  in pancreatitis, 290, 291

Diet—*Continued*
  in urolithiasis, 328
  urolithiasis and, 325
Diethylcarbamazine, 140
Diethylstilbestrol, 333
Differential cyanosis, 106
Diffuse granulomatous meningoencephalitis, 23
Digitalis
  for atrial fibrillation, 113
  for dilated cardiomyopathy, 112
Digoxin
  in heart failure, 86, 90
  in heartworm disease, 137
  in mitral valve disease, 68-69
  in pericardial disease, 76-77
Dihydrostreptomycin, 347
Dihydrotachysterol, 255
Dilated cardiomyopathy, 107-114. *See also*
    Cardiomyopathy, dilated
Dimenhydrinate, for vomiting, 262
Diphenoxylate
  for diarrhea, 265
  for tracheal collaspe, 179
Dipropionate, 21
Direct antiglobulin test, 382
*Dirofilaria immitis,*125
Dirofilaria reconditum, 130, 130t
Dirofilariasis, 125-141. *See also* Heartworm
    disease
Discharge
  in distemper, 399
  in pyometra, 342
  in rhinitis, 143
Discography in lumbosacral spondylomyelopathy,
    45
Discospondylitis, 46-49
  lytic lesion in, 52f
Disseminated intravascular coagulation, 385-386
  in gastric dilation volvulus, 282
Distemper, 194-195, 399-401
  clinical manifestations of, 399
  diagnosis of, 400
  diagnostic tests for, 397t
  encephalitis in, 27-29
  etiology of, 399
  pathogenesis of, 399
  prevention of, 400-401
  treatment of, 400
Distension in gastric dilation volvulus, 280
Diuresis, 311
Diuretic
  in acute renal failure, 309
  for dilated cardiomyopathy, 112
  in heart failure, 69, 90
  in heartworm disease, 137
  in pericardial disease, 76-77
DKA (diabetic ketoacidosis), 234-237
DM (degenerative myelopathy), 43-44
Doberman Pinscher
  cardiomyopathy in, 108
  cervical spondylomyelopathy in, 41

Doberman Pinscher—*Continued*
  copper storage disease in, 298
  hepatitis in, 297
  pimobendan in, 90
  primary ciliary dyskinesia in, 189
Dobutamine, 86
DOCP (desoxycorticosterone pivalate), 239
Domino effect in cervical spondylomyelopathy, 43
Dopamine, 310
Doppler study
  in mitral regurgitation, 64-66, 65f
  in patent ductus arteriosus, 97
  in subvalvular aortic stenosis, 99-100, 100f
  in ventricular septal defect, 103
Dorsoventral tracheal collapse, 177
Double-contrast cystography, 333
Doxapram, 172
Doxorubicin, 225
Doxycycline
  in ehrlichiosis, 406
  for respiratory infection, 196
  in Rocky Mountain spotted fever, 407
  for salmon poisoning, 408
Drainage
  pleural space, 216
  of pyothorax, 215
Drug-related liver disease, 299, 299t
Drug therapy
  for bronchitis, 186t
  immune-mediated hemolytic anemia and, 381
  for liver disease, 297
  for mitral valve disease, 66-69
  for nasal tumor, 165-166
  pancreatitis caused by, 288-289
  in pneumonia, 202
  renal failure caused by, 308
  for seizure, 9-14
  thyroid function and, 238
  for tracheal collapse, 179, 180t
  for vomiting, 261-262, 261t
Drug toxicity, hepatic, 299
Duct, bile, 304
Ductal occlusion, transcatheter, 97-99
Dyskinesia
  ciliary, 155
  primary ciliary, 189-190
Dysphagia, regurgitation and, 261
Dysplasia
  microvascular, 303
  tricuspid valve, 104-105

E
Echocardiography
  in dilated cardiomyopathy, 111, 111f
  in heartworm disease, 133
  in hypertrophic cardiomyopathy, 115
  in infective endocarditis, 121
  in mitral regurgitation, 63-65, 64f, 65f
  in patent ductus arteriosus, 96, 96f, 97
  in pericardial disease, 74, 75f, 76
  in pericardioperitoneal diaphragmatic hernia, 71

Echocardiography—*Continued*
  subvalvular aortic stenosis in, 99-100, 100f
  in ventricular septal defect, 103
Edema, 362-363
Edrophonium chloride, 18
Effusion
  pericardial, 72-73
    neoplastic, 78, 79
  pleural, 211-218
    pericardial versus, 74
Ehrlichiosis, 21, 404-406
Eisenmenger's syndrome, 105
Ejaculate, collection of, 349
Electrical alternans, 76
Electrocardiography
  in dilated cardiomyopathy, 111
  in heartworm disease, 133
  in infective endocarditis, 123
  in mitral valve degeneration, 66
  in pericardioperitoneal diaphragmatic hernia,
    71-72
Electrolyte in ketoacidosis, 235
Embolic myelopathy, fibrocartilagenous, 54-55
Embolism
  in heartworm disease, 131
  in infective endocarditis, 125
Emergency treatment
  of gastric dilation volvulus, 280-281
  of hypercalcemia, 252
  of hypoglycemia, 256-257
Empirical therapy for heart failure, 87
Enalapril
  for dilated cardiomyopathy, 112
  in mitral valve disease, 67
Encephalitis
  canine distemper viral, 27-29. *See also*
    Distemper
  meningoencephalitis, 18-29. *See also*
    Meningoencephalitis
  old dog, 29
  pug, 24-25
Encephalopathy, hepatic, 299-300
End-stage heart disease, 107-108
Endocarditis, infective, 118-125
  antibiotics for, 123-124
  anticoagulants in, 125
  bacteremia versus, 120
  breed affected by, 118
  causes of, 118-119
  congestive heart failure in, 124
  definition of, 118
  diagnosis of, 120-122
  echocardiography in, 123
  prevention of, 125
  sequelae to, 122-123
Endocrine disorder
  central diabetes insipidus as, 258-260
  diabetes mellitus as, 229-237. *See also* Diabetes
    mellitus
  hyperadrenocorticism as, 241-246
  hypercalcemia as, 250-253

Endocrine disorder—*Continued*
  hypoadrenocorticism as, 237-240
  hypoglycemia as, 255-257
  hypothyroidism as, 246-249
Endometrial hyperplasia/pyometra complex, 341-343
Endoscopy
  for diarrhea, 264
  for foreign body, 168
Endothelin, 91
Endotoxin, *Clostridium botulinum,* 16-17
Enema in hepatic encephalopathy, 300
English Bulldog
  brachycephalic airway syndrome in, 169
  pulmonic stenosis in, 101
  urolithiasis in, 326, 327
English Setter
  conformational disorder in, 155
  primary ciliary dyskinesia in, 189
English Springer Spaniel
  bronchiectasis in, 187
  immune-mediated hemolytic anemia in, 382
Enilconazole, 150, 391t
Enrofloxacin
  for infective endocarditis, 124
  for pyothorax, 215
  in urinary tract infection, 339
Enteritis
  eosinophilic, 271
  hemorrhagic, 266
Enterobacter, 337
Enterococcus, 303
Enterocolitis, uremic, 315
Enteropathy, protein-losing, 271-272
Enzyme
  in exocrine pancreatic insufficiency, 293
  hepatic, 295-296
    in adenovirus infection, 402
    in heartworm disease, 132
  in portosystemic shunt, 301
Enzyme-linked immunosorbent assay, 395
  in heartworm testing, 130
Eosinophilic enteritis, 271
Ephedrine, 333
Epidurography, 45
Epilepsy, 9. *See also* Seizure
Erosive polyarthritis, 360
Erythromycin, 262
Escherichia coli
  cholecystitis and, 303
  diarrhea and, 268
  pneumonia caused by, 197
  pyometra and, 342
  in pyothorax, 213
  urinary tract infection and, 337
Esophageal disease, 275-278
  regurgitation in, 261
Esophagitis, 277
Estrogen
  pyometra and, 341
  for urinary incontinence, 333

Estrous cycle, 344-345
Ethylene glycol toxicity, 307
Eucoleus aerophilus, 204
Excretory urography, 333
Exercise in diabetes mellitus, 230
Exocrine pancreatic insufficiency, 292-293
Extensor carpi radialis response, 3
Extensor postural thrust, 2
Extracellular fluid, 362-363
Extranodal lymphoma, 367
Exudate
  ascites and, 273
  pericardial, 72
Eye
  in adenovirus infection, 401
  in granulomatous meningoencephalitis, 23
  in Rocky Mountain spotted fever, 406

F
Facial nerve, 5-6
False-negative test for heartworm, 129
False-positive test for heartworm, 128-129
FCE (fibrocartilagenous embolic myelopathy), 54-55
Fecal flotation in salmon poisoning, 408
Feeding. *See* Diet
Felbamate, 13
Felbetrol, 13
Female infertility, 343-345
Femoral pulse in patent ductus arteriosus, 96
Fenbendazole
  dosages of, 207t
  for nasal mites, 152
Fenestration for intervertebral disc disease, 40-41
Fentanyl in pancreatitis, 291t
Fever
  definition of, 355
  in infective endocarditis, 122
  in neoplastic disease, 365
  Rocky Mountain spotted, 406-407
  treatment of, 357
  of unknown origin, 355-357
Fibrocartilage, vertebral, 54
Fibrocartilagenous embolic myelopathy, 54-55
Fibrosis, liver, 297
Filaroides osleri, 204, 206
Finasteride, 351
Fine needle aspiration biopsy
  of lung, 202, 220
  in plague, 412
Fish-borne disease, 407-408
Fistula
  bronchoesophageal, 190
  perianal, 287
Flail chest, 157-158
Flea-borne disease, plague, 396t, 412
Flexor reflex, 3
Fluconazole, 391t
  for cryptococcosis, 420
  for histoplasmosis, 421
  in phaeohyphomycosis, 22, 23

Flucytosine, 22, 390t-391t
Fludrocortisone, 240
Fluid
  ascitic, 273-275
  cerebrospinal. *See* Cerebrospinal fluid
  edema and, 362-363
  pericardial, 72-73
    pericardiocentesis for, 77-79
  pleural, 211-218
  prostatic, 349
  in syringohydromyelia, 35-36
Fluid therapy
  in acute renal failure, 309
  in chronic renal failure, 317
  in diarrhea, 265
  in heart failure, 87
  in hypercalcemia, 252-253
  in hypoadrenocorticism, 238
  in ketoacidosis, 235
  in pancreatitis, 290
  in pneumonia, 202-203
Fluke
  lung, 204
  in salmon poisoning, 407-408
Fluorescent antibody test, 395
  for rabies, 404
Fluoroquinolone
  in bacterial meningoencephalitis, 20
  for infective endocarditis, 123
  in Rocky Mountain spotted fever, 407
Fluoroscopy
  in pericardial disease, 76
  in pericardioperitoneal diaphragmatic hernia, 71
Focal granulomatous meningoencephalitis, 23
Food, adverse reaction to, 270
Foreign body
  esophageal, 277-278, 277f, 278f
  in upper airway, 167-168
Francisella tularensis, 413-414
Fructosamine, 232
Functional pulmonic stenosis, 103
Fungal infection, 414-421
  antifungal therapy for, 389, 390t-393t, 394
  aspergillosis as, 145-150, 147f, 148f, 149f
  blastomycosis as, 414-416
  coccidioidomycosis as, 416-418, 418f
  cryptococcosis as, 418-420
  histoplasmosis as, 420-421
FUO (fever of unknown origin), 355-357
Furosemide
  in acute renal failure, 309
  for dilated cardiomyopathy, 112
  for heart failure, 90
  in heartworm disease, 137
  in hypercalcemia, 253
  for hypoglycemia, 257
  in pericardial disease, 76-77
Furunculosis, anal, 287
Fusobacterium, 213

G
Gabapentin, 13
Gait
  in neurological disorder, 1
  in spinal cord disease, 31t
Gallbladder, 303-304
  in portosystemic shunt, 301
Gallstone, 303-304
Gastric dilation volvulus, 279-282
Gastric disorder, 279-285
  gastric dilation volvulus as, 279-282
  Helicobacter pylori causing, 282-284
  malignant, 282
  motility, 284-285
Gastroenteritis, hemorrhagic, 266
Gastrointestinal disorder
  in chronic renal failure, 314-315
  diarrhea as, 263-272. *See also* Diarrhea
  in distemper, 399
  esophageal, 275-278
  of liver, 293-303. *See also* Liver disease
  pancreatic, 288-293. *See also* Pancreas;
    Pancreatitis
  of rectum and anus, 285-287
  regurgitation and, 261
  of stomach, 279-285
    gastric dilation volvulus as, 279-282
    Helicobacter pylori causing, 282-284
    malignant, 282
    motility, 284-285
  vomiting in, 261-263
Gastropathy, uremic
  in acute renal failure, 310
  in chronic renal failure, 315, 317
GDV (gastric dilation volvulus), 279-282
Genetic disorder. *See* Hereditary disorder
Genetic testing in globoid cell leukodystrophy, 35
Gentamicin
  in gastric dilation volvulus, 282
  renal failure caused by, 306
German Shepherd
  aspergillosis in, 147
  conformational disorder in, 155
  congenital heart disease in, 93
  degenerative myelopathy in, 44
  exocrine pancreatic insufficiency in, 292
  infective endocarditis in, 118
  lymphoplasmacytic rhinitis in, 153
  subvalvular aortic stenosis in, 99
  urolithiasis in, 326
Giardia, 270
Gland, parathyroid, 252
Globoid cell leukodystrophy, 34-35
Glomerular disease, 319-324
  amyloidosis in, 322
  causes of, 320
  complications of, 323-324
  diagnosis of, 321-323
  prognosis for, 324
  renal anatomy in, 319-320
  treatment of, 323

Glomerulonephritis
  classification of, 320
  diseases with, 320-321
Glomerulonephropathy in ehrlichiosis, 405
Glomerulus, 319
Glossopharyngeal nerve, 6
Glucocorticoid
  for allergic rhinitis, 151
  in hyperadrenocorticism, 241
  in hypoadrenocorticism, 240
  thyroid function and, 238
Glucose
  diabetes mellitus and, 229-237
  in hypoadrenocorticism, 238
  hypoglycemia and, 255-257
  in pancreatitis, 289-290
Glucose curve, 231-233
Glycosuria, 229
Glycosylated hemoglobin, 232
GME (granulomatous meningoencephalitis), 23-24
Golden Retriever
  cardiac tamponade in, 75f
  ciliary dyskinesia in, 189
  conformational disorder in, 155
  infective endocarditis in, 118
  subvalvular aortic stenosis in, 99
  urolithiasis in, 327
Gordon Setter
  conformational disorder in, 155
  primary ciliary dyskinesia in, 189
Grading of intervertebral disc disease, 40
Granulocyte-colony stimulating factor in
    neutropenia, 377-378
Granulomatosis, lymphomatoid, 220, 223
Granulomatous meningoencephalitis, 23-24, 24f
Great Dane
  cardiomyopathy in, 108
  cervical spondylomyelopathy in, 41
  dilated cardiomyopathy in, 109
  urolithiasis in, 326

H
Hagedorn insulin, 230
Hansen classification of Intervertebral disc disease,
    37
HCM (hypertrophic cardiomyopathy), 114-117
HDDST (high-dose dexamethasone suppression
    test), 243
Head tilt, 5
Heart
  size of, in mitral valve disease, 62-63, 63f
  tumor of, 72, 75f, 79
Heart disease
  cardiomyopathy as
    dilated, 107-114
    hypertrophic, 114-117
  congenital, 93-106
    atrial septal defect as, 105
    cyanotic, 105-106
    definition of, 93
    diagnosis of, 94

Heart disease—*Continued*
  congenital—*Continued*
    genetics of, 93
    infective endocarditis and, 118
    patent ductus arteriosus as, 95-99
    pulmonic stenosis as, 100-101
    signs of, 93-94
    subvalvular aortic stenosis as, 99-100, 100f
    treatment of, 94
    tricuspid valve dysplasia as, 104-105
    ventricular septal defect as, 101-103, 104f
Heart failure, 81-92
  acute versus chronic, 88
  afterload in, 85
  causes of, 81-82
  clinical findings in, 82
  definition of, 81
  diagnosis of, 82-83
  drugs for, 84, 85-86, 89-91
  empirical therapy for, 87
  fluid therapy in, 87
  in heartworm disease, 137
  in mitral valve disease, 67, 68-69
  monitoring of, 87-88
  neuroendocrine activation in, 88
  preload in, 84, 85
  renin-angiotensin-aldosterone system in, 88
  tachycardia in, 86
  treatment goals for, 84
Heart murmur. *See* Murmur
Heart rate, in heart failure, 86
Heartgard, 134, 139-140, 140t
Heartworm disease, 125-141
  classification of, 130-131, 131t
  clinical findings in, 131-133
  damage caused by, 128
  demographics of, 126
  development of, 127
  diagnosis of, 133
  microfilariae and, 137-139
  occult, 126
  prophylaxis for, 139-140
  pulmonary artery disease in, 127-128
  testing for, 128-130
  thromboembolism prevention in, 136
  transmission of, 126
  treatment of, 133-137
Helicobacter pylori infection, 282-284
Helminth infection, 269-270
Hemangiosarcoma, 79, 370-371
  metastatic, 52f
Hemistanding, 2
Hemiwalking, 2
Hemodialysis, 311
Hemodynamics in thromboembolism, 209
Hemoglobin, glycosylated, 232
Hemoglobinuria, 137
Hemolymphatic disorder, 367-388
  anemia as, 373-375
    in chronic renal failure, 316, 317
  bleeding and, 372-373

Hemolymphatic disorder—*Continued*
  coagulopathy as, 384-388
  hemangiosarcoma as, 370-371
  immune-mediated hemolytic anemia as,
      381-384
  lymphoma as, 367-369
  neutropenia as, 377-378
  polycythemia as, 375-376
  thrombocytopenia as, 378-381
Hemolytic anemia, immune-mediated, 381-384
Hemorrhage in Rocky Mountain spotted fever, 406
Hemorrhagic effusion, pericardial, 72, 78
Hemorrhagic gastroenteritis, 266
Hemorrhagic myelomalacia, 56
Hemorrhagic pleural effusion, 217
Hemothorax, 217
Heparin
  in heartworm disease, 133, 137
  for infective endocarditis, 125
Hepatic encephalopathy, 299-300
Hepatic enzyme in adenovirus infection, 402
Hepatic failure, 256
Hepatic function, phenobarbital and, 11
Hepatic icterus, 294
Hepatic toxicity, 299
Hepatitis, 296-297
  diagnostic tests for, 397t
Hepatopathy, copper storage, 297-299
Hereditary disorder
  heart disease as, 93-106. *See also* Heart disease
  hemophilia as, 386-387
  hypertrophic cardiomyopathy as, 115
  of peripheral nerves, 17
  of spinal cord, 32-36
  von Willebrand's disease as, 387-388
Hernia, pericardioperitoneal diaphragmatic, 71-72
Herpesvirus infection, 194, 195
  pseudorabies as, 402-403
Hetastarch for gastric dilation volvulus, 280
HGE (hemorrhagic gastroenteritis), 266
High-dose dexamethasone suppression test, 243
Histiocytic sarcoma, 223-224
Histiocytic ulcerative colitis, 271
Histopathology of laryngeal tumor, 174
Histoplasma, 397, 420-421
  gastrointestinal infection with, 269
  liver disease and, 296
HM (hemorrhagic myelomalacia), 56
Hookworm, 269
  pulmonary migration of, 206
Hormone
  in hypoadrenocorticism, 238
  parathyroid
    chronic renal failure and, 316
    hypercalcemia and, 251-252
    in hypocalcemia, 254
  thyroid, 238. *See also* Thyroid disorder
    for urinary incontinence, 333
Hospitalization for diabetes, 233
HSA (hemangiosarcoma), 370-371
HW (heartworm), 125-141. *See also* Heartworm

Hydralazine
  heart failure and, 89
  in heartworm disease, 137
  in mitral valve disease, 67
Hydration. *See* Fluid therapy
Hydrocodone
  for bronchitis, 186t
  for tracheal collapse, 180t
Hydrocortisone, 238
Hyperadrenocorticism, 241-246
  causes of, 241
  clinical signs of, 241
  diagnosis of, 241-244, 242-244
  treatment of, 244-246
  urolithiasis in, 330-331
Hyperbilirubinemia, 293-294
Hypercalcemia, 250-253
  in cancer, 364
  in chronic renal failure, 317
Hypercoagulability, 323-324
Hyperhistaminemia, 364-365
Hyperkalemia
  in acute renal failure, 310
  in hypoadrenocorticism, 238
Hyperlipidemia, 323-324
Hyperparathyroidism, chronic renal failure and,
    316
Hyperpathia
  in discospondylitis, 47
  spinal, degenerative myelopathy and, 44
Hyperphosphatemia
  in chronic renal failure, 316
  in hypercalcemia, 251
Hyperplasia
  benign prostatic, 350-351
  cystic endometrial, 341-343
Hypertension
  chronic renal failure and, 315-316, 317
  pulmonary, in heartworm disease, 127-128
Hypertrophic cardiomyopathy, 114-117
Hypertrophic osteopathy, 365
Hypertrophy, antral pyloric, 284-285
Hyperventilation in thromboembolism, 209
Hypoadrenocorticism, 237-240
  causes of, 237
  clinical signs of, 237-238
  diagnosis of, 238-239
  electrocardiography in, 238
  electrolyte abnormality in, 238
  hypoglycemia and, 255
  treatment of, 238-240
Hypocalcemia, 253-255
  in chronic renal failure, 317
  status epilepticus and, 13
Hypocholesterolemia, 296
  in glomerulonephritis, 323-324
Hypoglossal nerve, 6
Hypoglycemia, 255-257
  in diabetes mellitus, 234
  in insulinoma, 365
  status epilepticus and, 13

Hypoglycemic drug, 230
Hypokalemia in acute renal failure, 311
Hypophosphatemia
in hypercalcemia, 251
in ketoacidosis, 236
Hypoplastic trachea, 155, 180-182, 181t, 182f
Hypotension in gastric dilation volvulus, 281
Hypothyroidism, 246-249
laryngeal paralysis and, 171
Hypoviscosity syndrome, 364
Hypoxemia in thromboembolism, 209

I

Icterus, 293-295
Idiopathic pericarditis, 79
IE (infective endocarditis), 118-125
IgG antibody, 407
Imaging. *See also* Computed tomography;
    Magnetic resonance imaging;
    Radiography
in liver disease, 296
in pancreatitis, 289
of portosystemic shunt, 302
in urinary tract infection, 338-339
in urolithiasis, 326
IMHA (immune-mediated hemolytic anemia),
    381-384
Imidocarb, 21
Imipramine, 334
Immiticide, 134-137, 135t
Immune-mediated disorder
glomerular, 320
hemolytic anemia as, 381-384
nonerosive polyarthritis as, 360-361
thrombocytopenia as, 379-380
Immunity
in distemper, 401
to Rocky Mountain spotted fever, 407
Immunoglobulin
in leptospirosis, 409
in Rocky Mountain spotted fever, 407
Immunoreactivity in pancreatitis, 290
Immunosuppressive agent
for granulomatous meningoencephalitis, 24
for immune-mediated hemolytic anemia, 383
for perianal fistula, 287
for pug encephalitis, 25
in steroid responsive meningitis-arteritis, 50
in thrombocytopenia, 380
IMPA (immune-mediated polyarthritis), 360-361
Incontinence, urinary, 331-334
Infection, 389-422
antifungal therapy for, 389, 390t-393t, 394
bacterial, 409-414
leptospirosis as, 409-410
Lyme disease as, 410-411
plague as, 411-412
respiratory, 196-204
tetanus as, 412-413
tularemia as, 413-414
brucellosis, 345-348

Infection—*Continued*
diagnosis of, 394-395, 396t-397t, 398-399
discospondylitis as, 46-49
fungal, 414-421. *See also* Fungal infection
of gallbladder, 303
heartworm, 125-141. *See also* Heartworm
    disease
Helicobacter pylori, 282-284
immune-mediated hemolytic anemia and, 381
meningoencephalitis as
bacterial, 19-20
protozoal, 25-27
pericardial, 72-73
polyarthritis in, 360
prostatic, 351-352
renal failure caused by, 307
rhinitis as
bacterial, 145-146
mycotic, 146-150, 147f, 148, 149f
rickettsial, 404-408
urolithiasis and, 325, 330
viral, 399-404. *See also* Viral infection
Infectious tracheobronchitis, canine, 194
Infective endocarditis, 118-125. *See also*
    Endocarditis, infective
Infertility in female, 343-345
Infiltrative lymphadenopathy, 358
Inflammation
liver, 297
pericardial, 79
Inflammatory disease
discospondylitis as, 47-49
hepatitis as, 296-297
intracranial, 18-29. *See also* Intracranial disease,
    inflammatory
Influenza, canine, 194
Infusion
for aspergillosis, 149
in hypoglycemia, 257
Inhalation therapy for pulmonary metastasis, 225
Inhaler, 151
Injury. *See* Trauma
Inotropic drug for heart failure, 86, 91-92
Insulin
in diabetes, 230-231
in hypoadrenocorticism, 238
in ketoacidosis, 236, 237
resistance to, 234
Insulinoma, 257
hypoglycemia and, 255-256, 365
Interceptor, 138, 139-140, 140t
Intermittent lameness in infective endocarditis,
    122
Intervertebral disc disease, 36-41
Intestinal parasite, 206
Intolerance, food, 270
Intoxication, rodenticide, 386-387
Itraconazole, 22
Intracranial disease, 7
inflammatory, 18-29
canine distemper viral encephalitis as, 27-29

Intracranial disease—*Continued*
  inflammatory—*Continued*
    meningoencephalitis as, 18-29
      bacterial, 19-20
      granulomatous, 23-24, 24f
      protozoal, 25-27
      pug encephalitis, 24-25
    mycotic
      cerebral phaeohyphomycosis as, 22-23
      cryptococcosis as, 21-22
    rickettsiosis as
      ehrlichiosis as, 21
      Rocky Mountain spotted fever, 20-21
    viral, 27-29
Intrapericardial fluid pressure, 73
Intraspinal fluid, in syringohydromyelia, 35-36
Intrathoracic tracheal collapse, 177
Irish Wolfhound, dilated cardiomyopathy in, 109
Irritable bowel disease, 270-271
Ischemic myelopathy, 54-55
Islet cell neoplasia, 255-256
Itraconazole, 392t
  for aspergillosis, 150
  for blastomycosis, 415
  for histoplasmosis, 421
Iverheart, 139-140, 140t
Ivermectin
  dosages of, 207t
  for nasal mites, 152

J
Joint disease, 359-362
Juvenile hypoglycemia, 255
Juxtapulmonary receptor, 61

K
Kaolin, 265
Kartagener's syndrome, 157
Keppra, for seizure, 13
Ketoacidosis, 234-237
Ketoconazole, 391t
  for aspergillosis, 150
  in cryptococcosis, 22
  in hyperadrenocorticism, 245-246
Ketone, 230
Kidney. *See* Renal failure; Urinary system disorder
Kinetics in lumbosacral spondylomyelopathy, 45
Klebsiella
  pneumonia caused by, 197
  in urinary infection, 337
Klebsiella pneumoniae, 196

L
Labrador Retriever
  aspergillosis in, 147
  dilated cardiomyopathy in, 110f
  infective endocarditis in, 118
  laryngeal paralysis in, 171
  lymphoplasmacytic rhinitis in, 153
  urolithiasis in, 327
Laceration, tracheal, 182-183

Lactate in gastric dilation volvulus, 280
Lactulose, 300
Lameness
  in infective endocarditis, 122
  in Lyme disease, 410
Laminectomy, 46
Large airway disorder, 177-184. *See also* Airway
    disorder
Large-bowel diarrhea, 263, 264t
Laryngeal paralysis, 171-173
  congenital, 155
  in hypothyroidism, 247
Larynx
  conformational disorder of, 154
  tumor of, 173-175
Latex agglutination, 395
Lavage
  in aspergillosis, 148
  in pneumonia, 201
LDDST (low-dose dexamethasone suppression
    test), 242-243
Left atrial enlargement, 61, 68
Left-sided heart failure, 82
Leg lameness in infective endocarditis, 122
Leptospirosis, 409-410
  diagnostic tests for, 396t
  liver disease and, 296
  renal failure caused by, 307
Leukodystrophy, globoid cell, 34-35
Leukogram, 49
Leukopenia, 400
Levamisole, 207t
Levatracim, 13
Levothyroxine, 248-249
Lhasa Apso
  immune-mediated hemolytic anemia in, 382
  urolithiasis in, 327
Lilium, renal failure caused by, 307
Lipase in pancreatitis, 290
Lipid in glomerulonephritis, 323-324
Lithotripsy, 330
Liver, phenobarbital and, 11
Liver disease, 293-303
  biochemical profile in, 295-296
  chronic inflammatory, 296-297
  clinical signs of, 295
  coagulopathy in, 386
  copper storage hepatopathy, 297-299
  diagnosis of, 296
  drug-related, 299, 299t
  encephalopathy with, 299-300
  icterus and, 293-294
  imaging in, 296
  portosystemic shunt and, 300-303
Liver enzyme, in heartworm disease, 132
Lobectomy, lung, 222
Localization of lesion
  cranial, 5-7
  spinal, 1-5, 30
    of postural reaction deficit, 7
Loperamide, 265

Low-dose dexamethasone suppression test, 242-243
Lower motor neuron disorder, 332
Lower respiratory tract tumor, 219-226. *See also* Lung tumor
LPR (lymphoplasmacytic rhinitis), 152-154
Lufenuron, 393t
Lumbosacral spondylomyelopathy, 44-46
Lumbosacral stenosis, 44-46
Lumen, tracheal, 181, 181t
Lung, conformational disorder of, 154
Lung tumor, 219-226. *See also* Pulmonary disorder
  clinical signs of, 219
  diagnosis of, 219-221
  differential diagnosis of, 219
  histiocytic, 223-224
  location of, 219
  lymphomatoid granulomatosis and, 223
  metastatic, 224-225
  paraneoplastic disorder with, 223
  staging of, 221
  treatment of, 222
Lungworm, 204
Lyme disease, 410-411
  renal failure caused by, 307
Lymph node
  aspiration of, 395
  in ehrlichiosis, 405
  lymphoma and, 367-369
Lymphadenitis, 358
Lymphadenopathy, 358-359
Lymphangiectasia, 271-272
Lymphedema, 363
Lymphocytic/plasmacytic irritable bowel disease, 271
Lymphoma, 222, 225, 367-369
Lymphomatoid granulomatosis, 220, 223
Lymphoplasmacytic rhinitis, 152-154
Lytic lesion, spinal, 52f

M
Macroadenoma, pituitary, 241
Magnetic resonance imaging
  in cervical spondylomyelopathy, 43
  in cryptococcosis, 22
  in discospondylitis, 48
  in Intervertebral disc disease, 38, 38f
  in lumbosacral spondylomyelopathy, 45
  for lung tumor, 219-220
  of nasal tumor, 164
  in phaeohyphomycosis, 23
  in syringohydromyelia, 36
  of tumor, 50
Malignancy, nasal, 159-166
Maltese
  patent ductus arteriosus in, 94
  tracheal collapse in, 177
  urolithiasis in, 327

Mannitol
  in acute renal failure, 310
  for hypoglycemia, 257
Mapping, Doppler, in mitral regurgitation, 64-66, 65f
Mast cell stabilizer, 152
MR (mitral regurgitation), 60-70
Mediastinal lymphoma, 367
Mediator in glomerular injury, 320
Medulla, 6
Megaesophagus, 275-276
  in hypothyroidism, 247
  laryngeal paralysis and, 172
Membranoproliferative glomerulonephritis, 320
Membranous glomerulonephritis, 320
Meningitis-arteritis, steroid responsive, 49-50
Meningoencephalitis
  bacterial, 19-20
  causes of, 18-19
  definition of, 18
  diagnosis of, 18-20
  granulomatous, 23-24, 24f
  protozoal, 25-27
  pug encephalitis, 24-25
  signs of, 18
Mestinon, 18
Metabolic acidosis in renal failure, 310
Metabolism of bilirubin, 294-295
Metastasis
  of hemangiosarcoma, 52f, 370
  hypertrophic osteopathy and, 365
  of lung tumor, 220
  pulmonary, 224
Metered-dose inhaler, 151
Methylprednisolone sodium succinate, 53
Metoclopramide
  in acute renal failure, 310
  for vomiting, 262
Metronidazole
  in bacterial meningoencephalitis, 20
  for *Giardia* infection, 270
  in *Helicobacter pylori* infection, 284
  for irritable bowel disease, 271
  for rhinitis, 145
Microalbuminuria
  in acute renal failure, 314-315
  in glomerular disease, 322
Microfilariae
  heartworm and, 126-127
  testing for, 128-130
  treatment for, 137-139
Microvascular dysplasia, 303
Midbrain, lesion of, 6
Midsystolic click, 61-62
Milbemycin oxime, 207t
Milrinone, 86
Mineralization
  bronchial, 190
  of disc, 40
Miniature Poodle
  conformational disorder in, 155

Miniature Poodle—*Continued*
  heart disease in, 93
  primary ciliary dyskinesia in, 189
  urolithiasis in, 327
Miniature Schnauzer
  pancreatitis in, 288-289
  urolithiasis in, 327
Minocycline
  for brucellosis, 347
  in ehrlichiosis, 21, 406
  in Rocky Mountain spotted fever, 407
Mite, nasal, 152, 204
Mitotane, 244-245
Mitoxantrone, 225
Mitral chorda tendinae rupture, 69
Mitral valve
  infective endocarditis and, 118
  systolic anterior motion of, 114
Mitral valve degeneration, 59-70
  ascites in, 70
  causes of, 59-60
  in Cavalier King Charles spaniel, 60
  consequences of, 60-61
  cough in, 61-62
  deterioration in, 69-70
  drugs for, 66-69
  echocardiography in, 62, 63f, 64-65, 65f
  electrocardiography in, 66
  heart failure in, 82
  heart failure with, 82
  heart size in, 62-63
  midsystolic click in, 61-62
  murmur in, 61
  normal, 59
  radiography in, 62, 63f
  signs of, 60
  surgery in, 69
Mitral valve regurgitation, 60-70
  ascites with, 70
  as consequence of valvular degeneration, 60
  cough in, 61-62
  drug therapy for, 66-68
  echocardiography in, 63-65, 64f, 65f
  midsystolic click and, 61
  murmur with, 61, 82
  in patent ductus arteriosus, 95
  radiography in, 62
  respiratory sinus arrhythmia and, 62
  severity of, 65-66
Monitoring
  in gastric dilation volvulus, 281
  glucose, 231-234
  of heart failure, 87-88
  of hypothyroidism, 249
  in immune-mediated hemolytic anemia, 383-384
  in parenchymal disease, 193
Monoparesis, 15-17
Mortality
  of infective endocarditis, 125
  lymphoma and, 369
Motility disorder, gastric, 284-285

Motor neuron paraparesis, 34
MRI. *See* Magnetic resonance imaging
Mucocele, 303
Mucoid nasal discharge, 143
Mucopurulent nasal discharge, 143
Mucosal bleeding time, buccal, 373
Mucosal damage in diarrhea, 266
Multicenter Spaniel Trial, 109
Multicentric lymphoma, 367
Murmur
  in hypertrophic cardiomyopathy, 115
  in infective endocarditis, 121
  in mitral valve disease, 60-61, 82
  in pulmonic stenosis, 101, 103
  in subvalvular aortic stenosis, 99
Muscle
  neosporosis, 26f
  in spinal cord disease, 31t
Muscle versus peripheral nerve disease, 15
MVD. *See* Mitral valve degeneration
Myasthenia gravis, 17-18
Mycotic infection
  cerebral phaeohyphomycosis as, 22-23
  cryptococcosis as, 21-22
Mycotic rhinitis, 146-150, 147f, 148, 149f
Myelodysplasia, 35
Myelography
  in cervical spondylomyelopathy, 43
  in chronic paraparesis, 52f
  in discospondylitis, 48
  in intervertebral disc disease, 38-39
  in lumbosacral spondylomyelopathy, 45
  in spinal cord disorder, 32
  in syringohydromyelia, 36
Myelomalacia, hemorrhagic, 56
Myelopathy
  degenerative, 43-44
  fibrocartilagenous embolic, 54-55
  ischemic, 54-55
Myocardial disease, 107-117
  cardiomyopathy as
    dilated, 107-114
    hypertrophic, 114-117
Myoclonus
  canine distemper viral encephalitis, 28
  in canine distemper viral encephalitis, 28
Myxomatous valvular degeneration, 59

N
Nanophyetus salmincola, 407-408
Narcotic analgesic, for diarrhea, 265
Nares, stenotic, 155
Nasal aspergillosis, 146-150, 147-148, 147f, 148, 149f
Nasal dermoid sinus cyst, 155
Nasal discharge
  in distemper, 399
  in rhinitis, 143
Nasal lavage in aspergillosis, 148
Nasal tumor, 159-166
  chemotherapy for, 165

Nasal tumor—*Continued*
  differential diagnosis of, 160
  nonsteroidal antiinflammatory drug for, 165-166
  prognosis of, 166
  radiation therapy for, 164-165
  radiography of, 160-162, 161f, 162f
  signs of, 160
  surgery for, 165
Nasopharyngeal foreign body, 167-168
Natriuretic peptide, 91
Nebulization, 203
Neck brace for atlantoaxial instability, 33
Needle aspiration of lung, 202, 220
Nematode, 204-206
Neomycin
  in hepatic encephalopathy, 300
  renal failure caused by, 306
Neonatal hypoglycemia, 255
Neonatal immune-mediated hemolytic anemia, 381-382
Neoplasm. *See* Tumor
Neoplastic pericardial effusion, 72, 78, 79
Neorickettsia helminthoeca, 396t, 407-408
Neospora caninum, 207
Neosporosis, 25-27, 26f
Nephrolith, 329
Nephron, 319
Nephrotic syndrome, 320, 321
Nephrotoxicity
  of drug, 306
    of amphotericin B, 389
  of toxin, 307
Nervous system in hypoglycemia, 256. *See also* Neurological *entries*
Neuroendocrine activation in heart failure, 88
Neurological disorder
  in adenovirus infection, 401
  in distemper, 399
  examination for, 1-7
  in hypothyroidism, 246-247
  inflammatory intracranial, 18-29. *See also* Intracranial disease, inflammatory
  peripheral nerve, 14-18
  seizure with, 8-14
  spinal cord, 30-57. *See also* Spinal cord disease
  urinary incontinence with, 331-332
Neurological examination, 1-7
  gait in, 1-2
  localization of brain lesion in, 5-7
  reflexes in, 2-5
Neurontin, 13
Neuropathy
  hypoglycemia and, 256
  in hypothyroidism, 246-247
Neurotoxin, tetanus, 412-413
Neutropenia, 377-378
Newfoundland
  conformational disorder in, 155
  heart disease in, 93
    dilated cardiomyopathy, 109
    subvalvular aortic stenosis, 99

Newfoundland—*Continued*
  primary ciliary dyskinesia in, 189
Nikkomycin, 393t
Nitrate, in heart failure, 84
Nitroglycerin, 84
Nitroprusside, 85
Nocardia, 213
Node, lymph. *See* Lymph node
Nodular airway disease, 157
Nonerosive immune-mediated polyarthritis, 360-361
Nonsteroidal antiinflammatory drug
  for fever, 357
  for nasal tumor, 165-166
  renal failure caused by, 306
Norwegian Elkhound, 189
Norwegian Lundehund, 272
Noxafil, 392t
NPH insulin, 230
NPO status in pancreatitis, 291
NSAID. *See* Nonsteroidal antiinflammatory drug
Nutrition. *See* Diet

O
Obstruction
  biliary, 303-304
  gastric, 284
Occlusion, transcatheter ductal, 97-99
Occult disease
  dilated cardiomyopathy, 108-109, 112
  heartworm, 126
Ocular discharge in distemper, 399
Ocular disorder
  in adenovirus infection, 401
  in granulomatous meningoencephalitis, 23
  in Rocky Mountain spotted fever, 406
Oculomotor nerve, 5
Old dog encephalitis, 29
Old English Sheepdog
  conformational disorder in, 155
  degenerative myelopathy in, 44
  immune-mediated hemolytic anemia in, 382
  urolithiasis in, 326
Oliguria, 308, 309
Oncocytoma, laryngeal, 173
Ondansetron, 262
Open pneumothorax, 216-217
Open pyometra, 341-342
Opiate for diarrhea, 265
Optic nerve, 5
Oral hypoglycemic drug, 230
Orthopedic injury, tumor versus, 15
Oslerus osleri, 204, 206
Osmotic agent in renal failure, 310
Osmotic diarrhea, 263
Osteodystrophy, renal, 316
Osteopathy, hypertrophic, 365
Ovariohysterectomy for pyometra, 342
Overflow incontinence, 331
Overgrowth, bacterial, 268
Oversaturation, urine, 325

Oxygen in parenchymal disease, 193
Oxymorphone, 291t
Oxytetracycline
  in ehrlichiosis, 21, 406
  in Rocky Mountain spotted fever, 407
  for salmon poisoning, 408
Oxytrema silicula, 407

P
Packed red cell volume, 372
Pain
  generation of, 32
  in intervertebral disc disease, 41
Palate, conformational disorder of, 154
Palliation, brachycephalic airway and, 170-171
Pancreas. *See also* Pancreatitis
  autodigestion and, 288
  function of, 288
  hypoglycemia and, 255-256
  tumor of, 292
Pancreatic insufficiency, exocrine, 292-293
Pancreatic islet cell
  in diabetes mellitus, 229
  neoplasia of, 255-256
Pancreatitis, 288-292, 291t
  autodigestion and, 288
  clinical signs of, 289
  complications of, 291
  diagnosis of, 289-290
  imaging of, 289
  potassium bromide and, 12
  risk factors for, 288-289
  treatment of, 290-291, 291t
Paradoxical incontinence, 331
Paragonimus kellicotti, 204, 206
Paralysis
  congenital laryngeal, 155
  of four limbs, 5
  laryngeal, 171-173
    in hypothyroidism, 247
  tick, 16
Paranasal sinus, tumor of, 159-166
Paraneoplastic disorder, 223, 364-366
Paraparesis
  in degenerative myelopathy, 44
  myelography, 52f
  upper motor neuron, 34
Parasitic disease
  gastrointestinal, 269-270
  respiratory, 204-208
Parathyroid gland
  in hypercalcemia, 251-252
    removal of, 253
  in hypocalcemia, 253-255
Parathyroid hormone
  chronic renal failure and, 316
  hypercalcemia and, 251-252
  in hypocalcemia, 254
Parathyroid hormone-related peptide, 252
Parenchymal pulmonary disorder, 192-208
  bacterial, 196-204

Parenchymal pulmonary disorder—*Continued*
  overview of, 192-194
  parasitic and protozoal, 204-208
  viral, 194-195
Parvovirus, 266-267
Pasteurella, 213
Pasteurella multocida, 196, 197
  rhinitis and, 145
Patent ductus arteriosus, 93, 95-99
PCD (primary ciliary dyskinesia), 189-190
PDH (pituitary-dependent hyperadrenocorticism),
  241, 243-244
Pectus excavatum, 157-158
Pekingese
  brachycephalic airway syndrome in, 169
  urolithiasis in, 327
Pelvic bladder, 332
Pelvic limb reflex, 3
Penicillin for salmon poisoning, 408
Pentobarbital for status epilepticus, 13
Perfusion in thromboembolism, 210
Perianal adenoma, 286
Perianal fistula, 287
Pericardial cyst, 71
Pericardial disease, 71-81
  cardiac tamponade and, 73-74, 76-78
  congenital, 71
  constrictive, 79-80
  echocardiography in, 74, 75f, 76
  electrical alternans in, 76
  electrocardiography in, 76
  fluoroscopy in, 76
  infectious, 72-73
  pericardiocentesis for, 77-79
  pericardioperitoneal diaphragmatic hernia and,
    71-72
  pneumopericardiography in, 76
Pericardial effusion
  hemorrhagic, 78
  neoplastic, 72, 78, 79
  pleural effusion versus, 74
Pericardiectomy
  for constrictive disease, 80
  in neoplastic disease, 79
Pericardiocentesis, 77-79
Pericardioperitoneal diaphragmatic hernia, 71-72
Perineal hernia, 285-286
Peripheral blood, microfilariae in, 127
Peripheral nerve disease, 14-18
  breed-related, 17
  causes of, 15-17
  myasthenia gravis and, 17-18
  signs of, 14-15
Peripheral neuropathy, 256
Peripheral pulse in infective endocarditis, 121
Peritoneal dialysis, 311
Phaeohyphomycosis, cerebral, 22-23
Pharyngeal conformational disorder, 154
Phenobarbital, 10, 11
Phenothiazine, 262
Phenylpropanolamine, 333

Phlebotomy in polycythemia, 376
Phosphate
  in chronic renal failure, 316
  in hypercalcemia, 251
  in ketoacidosis, 236
Pimobendan
  for dilated cardiomyopathy, 114
  for heart failure, 90
Pinch biopsy in diarrhea, 264
Pitting edema, 362
Pituitary-dependent hyperadrenocorticism, 241,
    243-244
Pituitary macroadenoma, 241
Placing, visual and tactile, 2
Plague, 396t, 411-412
Plaque in aspergillosis, 148
Platelet, thrombocytopenia and, 378-381
Pleural effusion, 74, 211-214
Pleural space disease, 211-218
  chylothorax as, 213-214, 214f, 217
  hemothorax as, 217
  pneumothorax as, 216-217
  pseudochylothorax and, 217-218
  pyothorax as, 213-216, 213f, 215f
Pneumatocele, 158
Pneumonia
  bacterial, 196, 197, 198f
  diagnosis of, 201-202
  treatment of, 202-203
Pneumonyssoides caninum, 204, 206
Pneumopericardiography, 76
Pneumothorax, 216-217
Pointer, conformational disorder in, 155
Poisoning, salmon, 407-408. *See also* Toxicity
Polyarthritis
  infectious, 360
  nonerosive immune-mediated, 360-361
  rickettsial, 360
Polycythemia, 375-376
Polydipsia
  in diabetes insipidus, 258
  in hypercalcemia, 251
  in pyometra, 342
Polymerase chain reaction, 395
  in canine distemper viral encephalitis, 29
  in leptospirosis, 409-410
Polysystemic disorder
  edema as, 362-363
  fever as, 355-357
  joint disease as, 359-362
  lymphadenopathy as, 358-359
  paraneoplastic, 364-366
Polyuria
  in diabetes insipidus, 258
  in hypercalcemia, 250, 251
  in pyometra, 342
Pomeranian
  patent ductus arteriosus in, 94
  tracheal collapse in, 177
  urolithiasis in, 327
Pons, 6

Poodle. *See also* Miniature Poodle
  immune-mediated hemolytic anemia in, 382
  pancreatitis in, 288-289
  tracheal collapse in, 177
Portosystemic shunt, 300-303
Positioning for pericardiocentesis, 77
Posthepatic icterus, 294-295
Postmortem appearance of degenerative valvular
    disease, 59
Postural reaction, 31t
Postural reaction deficit, 7
Postural thrust, extensor, 2
Potassium
  in acute renal failure, 310, 311
  in hypoadrenocorticism, 238
  in ketoacidosis, 235
Potassium bromide, 10, 11-12
Potassium iodide, 392t
PPDH (pericardioperitoneal diaphragmatic hernia),
    71-72
Praziquantel, 207t
Prednisolone
  for allergic rhinitis, 151
  for lymphoplasmacytic rhinitis, 154
Prednisone
  for bronchitis, 186t
  in hypoadrenocorticism, 240
  for immune-mediated hemolytic anemia, 383
  in lymphoma, 369
  in steroid responsive meningitis-arteritis, 50
  for tracheal collapse, 180t
Pregnancy, brucellosis in, 346
Prehepatic icterus, 294, 295
Preload in heart failure, 83-84, 84
Premature contraction, ventricular, 281
Prerenal azotemia, 305
Pressure
  blood
    chronic renal failure and, 315-316
    in gastric dilation volvulus, 281
  central venous, 76
  intrapericardial fluid, 73
Prevention
  of adenovirus infection, 402
  of dermoid sinus, 34
  of distemper, 400-401
  of heartworm disease, 138-140, 140t
  of infective endocarditis, 125
  of leptospirosis, 410
  of protozoal disease, 27
  of rabies, 404
  of Rocky Mountain spotted fever, 407
  of viral infection, 195
Primary ciliary dyskinesia, 189-190
Primary epilepsy, 9
Primidone, 10-11
Prioxicam, 152
Proestrus/estrus, prolonged, 345
Progesterone, pyometra and, 341
ProHeart, 139-140, 140t
Prolapse, rectal, 286

Prophylaxis, heartworm, 138-140
Propofol, 13
Prostaglandin F$_{2a}$, 343
Prostatic disease
  bacterial infection as, 351-352
  benign hyperplasia as, 350-351
  categories of, 348
  common features of, 348
  cystic, 352-353
  diagnosis of, 348-350
  neoplastic, 352-353
Prostatic hyperplasia, benign, 350-351
Prostatic wash, 349-350
Protein in pleural transudates, 212
Protein-losing enteropathy, 271-272
Protein:creatinine ratio, 321-322
Proteinuria, 322
  in ehrlichiosis, 405
  in heartworm disease, 132-133
  in pyometra, 342
  reduction of, 323
Proteus, 325
Proteus mirabilis, 337
Protozoal disease
  meningoencephalitis, 25-27
  prevention of, 27
  respiratory, 204-208
PS (pulmonic stenosis), 100-101
Pseudochylothorax, 217-218
Pseudoephedrine, 333
Pseudomonas aeruginosa, 145
Pseudoneutropenia, 377
Pseudorabies, 402-403
  diagnostic tests for, 397t
PSS (portosystemic shunt), 300-303
Ptyalism, 402-403
Pug, brachycephalic airway syndrome in,
    169
Pug encephalitis, 24-25
Pulmonary artery, heartworm in, 127, 128
Pulmonary cavitary lesion, 158
Pulmonary disorder
  in adenovirus infection, 401
  of airway, 177-184
    bronchial, 184-189
    nodular, 157
    tracheal, 177-184
      collapse as, 177-179, 180f, 180t
      hypoplastic, 180-182, 181t, 182f
      laceration as, 182-183
    upper, 167-173
      brachycephalic airway syndrome as,
        168-171
      foreign body causing, 167-168
      laryngeal paralysis as, 171-173
      laryngeal tumor as, 173-175
      tracheal tumor as, 175-176
  conformational disorder causing, 154-159
  lung tumor as, 219-226. *See also* Lung tumor
  nasal tumor as, 159-166
  parenchymal, 192-208

Pulmonary disorder—*Continued*
  parenchymal—*Continued*
    bacterial, 196-204
    overview of, 192-194
    parasitic and protozoal, 204-208
    viral, 194-195
  of pleural space, 211-218
  rhinitis as, 143-154. *See also* Rhinitis
  thromboembolism, 208-210
Pulmonary hypertension in heartworm disease,
    127-128
Pulmonary metastasis, 224
Pulmonary thromboembolism, 208-210
  in heartworm disease, 131
Pulmonary vascular resistance, 102
Pulmonic stenosis, 94, 100-101
  ventricular septal defect with, 102
Pulse
  in infective endocarditis, 121
  in patent ductus arteriosus, 96
Pulsed-wave Doppler echocardiography, 64-65,
    65f
Pulsus paradoxus, 74
Pyelonephritis, 336
  imaging in, 339
  pyometra and, 342
Pyloric hypertrophy, 284-285
Pyometra, 341-343
Pyridostigmine bromide, 17
Pyrimethamine, 27
Pyothorax, 213-216, 215f, 213f
Pythiosis, 268-269

R
Rabies, 403-404
  diagnostic tests for, 397t
Radiation therapy
  for laryngeal tumor, 174-175
  for lung tumor, 222
  for nasal tumor, 164
  of tracheal tumor, 176
Radiography
  in atlantoaxial instability, 33
  in blastomycosis, 415, 416f, 417f
  of bronchiectasis, 187-188, 188f
  in bronchitis, 185, 185f
  in cervical spondylomyelopathy, 42f
  in coccidioidomycosis, 417, 418f
  of dilated cardiomyopathy, 110-111, 110f
  in discospondylitis, 47, 47f
  of foreign body, 167
  in gastric motility disorder, 284
  in heart failure, 83, 83f
  in heartworm disease, 132
  in hemangiosarcoma, 371
  in hypercalcemia, 251
  hypoglycemia and, 256
  of hypoplastic trachea, 181
  in Intervertebral disc disease, 37, 37f
  in intervertebral disc disease, 40
  in liver disease, 296

Radiography—*Continued*
  in lumbosacral spondylomyelopathy, 45
  of lung tumor, 220
  in lymphoplasmacytic rhinitis, 153
  of megaesophagus, 276
  in mitral valve disease, 62-63, 63f, 66
  of nasal tumor, 160-162, 161f, 162f
  in pancreatitis, 289
  in parenchymal disease, 192-194
  in pericardial disease, 74, 80
  in pericardioperitoneal diaphragmatic hernia, 71
  of pleural effusion, 211-212, 214
  of pulmonary metastasis, 225
  in rhinitis, bacterial, 145
  in thromboembolism, 209
  of tracheal collapse, 178
  of tracheal tumor, 176
  of tumor, 50
  in urolithiasis, 326, 328
Ratio
  cortisol:creatinine, 242
  protein:creatinine, 321-322
  ventilation-perfusion, 208-209
Reactive lymphadenopathy, 358
Receptor, juxtapulmonary, 61
Recombinant granulocyte-colony stimulating
      factor in neutropenia, 377-378
Rectal disorder, 285-287, 286t
Rectal scraping, 398, 398f
Recurrent urinary tract infection, 339
Reflex
  abnormal, 4
  degenerative myelopathy in, 44
  pelvic limb, 3
  spinal, testing of, 2-5
  in spinal cord disease, 31t
Reflex incontinence, 331
Regenerative anemia, 374
Regurgitation, 261
  in esophageal disease, 275-278
  gastric dilation volvulus and, 279
  mitral valve, 59-70. *See also* Mitral valve
      regurgitation
Rehydration
  in acute renal failure, 309
  in hypercalcemia, 252-253
  in ketoacidosis, 235
Reinfection, urinary tract, 339
Remission of lung cancer, 222
Renal biopsy, 322-323
Renal disorder, 305-340. *See also* Renal failure;
      Urinary system disorder
Renal failure
  acute
    causes of, 306-308
    clinical signs of, 308
    definition of, 305
    differential diagnosis of, 308
    management of, 308-311
    phases of, 305-306
    prognosis for, 311-312

Renal failure—*Continued*
  chronic, 312-319
    anemia in, 316, 317
    azotemia in, 313
    causes of, 312-313
    clinical course of, 313
    clinical findings in, 314
    definition of, 312
    diet in, 318
    hyperparathyroidism with, 316-317
    hypertension and, 315-316
    macroalbuminemia in, 314-315
    management of, 318
    prognosis for, 318-319
    stages of, 313
    uremia in, 313-314
Renal tumor, 334-335
Renin-angiotensin-aldosterone system
  in dilated cardiomyopathy, 107-108
  in heart failure, 88
  in mitral valve disease, 67
Reproductive disorder, 341-354
  brucellosis as, 345-348
  cystic endometrial hyperplasia/pyometra
      complex as, 341-343
  hypothyroidism and, 247
  infertility, 343-345
  prostatic, 348-354. *See also* Prostatic disease
Resistance
  insulin, 234
  vascular, 85
Respiratory disease. *See* Pulmonary disorder
Respiratory distress in mitral valve disease, 61
Respiratory infection, viral, 194-195
Respiratory sinus arrhythmia
  heart failure and, 82
  in mitral valve disease, 62
Retrograde urohydropulsion, 328-329
Retrograde vaginourethrography, 333
Revolution, 139-140, 140t
Rheumatoid arthritis, 360
Rhinitis, 143-154
  allergic, 151-152
  bacterial, 145-146
  definition of, 143
  diagnostic testing for, 143-145
  lymphoplasmacytic, 152-154
  mycotic, 146-150, 147f, 148f, 149f
  nasal discharge in, 143
Rhinoscopy, 144
  in aspergillosis, 147, 148
  for nasal tumor, 164
Rhinotomy, for aspergillosis, 150
Rhodesian Ridgeback
  degenerative myelopathy in, 44
  dermoid sinus in, 34
Rickettsial infection, 404-408
  diagnostic tests for, 396t
  ehrlichiosis, 404-406
  polyarthritis in, 360
  in rhinitis, 144

Rickettsial infection—*Continued*
  Rocky Mountain spotted fever, 406-407
  salmon poisoning disease as, 407-408
Rickettsiosis, 20-21
Right atrial wall, 75f
Risk factors
  for bronchitis, 186
  for renal failure, acute, 307
  for urinary incontinence, 332
  for urolithiasis, 325
Rocky Mountain spotted fever, 20-21, 406-407
Rodenticide intoxication, 386-387
Rottweiler
  aspergillosis in, 147
  conformational disorder in, 155
  infective endocarditis in, 118
  laryngeal paralysis in, 171
  primary ciliary dyskinesia in, 189
  subvalvular aortic stenosis in, 99, 100f
  urolithiasis in, 326
Roundworm, 269-270
  pulmonary migration of, 206
Rupture
  of mitral valve chorda tendineae
    deterioration caused by, 69
    heart failure and, 82
  splenic, 370
Rutin for chylous effusion, 217

S
Saline slide agglutination test, 382
Salivation, vomiting and, 261
Salmon poisoning, 407-408
Salmonella, diarrhea caused by, 267-268
Sarcoma
  hemangiosarcoma, 370-371
  histiocytic, 223-224
SAS (subvalvular aortic stenosis), 99-100, 100f
Saturation, urine, 325
Schiff-Sherrington sign, 30
Schnauzer
  pancreatitis in, 288-289
  urolithiasis in, 327
Schnauzer/Poodle mix, cardiac tamponade in, 75f
Scintigraphy, 209
Scottish Terrier, prostate in, 348
Scraping
  conjunctival, 395
  rectal, 398, 398f
Screening for brucellosis, 347
Secondary epilepsy, 9
Secretory diarrhea, 263
Sedation
  in heart failure, 87
  for laryngeal paralysis, 172
  with phenobarbital, 11
Seizure, 8-14
  causes of, 8, 8t
  definition of, 8
  drugs for, 9-14
  in epilepsy, 9

Seizure—*Continued*
  significance of, 7
  types of, 9
Selegiline, 245
Septal defect
  atrial, 105
  ventricular, 94, 101-103, 104f
Septic effusion, pleural, 213-214, 213f
Serous nasal discharge, 143
Shar-Pei
  conformational disorder in, 155
  primary ciliary dyskinesia in, 189
Shetland Sheepdog, bladder tumor in, 335
Shifting leg lameness, in infective endocarditis,
    122
Shih Tzu
  brachycephalic airway syndrome in, 169
  conformational disorder in, 155
  immune-mediated hemolytic anemia in, 382
  urolithiasis in, 327
Shunt
  portosystemic, 300-303
  in ventricular septal defect, 102
Siberian Husky
  bronchiectasis in, 187
  conformational disorder in, 155
  laryngeal paralysis in, 171
Sign, Schiff-Sherrington, 30
Silica urolith, 328
Sinus
  dermoid, 33-34
  paranasal, tumor of, 159-166
Sinus arrhythmia, respiratory
  heart failure and, 82
  in mitral valve disease, 62
Sinus cyst, nasal dermoid, 155
Sinusotomy, 150
Skin
  in distemper, 399
  in hypothyroidism, 246
  potassium bromide and, 12
Skye Terrier, copper storage disease in,
    298
Small-bowel diarrhea, 263, 264t
Small-intestine bacterial overgrowth, 268
Sodium bicarbonate
  in acute renal failure, 310
  in hypoadrenocorticism, 238
Sodium bromide, 12
Sodium in ketoacidosis, 235
Sodium iodide, 392t
Soft-coated Wheaten Terrier, 272
Spinal cord, lesions of, 3-4
Spinal cord disease, 30-57
  congenital or hereditary, 32-36
    atlantoaxial instability as, 32-33
    dermoid sinus as, 33-34
    globoid cell leukodystrophy as, 34-35
    myelodysplasia as, 35
    syringohydromyelia as, 35-36
  conservative management of, 32

Spinal cord disease—*Continued*
  degenerative, 36-46
    cervical spondylomyelopathy as, 41-43
    of intervertebral disc, 36-41
    lumbosacral stenosis as, 44-46
    myelopathy as, 43-44
  inflammatory, 47-51
    discospondylitis as, 47-49
    steroid responsive meningitis-arteritis as, 49-50
  injury and, 52-54, 52f
  localization in, 30, 30t, 31t, 32
  neoplastic, 50, 51t, 52f
  signs of, 30t, 31t
  vascular, 54-56
    hemorrhagic myelomalacia as, 56
    ischemic myelopathy as, 54-55
Spinal hyperpathia, 44
Spinal reflex, 2-5
Spironolactone, 69
Splenectomy in hemangiosarcoma, 371
Splenic rupture in hemangiosarcoma, 370
Spondylomyelopathy
  cervical, 41-43
  lumbosacral, 44-46
Spontaneous pneumothorax, 217
Spotted fever, Rocky Mountain, 406-407
Spray
  for allergic rhinitis, 151
  for lymphoplasmacytic rhinitis, 154
SRMA (steroid responsive meningitis-arteritis), 49-50
Staffordshire Bull Terrier
  conformational disorder in, 155
  primary ciliary dyskinesia in, 189
Staging
  hemangiosarcoma, 370
  of lung tumor, 221
  of nasal tumor, 164
Staphylococcus
  pyometra and, 342
  rhinitis and, 145
  urinary tract infection and, 337
  urolithiasis and, 325
Status epilepticus, 13
Stenosis
  pulmonic, 94, 100-101
    ventricular septal defect with, 102
  subvalvular aortic, 94, 99-100, 100f
    hypertrophic cardiomyopathy versus, 115-116
Stenotic nares, 155
Sternum, 155
Steroid
  in chronic renal failure, 318
  for intervertebral disc disease, 40
Steroid responsive meningitis-arteritis, 49-50
Stomach disorder, 279-285
  gastric dilation volvulus as, 279-282
  Helicobacter pylori causing, 282-284
  malignant, 282
  motility, 284-285

Stomatitis, uremic, 315
Stone, urinary, 324-331. *See also* Urolithiasis
Storage disease, copper, 298-299
Streptococcus
  pneumonia caused by, 197
  in pyothorax, 213
Stricture, esophageal, 278
Strongyloides stercoralis, 206
Struvite urolith
  composition of, 325
  infection and, 330
  management of, 327-328
Stump pyometra, 343
Subaortic stenosis, 118
Subvalvular aortic stenosis, 94, 99-100, 100f
  hypertrophic cardiomyopathy versus, 115-116
Sudden death in cardiomyopathy, 116
Sulfapyridine, 271
Sulfonamide
  in bacterial meningoencephalitis, 20
  for protozoal meningoencephalitis, 27
  for salmon poisoning, 408
  thyroid function and, 238
Supersaturation, urine, 325
Surgery
  for aspergillosis, 150
  for cervical spondylomyelopathy, 43
  for cyanotic heart disease, 106
  for dermoid sinus, 34
  for discospondylitis, 48-49
  for foreign body, 168
  for gastric dilation volvulus, 281
  in hemangiosarcoma, 371
  in hypercalcemia, 253
  for hyperthyroidism, 250
  for intervertebral disc disease, 38, 40
  for laryngeal paralysis, 172-173
  of laryngeal tumor, 174
  in lumbosacral spondylomyelopathy, 46
  for mitral valve degeneration, 69
  for nasal tumor, 165
  for patent ductus arteriosus, 98
  pericardial, 79, 80
  for pericardioperitoneal diaphragmatic hernia, 72
  of portosystemic shunt, 302
  in pulmonic stenosis, 101
  for pyometra, 342
  for pyothorax, 216
  in spinal trauma, 53-54
  in thromboembolism, 210
  of tracheal tumor, 176
  for ventricular septal defect, 103
Syndrome of inappropriate secretion of antidiuretic hormone, 365
Syringohydromyelia, 35-36
Systemic disease, peripheral nerve disorder in, 17
Systolic anterior motion of mitral valve, 114
Systolic murmur
  in pulmonic stenosis, 101
  in subvalvular aortic stenosis, 99

T

T3, 248
T4
  in hyperthyroidism, 249-250
  in hypothyroidism, 247-248
Tachycardia, 86
Tacrolimus for perianal fistula, 287
Tactile placing, 2
Tamponade, cardiac, 73-74
Tap, pericardial, 77-79
Taurine, 109
Temperature, body, 355-357
Terbinafine, 392t
Terbutaline
  for bronchitis, 186t
  for tracheal collapse, 180t
Terrier, dermoid sinus in, 34. *See also specific breed*
Tetanus, 412-413
Tetracycline
  in ehrlichiosis, 21, 406
  in Rocky Mountain spotted fever, 406
  for salmon poisoning, 408
Tetralogy of Fallot, 105
Thalamus, lesion of, 6
Theophylline
  for bronchitis, 186t
  for tracheal collapse, 180t
Thermoregulatory set point, 355
Thiazide diuretic, 69
Thoracic wall, conformational disorder of, 155
Thoracocentesis, 212
  for hemothorax, 217
Thoracolumbar spinal disc disease, 39
Thoracostomy tube, 216
  in pneumothorax, 217
Thoracotomy, 221
Thrombocytopenia, 378-381
  immune-mediated, 379-380
  immune-mediated hemolytic anemia and, 382
  in Rocky Mountain spotted fever, 406
Thromboembolism
  in glomerulonephritis, 323-324
  in heartworm disease, 136
  pulmonary, 208-210
    in heartworm disease, 131
Thrombolytic therapy, 210
Thymic lymphoma, 367
Thyroid disorder
  hyperthyroidism, 249-250
  hypothyroidism, 246-249
  tumor and, 250
Thyroidectomy, 255
Thyroxine (T4), 247-248
Ticarcillin, 123
Tick-borne disease, 410
  renal failure caused by, 307
Tick paralysis, 16
Tilt, head, 5
Tissue aspiration, 395
Tolerance test, ammonia, 301

Topical therapy for aspergillosis, 149
Total calcium concentration, 250
Toxic liver disease, 299
Toxicity
  of amphotericin B, 389
  of Immiticide, 136-137
  renal failure caused by, 306-307
  rodenticide and, 386-387
  vitamin D, 251
Toxin
  in hepatic encephalopathy, 300
  in tetanus, 412-413
Toxocara canis, 206
Toxoplasma gondii, 207
Toxoplasmosis, 25-27
Trachea, 177-184
  collapse of, 177-179, 180f, 180t
  conformational disorder of, 154
  hypoplastic, 155, 180-182, 181t, 182f
  laceration of, 182-183
Tracheal tumor, 175-176
Tracheal wash, 398
Tracheobronchitis, canine infectious, 194
Transcatheter ductal occlusion, 97-99
Transmission of heartworm, 126
Transnasal core biopsy, 163
Transplantation, renal, 318
Transthoracic fine need lung aspiration, 202
Transtracheal aspiration, 199
Transudate
  ascites and, 273-274
  pericardial, 72
  pleural, 212
Trauma
  peripheral nerve, 15-16
  pneumothorax caused by, 216-217
  spinal, 52, 53f, 53-54
  tracheal, 182-183
Triazole, 389, 391t-392t, 394
Triceps reflex, 3
Tricuspid valve dysplasia, 104-105
Trigeminal nerve, 5
Triiodothyronine (T3), 248
Trimethoprim-sulfamethoxazole
  for protozoal meningoencephalitis, 27
  for respiratory infection, 196
Triple diuretic therapy, in heart failure, 69
Trochlear nerve, 5
Trypsin-like immunoreactivity
  in exocrine pancreatic insufficiency, 293
  in pancreatitis, 290
Tube
  chest
    for pyothorax, 215
    removal of, 216
  thoracostomy, 216, 217
Tularemia, 413-414
Tumor
  adrenal, 246
  anal, 286·
  bladder, 335-336

Tumor—*Continued*
  cachexia and, 365-366
  fever with, 365
  gastrointestinal, 272
  glomerulonephritis and, 320
  of heart, 72, 75f, 79
  hypercalcemia and, 251-252, 364
  hyperhistaminemia in, 364-365
  hypertrophic osteopathy in, 365
  hyperviscosity syndrome in, 364
  hypoglycemia and, 255-256
  insulinoma and, 365
  laryngeal, 173-175
  lung, 219-226. *See also* Lung tumor
  nasal, 159-166. *See also* Nasal tumor
  orthopedic injury versus, 15
  pancreatic, 292
  pituitary macroadenoma, 241
  prostatic, 353-354
  renal, 334-335
  spinal, 50, 51t
  of stomach, 282
  syndrome of inappropriate secretion of
       antidiuretic hormone with, 365
  thyroid, 250
  tracheal, 175-176
  of urinary tract, 334-336
Turkish Shepherd, 298
Tylosin, 271

U
Ulcerative colitis, histiocytic, 271
Ultrasound
  of gallbladder, 303
  in hypoglycemia, 256
  in pancreatitis, 289
  of tracheal collapse, 178
  in urinary incontinence, 333
Unconjugated bilirubin, 294
Upper airway disorder
  brachycephalic airway syndrome as,
       168-171
  foreign body causing, 167-168
  laryngeal paralysis as, 171-173
  laryngeal tumor as, 173-175
  tracheal tumor as, 175-176
Upper motor neuron paraparesis, 34
Urate urolith, 328, 330
Ureaplasma, 325
Uremia, 313-314
Uremic gastropathy
  in acute renal failure, 310
  in chronic renal failure, 315, 317
Uremic stomatitis, 315
Ureterolith, 329
Urethral disorder, 332
Urge incontinence, 331
Urinalysis
  in acute renal failure, 308
  in diabetes, 229
  in hyperadrenocorticism, 241

Urinalysis—*Continued*
  in portosystemic shunt, 301
  in urinary tract infection, 337
Urinary incontinence, 331-334
Urinary system disorder
  in adenovirus infection, 401
  glomerular, 319-324
  incontinence as, 331-334
  infection as, 336-340
  renal failure. *See also* Renal failure
    acute, 305-312
    chronic, 312-319
  tumor as, 334-336
  urolithiasis as, 324-331. *See also* Urolithiasis
Urinary tract infection, 336-340
  antibiotics for, 337
  diagnosis of, 338
  disease with, 337-338
  failure of therapy for, 339
  imaging in, 338-339
  incidence of, 337
  localization of, 336
  organisms causing, 337
  signs of, 336
  urinalysis in, 337
  urolithiasis and, 330
Urine
  blastomycosis and, 415f
  urobilinogen in, 294
Urine cortisol:creatinine ratio, 242
Urine culture
  in brucellosis, 347
  in infective endocarditis, 121
Urine glucose, 231
Urine protein:creatinine ratio, 321-322
Urobilinogen, 294
Urohydropulsion, 328-329
Urolithiasis, 324-331
  clinical signs of, 324
  crystalluria in, 324
  diagnosis of, 326-327
  diseases associated with, 330-331
  formation of, 325
  imaging of, 326
  lithotripsy for, 330
  treatment of, 327-329
  types of, 325-326
  urinary tract infection and, 330
  urolith analysis in, 329
Ursodiol, 297

V
Vaccination
  distemper, 400-401
  for rabies, 404
  for viral infection, 195
Vagina, artificial, 349
Vaginal discharge, 342
Vaginourethrography, retrograde, 333
Vagus nerve, 6
Valve dysplasia, tricuspid, 104-105

Valvular disease
  infective endocarditis as, 118-125. *See also* Endocarditis, infective
  mitral, 59-70. *See also* Mitral valve
Vascular disorder, spinal, 54-56
Vascular resistance, 85
Vasodilator
  in heart failure, 85
  in mitral valve degeneration, 66-68
  in pericardial disease, 76-77
Vasopressin, 91
Venous pressure, central, 76
Ventilation-perfusion ratio, 208-209
Ventricular filling, 79
Ventricular premature contraction, 281
Ventricular septal defect, 94, 101-103, 104f
Vertebra
  fibrocartilagenous embolic myelopathy of, 54-55
  tumor of, 50
Vestibular disease, 7
Vestibulocochlear nerve, 6
Vfend, 392t
Vincristine, 380
Vinorelbine, 222
Viral infection, 399-404
  adenovirus, 401-402
  diagnostic tests for, 397t
  distemper as, 27-29, 399-401
  gastrointestinal, 266-267
  pseudorabies, 402-403
  rabies, 403-404
  respiratory, 194-195
Virchow's triad, 208
Visual placing, 2
Vitamin D
  in hypercalcemia, 251
  for hypocalcemia, 254-255
  renal failure caused by, 307
Vitamin E, 297
Vitamin K-dependent coagulation factor deficiency, 384-385
Voiding urohydropulsion, 329
Vomiting, 261-263
  in acute renal failure, 310
  in chronic renal failure, 315

Vomiting—*Continued*
  in gastric dilation volvulus, 281
  in gastric motility disorder, 284
Von Willebrand's disease, 387-388
VSD (ventricular septal defect, 101-103, 104f

W
Wall, atrial, 75f
Wash
  prostatic, 349-350
  tracheal, 398
Washing, transtracheal, 199
Water deprivation test, 258
Weimaraner
  degenerative myelopathy in, 44
  myelodysplasia in, 35
West Highland White Terrier
  bronchiectasis in, 187
  copper storage disease in, 298
  hepatitis in, 297
Wheelbarrowing, 2
White matter in leukodystrophy, 34
Wildlife species, rabies in, 403
Wobbler syndrome, 41-43
World Health Organization, cardiomyopathy and, 107
Worm infestation, heartworm. *See* Heartworm disease

X
Xanthine urolith, 326
Xylophypha infection, 22

Y
Yersinia pestis, 396t, 411-412
Yorkshire Terrier
  lymphangiectasia in, 272
  pancreatitis in, 288-289
  tracheal collapse in, 177
  urolithiasis in, 327

Z
Zinc, in copper storage disease, 298
Zonisamide, for seizure, 13
Zoonosis, parasitic, 269-270
  brucellosis as, 347